I0763111

WOUND MAN

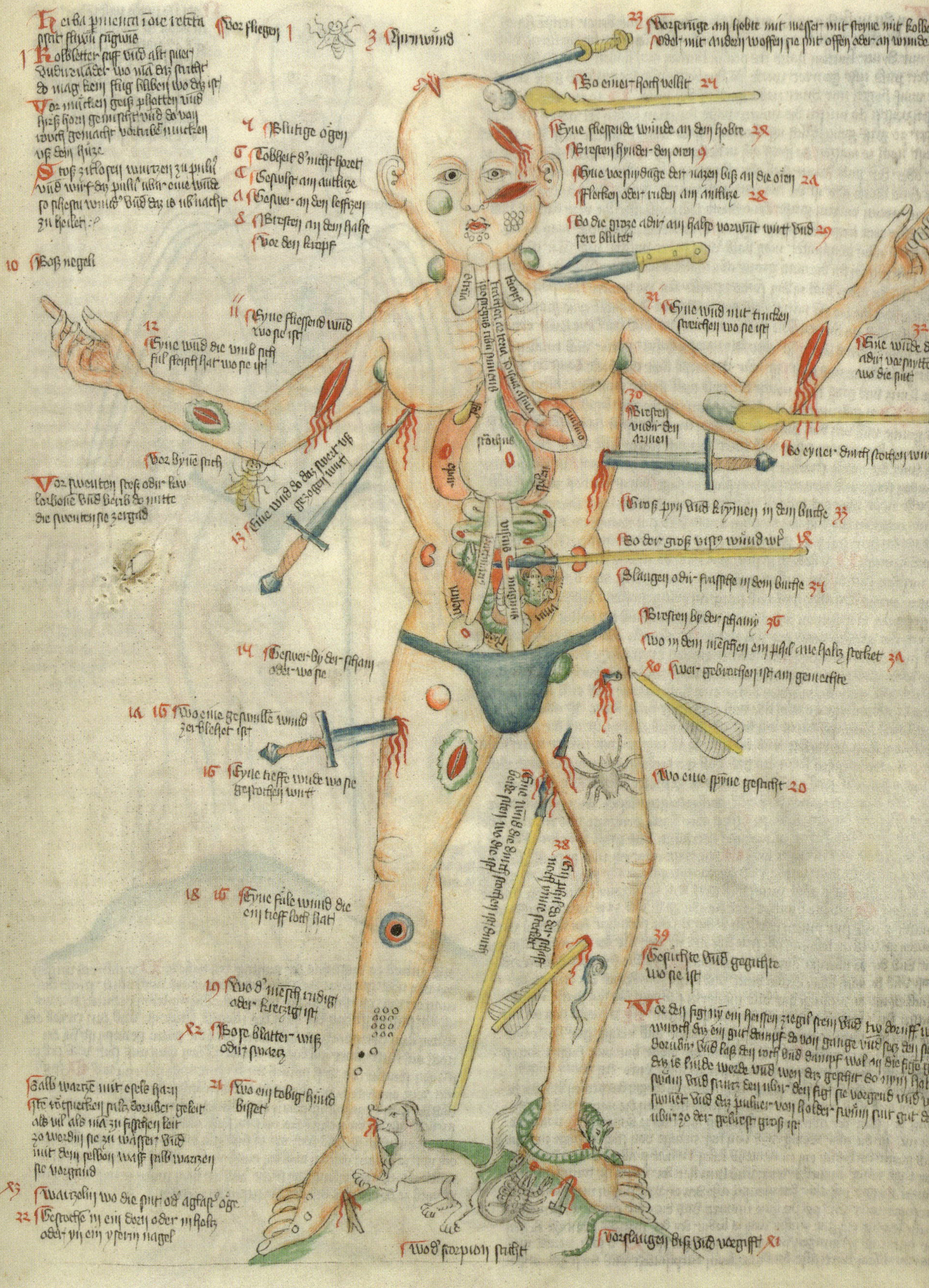

Wound Man

THE MANY LIVES OF A SURGICAL IMAGE

Jack Hartnell

PRINCETON UNIVERSITY PRESS · PRINCETON AND OXFORD

Published by Princeton University Press, 41 William Street, Princeton, New Jersey 08540

In the United Kingdom: Princeton University Press, 99 Banbury Road, Oxford OX2 6JX

GPSR Authorized Representative: Easy Access System Europe - Mustamäe tee 50, 10621 Tallinn, Estonia, gpsr.requests@easproject.com

press.princeton.edu

Front of jacket images: (top) Wound Man, c.1485, possibly Regensburg (Munich, Bayerische Staatsbibliothek, Cgm 597, fol. 244r); (left) Wound Man, after 1491, probably England (London, Wellcome Collection, MS 290, fol. 53v); (right) Wound Man, c. 1580, Vienna (Los Angeles, UCLA, Louise M. Darling Medical Library, MS Benjamin 8, fol. IVv).

Back of jacket image: Wound Man, c. 1559, Germany (Ljubljana, Semeniška knjižnica, SKLJ Rkp. 2, fol. XLIIIr).

Frontispiece: detail of Wound Man, c. 1420–30, possibly Thuringia. Ink and paint on parchment, 40 x 30 cm. London, Wellcome Library, MS 49, fol. 35r.

ISBN 978-0-691-24348-1
ISBN (ebook) 978-0-691-27445-4

Library of Congress Control Number: 2025930827

British Library Cataloging-in-Publication Data is available

Editorial: Michelle Komie and Annie Miller
Production Editorial: Mark Bellis
Text and Jacket Design: Monograph / Matt Avery
Production: Steve Sears
Publicity: Jodi Price and Charlotte Coyne
Copyeditor: Cynthia Buck

This book has been composed in Lyon and Chassi

Printed in Italy

10 9 8 7 6 5 4 3 2 1

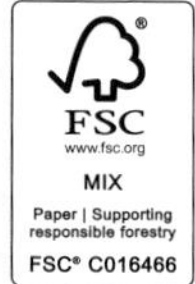

Contents

WOUND MAN

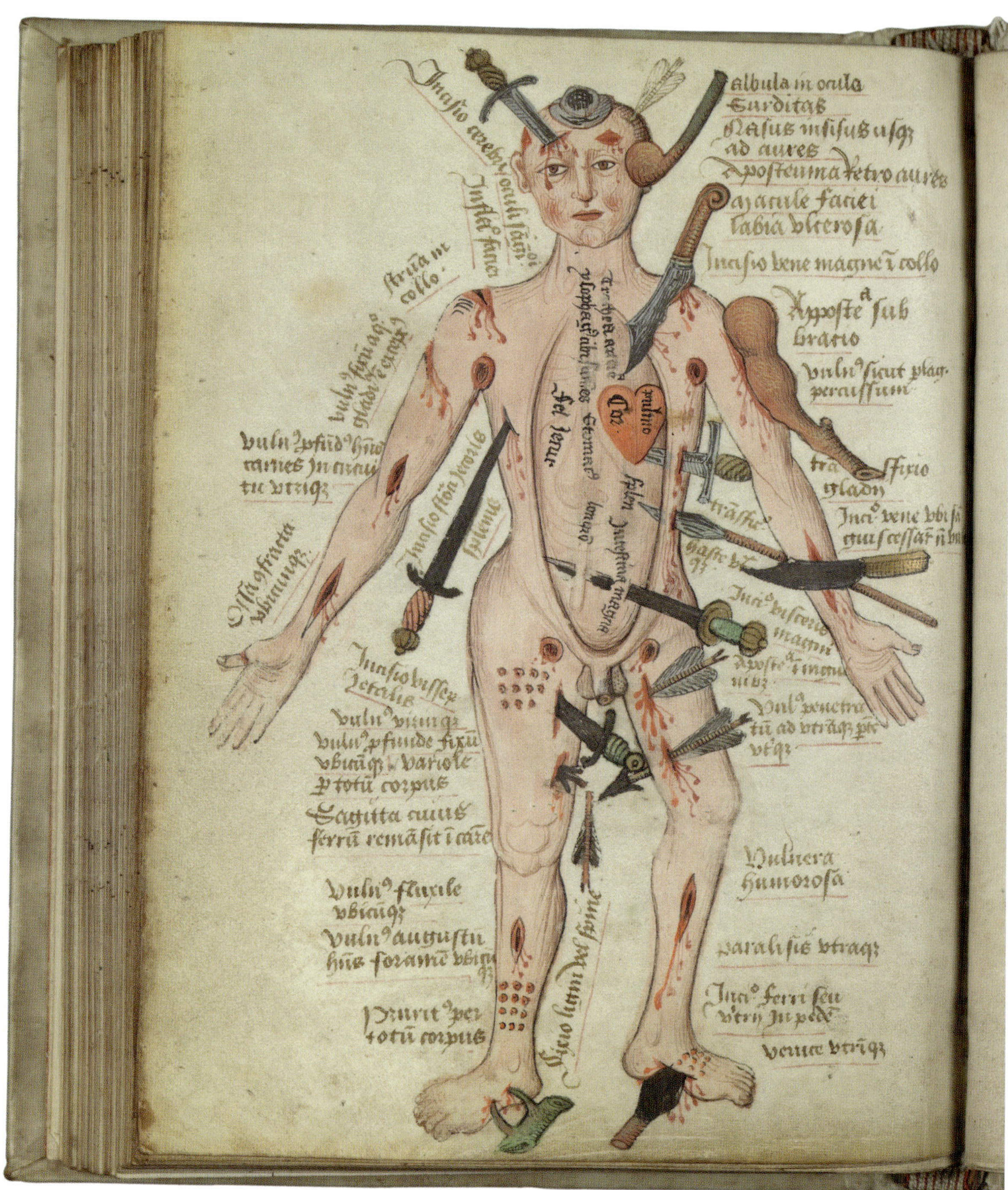

Fig. 0.1. Wound Man, after 1491, probably England. Ink and paint on parchment, 18 x 13 cm. London, Wellcome Library, MS 290, fol. 53v.

INTRODUCTION

Long, Strange Histories

The Wound Man is an image at once troubling and enigmatic (fig. 0.1). A male figure looks out from the parchment page bearing a multitude of graphic wounds. His skin is covered in bleeding cuts and lesions, stabbed and sliced by elaborately detailed knives, spears, and swords of varying sizes, many of which remain stuck threateningly in his body. His head and thighs are pierced with arrows, some intact, some snapped down to just their heads or shafts, their fletch feathering his form. A club metes out blunt trauma at his shoulder, while inside his chest—rendered eerily transparent so as to reveal the structure of his intestines, lungs, spleen—the tip of a dagger punctures his heart. As well as weapons of war and affray, the figure bears traces of more quotidian accident. His shins and feet are clustered with thorn scratches and trod-upon blades. He is peppered with itchy insect bites. And to compound his appalling, cumulative misfortune, the Wound Man is also deeply unwell. His armpits and groin sport rounded, dark red buboes. A label tells us he is beset by "*pruritus per totum corpus*" (itching all over the body), which alongside the depicted rashes and swellings suggests the contraction of multiple diseases. The violence and illness rendered unto his body is total and all-consuming. Yet, despite such a horrendous barrage, the figure's expression is unnervingly resolute. He stands with eyes wide open, very much still alive, and in this simple act the image's purpose crystallizes. For despite its gratuitous display, the Wound Man was not a figure originally designed to inspire fear or to menace. Instead, it represented something altogether more hopeful: an imaginative and arresting reminder of the powerful knowledge that could be channeled and dispensed through the practice of premodern medicine.

Consider, though, the different levels of description and categorization we are required to slip and slide between in order to capture the Wound Man's many simultaneous aspects in words. The image's abundance necessitates leading with an ekphrastic register, descriptions that parse the essential details of the figure's body and its penetrating objects, hinting also at the materiality of the page. And at the same time, the image inevitably invites other forms of language: medical discussions of anatomy and diagnostics, the

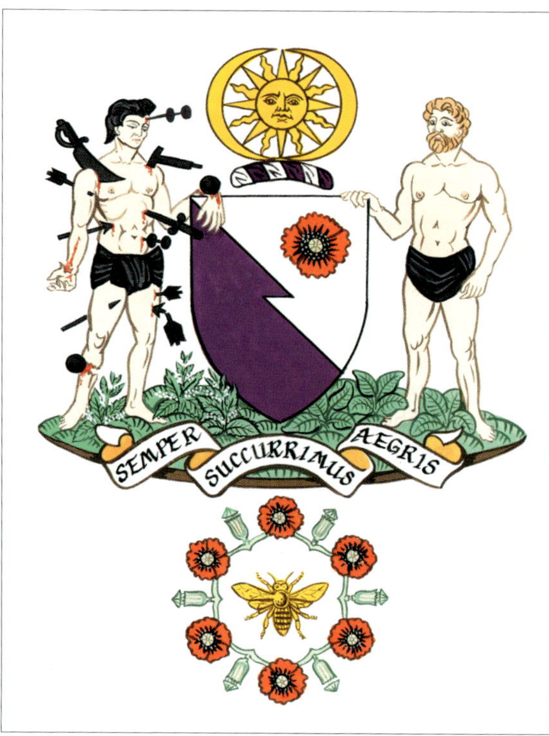

Fig. 0.2. Coat of arms of the Royal College of Emergency Medicine, adopted November 2, 1995. Ink on paper. London, College of Arms, MS Grants 162.

employment of technical descriptors to diagnose the figure's diagrammatic innards and brimming diseases, and even far more nebulous yet fundamental questions over what the figure is doing to the viewer emotionally, spiritually, hovering somewhere between surprise and salvation. Amid this scuffle for critical angles, the Wound Man aggressively resists clear interpretation.

A major consequence of this complexity is that today the image lives out an empty, exclusively spectacular life. Recently, his broken body has provided a grotesque lure to a diverse and somewhat bizarre variety of modern constituents. In 1995, the figure was included as part of the new official coat of arms of the United Kingdom's Royal College of Emergency Medicine, reworked with rippling abs and Ken-doll hair to conveniently present in a single body the many trauma injuries that the college's members were equipped to tackle (fig. 0.2).[1] For the administrators of Mont Orgeuil Castle, a thirteenth-century fortress overlooking the port of Gorey on the island of Jersey, the Wound Man was a more playful thing, a fitting inspiration for a sculpture by the artist Owen Cunningham, who produced a giant three-dimensional likeness of the figure for the gleeful, gross-out delight of visitors. This same gruesome sensibility, revived and mercilessly amplified, ushered the image onto TV screens, gracing the desk of Mads Mikkelsen's eponymous cannibalistic doctor Hannibal Lecter in the 2013 NBC series *Hannibal*, a show in turn based on Thomas Harris's 1981 novel *Red Dragon*. Harris drew on the Wound Man as a model for several of his book's particularly spectacular murders, but he was not the first writer to cite the figure as their muse. Back in 1957, no less a literary luminary than Ian Fleming had written to his publisher to suggest that instead of its current title, *Dr. No*, perhaps the sixth book in his

James Bond series of spy thrillers should be renamed *The Wound Man*, after a historical picture he had recently come across in a pamphlet and for which he claimed to have great affection.[2] The publisher declined. In the last decade or so, the image has inspired music from a heavy metal band, a book of Scots poetry, a piece of one-man storytelling theater entitled *The Adventures of Wound Man and Shirley*, an anarchist tea-towel protesting corporate profiteering, and a diagram in a respected veterinary journal outlining commonly sustained wounds among dueling cats.[3]

Academic studies have for the most part mirrored this surface-level pop prominence, albeit less often. The Wound Man is not new to the scholarly understanding of medicine's past, first brought to the attention of the academy some time ago, in 1907, by the German historian of medicine and medical images Karl Sudhoff.[4] A highly problematic yet pioneering academic in the emerging field during the first decades of the twentieth century, Sudhoff conducted exhaustive historical research in the grand libraries of interwar Europe that greatly expanded the understanding of much premodern European medical practice.[5] In the case of the Wound Man, he gathered together, for the first time in a single space, what was then only a handful of known examples and offered detailed codicological commentary on their origins and the texts they appeared alongside. Yet since Sudhoff, specific studies of the Wound Man have largely been restricted to niche medical-historical subfields, and more importantly, they have only been brief: a journal article from 1965 and a book chapter from 1993 again focus primarily on the texts circulating in the orbit of the figure, while a medical dissertation from 1982 adds several further Wound Men to Sudhoff's short list of examples.[6] A number of recent academic publishers, keen to display a dramatic dust jacket, have presented the figure as a full-on frontispiece to books on various aspects of the Middle Ages and early modernity. But the contents of these publications rarely dedicate more than a footnote to the Wound Man himself, and in many the injured figure who violently bestrides their covers goes entirely unmentioned.[7]

The central contention of this book is that the Wound Man is far more than spectacle. In fact, the image demands a new kind of thinking to keep pace with its exciting, multifaceted vastness, a scope that straddles manifold arenas of both the premodern world and modern scholarship. The spine of this approach lies in the first-ever detailed excavation of the figure's material history, an account that in the chapters to come traverses a broad sweep of more than three hundred years. Known from at least fifteen late medieval manuscripts and over thirty early modern printed books reproduced in hundreds of editions, the Wound Man appeared as a constant in medical and nonmedical works from fourteenth-century Central Europe to eighteenth-century East Asia. These items are this book's historical core, requiring the examination of materials held in roughly eighty libraries and archives, principally in Europe but also at an increasing remove from the lands of the Wound Man's origin, as far afield as collections in North America and Japan. Some of these images have been known to scholarship since Sudhoff's day, but the majority have not previously been examined, among them works from outside of institutional collections that have surfaced on the rare books market as recently as 2023. In all, ninety-three Wound Men are gathered here to plot the coordinates of a complex collective life.

This book is no catalog, however. From the very moment of its inception, the Wound Man was an image intimately tied to actual practice. As such, to chart a history of the figure is also to chart a history of the medical ideas, literary interests, technological shifts, and artistic currents that it emerged alongside: their documentation, debate, distribution, evolution, and in some cases collapse. This book deals as much with cutting, bleeding, and suturing as it does with drawing, painting, and printing, showcasing how the Wound Man helps us bring together historical areas of cultural production that interpreters today far too often claim as entirely discrete. In this sense, to track the Wound Man's history is also to explore a developing cast of characters who interacted with the image from different vantage points across its busy chronological and geographical sweep. Engaged by healers and patients alike, but also by printmakers and poets, scribes and students, nuns and monks, this was a figure of the utmost importance for premodern users from both literate and nonliterate worlds, stretching from learned academic elites to workshop artisans who generated their knowledge not through writing texts but through hands-on craft. The chapters to come thus aim both to illuminate the Wound Man's image and to revive his deep context, restoring the captivating presence that the figure once held for a wide range of medieval and early modern people.

Finally, as well as working to make the image of the Wound Man more familiar—explaining the details of its appearance, its purpose, its makers, its users—this book sets in motion another set of arguments that look to do the opposite: to allow the Wound Man to remain strange. At almost precisely the same time as Karl Sudhoff was publishing the first academic outlines of the Wound Man's medicine, he struck up an epistolary relationship with another German scholar more familiar to historiographers of the visual, the cultural historian Aby Warburg.[8] Both were deeply interested in the long histories of similar medieval and early modern images, writing in letters of their "*Paralleler Hinreisen*" (parallel paths). But where Sudhoff's approach was unashamedly historical, focusing on what he saw as rigorous matters of provenance, technicality, and cause, Warburg's engagement with the same material could be characterized as far more fluid and philosophical, even bordering on the mystical.[9] Take the so-called Panel B of Warburg's unfinished yet famed *Bilderatlas Mnemosyne*, a grand project running from 1927 until his death in which he gathered black-and-white reproductions pinned to large-scale boards in order to trace recurring visual patterns running from antiquity to early modernity (fig. 0.3). In Panel B, Warburg was exploring notions of what we might call proto-science, specifically the metaphysical imbrication of the human body and the cosmos through a suite of astrological images. On the surface, the panel emphasizes direct similarity. Showing multiple idealized male figures set into correspondence with discs of zodiacal signs and circuits, it draws our attention to the simple yet undeniable fact that makers across periods maintained a keen interest in visualizing humankind's relation to the stars. Yet in presenting an art historical argument in pictorial form, Warburg was less interested in matters of concrete lineage—that the artist of

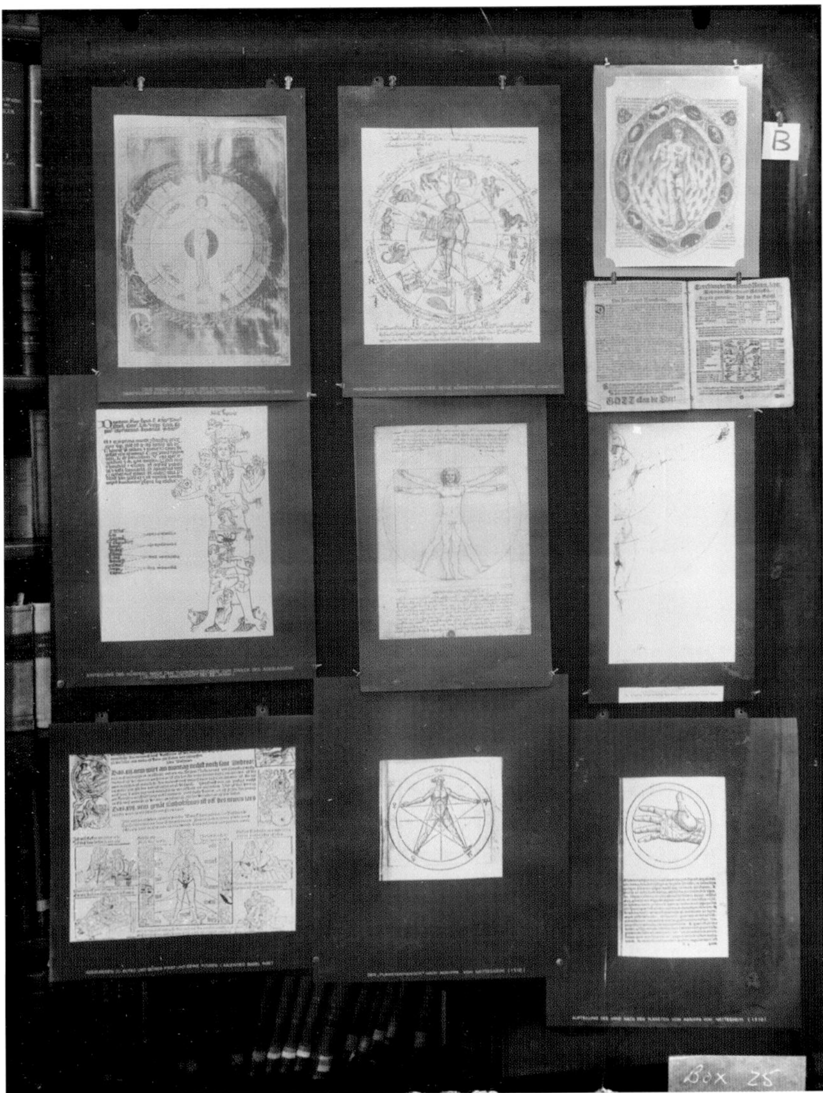

Fig. 0.3. "Panel B" of Aby Warburg's *Bilderatlas Mnemosyne* in its so-called Final Version, 1929, Hamburg. Photograph. London, Warburg Institute Photographic Collection.

one image had directly seen and was trying to emulate another pictured on the board—than he was in their collective presence, a cultural through line of epistemically potent objects that together were complicit in the production and transmission of ideas. The Wound Man himself never featured directly in Warburg's *Bilderatlas*, yet in conveying the shared intellectual stakes and sweeping aesthetics of its many versions, this book advocates that we take the image seriously on precisely these abstracted yet bewitching terms. Doing so requires not only looking contextually across periods for the Wound Man's role in reflecting medical knowledge and personnel but also looking at the image more obliquely, alert to its subsurface associations with contemporary patterns of religious discourse, literary practices of legal compunction and fantastical violence, paradigm shifts in media landscapes, and cross-cultural currents of artistic flare that could be deployed to multiple audiences around the world.

In short, this book mobilizes the Wound Man for inspiration in expanding the fundamentals of what can be done with medical images made before the modern era. This broad category of picture has for the most part languished. Once among the past's most active and engaging images, they now find themselves stalled in a niche between disciplines, overlooked both by historians of art unable to sufficiently parse their curative contents and historians of medicine unable to sufficiently contextualize their visual structures. The creative friction between these and other fields, however, can also act with reanimating force. To start this process, the five chapters that follow develop from one another chronologically, charting the course of the Wound Man's history from its later medieval backgrounds and origins through to its multiple early modern lives. But they also develop conceptually, each showcasing how the Wound Man can in turn act as a prompt to various scholarly fields: diagrammatics, medicine, literature, technology, and art history. In this sense, they take the interdisciplinary and transcultural ideas of today's historical writing and explore them not as methodologies but as maneuvers that image-makers and medics were themselves making long before modern historians.

Chapter 1, "Diagram: Ambitious Figures," begins the book by setting the scene for the Wound Man, introducing the various contexts for diagramming the body that emerged in European book culture during the later Middle Ages and exploring contemporary attitudes toward epistemic function, artistic figuration, and the medical audiences of images. First, it surveys a host of materials from across medical and nonmedical contexts that help us grapple with the fuzzy modern term "illustration," a word that, on the one hand, leans toward aesthetic ideas of art, ornament, and embellishment, and on the other, toward more intellectual models of explanation, images that differentiated and made tangible the intricacy of complex ideas. Thereafter focusing on material from fourteenth- and fifteenth-century physicians' notebooks and surgical manuscripts, the chapter demonstrates how makers of medical books were constantly playing with diagrammatic tensions in their work, especially in images of their patients, which they used to simultaneously generate and distribute medical understanding. It concludes by offering an extended analysis of one medical predecessor of the Wound Man in detail, so-called bloodletting figures, which from the fourteenth century onward offered diagrammatic accompaniment to widely circulated texts on the practice of phlebotomy. Bringing to light many previously unknown examples from late medieval Germany, Bohemia, France, Italy, England, Wales, Ireland, and Spain, the chapter maps out the key visual coordinates and medical circumstances for understanding the Wound Man itself.

Chapter 2, "Medicine: Wound Mechanics," turns from matters of backdrop to the specifics of the Wound Man's own origins, explicating the figure's emergence in late medieval European medical culture by examining the eight earliest surviving examples of the figure, found in a group of surgical books from fifteenth-century Bohemia and southern Germany. Known to the few historians of medicine who have considered them as manuscripts of the *Dreibilderserie* (Three-Picture Series), these were flexible works whose changeable medicine addressed a tripartite agenda—disease, gynecology, and wound surgery—and whose shared characteristic was the marshaling of their contents not through fixed titles or concretized cures but through medical diagrams. The chapter offers the first holistic close reading of these images, known respectively as the Disease Man, the Disease Woman, and of course the Wound Man, although, intriguingly, all three were in part intended for the treatment of both male and female bodies. It then goes on to specifically unpack the Wound Man's complex taxonomic armature in these works, showing how the figure's envelopment in individuated catchphrases and number keys linked his respective injuries to an accompanying list of surgical procedures and pharmaceutical recipes, each carefully designed to heal his many woes. Presenting the figure as an all-too-vivid table of surgical contents, we come to understand the Wound Man's fundamental grounding, at once a unique, encyclopedic catalog of the late medieval profession's craft and a visual reflection of the increasingly prominent social positioning of surgeons within contemporary medical culture.

Having traced the medical origins of the Wound Man in a world of hands-on surgical practice, the book turns in chapter 3, "Affect: Wounds in the World," to consider the powerful emotional qualities that the figure's bruised and battered body could also communicate to readers. Building on both medieval and modern theories of pain as a communal yet fundamentally uncommunicable phenomenon, the chapter considers how the Wound Man's distressing emotional power exemplified the strong links between medical and nonmedical fields in fifteenth-century Europe, in particular in the German-speaking lands from which the figure emanated. Creating a detailed affective framework for the Wound Man, the chapter gradually weaves a rich contemporary "woundscape" from many strands: the visual legal testimony used to indict murder suspects; the bloody treatment of literary heroes in poetic epics; the aggressive masculinity of illustrated fight manuals; and contemporary religious discourses around wounded holy bodies, from strong saintly precedent—Saint Sebastian riddled with arrows, the stoning of Saint Stephen, the gruesome torture of Saint Barbara—to expiatory forms of Christological pain that heralded the promise of healing through a familiar devout model of spiritual sickness and cure. By effectively developing a personhood for the Wound Man, the chapter concludes, conflation with these points of cultural resonance activated a backstory for the figure, something that contemporary medical discourses in turn saw as key to his effective healing.

Chapter 4, "Into Print: International Intermediality," heralds a chronological shift in the book, moving away from the Wound Man's origins to consider the figure's changing fortune across an expansive late medieval and early modern life. Most traditional accounts of illustrated printed medical books in Europe tend to start with the highly detailed and decorated output of the sixteenth century, but this chapter instead begins by demonstrating that many illustrative traditions of early modern medicine were in fact flourishing in print well before 1500, bringing to light a range of previously undiscussed figures used in bodily diagnosis, astronomical prognosis, surgical procedure, and natural philosophical discussions of anatomy. The image of the Wound Man was a crucial element among these illustrated medical incunabules, first appearing as part of the wildly successful *Fasciculus medicinae* (Little Bundle of Medicine) published in 1491 by the Venetian printers Giovanni and Gregorio de Gregori. Through a close analysis of the images and texts of the *Fasciculus*, the chapter addresses the innovative printing techniques and editorial syntheses needed to realize the Wound Man in this new technological medium. It also examines the role of print in ensuring the figure's immense popularity throughout the sixteenth century, tracking the Wound Man's reworking across subsequent editions, translations, and reimaginings of the book made in Zaragoza, Burgos, Pamplona, Milan, Antwerp, Seville, Strasbourg, Frankfurt, Augsburg, Mainz, and Basel. It was through these multiple printed appearances that a number of contemporary European artists were also inspired to capture their own versions of the painful figure, producing extravagant hand-illustrated copies of the *Fasciculus* Wound Man and his printed ills. As a result, the chapter argues, the figure testifies to both the movement of manuscript medical imagery into international print circuits and an altogether more unusual and interesting phenomenon only recently beginning to be identified by print scholars: intermedial images that could bounce back and forth between the different technologies of early modern books.

Having considered the widespread implications of the Wound Man's initial appearance as a printed medical phenomenon, the book's fifth and final chapter, "Image: Wound Man Aesthetics," argues for the figure's emergence among an increasingly transnational set of early modern aesthetic networks. With its unusual combination of eye-catching violence and curative potency, the Wound Man was featured regularly in a new wave of groundbreaking surgical treatises as a visually striking medical title page, starting with printed surgical works by German authors writing around 1500, such as Hieronymus Brunschwig and Hans von Gersdorff. Here the chapter explores how the figure was put to increasingly abstract, artistic use by authors and printers, conjured to both market a book's surgical contents and, in an intriguing poetic turn, literally speak in favor of particular surgeons and their work. From this springboard, the chapter considers the detail of three early modern moments in which the Wound Man's image, rather than his specific medicine, took on particular local import: in sixteenth-century France, seventeenth-century England, and eighteenth-century Japan. By tracing the lines of these many early modern Wound Men as they evolved into almost stand-alone artworks, this chapter emphasizes the figure's strange yet recurrent slippage between cultures, contexts, and technologies. The Wound Man's medico-artistic potential more often than not dwelled in its ability to speak for the surgical craft as a whole: a totemic emblem of the profession through which we can map both the developing expertise and cultural positioning of its many surgical participants.

Today the overarching discipline of the Medical Humanities tries to keep up a parity between the methods of history and the materials of health. Yet as with many aspects of the historical field, the rich Medical Humanities of modernity and the present day—explorations of X-rays, robotics, genomics, artificial intelligence—are all too often allowed to overpower the important contributions of medical visual culture from a more distant era. Together, these chapters make the case that medieval and early modern voices must be kept loud and strong in evolving discussions of medicine's relation to images and objects, presenting the Wound Man's many aspects as an ideal point of departure for dialogue between past and present. Utilizing the image's exceptional complexity and intensity, this book reveals a process of medico-artistic entanglement that transports the reader beyond the specifics of bodily injury and allows the Wound Man to emerge as an intricate, unique site of contact: between sickness and cure, painting and print, suffering and sanctity, and ultimately between art, society, and healing.

CHAPTER ONE

Diagram: Ambitious Figures

Fieri autem potest, ut recte quis sentiat, et id, quod sentit, polite eloqui non possit. Sed mandare quemquam litteris cogitationes suas, qui eas nec disponere, nec illustrare possit, nec delectatione aliqua allicere lectorem, hominis est intemperanter abutentis et otio, et litteris.

It may happen that a man can think rightly, yet cannot express elegantly what he thinks. But committing thoughts to writing without being able to arrange or explain them, or at all amuse the reader, is for a person who unreasonably abuses both leisure and learning.

CICERO, *Tusculan Disputations*

Before turning to the Wound Man's late medieval specifics, it is important to understand the image's medico-visual context, its ambitious predecessors and their processes. To do so, however, is to straight away be thrown into a conceptual gray area neatly encompassed by the modern term "illustration," a word whose meanings pull in two directions at once. On the one hand, the term conjures aesthetic ideas of representation: a sense of ornament and embellishment, decorative details that beautify and excite the page. On the other, it leans toward more epistemic models of explanation: serious images that help to elucidate complex concepts, visualizing individual elements of ideas and their intricate connections. To put it in more premodern terms, we might borrow a formulation from the *Tusculan Disputations* cited in this chapter's epigraph—a rhetorical dictum well known to European intellectuals of the later Middle Ages—which acknowledges that *illustrare* always sits in delicate pact with *delectatione*.[1] To illustrate is sometimes to enlighten, sometimes to enliven, and sometimes both.

A tension between these two etymological poles can be found in a wide group of images from medieval Europe, ranging from religious, philosophical, and legal contexts to astronomical, mathematical, and cartographic visual culture. But medical pictures from the European Middle Ages represent a particularly complex and creative approach to illustration's extremes. Knotting together highly diverse concepts of the visual with highly diverse concepts of bodily cure, they emerge more often than not as sites of distinctly paradoxical image-craft. Their visual leisure and their visual learning, to again use Cicero's words, are sometimes synthesized but also often

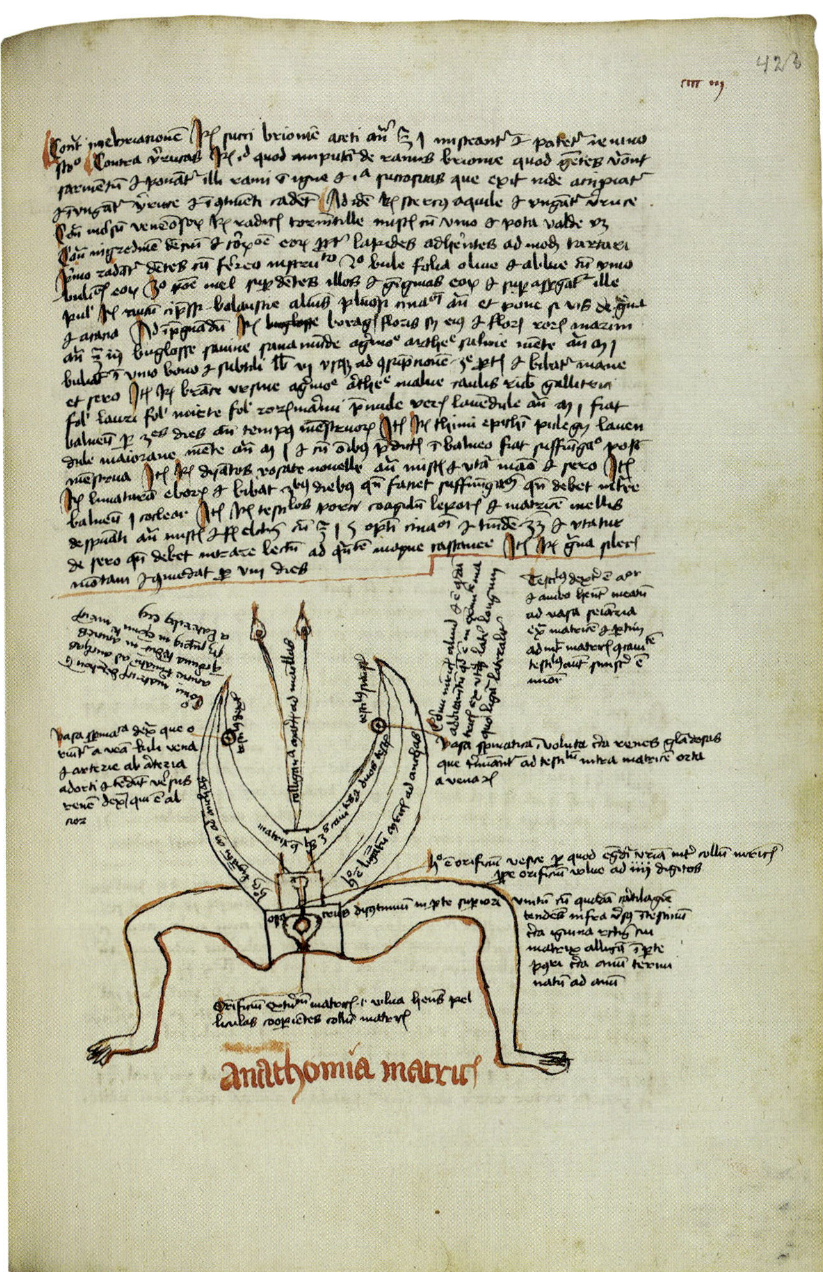

Fig. 1.1. Diagram of the womb sketched by the Heidelberg physician Erhard Knab, c. 1460, Heidelberg. Ink on paper, 31 x 22 cm. Vatican City, Biblioteca Apostolica Vaticana, MS Pal. Lat. 1225, fol. 423r.

staged antagonistically, so much so that they quickly generate difficulties of categorization and interpretation for a modern reader attempting to understand past relationships between image, knowledge, and the human body.

Consider by way of introduction to this problem a particularly unusual image from a chunky medical notebook written at some point around the year 1462 by a physician and high-ranking master at the University of Heidelberg named Erhard Knab (fig. 1.1).[2] Knab's notebook as a whole is a typical piece of late medieval academic work. Across nearly five hundred folios, an eclectic assortment of treatises and recipes have been reproduced in a thin black hand with occasional red flourishes, all drawn from Knab's wide-ranging medical reading. He lists digestive medicines and laxatives cribbed from the fourteenth-century French surgeon Gui de Chauliac; he cites treatments for plague drawn from Chauliac's contemporary, the Italian physician Pietro da Tossignano; and he situates excerpts such as these by esteemed medieval experts alongside his own suite of original commentaries on apostemes, ulcers, wound management, uroscopy, and a variety of other topics. The notebook is typical too in its infrequent use of images, with only one large-scale drawing sandwiched by Knab toward the back of the book between a treatise on healing kidney stones and a multifaceted text on various diseases such as fever, asthma, and reproductive health.

Although singular, the image is nonetheless striking. Above a bold red label reading "*anathomia matricis*" (anatomy of the womb), a close-packed set of graphical elements outline key parts of the female reproductive system. At its lower center, two rectangular blocks stacked one atop the other are identified in Knab's highly abbreviated Latin as the mouth of the womb and the womb itself, the former shown as a pair of large concentric ovals and the latter sitting above it, looking like a miniaturized lightbulb in a box. A pair of arching bands spring upward from these blocks to the left and right representing the uterine ligaments, muscular components that Classical writers had long described as loosely anchoring the womb within the body. Here they also forge anatomical connection between the uterus and a pair of small round circles labeled both "*vasa spermatica*" and "*testes*," organs that today we would call the ovaries, but which in medieval generative thinking were conceived as direct correspondents to the male testicles, even to the point of providing a form of female sperm for reproduction.[3] Adding even more to the upward sweep of the image, another twin set of anatomical elements shoot vertically from the center, depicted almost as a pair of eyes overlooking the scene. These in fact are the breasts, labeled "*mamillas*," organs that, despite their linking lines, were thought only to hold conceptual rather than physical connection to the uterus, processing the humoral excess of menstrual blood into milk for nursing.[4] Lastly—and most unnervingly—a pair of realistic legs sprout outward from the bottom of this core cluster, complete with carefully rounded calves and individuated toes. They anchor the accumulated apparatus firmly to the ground, as if it were standing still in a half-squat in front of the reader, yet somehow at the same time they communicate a disturbing capacity for movement. We get the sense that this entire accumulated ensemble could at any moment stand up and scuttle sideways off the page.

It is unclear what exactly to make of this contradictory image. On first impression, its scratchy forms feel rather hastily sketched, the shaky work of a penman more familiar with small-scale letters than long sweeping lines. Yet there has still been considerable care taken in building up the pointed curves of elements like the uterine ligaments, underscoring the legs and breasts in red, and delicately plotting the image's labels in an elegant spiral around the central body, each one reproduced without error, unlike the multiple strike-throughs of the messy treatise above the image. It is also contradictory in a more conceptual sense, stuck between illustration's two poles. In its upper portion, explanation clearly takes the reins, employing a familiar technical vocabulary of simple shapes, linking lines, and textual labels for the principal purpose of clarifying its different anatomical elements to the reader. Below, though, naturalistic legs bring alarming personality to this otherwise mechanical image. If in its top half the image is giving form to anatomical ideas, outlining organs and their theoretical connections, then what is coming into shape in the bottom half? Is this schematic caught in the process of becoming a person, a patient? Standing at the precipice between epistemics and aesthetics, Knab's image feels no need to provide a clear answer.

Diagrammatic Perspectives

Images in medical manuscripts such as Knab's figure—and, as we shall see, the figure of the Wound Man too—are often classified in catalogs, archives, and scholarly texts as diagrams. Yet as the historian of science Faith Wallis has recently noted, her tongue firmly in cheek, "Many medievalists, it seems, know a diagram when they see one; but few are prepared to agree on what qualifies as a diagram and why."[5]

The idea that scholars of the Middle Ages might be particularly attuned to the diagrammatic in part reflects the place of such images in late medieval European visual culture itself. In this set of traditions, the subtle explanatory power of visualized information was regularly evoked, especially in medieval books. Whether leafing through the folios of an eleventh-century monastic treatise on the weather, a thirteenth-century legal argument on the limits of intermarriage, or a fifteenth-century religious work outlining the simultaneous oneness and infinitude of God, a medieval reader would frequently find their texts interspersed with eloquent trees, wheels, grids, tables, and mappings of myriad types. Not that "diagram" is the term they would have used to describe such images. In most European vernaculars this word—coined from the Greek roots *dia-* (through) and *graphein* (writing, drawing, painting, describing)—was only popularized by scholars in the seventeenth century, while its premodern Latin iteration, *diagramma*, was mostly limited to the specific technical vocabulary of land surveyors to describe their designs. Instead, in medieval European works such images are noted variously as *figura*, *schema*, *forma*, *imago*, *rota*, *nota*, *descriptio*, *caracter*, צורה (tzeura), תבנית (tavnit), صور (ṣuwar), جداول (jadāwil), or أشكال (ashkāl).[6]

It is the sheer vastness of this scope, etymologically but also formally, that has left scholars who try to pin down the medieval diagram with a broad lexicon of conflicting definitions and blurred categorizations. Michael Evans was surely right when he argued in his pioneering 1980 essay "The Geometry of the Mind"—one of the earliest attempts to collate this loose group of images and their implications—that the problem is at least in part one of neglect through disciplinary boundaries.[7] For much of the twentieth century, art historians deemed the simplistic aesthetics of medieval diagrammatic images too insubstantial for serious study, while their accompanying words and labels never quite seemed sizable enough to reach the independent status of a text, the bar often necessary for literary scholars to sit up and take notice. In the wake of work by Evans and others, however, the diagrammatic mode has now become of central interest to a number of strands of medieval and early modern studies and the subject of several important recent volumes. For our exploration of the Wound Man, it is important to tease apart the significant multidisciplinary arsenal amassed by recent scholars for elaborating these deceptively simple pictures.[8]

Historians of science and technology have largely led the charge in tackling such diagramming, their commentary coalescing in particular around what they see as these images' unique capacity to argue.[9] This idea essentially proceeds from observations made by scholars of older scientific traditions, who note that in the Classical writings of Plato, Pappus, Proclus, and others, the term *diagramma* tended to describe an image presented alongside a scientific proof but was also used more synecdochally to infer the intellectual content of that same scientific proof itself, as well as sometimes even describing the entire discipline to which the proof was contributing. To paraphrase the historian of Classical mathematics Reviel Netz, this early science conflated talk *about* diagrams with the talk *of* diagrams, synthesizing the apparatus of argumentation with an argument's conclusions.[10]

Much the same has been maintained of medieval diagrammatic images, principally through their participatory logic. We can see this even in the very simplest forms of visual argumentation to survive from the Middle Ages: stemmatic analyses, whose clearly defined structural armatures laid out a series of demonstrative paths for the reader to follow. Whether these images were individuating groups of Aristotelian predicates or different aspects of whole scholastic disciplines organized by their varied parallel branches, by running one's eyes back and forth along their multiple diagrammatic routes it was possible to both absorb their primary information and, at the same time, model progressive stages of connected logic.[11] This was the case for these divergent images both when speedily sketched in the margins of a manuscript and when given a more thoughtful, even luxurious life. They could certainly appear grand. Think, for instance, of the spectacular series of images produced in monastic communities across Europe that outlined respective modes of good Christian deeds, not in simple line but by showing each as discrete colorful feathers on a mystical cherub's enormous wings, the flapping whole intertwining pious actions today with apocalyptic judgment tomorrow (fig. 1.2).[12] Yet regardless of their degree of visual eloquence, if, as Aristotle claimed, it is "not possible to think without an image," then by reading any such diagram, artistically executed or not, the reader unavoidably participated in its argumentative logic.[13] Indeed, historians of science have suggested that such diagrammatic images argued not merely by replicating textual processes of thinking but by going above and beyond them. Scholars like Kathrin Müller and Barbara Obrist have convincingly shown that as certain historical shifts took place in the fundamentals of scholastic logic over the course of the Middle Ages, the diagrammatic function of images presented alongside scholarly texts also evolved.[14] By the later medieval period, such pictures had grown to become far more active and autonomous participants in persuasive reasoning, to the extent that we find figures such as the cherub bundled together with all sorts of related schematics and tables to form discrete, entirely diagrammatic booklets. With no need for

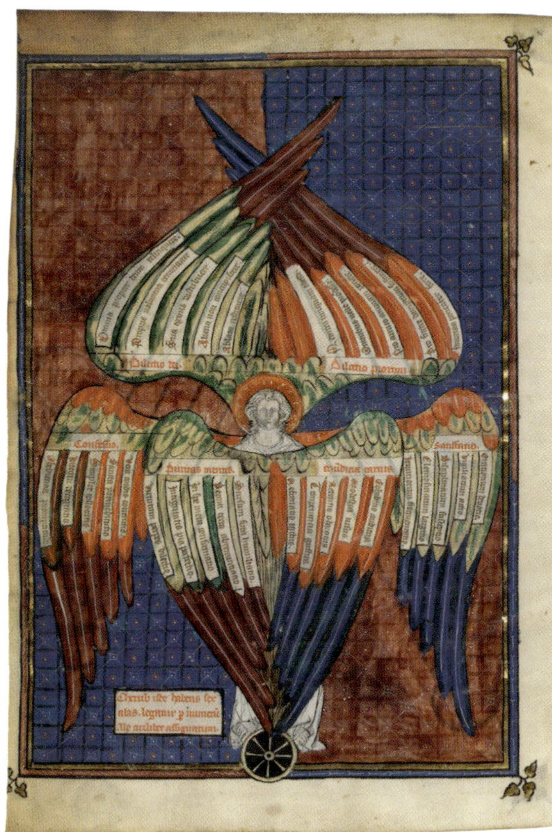

Fig. 1.2. A branching diagram in the form of a six-winged cherub whose feathers individuate different elements of Christian religious virtues, c. 1300, France. Ink and paint on parchment, 28 x 21 cm. Paris, Bibliothèque de l'Arsenal, MS 1037 Rés., fol. 6v.

accompanying explanatory treatises, such images presented what Müller has termed their own unique "visual gloss" on what could be highly complex concepts, arguing novel points of view from an entirely independent epistemic footing.[15]

If viewing these medieval images might therefore be tantamount to thinking through arguments, could they also spark other kinds of mental processes? This is the parallel jumping-off point for another group of medievalists, historians of memory, who have addressed the significant role played by diagramming in conditioning premodern practices of learning, narrative, and creative recall. As Mary Carruthers has most extensively argued, both Classical and medieval methods of *memoria* understood that images could form central prompts for mental recollection and reconstitution.[16] Such prompts work not only in the dry sense that we might be familiar with from modern memory techniques, where pictures stand in as mental substitutes for objects or terms in a straightforward one-to-one manner, although we do find entire late medieval Bibles written in this manner.[17] Rather, for thinkers as diverse as Thomas Aquinas, John Garland, and Ramon Llull, among many others, images both real and imagined could also trigger more meditative and rhetorical forms of thinking that actively unfolded across a viewer's consciousness.

Take the case of the twelfth-century Benedictine author Hugh de Fouilloy, who regularly combined notions of diagrammatic argument and diagrammatic memory in his work, producing eloquent combinations of image and

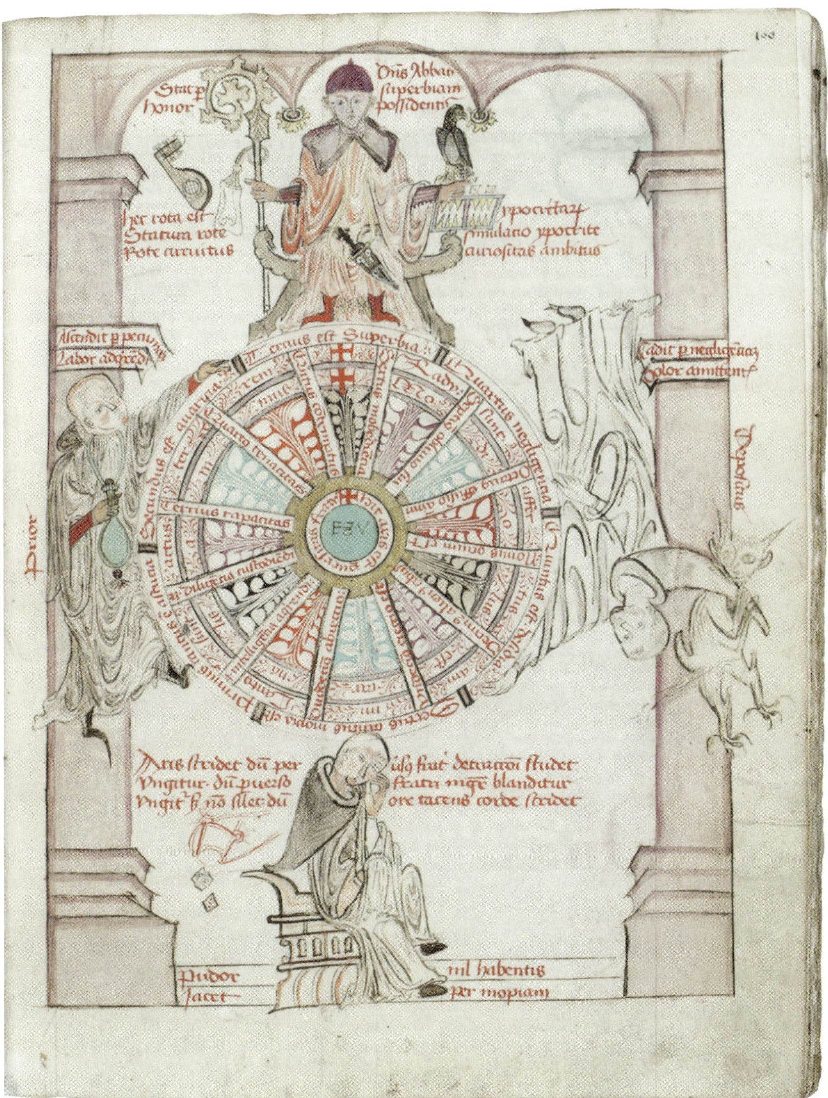

Fig. 1.3. Hugh de Fouilloy's "Axis of Brotherly Perversion," showing the fortunes of a corrupt monk, 1435, probably Austria. Ink and paint on parchment, 29 x 22 cm. Melk, Stiftsbibliothek, Cod. 737 (23, A 26), fol. 100r.

text.[18] Typical of this is his *Liber de rota verae et falsae religionis* (Book of the Wheel of True and False Religion), a treatise that reworks the much-favored Classical metaphor of Fortune's Wheel into a pair of good and bad models for medieval monastic ethics, its eponymous *rotae*.[19] In an Austrian copy of the work now in Melk Abbey, one of these circular images is preserved particularly well (fig. 1.3).[20] This is Hugh's "Axis of Brotherly Perversion," chronicling the rise and fall of one monk's dastardly fortunes around a circular wheel. On the far left of the page we enter the cycle *in medias res* with the wheel's central character on the up: "*ascendit per pecuniam*" (he ascends through money), a marginal note observes. Drawn skyward by the spinning wheel, a quarter turn clockwise we find the same man with purse in hand, comfortably ensconced in a double-headed throne, promoted from mere bad monk to a full-fledged bad abbot. The ill-gotten nature of this office is stressed by a nearby label discussing his "*superbia*" (pride), while alongside his sacred crozier he wields more frivolous worldly possessions: a hunting hawk and a backgammon board. The cycle of evil pauses for no one, however, and with a further quarter turn, the figure is soon set spinning downward. We read "*Cadit per negligentiam*" (He falls through negligence) and see the man whisked by the wheel so quickly from his throne that a gray devil catches a ride on his hood and saps the washed-up, washed-out monk's entire body of color.[21] Finally, at the bottom of the ensemble, he reaches rock bottom, "*iacet per inopiam*" (he is cast down by poverty), with even his gambling dice flung uselessly to the side.

On an immediate level, the image as a whole vividly animates Hugh's central message to the reader: sin has a cyclical, runaway quality to it, where one bad action inevitably generates another as the wheel turns interminably. Yet at the same time, the circular configuration here serves as a more mnemonic form of ward for the reader. As Carruthers has noted, Hugh himself described his varied investments in images, arguments, and memorization using a wide range of terms, including both *pingere* (to paint) and *decrescere* (to reduce in size).[22] Enacting precisely this combination, the *rota* is a visual commemorative compression whose twelve spokes are also each neatly labeled and numbered with a different specific stage in its story of sin: *rapacitas* (rapaciousness), *contemptus* (contempt), *oblivio sui* (forgetfulness of self), and so on. In fusing mnemonics with narrative to elaborate its central claims, this image's circling terms aid the reader in fully appreciating the gamut of these monastic perils and offer the best possible chance of recognizing such temptations in their own lives.

The *Liber de rota* unquestionably contains serious diagrammatic images with serious consequences. But other historians have suggested that even such seemingly sober systems were, in their own way, drawing upon yet another potential resonance of medieval diagrammatic pictures: their capacity for puckishness and play. Steffen Bogen has unpacked these ludic qualities most recently in relation to the so-called *Libro de axedrez, dados, e tablas* (Book of Chess, Dice, and Table Games), written for the Spanish King Alfonso X in the mid-thirteenth century.[23] The book describes rules, practice problems, and even board- and piece-making methods for a number of different games of skill and chance, all vividly illustrated in more than 150 colorful painted miniatures. The games imaged for Alfonso vary, from chess—"*assessegado iuego e onrrado*" (a noble and honored game)—through to lowlier entertainments such as checkers, backgammon, and dice, as well as several unusual iterations of each, such as *Acedrex de las diez casas* (Chess on a ten-sided board) or *Cercar la liebre* (Corner the Hare, played on a Twelve Men's Morris board).[24] And on a formal level alone the manuscript's colorful images of games strike particularly persuasive parallels with the medieval diagrammatic tradition, perhaps none more so than the penultimate image in the book, which bears an interesting resemblance to Hugh's circular *rotae* (fig. 1.4).[25]

It outlines a remarkable seven-player version of draughts "*que se iuegan por Astronomia*" (that is played by astronomy), with each player taking on the personification of a different planet to simultaneously model their skill in the game and their knowledge of the stars. As with all depictions in the book,

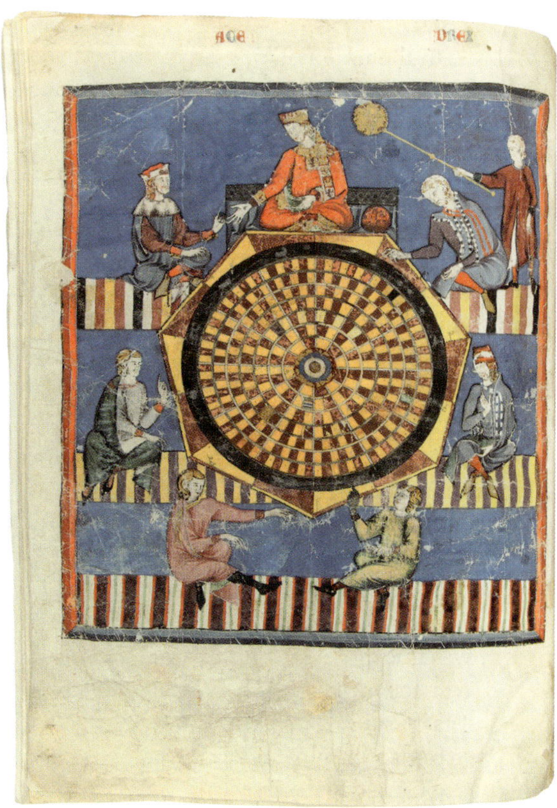

Fig. 1.4. Game of draughts "played by astronomy" from the *Libro de axedrez, dados, e tablas* written for King Alfonso X of Spain, 1283, Seville. Ink and paint on parchment, 40 x 28 cm. Madrid, Real Biblioteca del Monasterio de El Escorial, MS T-I-6, fol. 96v.

the action is presented to the reader within a semi-realistic environment. Seven well-dressed players sit cross-legged around a grand circular board, the miniature's striped backdrop evoking the lush, carpeted surrounds of an elite household, just as the fancy chair and attentive servant belonging to the player dressed in heraldic robes at the table's top evoke Alfonso himself. The board at which the figures play, however, is differently rendered, modeled not in three dimensions but schematically, as if viewed directly from above. This is primarily an attempt at communicative clarity. It is far easier to appreciate the specific details of starting positions and to differentiate board design or other details when games are shown square-on in this manner. But as Bogen subtly notes, in choosing to present the accoutrements of the game this way, such an image might also be trying to harness a more fundamental aspect of the diagrammatic image's potential. Despite the apparent animation of the figures sitting around these bird's-eye boards—pointing hands, leaning shoulders, flapping fans—no games in the *Libro* are ever actually in progress. Pieces either hover in opening positions, awaiting play, or, as in the case of astronomical draughts, are yet to even be placed on the table. Unlike their realistic surrounds, these diagrammed boards instead present a frame for the game with a more universal, prospective eye. John Bender and Michael Marrinan, discussing modern visual tropes, have suggested something similar when they argue that diagrams do not simply describe objects or ideas but try to capture multiple moments in the potential unfolding of a process. As they put it, diagrams are "closer in kind to a Jackson Pollock than to a Rembrandt."[26] Just as with the mnemonic reader who spins their way around Hugh de Fouilloy's *rotae*, viewers of Alfonso's book could also be drawn into projecting the pleasure of future games onto these outlined boards. More than a mere static rulebook, these images can be seen as an invitation, a prompt to go out and play.

Several conceptual strands, then, are beginning to emerge from the eclectic body of diagrammatic thinking assembled here, each of which ascribes to what we might anachronistically call diagrams from across later medieval Europe a slightly different set of abilities: they could make arguments, structure mnemonic narratives, and present as playful challenges. Yet to separate out even just these three emphases from one another is clearly something of an artificial construct. While individual medieval readers might have arrived at the page with specific facets of a specific image in mind, it is vital not to disaggregate the multiple capacities of these diagrammatic things but instead to embrace the sheer vastness of their visual ambition as we consider the layered nature of their interconnected lines and labels.

Medieval diagrammatic images were, after all, often deliberately excessive things that attempted to represent far more than the mere sum of their individual parts. Nowhere was this more apparent than in the religious realm, where the potential of such schematics to simultaneously connect readers with multiple grand truths of spiritual thought was utilized to the very fullest.[27] Jeffrey Hamburger brings this out most clearly in his recent analysis of a highly original series of Christian images associated with the *De missarum mysteriis* (On the Mysteries of the Mass), written in the mid-1190s by Lothar of Segni, known from 1198 as Pope Innocent III.[28] Surviving in several copies made between the thirteenth and fifteenth centuries, Lothar's textual discussion of religious practice is reinforced by a graphically punchy spread of forty-two individual pictures that rework conceptual, causal, temporal, and spiritual relationships between religious elements into meshes of dense pattern (fig. 1.5). These images held the impressive ability to both focus Christian thought and, paradoxically, radically untether it from the ordered armatures represented. On the one hand, they function as highly specific maps of ritual practice: one plots the disposition of religious personnel in front of the high altar during the Mass, another the various sacred uses of incense, yet another the different forms of kiss given during such ritual performances, and so on. But on the other hand, Lothar's images also begin to accrue ritual elements one atop each other in time and space to form grand webs of increasingly universalizing doctrine. Guiding the viewer toward a far more ineffable set of forces at work within the world, it is as if the treatise is laying out "the intricate gears of a mysterious machine," to use Hamburger's words, just as contemplation of the smallest network of atoms might prompt thoughts of how entire galaxies are constituted.[29] In performing this remarkable bifocal flip from microscopic to macrocosmic, Lothar's images demonstrate a faculty true to all types of medieval diagrammatic images: that they might mystify just as much as they clarify.

Such diagrams were not always entirely successful in this grand aim. As Hamburger notes, Lothar's seemingly unflappable sense of Christian order

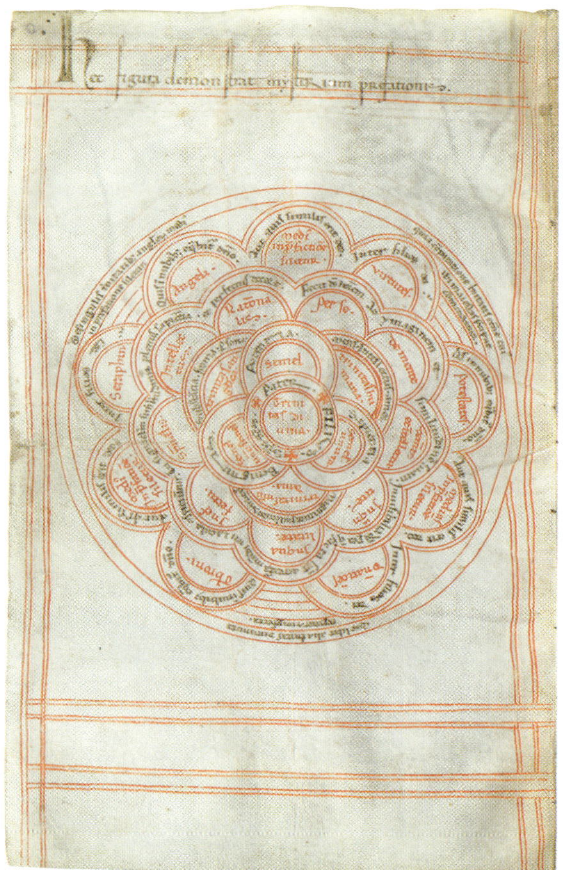

Fig. 1.5. Diagram depicting interconnected Christian mysteries from Lothar of Segni's *De missarum mysteriis*, c. 1250–75, probably Italy. Ink on parchment, 23 x 15 cm. Munich, Bayerische Staatsbibliothek, Clm 28609, fol. 6v.

could on occasion be undercut through miscopied details or clumsy reconfigurations that left their contents confused or simply incorrect. Yet regardless of their success, this observation draws our attention to a final aspect of medieval diagrammatic thinking that is often overlooked by modern commentators, one essential to understanding not just their internal mechanisms but their social presence in the medieval world. This is the idea that, perhaps more than anything, thinkers, writers, and artists of the European Middle Ages saw diagrams as objects of communication. In his recent book *Thing Knowledge*, the philosopher of science Davis Baird writes that, historically speaking, scientific instruments—of which diagrams are a branch—tend to develop principally in contexts where ordinary language somehow fails as a vehicle for communicating knowledge.[30] When technical vocabularies fall short in explaining ideas, objects and images are deployed to take up the epistemological reins as a kind of scientific interlocutor unto themselves.

The last place we might expect to find Baird's twenty-first-century idea affirmed is in thirteenth-century poetry, yet communication through diagrammatic imagery appears to be precisely what the Friuli-born writer Thomasin von Zerclêre had in mind when crafting his grand didactic poem *Der Welsche Gast*.[31] Translated variously as *The Italian Guest* or *The Romance Stranger*, Thomasin's work is a poetic stroll through ethical conduct for courtly gentlemen and gentlewomen, schooling the reader in aristocratic virtues, vices, and niceties, complete with secular and spiritual exemplars taken from Thomasin's world. In *Der Welsche Gast*'s seventh book, for instance, Thomasin turns specifically to the edification of the soul, which, he argues, is a two-part process. First, a courtier's soul might be nourished through the cultivation of inherently heavenly attributes, such as common sense or reasoning. But the soul is equally fueled by a dedication to earthly learning—"*wir wellen sîn alle wîs*" (we all want to be wise), as the poet puts it—and key to this, according to Thomasin, is knowledge of the finest historical thinkers from across the Seven Liberal Arts.[32] The ensuing poetic roll call lists the ancient names that dominated academic discourse of the day, alongside which several manuscripts of *Der Welsche Gast* also preserve a set of images to develop Thomasin's point.[33] We might assume that these pictures, like the text, show portraits of the great figures in question, and this is indeed how they are labeled: Priscian is paired with Grammar, Euclid with Geometry, Pythagoras with Arithmetic, Aristotle with Dialectics, Milesius with Music, Ptolemy with Astronomy, and Cicero—whose words began this chapter—with Rhetoric. Yet the illustrations in fact present a number of ordinary individuals, female and male, rich and poor, all exchanging giant diagrams (fig. 1.6).[34] Two men pass an outsize Aristotelian Square of Opposition between each other, its counterbalanced lines labeled in Latin with dialectical terms. A pair of crowned figures discourse together on astronomy by hoisting large interlocking circles into the air, an image drawn from Ptolemy's works on planetary orbit. And two figures enacting musical exchange come across as the most dynamic of all: they hold

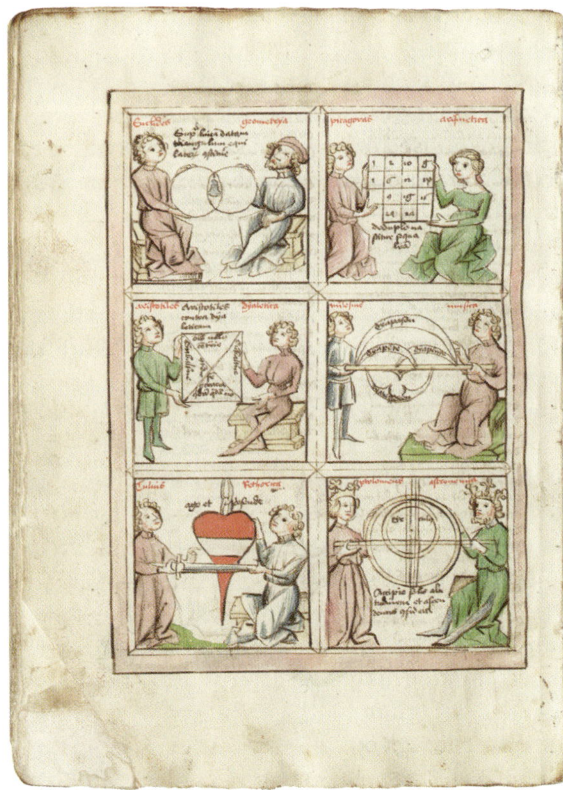

Fig. 1.6. Communicative diagrams of the Seven Liberal Arts from Thomasin von Zerclêre's *Der Welsche Gast*, c. 1450–75, Swabia. Ink and paint on paper, 31 x 21 cm. Munich, Bayerische Staatsbibliothek, Cgm 571, fol. 70v.

opposite ends of a realistically rendered thick wooden staff, from which burst the different intervals of Classical music theory—*diatessaron*, *diapente*, *diapason*—as if these technical elements were actually springing forth from this quotidian object, a tangible diagrammatic presence conjured into being during the process of intellectual communion.

As well as the vividness of seeing such images brought to life, their presence within this explicitly moralizing work steers us toward an important point, in some ways the most crucial lesson of these medieval diagrams for explorations of the Wound Man in the chapters to come. Thomasin's concern with these diagrammatic arts is not merely an intellectual exercise: it is explicitly ethical. In *Der Welsche Gast*, knowledge's true value is as a moral force, one that can help in telling "*daz slehte vome krumben, die wârheit vom valsche*" (the straight from the crooked, truth from falsehood). And in the process of making diagrammatic images real, Thomasin's illustrators come to echo the one medieval profession that actually did use the term *diagramma*: land surveying, a discipline that regularly utilized images to create physical boundaries in the landscape. Steffen Bogen and Felix Thürlemann have drawn attention to this by examining in detail the sixth-century scholar Magnus Aurelius Cassiodorus's description of an early medieval land surveyor at work.[35] Clomping his way through woods and groves with instruments and images in hand, Cassiodorus suggests that anyone coming across a surveyor in reality might well mistake him for a madman desperately lost in a forest. Yet this individual's diagrams, he reminds us, are the most potent of all, because they form a graphical template for imposing the law equitably and uniformly onto the complexities of sociopolitical space. Kathrin Müller has termed this capacity of medieval images "*visuelle Weltaneignung*," a direct appropriation of the world through the visual.[36] If, as we have seen, diagrams from the European Middle Ages were proponents of argument, narrative, play, mystery, and communication, what better tools could there be for those wishing to make their own claims to power and to knowledge?

Figura and the Problem of Medicine

Most diagrammatic images found across later medieval Europe exhibit a strong analogical streak. This is to say that, as well as utilizing what we might term a shared schematic vocabulary—lines leading to circles, labels surrounding squares, arrows gesturing across grids, and so on—artists and writers of the period were keen to move beyond this simple informational texture and employ more creative tropes when crafting their visual explanations. A stemma presenting spiritual tenets could have remained a branching bundle of texts and lines rather than transform into an elaborate cherub with labeled feathers. Hugh's *rotae* could have stayed as plain numerated circles rather than germinate into human-scaled spinning wheels peopled with crooks and hellish caricatures. But they did not. Instead, these images were extended into complex analogical structures: full-fledged visual ecosystems built from multiple metaphorical connections.

This accumulative style of visual thinking was very much in keeping with broader developments unfolding across contemporary models of thought.

It resonated with the growing intellectual penchant of medieval European scholars for *concordia*—the rhetorical potential of thinking by grand association—and it resonated too with such theoreticians' increasing engrossment with ideas of equilibrium, the strong sense present from the thirteenth century onward that totalizing balance was the ultimate goal of legal, religious, economic, and medical systems alike.[37] Visually speaking, a cluster of analogical refrains also emerged as particularly popular with authors and image-makers thinking in this mold. The organic, root-and-branch forms of trees, for instance, matched neatly with the carefully stratified nature of much scholastic thought.[38] The image of the house was likewise a common analogy, doubly handy for making available both a host of interconnected architectural metaphors—foundations, walls, roofs, gardens—and more affective concepts of home, safety, and custodianship.[39] Even so, the most common and most versatile of the visual forms these thinkers utilized was that of the human body, the figure, a piece of analogical apparatus par excellence.

In part this was an inheritance from the Classical world, where a substantial repertoire of literary and visual personifications had been built up over the centuries.[40] As Erich Auerbach has observed, the Latin word *figura* condensed a complex series of inferences into a single term.[41] Beginning with the generalized rhetorical allusions of early authors such as Quintilian, the word grew to take on an increasingly prophetic, prefigurative quality in the writing of Christian thinkers such as Tertullian and Augustine, while throughout retaining its chameleon-like capacity to signify a multitude of everyday ideas: a number, a quantity, an image, a physique, and of course an actual body. Figurative allusions of this kind resonated particularly with European medieval readers, who regularly encountered the Elements or Cardinal Directions, the Liberal Arts or the Four Seasons, all taking on human form in the pages of their books.[42]

Personification, though, was only the first and arguably the most superficial of corporeal tools in the medieval analogist's arsenal. More useful was the body's structure itself, whose somatic correspondences lent strong conceptual coherence to all sorts of parallel ideas when diagrammed on the page. At its simplest, these correspondences cohered in a modular sense, with individual body parts acting in the stead of more typical schematic elements (fig. 1.7). In a well-known twelfth-century diagrammatic image accompanying Honorius Augustodunensis's *Clavis physicae* (The Key of Natural Philosophy), a text summarizing and synthesizing Neoplatonic philosophy, twelve individually labeled arms run up, down, and across the page, their grasping hands and ruffled sleeves used to clarify the interconnected qualities of the scheme's different conceptual parts.[43] In an even more tactile example from several centuries later, an English *rota* for calculating the date of Easter and other important calendar events comes complete with a figural volvelle at its center.[44] Labeled "*Digito noto pascha*" (Finger denotes Easter), its right hand and foot function as a movable pointer to identify paired variables at different sites around the wheel. But more than its deconstructed parts, the body could also be made to stand for what Michael Camille astutely termed "any bounded system" of the European Middle Ages, regardless of complexity or magnitude.[45]

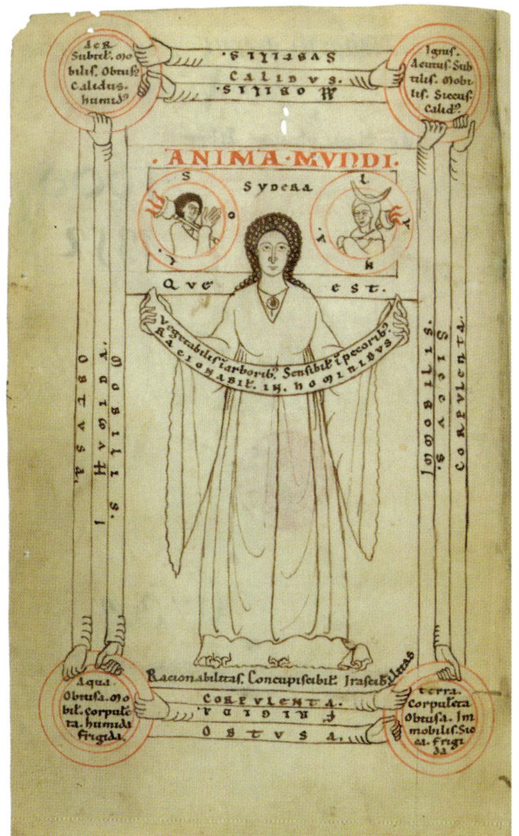

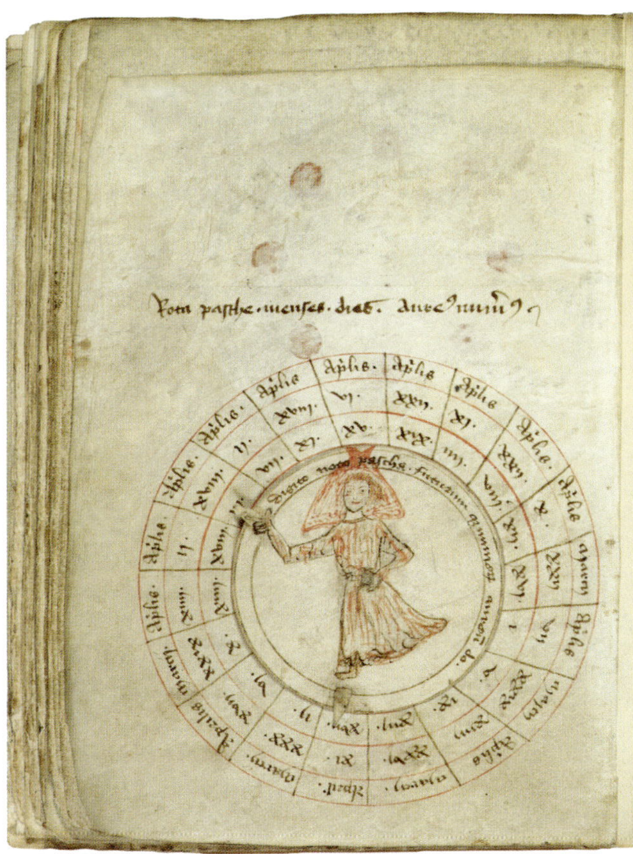

Fig. 1.7. Two pieces of corporeal diagrammatic technology. *Left:* Concepts connected by interlocking arms from Honorius Augustodunensis's *Clavis physicae*, 14th century, probably Meuse region. Ink on parchment. Paris, Bibliothèque nationale de France, MS Latin 6734, fol. 1v. *Right:* A figural volvelle, 15th century, probably Germany. Ink and paint on parchment with string attachments, 21 x 15 cm. London, British Library, Harley MS 941, fol. 29v.

At one end of this spectrum, we find the body elucidating extremely focused, small-scale concerns. For instance, in a prefatory image found at the beginning of one of the oldest medieval books to survive in Middle Dutch, Jacob van Maerlant's thirteenth-century *Der naturen bloeme* (The Flower of Nature), an author portrait of Jacob holding his book has been hybridized with a diagrammatic explanation of his various intellectual sources (fig. 1.8).[46] Clearly modeled on so-called Trees of Consanguinity—legal and religious diagrams designed to plot the limits of familial intermarriage—the portrait shows Jacob's interconnected learning cascading forward from his stomach like a dangling parasitic growth, each issued circle occupied by a different author cited in the work, from Philemon to Democritus to the cardinal point at the top of the tree held by Aristotle.[47] Meanwhile, at the other end of the spectrum we find the body giving bounds to something as unendingly enormous as the fundamental workings of the universe itself. In a scientific book roughly contemporaneous with Jacob's work, produced most likely in southern Germany, a single human form takes up the role of connecting an entire world-system (fig. 1.9).[48] The multiple elements of this "microcosmus," as it is labeled, come thick and fast, listed one by one atop the figure's body: its limbs are likened to months of the year and signs of the zodiac, it stands amid a four-part backdrop of the four cardinal elements, and labels fire out from its face declaring the names of the seven planets.[49] Not only does the

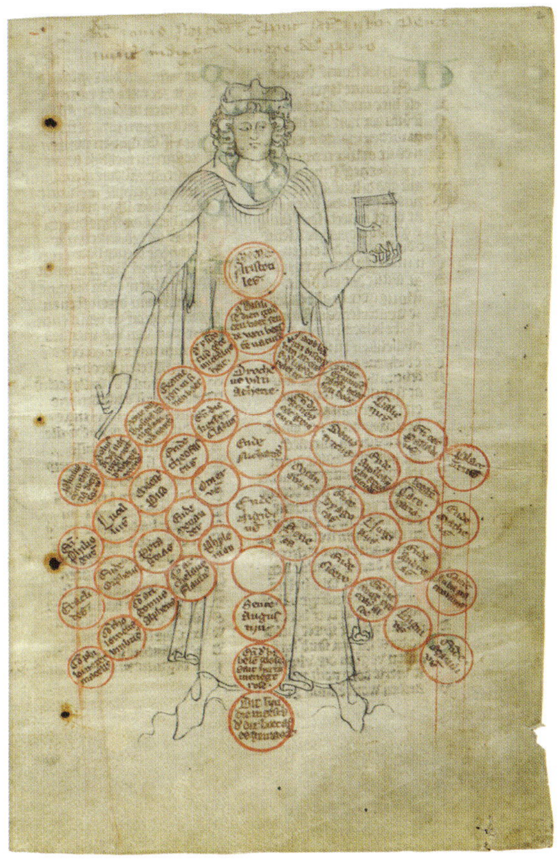

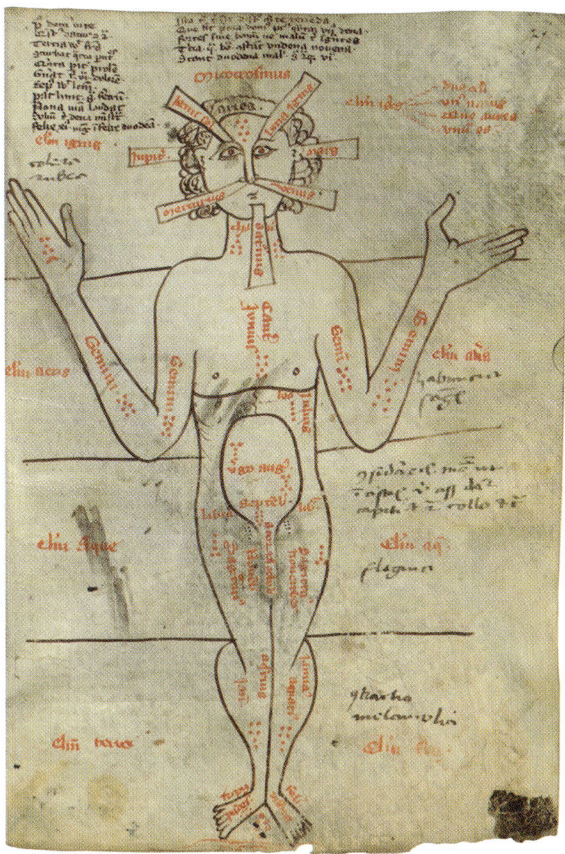

Fig. 1.8. Figural diagram of learned sources from Jacob van Maerlant's *Der naturen bloeme*, c. 1325, Belgium. Ink and paint on parchment, 24 x 15 cm. Brussels, Koninklijke Bibliotheek van België, MS 19546, fol. 2r.

Fig. 1.9. Microcosmic figure showing the correspondence of planets, elements, the zodiac, and the body, c. 1290, probably southern Germany. Ink on parchment, 21 x 15 cm. Vienna, Österreichische Nationalbibliothek, Cod. 2469, fol. 41r.

body here unite a disparate universe, but like all of these corporeal analogies, it lends a sense of inviolability and authority to its embodied ideas. Rewiring the knowledge contained in such figures would require a violent reconstituting of parts, the coherence of the scheme as a corporeal whole stewarded by protective figuration.

It was within the medical sphere, however, that this useful medieval habit of turning base information into bodies came up against a unique set of contradictions. Medical authors and image-makers of the later Middle Ages, just like their intellectual and artistic counterparts in other fields discussed earlier, were well aware of the intricacies of the diagrammatic mode and had been utilizing them frequently for centuries.[50] Among the earliest medical texts to be transported around the medieval Mediterranean in the busy exchange between Latin, Arabic, and Hebrew healing cultures were the so-called *Alexandrian Summaries*, a mixed commentary built around a core of sixteen books on Classical Galenic medicine whose contents were often shared in the form of branched trees of information to aid recollection.[51] As the period progressed, many other key medical concepts and practical procedures also soon found useful schematic form, with a single medical book often housing many such images at once. Theoretical understandings of the body's internal workings—grids contrasting the four elements, bodies marked with points for strategic humoral cautery with heated irons, the so-called Zodiac Man plotting the influence of the stars on human health—could all be clarified through tables and maps that neatly visualized their distinctions and correspondences.[52]

Other more active diagrammatic images were mobilized directly in the process of diagnosis, the most common being Urine Wheels in which the color of a patient's urine—a key indicator of their internal humoral balance—could be assessed against circular *rotae* describing and sometimes even imaging different colors of the micturitic spectrum.[53] Prognosis too could be divined through grids and circles, for instance onomantic images such as the *Spera de vita et morte* (Sphere of Life and Death), variously known as the Sphere of Pythagoras, the Sphere of Hippocrates, or the sphere of pretty much any other great scholarly name of the period.[54] Using a circular schematic packed with numbers, this image instructed the reader to reformulate the name of a patient into a series of numerical values, add to it various pieces of calendrical information regarding the date they fell ill, and then divide by thirty to achieve a final number that was itself cross-referenced against a key at the circle's center for a final dramatic prediction: life or death.

Nonetheless, when medieval medics wished to follow their fellow authors and image-makers in branching out from lines and circles into thinking by creative visual analogy, they encountered an obvious problem particular to their field. Unlike in discussions of cosmology or theology, mathematics or memory, legalese or literature, in medicine the subject of the field's theory and practice was one and the same as the period's dominant frame for elucidating theoretical and practical correspondence: both were bodies. One of the earliest and most influential theorists of the modern diagram, the nineteenth-century semiotician Charles Sanders Peirce, argued that a diagram's fluid function relied upon a clear differentiation between its frame and its content: "many diagrams resemble their objects not at all in looks; it is only in respect to the relations of their parts that their likeness consists."[55] Yet this relational separation is patently not always possible in medicine, where the distinction between analogical framework and informational content is instead collapsed into one.

Take an image presented on the penultimate page of an early fifteenth-century Hebrew manuscript, made in southern France or perhaps northern Italy (fig. 1.10).[56] We are shown a man with short, curly hair who wears a high-collared blue coat, the red of his undersleeves vanishing into a pair of pocket slits at the robe's front. But erupting from his face is a much-magnified image of an eye, plotted out entirely schematically so as to make clear the different parts of the ocular anatomy, mostly descriptions of different kinds of אומור (humor) and כתונת (tunic).[57] Could this exploded eye ever actually belong to the specific figure from which it emanates, to the singular, individual patient we see carefully depicted in flesh and blood? Or is it instead a universalized abstraction, an image whose relation to the actual object of a human eye is entirely theoretical, mapping instead how all fifteenth-century eyes were understood to function, and in turn transforming the robed figure into a conglomerate of all fifteenth-century men and women?

We have arrived back where this chapter began: at the two antagonistic concepts lashed together in the word "illustration," image as information

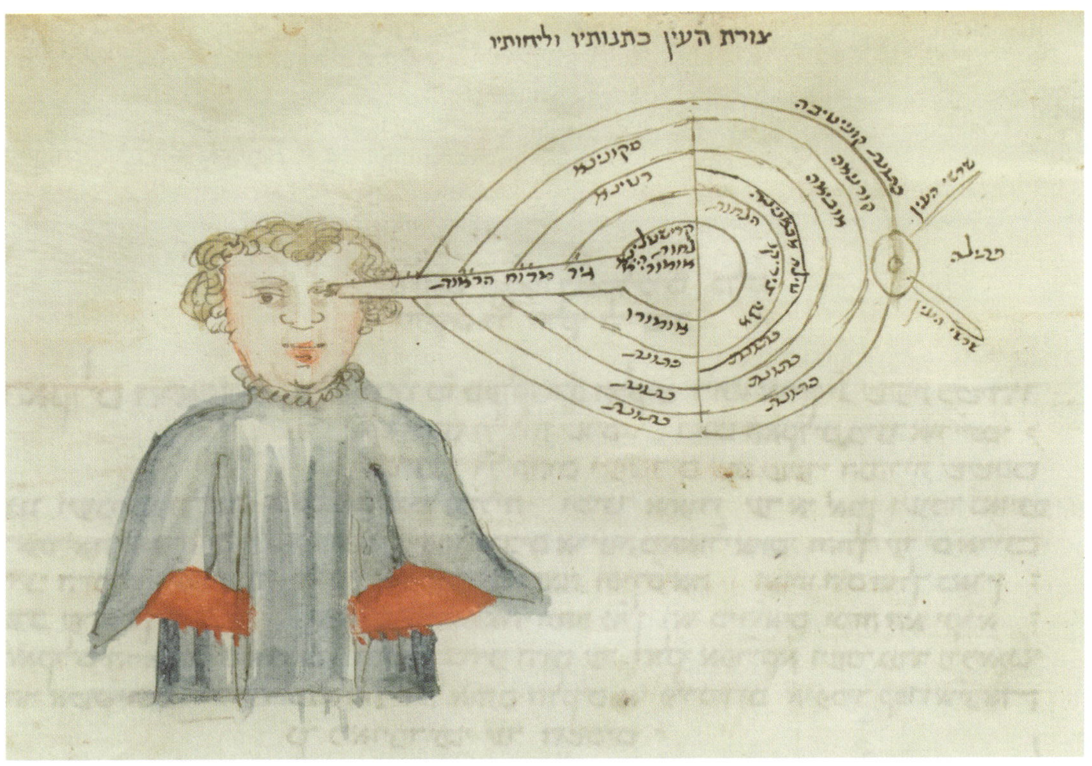

Fig. 1.10. Diagram of the eye from a Hebrew medical manuscript, 15th century, probably northern Italy. Ink and paint on parchment, 35 x 25 cm. Paris, Bibliothèque nationale de France, MS Hébreu 1181, fol. 265r.

and image as representation. So let us return as well to the unusual half-woman-half-diagram sketched by Erhard Knab in his Heidelberg notebook (see fig. 1.1). Given the impressive conceptual depth found across the varied late medieval diagrammatic contexts surveyed earlier, especially their epistemic back-and-forth between bodies at once ubiquitous and individuated, we are now better placed to understand this particular body's resistance to being either wholly a patient or wholly a schematic. After all, Knab was himself far from naive when it came to diagrammatic medical images and their different knowledge functions. We know this because an unusually high number of books associated with Knab survive today, owing in part to the wholesale transfer of Heidelberg's Palatine Library to Rome in 1634 following the Thirty Years' War.[58] Such a concentration of sources is perhaps unique in the medical world of the Middle Ages. As Peter Murray Jones reminds us, unlike their counterparts in the modern textbook, medieval medical images are almost never associated with named illustrators, designers, publishers, or even authors.[59] Instead, particular illustrative tropes bounced around freely from text to text. Being able to look broadly across Knab's Heidelberg books is thus a rare opportunity, and in them we find illustrations put to a highly varied number of uses. One manuscript from the later 1450s, for instance, presents the different divisions and subdivisions of the art of medicine plotted out by Knab as a typical tree diagram, much like those that had been used to illustrate the *Alexandrian Summaries* for centuries.[60] In another book from around 1460, Knab has copied out a canonical medical commentary on Galen by the early medieval author Ḥunayn ibn Isḥāq—known to medieval European physicians as Johannitius—alongside what appears to be his own glossed commentary on the text and, in the lower left-hand corner of one page, a diagram of the twelve winds, each personified with a large grotesque face not dissimilar to those in Hugh de Fouilloy's *rotae*.[61] And among the lines of yet another manuscript, this one completed in 1466, Knab has included a series of compact sketches of instruments to be used in different surgical operations, an illustrative idea whose pedigree stretched back at least three hundred years to the Arabic writings of the prolific Hispanic surgeon Abū'l Qāsim al-Zahrāwī.[62]

What is more, the evidence of Knab's collected manuscripts suggests that he was not only well versed in medieval traditions of medical imaging but also well aware of the social value of an illustrated book more generally in the intellectual climate of his age. Most of his manuscripts are rather chaotically collected notebooks completed in his own scrawly writing, but several of them include images that were no doubt commissioned from professional artists. In a manuscript from around 1470, Knab's hand leaves space at the opening of a text that he has copied—Abū ʿAlī al-Husayn ibn Sīnā's *Canon of Medicine*, a medieval medical classic—for a highly competent painter to insert a giant illuminated letter *S*, complete with swooping acanthus patterning and a subtly gilded black ground.[63] Later in this book, the same illuminator also provides a stretched floral bouquet across the bas-de-page beneath the opening of Ibn Sīnā's chapter on urine and egestion, as well as a rendering of a heraldic display beneath the opening of the *Canon*'s fourth book, including a knightly helm between the arms of the city of Heidelberg and the Palatinate.[64] Knab knew that an expensive illuminator's work could raise the professional cachet of a book significantly, connecting his writings with a broader network of artistic and intellectual patronage.

Most of all, though, Knab seems quite simply to have taken real joy in making images himself. Another of his autograph commentaries, this time addressing a uroscopy treatise by the thirteenth-century French royal physician Gilles de Corbeil, opens with an oversized figural initial of a man holding a book whose rough style, executed in the same red and black ink as the text, is surely the physician's own.[65] Even more playfully, in another manuscript from the 1450s, Knab has copied out a text on chiromancy—the popular medieval practice of divination by lines on the palms—illustrated on either side of the folio by a pair of five-fingered diagrams whose outline Knab has clearly produced by tracing carefully around his own hands (fig. 1.11).[66] This array of visual evidence in which Knab shifts between pictorial registers and almost revels in representative techniques suggests that he understood exactly the different modes he was straddling when creating his intriguing half-woman-half-diagram.

Fig. 1.11. Chiromantic hand diagrams sketched by the Heidelberg physician Erhard Knab using his own hands, c. 1450–55, Heidelberg. Ink on paper, 29 x 21 cm (each folio). Vatican City, Biblioteca Apostolica Vaticana, MS Pal. Lat. 1264, fol. 244r–244v.

Fig. 1.12. Bloodletting figure inserted opposite a tree diagram showing the "Entire Art of Medicine," 14th century (diagram) and early 15th century (figure), Germany. Ink on parchment, 41 x 32 cm (right folio). Vatican City, Biblioteca Apostolica Vaticana, MS Pal. Lat. 1181, inside cover and fol. 1r.

This was, we now recognize, a diagrammatic doubling of bodies as both medical subject and informational vehicle common to many medical makers of the day. Another book also conveyed from Heidelberg to Rome, produced by an unnamed author, clarifies the situation in a perfect snapshot. The manuscript is only short, a fourteenth-century treatise just nine folios long, yet it summarizes several popular scholastic medical works by condensing them into easily consumable tree diagrams (fig. 1.12).[67] The original opening

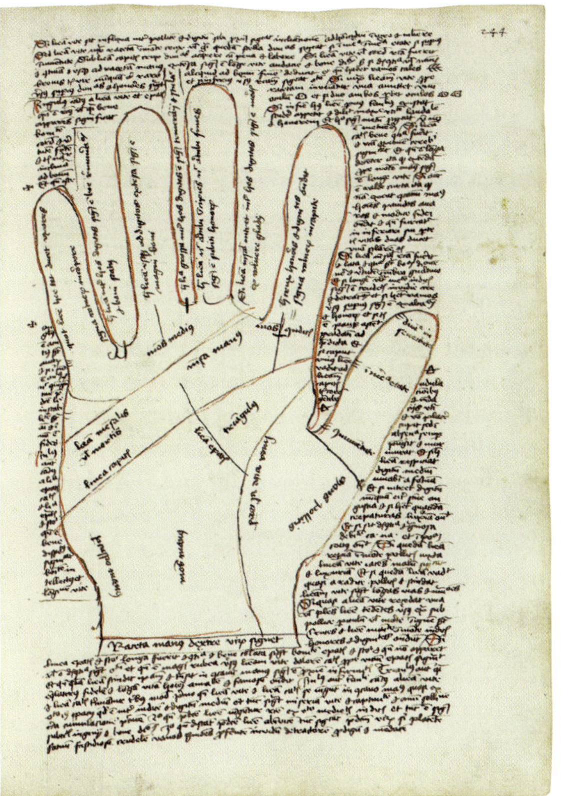

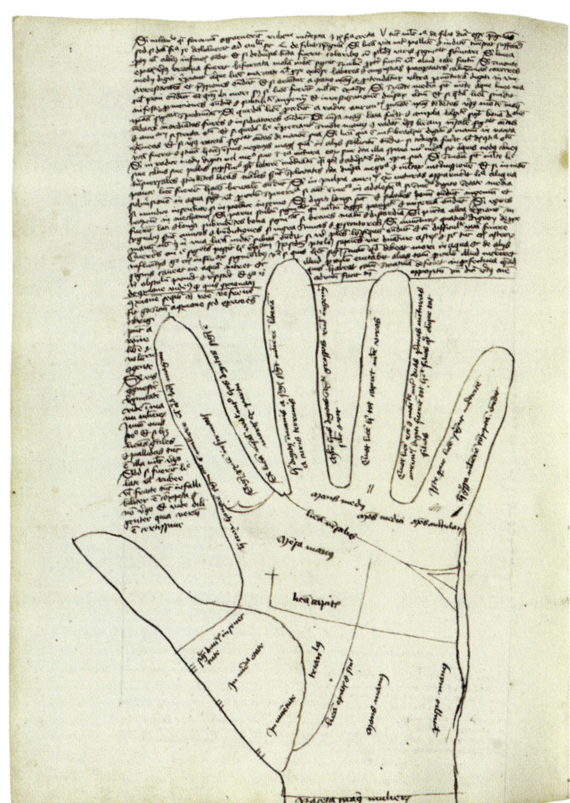

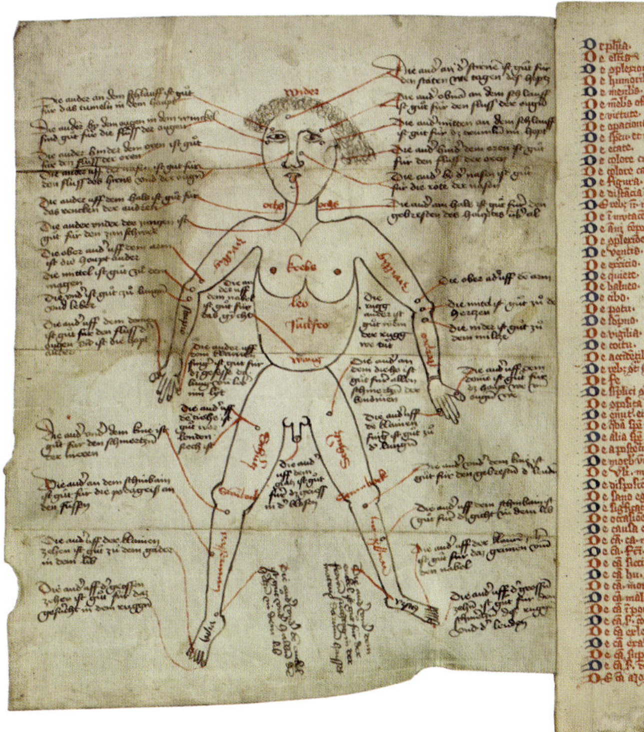

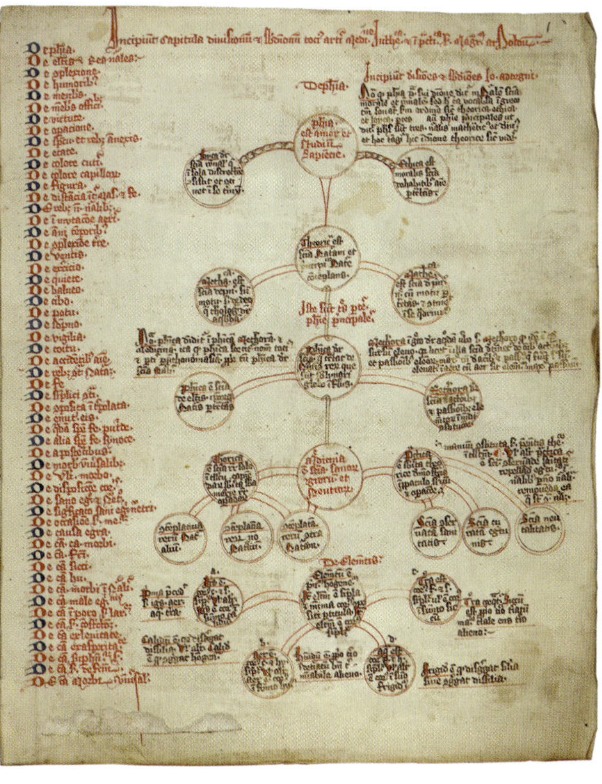

page of the book is typical of the work as a whole. At the top, we read the phrase "*Capitula divisionum et subdivisionum totius artis medicinae*" (Chapters of the divisions and subdivisions of the entire art of medicine). Below it, units of the eponymous medical art are laid out in connected circles indicating their relations, with bubbles representing theory and practice springing forth from medicine, which in turn takes its place amid a progressively all-encompassing tree showing different categories of knowledge. This tree, however, did not remain the booklet's opening page for long. To judge by the extant binding, another folio—a single parchment sheet showing the figure of a male patient, his body labeled from head to toe with locations for therapeutic bloodletting—was tipped in during the early 1400s to serve as a new entry point for the reader.[68] If this sketch was intended as a punchy new title page to the work, the insert fails, for it is the blank recto of this sheet that greets us as we hold the unopened booklet in our hands. Instead, the figure has been flipped so as to form a deliberate pair with the diagram of the Entire Art of Medicine, which now sits exactly across the gutter on the facing page at an almost identical height and width. With their shared branching limbs and floating paratexts, a map of the idealized patient and a map of the medical profession itself are being precisely aligned, a comparison that once more stages the correspondence between medical illustration's opposing ends: on the right, medical epistemics is enlivened through diagrammatic display, while on the left, a diagrammed body is enlightened by medicine's knowledge.

Blood and Words: The Wound Man's Double

The appearance of a figure outlining bloodletting in this diagrammatic manuscript is particularly pertinent given that medieval phlebotomical imagery provides a final important piece of staging for understanding the Wound Man's prehistory. A deep dive into the *figurae* of medieval European bloodletting, a body of images never before systematically explored, offers space for unpacking various key qualities of medieval medical images at large, revealing aspects of their fabrication, function, readership, and circulation. This was the Wound Man's world too, not just aesthetically speaking but also in the often overlooked social roles played by such images within and beyond the medical encounter. Moreover, this phlebotomical corpus has even keener links to the Wound Man, not only as a visual precursor but also as a conceptual double. Whereas images of the Wound Man, as we will soon discover, aided the enclosure of the body—its sealing through suturing, bandaging, and protection from the consequences of invading objects—bloodletting images facilitated the reverse: the therapeutic opening up of the body to bleed it. Bound by this inverted interest, these phlebotomical figures showcase better than any other diagrammatic antecedent of the Wound Man how medics and image-makers across Europe were mobilizing broader late medieval diagrammatic stances for their own means, innovating novel modes of medico-visual explanation that evolved across the period.

A manuscript from the Biblioteka Uniwersytecka in Wrocław, the excitingly named MS I F 334, is a good place to start, if for no other reason than its unusually long historiography. The earliest description of the book appears in a calligraphic catalog composed in the 1820s by the collection's first curator, Johann Christoph Friedrich.[69] Here he summarizes a parchment folio inserted toward the back of the paper manuscript in just four words: "*Medicina contra varios morbos*" (Medicine against various diseases). Simple enough. A little over a century later, the librarian Willi Göber and several of his colleagues in Wrocław updated and significantly extended Friedrich's catalog to better reflect the university's collections, expanding it from four volumes to a gargantuan twenty-six.[70] Göber summarizes the same page of the same book in similarly short but nonetheless quite different terms: "Doppelbl. mit Aderlaßmännchen" (Double page with Bloodletting Man). Friedrich and Göber are clearly only briefly noting the manuscript's contents. But still, for one librarian the page contains *medicina* (medicine), a formulation that in Friedrich's shorthand essentially means a medical text, and for the other it contains a *männchen* (a man or manikin), an image of a male figure.

It is only when looking at the Wrocław page itself that it becomes clear how these curatorial colleagues could describe the same thing so diversely (fig. 1.13). Sure enough, the folio is dominated by a male figure at its center, facing the reader with hands to the side and palms outstretched. A light pink wash flushes across its skin, while yellow shading and curly pen-work on its tufted bob endow the figure with peculiar life, a tangible presence on the page. Just as eye-catching, however, is the maelstrom of words in which the figure finds itself entangled: thick lines of red ink snake outward from its body in every conceivable direction to connect head, abdomen, and limbs with multiple gobbets of neatly inscribed text.

As Friedrich intimated, the *medicina* that surrounds this figure is directly curative, focusing specifically on the practice of phlebotomy, the therapeutic letting of blood. By the time this image was made in the early 1400s, the practice had been a mainstay of European medicine for centuries, stretching back at least as far as Classical Greek treatises that described the letting of blood as key to balancing internal bodily excess.[71] Blood was understood in this medical tradition to be both one of the quartet of corporeal humors—alongside phlegm, yellow bile, and black bile—and also the actual vehicle through which all four humors circulated within the body. Perhaps because of this structural potential, blood had long been considered to have strong medical and apotropaic properties, both diagnostically and as a prescriptive material in its own right.[72] Humorally speaking, evacuating the blood had the particularly valuable ability to realign the body in what contemporary writers described as an abnormal, overabundant state of *plethora* by removing potentially dangerous elements circulating within and returning the patient to a natural state of balance.

Stepping back from the Wrocław image for a moment, it is important to acknowledge that the specific mechanisms of this bloodletting practice were extremely complex and often depended heavily on a broadly circulating literature that outlined bloodletting's changing specifics for different medics in different contexts. The historian of medicine Pedro Gil-Sotres has neatly categorized medieval European phlebotomical writings into three broad stages.[73] First, the earlier Middle Ages saw a series of short texts emerge that drew principally on precedents from the Ancient Greek corpus, further

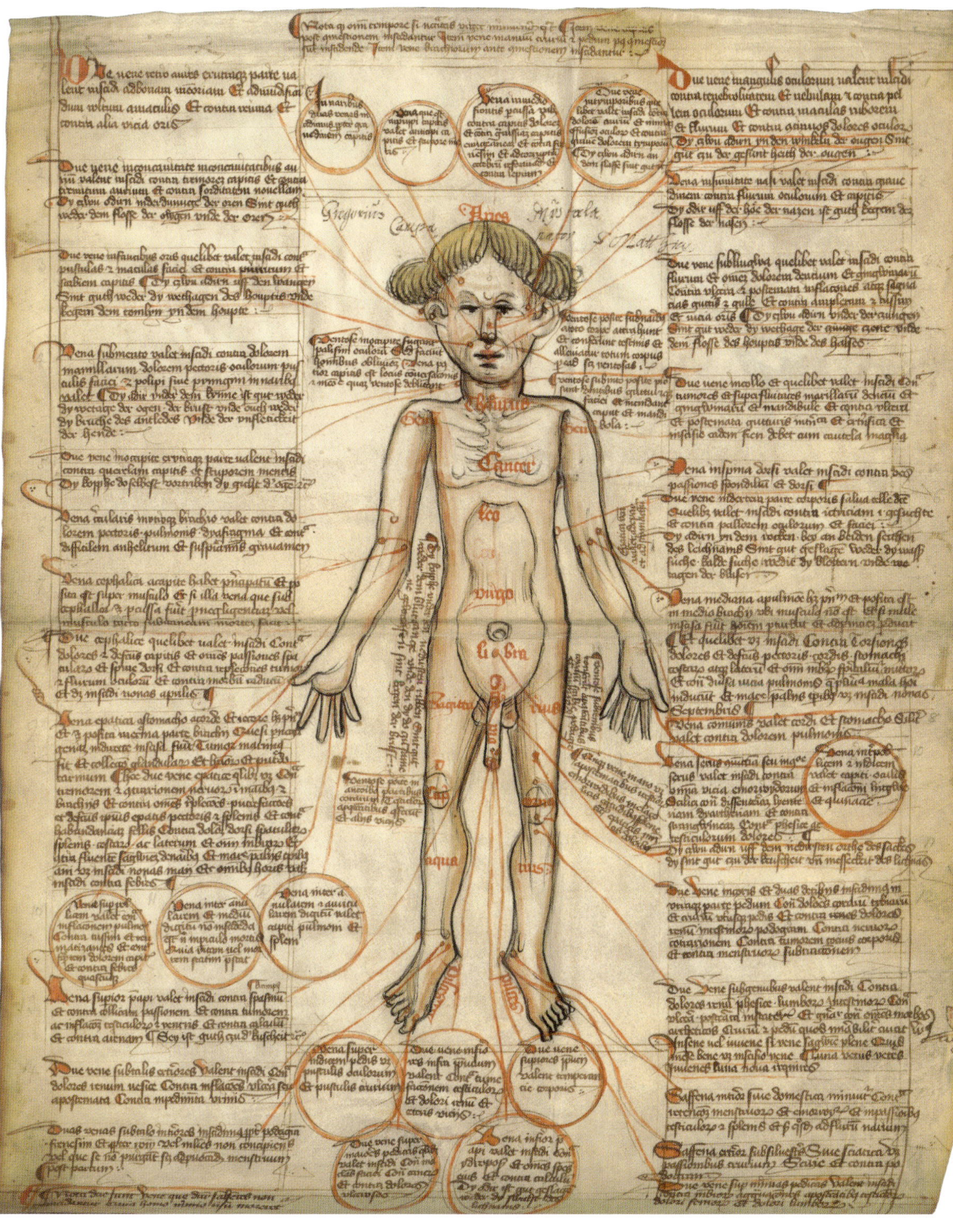

Fig. 1.13. Bloodletting figure, 15th century, Germany. Ink and paint on parchment, 60 x 42 cm (unfolded). Wrocław, Biblioteka Uniwersytecka, MS I F 334, inserted as fol. 262.

developed by medieval practitioners in major medical centers, especially Salerno. This widely circulated group of initial writings—most prominent among them the pseudo-Hippocratic *Epistula de phlebotomia* (Epistle on Bloodletting)—were primarily practical in nature, presenting bloodletting as an explicitly surgical concern closely linked to astrological readings of the heavens, through which the correct timing of an effective bloodletting cure could be gleaned.[74] From the late twelfth century, translations into Latin of previously unknown works, such as Ibn Sīnā's *Canon* and other Arabic commentaries on Galen, shifted the tenor of European phlebotomical practice into a second broad phase. In these writings, bloodletting's individual qualities were not isolated in a separate surgical tradition but rather synthesized more fully into increasingly encyclopedic medical treatises, where the practice sat alongside other purgative methods appropriate for a broad range of conditions.[75] A third and final phase developed from the late thirteenth century onward, when a new generation of scholastic medics based in Europe's emerging universities began to develop this therapeutic status even further. Writers such as Arnau de Villanova, Bernard de Gordon, and Jean de Saint-Amand produced extensive theoretical monographs on phlebotomy, uniting the practice's earlier surgical heritage with a newly enriched scholarly context. This distinctly academic work also bounced off a simultaneous explosion of writings on phlebotomy in various vernacular European languages, an often fragmented series of more practically oriented texts that were regularly recombined and reworked without clear authorship or recourse to grand theoretical traditions.[76]

Together, these interwoven strands popularized the practice of phlebotomy at all levels of medieval medical engagement, and by the later part of the period bloodletting was seen as a universalizing treatment recommended by European healers, both trained and untrained, whether specifically in times of sickness or as a more general prophylactic to protect against anticipated humoral change in the future. Texts associated with this phlebotomical corpus were therefore interested in communicating an extremely broad range of information: the type of patient for whom bloodletting might be appropriate (the vulnerable young and those of particularly advanced age were to be avoided); the qualities of a good bloodletter (keen eyesight and a steady hand); the timing of procedures in relation to astrological movements and times of day (both of which governed the internal humoral workings of the body); practical details (such as the identification of particular veins, the depth and direction of cuts, and proper inspection and interpretation of drawn blood); and further consideration of the aftercare of patients (including prescribing rest and certain diets, as well as encouraging a positive mental outlook, which was thought to aid recovery from treatments).

Images began to play a significant role within European phlebotomical practice from the thirteenth century onward, the last and busiest of Gil-Sotres's three phrases. Precisely what first moved makers of bloodletting works to convey information pictorially rather than just orally or textually is difficult to say with any certainty. The increasingly easy availability of paper in Europe may have played a material role by affording medical thinkers more

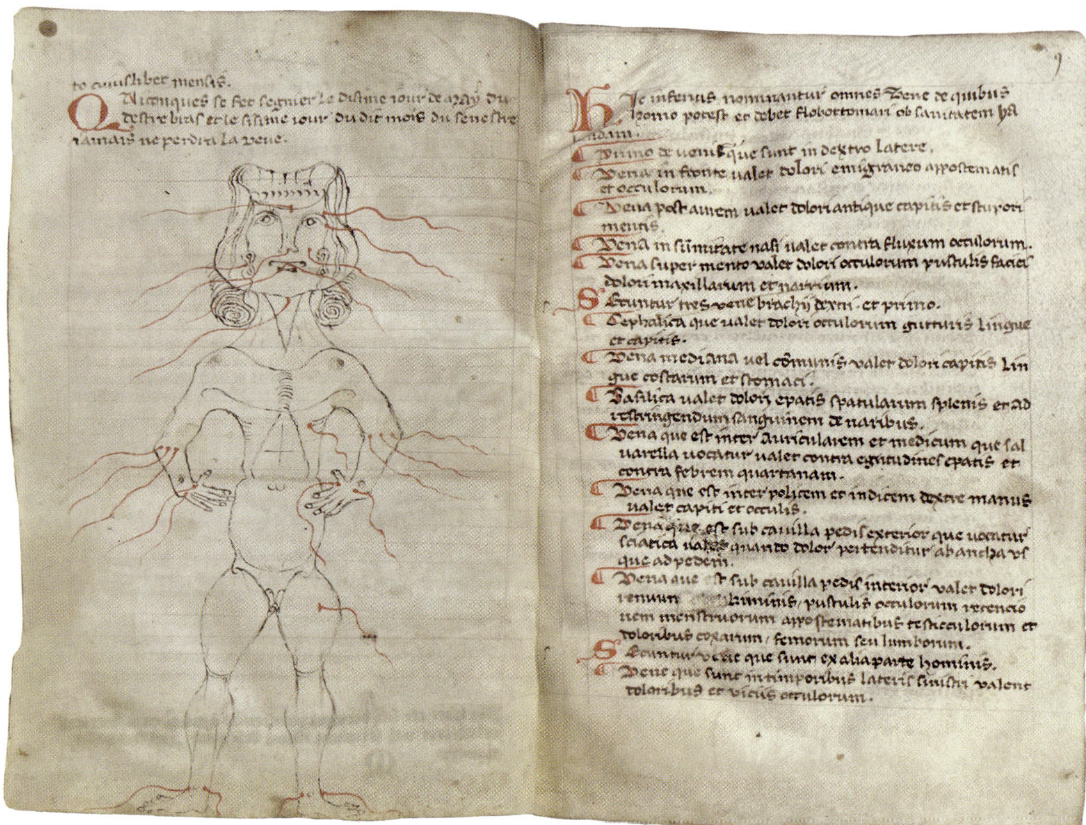

Fig. 1.14. Bloodletting figure opposite the opening of a phlebotomical treatise, 14th century, France. Ink on parchment, 21 x 14 cm (each folio). Paris, Bibliothèque nationale de France, MS Latin 15113, fols. 8v–9r.

and more space for the ample text and imagery they wished to include in their treatises.[77] Similarly, Helen Valls has convincingly argued that to navigate what were quickly becoming increasingly large and complex books, illustrative vignettes with naturalistic depictions of various procedures, bloodletting included, began to evolve as an important "visual rubric" in medical works, drawing the reader's attention to the specific contents of particular passages by bringing different forms of interaction between medics and patients to life.[78] Historians of medicine have also often vaguely gestured to images such as the Wrocław figure as following Antique prototypes, perhaps prompted by the likelihood that the phlebotomical theories they showcased had evolved from Classical models of thought. However, the sporadic nature of surviving early figures offers little evidence of this. Take one of the earliest-known bloodletting figures from medieval Europe, found in a medical compilation gathered at the Parisian abbey of Saint-Victor, whose bloodletting material may date back as early as the turn of the fourteenth century (fig. 1.14).[79] Here, phlebotomical knowledge and image are indeed paired across two folios: to the right, a short set of Latin sentences list veins for letting blood in the case of particular conditions, while opposite a rough and unevenly modeled figure with a bulbous, bowed forehead sprouts wiggling streams from a series of punctures. Yet, while this figure's bleeding spots certainly reflect several of the general phlebotomical areas mentioned in the text—veins in the head, arm, hands, groin, and feet—they are by no means exhaustive in relation to the paired treatise, which lists twenty-six veins against the figure's twenty-three squiggles. Nor are they particularly precise, spurting blood in only loose correlation to the Classicizing practice across the page.[80]

Rather than assuming the presence of distant, extinct historical models, we would do better to examine more contemporary medieval visual trends as the potential motivation behind such images, especially the increasingly diagrammatic discourse of the later Middle Ages with which practitioners in medical circles were particularly enchanted. Loren MacKinney has suggested that at the turn of the fourteenth century the French author and surgeon Henri de Mondeville began to illustrate his medical lectures at the University of Montpellier with large-scale schematic drawings of human anatomical elements, perhaps similar to the images that still survive accompanying early copies of his monumental anatomical treatise, the *Chirurgie* (Surgery).[81] A connection, at least in formal terms, might also be drawn with another group of pioneering medieval medical images known as the Nine-Figure Series, which had begun appearing in anatomical treatises around a century earlier in the late 1100s.[82] This set of contemporary figures visualized the body's internal circuits and organs, and they clearly exerted some influence on their phlebotomical cousins. Consider the range of visual relations between one early bloodletting figure, found attached to the front of a fourteenth-century dietetic text now in Dessau, and a parallel anatomical image plotting the body's veins, part of an English manuscript of the Nine-Figure Series (fig. 1.15).[83] Their shared squat poses are remarkably close, from their centrally parted hair to their out-turned feet, as well as the

Fig. 1.15. Schematic figures with matching abstract anatomies. *Left:* Bloodletting figure, 14th century, probably Germany. Ink on parchment, 33 x 23 cm. Dessau-Roßlau, Anhaltische Landesbücherei, Georg Hs. 271, fol. 1r. *Right:* Figure mapping the body's veins, late 12th century, England. Ink and paint on parchment, 21 x 15 cm. Cambridge, Gonville and Caius College, MS 190/223, fol. 2v.

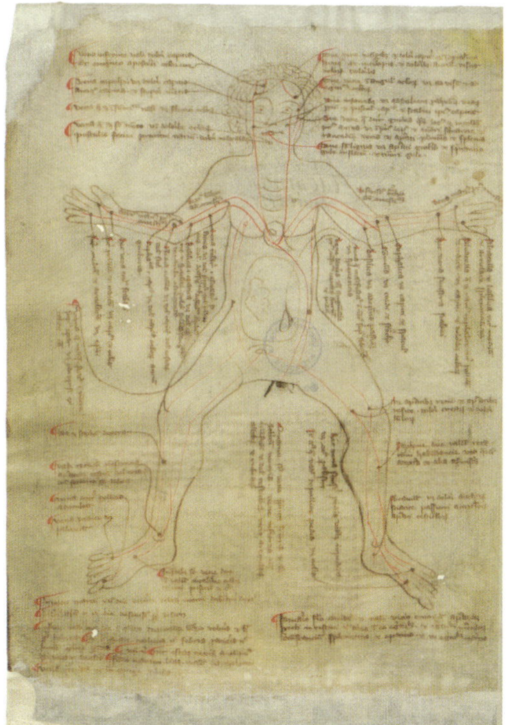

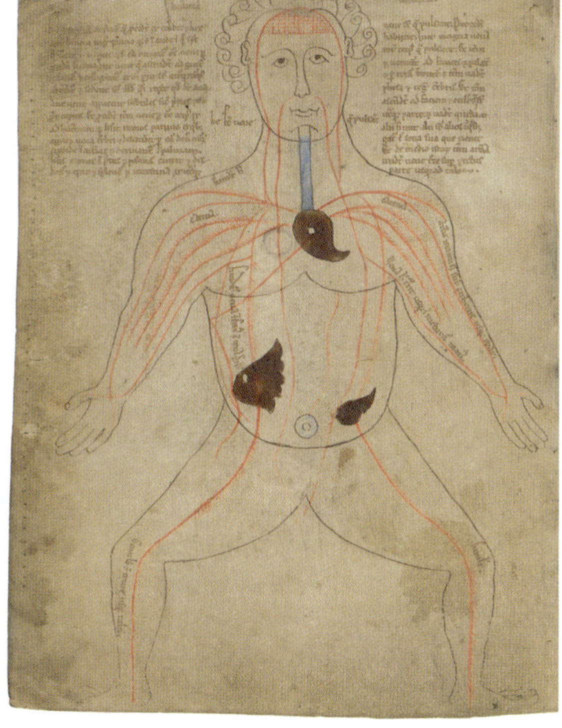

unusual inclusion of stylized internal organs such as a comma-shaped heart, multi-lobed liver, and teardrop spleen.

Whatever their specific origins, bloodletting figures of the sort on display in the Wrocław manuscript sharply increased in popularity toward the end of the Middle Ages, and if we begin to view this collection of images as a coherent rather than sporadic corpus, we can in fact ascertain a wide range of information on their users, makers, and explanatory visual methods. Popular across the continent, such bloodletting imagery circulated alongside multiple types of text.[84] Roughly half of the two hundred or so figures currently known feature in manuscripts written in Latin, suggesting academic connections to more scholarly forms of medicine.[85] Such is the case with the Wrocław figure, around which a standard Latin text on bloodletting has been broken down into individual phrases swarming the central body. The content of each textual gobbet follows a relatively consistent structure: first it lists the rough location or specific name of the vein to be found at a particular bodily point—to which it is linked by a snaking red line—and then it records the healing specialisms and practical concerns correspondent with letting blood from this particular site. So, for example, at points respectively linked to the forehead, arm, and foot, the user could trace outward from the Wrocław figure's body to read phrases such as:

> *Vena in medio frontis percussa valet contra capitis dolorem et contra gravissimam capitis emigraneam et contra frenesim et ad corruptum cerebrum reformandum et contra lepram.*
>
> A vein cut in the middle of the forehead is efficacious against headache and against severe migraine and against phrenitis and for the restoration of the damaged brain and against leprosy.
>
> *Vena cephalica a capite habet principatum et posita est super musculo et si illa vena que sub cephalica est percussa fuerit per negligenciam vel musculo tacto subitaneam mortem facit.*
>
> The cephalic vein originates in the head and is located above the muscle, and if that vein which is beneath the cephalic vein is cut through negligence, or else the muscle is touched, it will cause sudden death.
>
> *Vena super indicem pedis valet pustulis oculorum et pustulis aurium.*
>
> The vein above the index toe is efficacious for pustules of the eyes and pustules of the ears.

The other half of surviving bloodletting figures appear in books written in a variety of European vernaculars, indicating their simultaneous popularity in non-academic or at least non-Latinate circles (fig. 1.16). The occasional examples found with annotations in Czech, French, Hebrew, Italian, Irish, and Welsh often bear a close resemblance to their Latin counterparts, but with interesting regional variations: a French figure looms over a smaller seated man, who turns his back to the viewer to reveal points for cupping,

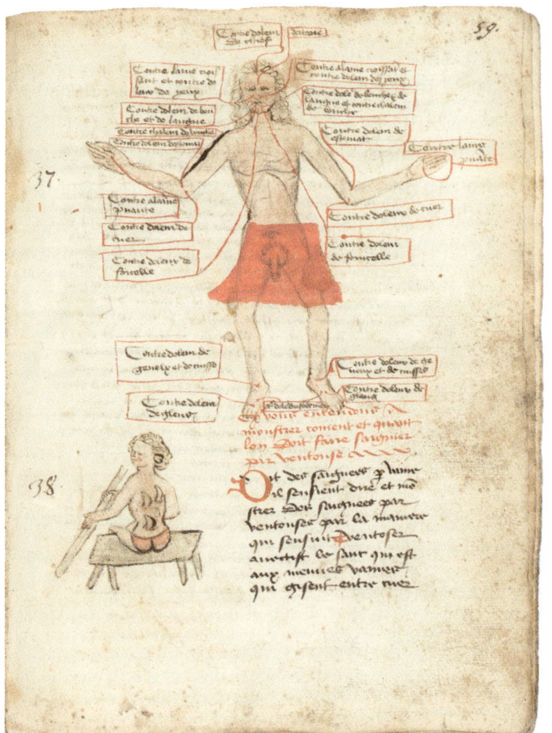

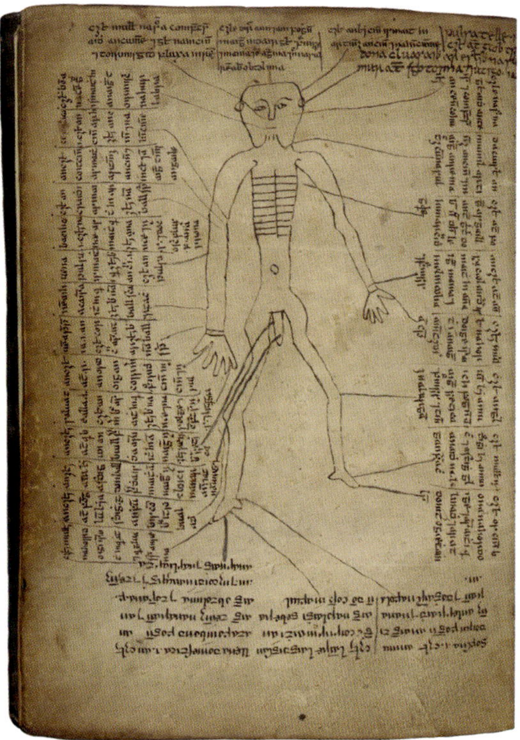

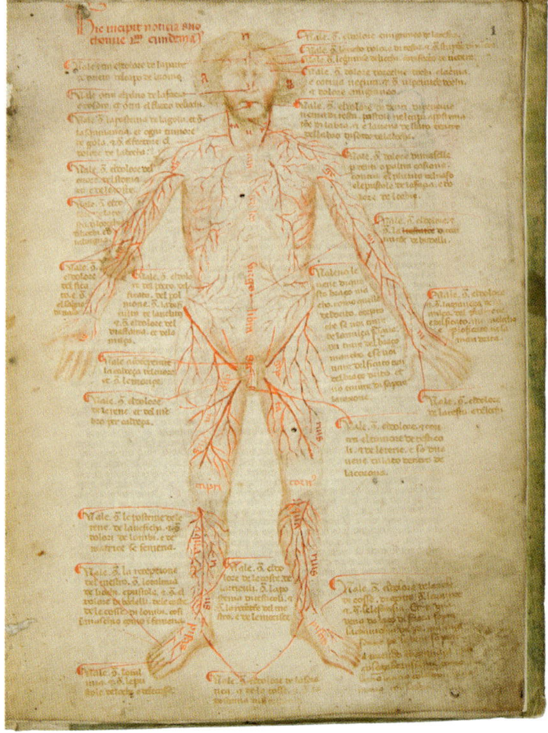

Fig. 1.16. Vernacular bloodletting figures in French, Irish, and Italian books. *(In clockwise order)*: Bloodletting figure alongside a figure demonstrating medicinal cupping, 15th century, France. Ink and paint on paper, 29 x 21 cm. Paris, Bibliothèque nationale de France, MS Arsenal 2894, fol. 59r. Bloodletting figure, early 16th century, Ireland. Ink on parchment, 22 x 15 cm. London, British Library, Additional MS 15582, fol. 61v. Bloodletting figure, 15th century, Padua. Ink and paint on paper, 28 x 20 cm. Padua, Biblioteca storica di Medicina e botanica Vincenzo Pinali e Giovanni Marsili, MS Fanzago 2,I,5,28, fol. 1r.

another technique for balancing the humors using upturned suction cups; an Irish example adopts an unusually square aesthetic, with long, piano-key ribs; and an Italian figure uniquely depicts an entire branching network of veins and arteries, each picked out in red atop the skin.[86] A slightly larger corpus survives from England, in part owing to the strong regional popularity of so-called Bat Books during the fifteenth century. These portable physicians' almanacs, mostly written in English, often included bloodletting figures with very simple legends alongside diverse calendrical materials, an inheritance of phlebotomy's status as a time-dependent, seasonal practice.[87] But by far the most substantive group appears in German manuscripts, annotated in various regional dialects of Mittelhochdeutsch. Following in the footsteps of Karl Sudhoff, generations of German medical historians have traced this regional phlebotomical tradition back to a circulating catalog of fourteenth-century practical vernacular texts, a body of work subsequently promulgated by the widely reproduced writings of the Würzburg surgeon Ortolf von Baierland.[88] Ortolf's much-copied *Pharmacopoeia* helped popularize several phlebotomical theories drawn from Ibn Sīnā, Abū Bakr al-Rāzī, and the pseudo-Hippocratic corpus by simplifying them into a pithy series of practically focused bloodletting directions. These abbreviated instructions and others like them must have been particularly useful for replication in limited space, hence their regular appearance crammed onto a single page in clusters around a central figure.

It is important not to see these different linguistic traditions as necessarily isolated from one another. Returning to the Wrocław figure once again, we find that its principal set of Latin vein descriptions are complemented with a short suite of German paratexts that also hug the figure's side, linked like the Latin to specific parts of the body using thin red lines, stating, for instance, that:

> *Dy czwu adirn yn den winkeln der ougen sint gut czu der gesunt heith der ougen.*
>
> The two veins in the corners of the eyes are good for the health of the eyes.
>
> *Dy adir vunder dem kynne ist gut weder dy wetage der ogen, der brust, unde ouch weder dy bruche des antledes unde der unfletickeit der hende.*
>
> The vein under the chin is good against pain in the eyes, the breast, and also against a broken complexion and a lack of manual dexterity.
>
> *Dy czwu adirn uff dem nedirsten orthe des sackes dy sint gut czu der keuscheit und messeckeit des lichnams.*
>
> The two veins on the lowest part of the scrotum they are good for the continence and moderation of the body.

In terms of balance, Latin certainly leads in this particular Wrocław example, but other bilingual figures present different weightings. A short eight-folio

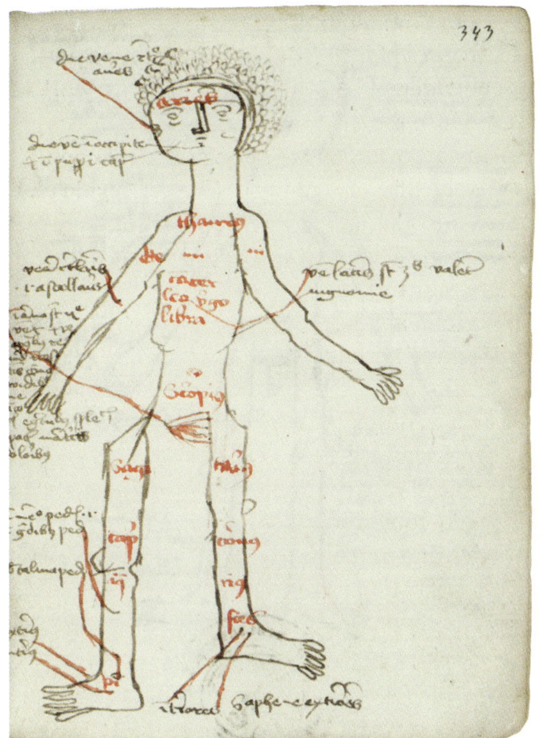

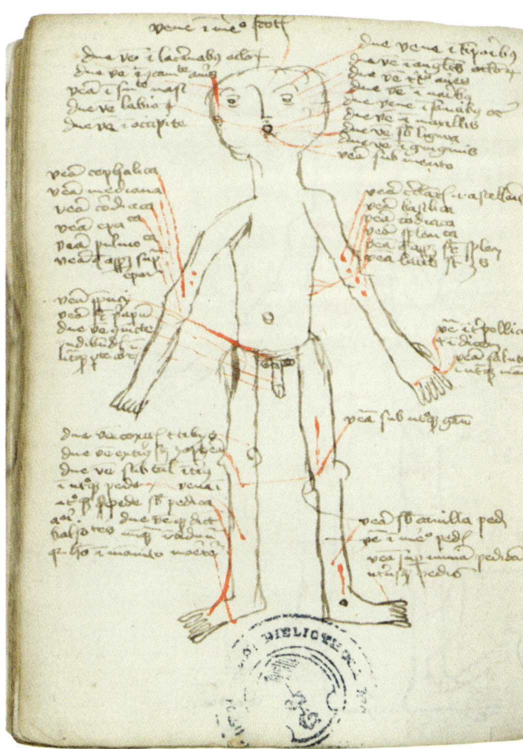

Fig. 1.17. Male and female bloodletting figures, 15th century, Austria. Ink on paper, 14 x 10 cm (each folio). Vienna, Schottenstift, Cod. 160 (Hübl. 257), fol. 343r–343v.

pamphlet of religious and medical material, probably made in a Bavarian Benedictine context during the 1440s, contains no fewer than four separate bloodletting figures, three labeled in German and only one in Latin.[89] And just as multiple languages might find connection sitting side by side around these floating figures, so too could discrete practices of healing. Several particularly polyvalent schematic bodies survive that coupled bloodletting information with instructions for treating plague buboes at the arms and groin, while others chose to pair phlebotomy with more general anatomical information by splitting their figures open at the chest to reveal various labeled organs beneath.[90]

Aesthetically, the figures of this multilingual corpus showcase dramatically different levels of investment in the detail of the human form, suggesting a diverse set of makers behind their individual designs. Some particularly rough and sketchy images were probably made by medical professionals or untrained scribes for whom quality of design was no real priority (fig. 1.17). Two figures in a manuscript now in Vienna, for instance, have a particularly childlike quality to them, with six-fingered hands and single-line hips, while another from a book now in Trier gives up at the arms, which trail off at the wrists into nothingness.[91] Others, by contrast, are clearly the work of talented professional artists (fig. 1.18). The tousled hair, built-up musculature, and subtle skin tones of one figure from a Bohemian manuscript give it real presence on the page, and although tightly hemmed in by its surrounding bloodletting text, its left foot still somehow finds room to gently toe the threshold of the page's ruled baseline, as if stepping out from its diagrammatic confines and into the reader's own space. Similarly, the artist of

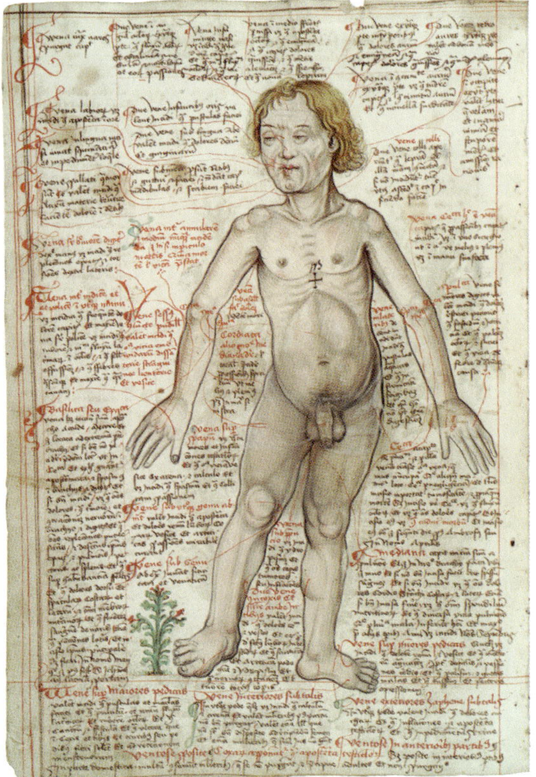

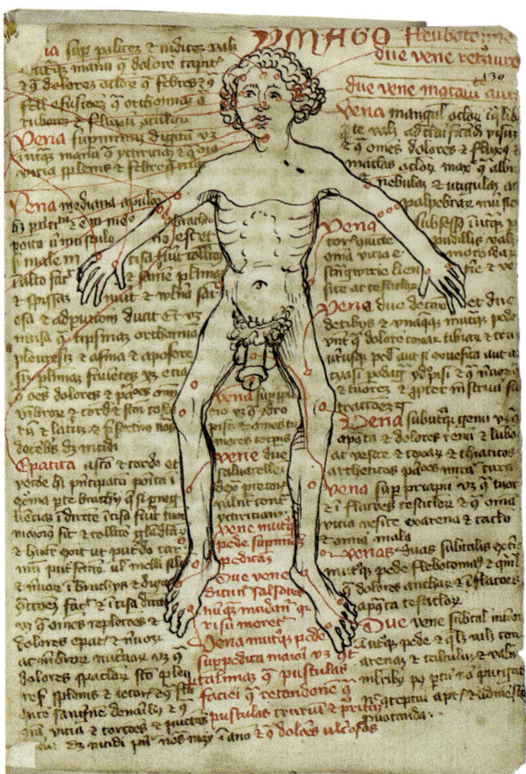

Fig. 1.18. Artistically accomplished bloodletting figures. *Left:* Bloodletting figure, c. 1498–1503, Bohemia. Ink and paint on paper, 31 x 21 cm. Prague, Národní knihovna České republiky, MS XVII D 10, fol. 41v. *Right:* Bloodletting figure, 15th century, Germany. Ink on paper, 21 x 15 cm. Vatican City, Biblioteca Apostolica Vaticana, MS Pal. Lat. 1305, fol. 130r.

another bloodletting figure—incorporated as part of a double-page spread appended to the back of a fifteenth-century German medical compilation—has employed extremely careful draftsmanship to imbue even this uncolored figure with life, from the assured single strokes that make up its expressive eyes and mouth to the neatly enunciated ridges demarcating individual toes.

Other material qualities shed further tantalizing light on the specifics of these figures' authorship. Beneath a slightly hairy-looking example now in Heidelberg we read the phrase "*hans grunawer picktoravit*" (Hans Grunawer painted this), although it is unclear if this legend is contemporary with the drawing. If so, Grunawer did not think much of his medical patrons, putting into his bloodletting figure's mouth the damning Latin phrase "*Credo quod ignorat medicorum contio tota*" (I believe that the entire medical establishment is ignorant).[92] Another fifteenth-century manuscript, possibly made in Kloster Maulbronn in southwestern Germany, contains a carefully drawn bloodletting figure whose surrounding labels are only half finished, maybe because the drawing and labeling of such figures were sometimes completed by different people, one a draftsman and the other a scribe.[93] Meanwhile, two contemporaneous English figures, both now in the collections of the Bodleian Library in Oxford, bear such similarity in execution that they seem almost certainly the work of the same artist, or at least copied in the same workshop: the pair sport identical shell-shaped locks, right-facing poses, and wide-eyed stares (fig. 1.19).[94] The structure and style of this pair in turn bear strong resemblance to the only surviving bloodletting figure annotated in Middle

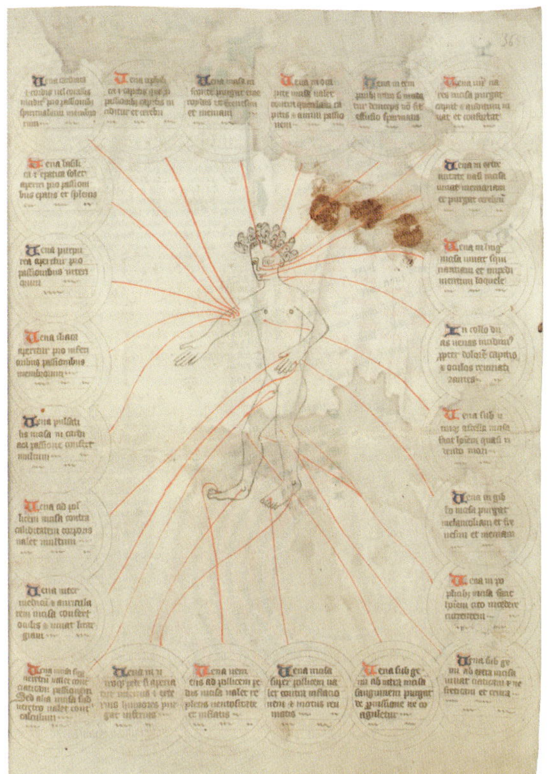

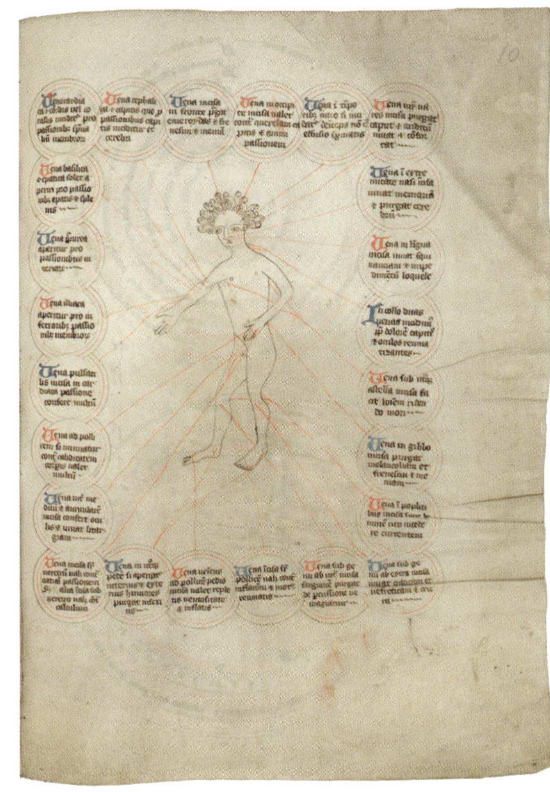

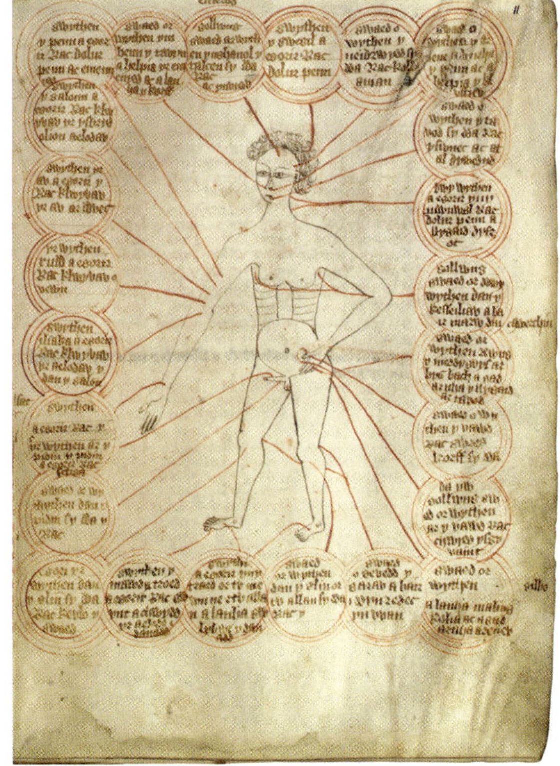

Fig. 1.19. Bloodletting figures from England and Wales. *(In clockwise order)*: Bloodletting figure, late 14th century, England. Ink on parchment, 28 x 21 cm. Oxford, Bodleian Library, MS Ashmole 789, fol. 365r. Bloodletting figure, late 14th century, England. Ink on parchment, 29 x 20 cm. Oxford, Bodleian Library, MS Saville 39, fol. 10r. Bloodletting figure, 15th century, Wales. Ink on parchment, 23 x 16 cm. Cardiff, National Library of Wales, MS 3026C, fol. 11r.

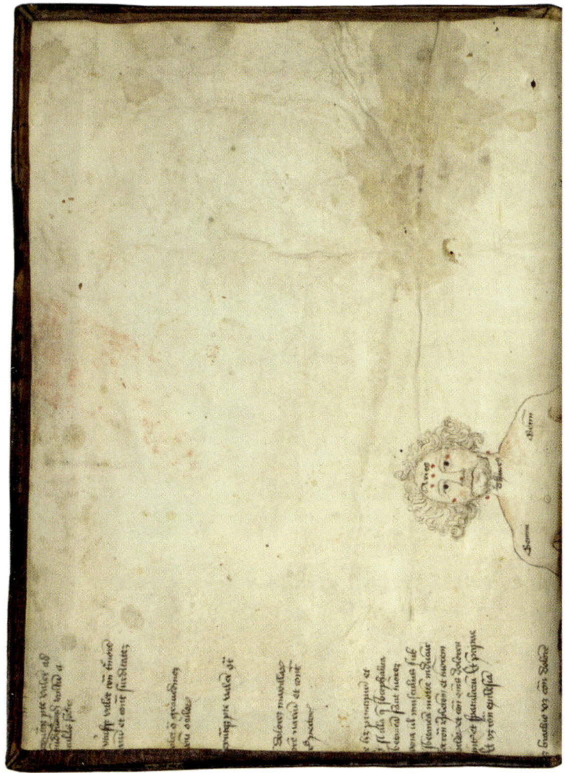
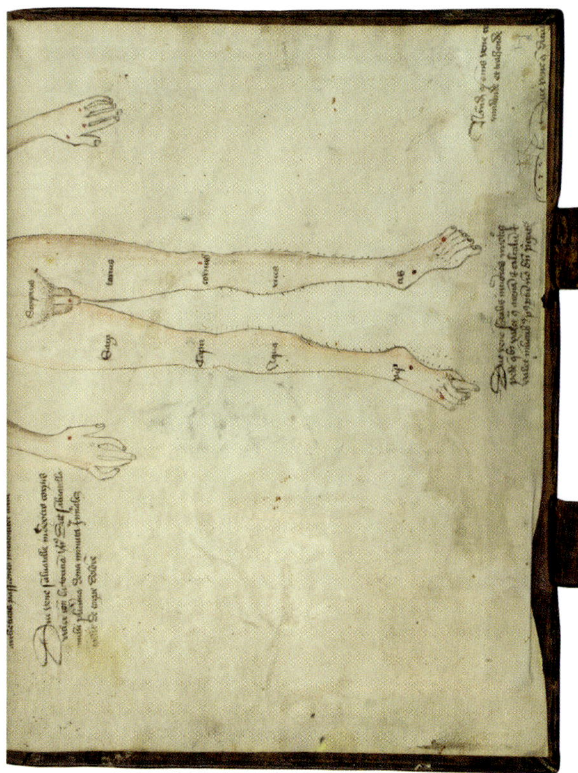

Fig. 1.20. Bloodletting figure used as binding material, before 1474, Austria. Ink and paint on parchment, 29 x 21 cm. Klosterneuburg, Augustiner-Chorherrenstift, Cod. 278, inside covers.

Welsh, suggesting that models for these images could be disseminated some distance along preexisting artistic networks.[95]

Indeed, the codicological lives of these figures are rarely straightforward, often intimating even busier processes of circulation and exchange. In a sizable number of cases, there is a material mismatch between a bloodletting figure and its immediate manuscript surrounds: paper figures are bound into parchment manuscripts and vice versa, with several clearly tipped in at either the very beginning or very end of a book to which they are evidently not original.[96] These appended figures are often of significantly larger scale than their host volumes—mostly twice the size, a single folio folded in half—raising the intriguing possibility that they originally circulated as discrete annotated objects before being bound up into other medical works. This certainly seems to be the case for at least five independent sheets that were reused as binding material for later books, leaving nothing but their upper or lower torsos to poke out from beyond the gutter (fig. 1.20).[97]

Taken together, this practical diversity paints a picture of widespread use. Present both as scrappy sketches in individual medical notebooks and as grander illustrative elements in higher-quality manuscripts, bloodletting figures were clearly mobilized by healing professionals from across the spectrum in a number of ways. After all, the information actually recorded in these figures is scant. Unlike the dense tomes they were often placed within, the *medicina* they immediately marshaled around them was short, deliberately digestible, and easily committed to memory. Given the regularity of bloodletting within the late medieval medical landscape, it seems highly unlikely that phlebotomists would need to repeatedly return to these images to remind themselves of basic daily particulars. Instead, a sense emerges of their value less as factual prompts than as an important part of a medic's broader intellectual toolkit. On the one hand, the more rough-and-ready of bloodletting images, recorded in personal-facing notebooks—just like those of Erhard Knab—reveal a network of individuals in the process of acquiring these figures' phlebotomical information. Some clearly found this work tedious, such as the student whose medical copybook bedecks its bloodletting figure with comic doodles: in its right hand is a penis, annotated with the phrase "*Du bist mein alle hoffnung*" (You are all my hope), and in its left is a vagina, noting "*Du mein aller liebster tröster*" (You are my dearest comforter) (fig. 1.21).[98] Others we can identify as more committed scholars. The paleographical sleuthing of Lucie Doležalová has identified the author of one such bloodletting figure as Crux of Telč, a cleric active in Třeboň in Bohemia, who sketched out the image alongside texts cribbed from important authors in the pages of his late fifteenth-century copybook.[99] Tiziana Pesenti identifies another figure in a contemporaneous manuscript owned by one Francesco Zurla da Brescia, an Italian barber-surgeon who prized the book so highly that it was bequeathed to his son Giovanni to use in his practice.[100] And a third is tucked toward the back of a manuscript known to have been in the early fifteenth-century collection of Amplonius Rating de Berka, the Elector

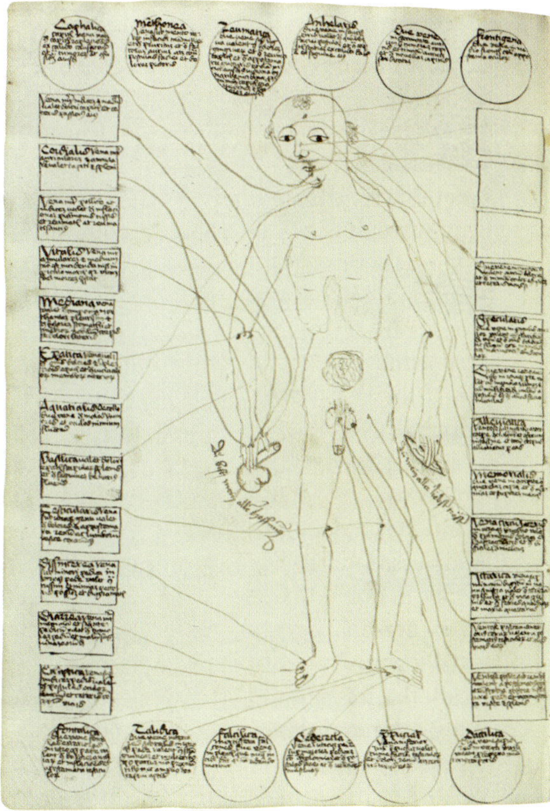

Fig. 1.21. Bloodletting figure holding a penis and a vagina, late 15th century, Leipzig. Ink on paper, 31 x 21 cm. Leipzig, Universitätsbibliothek, MS 1346, fol. 228v.

of Cologne's personal physician, who in 1412 donated over six hundred books to Erfurt's Collegium Porta Coeli for its scholars to study.[101] Acting in the well-established tradition of the medieval memory diagram, they evidence medics who were midway through absorbing information on theory and practice during their training, reading, and thinking.

By contrast, the presence of more elaborate bloodletting figures may have served a useful function beyond learning as part of the doctor-patient encounter. These high-quality illustrations, situated within precious books commissioned at significant cost, would also surely not have been consulted midway through the blood-spattered phlebotomical moment for live, step-by-step instruction.[102] As with many other objects of medieval medicine, it seems likely that they existed as markers of a more social form of expertise, mobilized as an impressive frame for consultation.[103] Bloodletting commentaries themselves return regularly to the importance of a patient's psychological state during the phlebotomical process, a common feature of medieval medical texts, which often address techniques of bedside manner to put patients at ease.[104] What better reassurance could be made of both the intellectual capacities of the practitioner and their prior success as a well-paid professional than the ownership of an expensive book, replete with detailed, impressively illustrated diagrams? To use modern parallels, these finer figures were part authoritative white coat, part neatly framed medical diploma, and part fancy waiting room.

It is also clear that the use of bloodletting figures extended some distance beyond exclusively professional healing networks and into various other types of what we might call phlebotomical communities. As Ortrun Riha and others have usefully observed, many such images are found in books from "para-medical" contexts that were intended to be consulted for medical information but not by expert healers.[105] Most common are those with close ties to monastic institutions, which stretched across the continent from the Kloster Sankt Emmeram in Regensburg to the Benedictine Schottenstift in Vienna or the monastery of Coupar Angus in eastern Scotland, to name only three.[106] Such communities had long been custodians of medical books, at times developing enormous libraries reflecting theoretical and practical concerns alike, and they also practiced phlebotomy on themselves on a regular basis during annual cycles of so-called periodic bloodletting, typically a three-day event wherein prophylactic bleeding was followed by rest and recovery.[107] One example, now attached to a booklet in Copenhagen that also incorporates the Wound Man, has been suggested from surviving pin holes to have originally hung in a monastic bathhouse.[108] Extant observable pin marks on another, painted on an enormous piece of parchment fifty-seven centimeters tall, make clear that such patterns of display were not uncommon.[109]

We also know that nonreligious professionals turned regularly to bloodletting figures in more secular and civic contexts. Take the example of one figure from Beilngries in Bavaria, found on a fifteenth-century folio repurposed as binding material for one of the town's later court registers from 1537. As Max Künzel has noted, in exactly the same year that this sixteenth-century register was produced, the town's account-book records the purchase of what

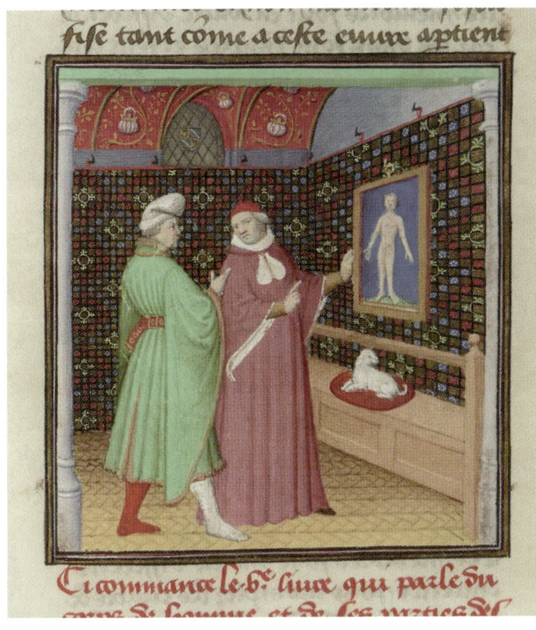

Fig. 1.22. Robed academic and wealthy layman discussing a framed bloodletting figure, from a French translation of Bartholomew the Englishman's *De proprietatibus rerum*, c. 1414, Paris. Ink and paint on parchment, 40 x 32 cm. Paris, Bibliothèque nationale de France, MS Français 9141, fol. 55r.

it calls a new *laßtafel* (bloodletting table), to be pinned up in the town hall for group reference by members of the municipal council.[110] This detail, he suggests, sheds light on how the older figure would also once have been used until its replacement. Displayed in semipublic space, it would have helped senior officials gauge what aspects of medical treatment townsfolk might require and, if necessary, prompt them to alert the nearest local practitioner in the sister municipality of Eichstatt, an eight-hour journey away.

We know that figures of a related consultative type were produced on a somewhat physically smaller scale in German-speaking lands as part of the tradition of so-called *Volkskalender*, or Iatromathematical Housebooks, a popular genre that combined calendrical, astronomical, and medical advice into a single useful tome.[111] Normally commissioned by urban, upper-class elites, the bloodletting figures in these books are of particularly high artistic quality, suggesting that while they could in theory have been used practically by those running a wealthy household—aiding with decisions over treatment and the summoning of local medical professionals—here they were far more likely to be leveraged for their social cachet.[112] One such figure appears in a 1482 book crafted by the Swiss medic and cartographer Conrad Türst for no less a civic personality than Johann Rudolf von Erlach, the high-ranking *Schultheiß* (municipal governor) of Bern. Sketched with exquisitely fine line and careful annotation, this figure incorporated bloodletting into Johann's bookish personal collection of beautified craft, transforming its learned, amateur owner into a proud possessor and custodian of phlebotomical knowledge.[113] Just such a model of performative consultation seems to be depicted in a contemporaneous vignette from a fifteenth-century French manuscript containing a translation of the Franciscan scholar Bartholomew the Englishman's popular encyclopedic work *De proprietatibus rerum* (On the Properties of Things) (fig. 1.22).[114] Opening Bartholomew's fifth book—"*qui parle du corps de l'homme et de ses parties*" (that addresses the body of man and its parts)—we see a scholar in full academic robes drawing the attention of a finely dressed layman to a large-scale picture hanging on the wall from a golden hook, a depiction of a naked man standing on a similar small hillock and with the same wide-armed pose as most surviving bloodletting figures: phlebotomical knowledge depicted in action.

In sum, bloodletting figures from across late medieval Europe show that medical images from the period can help us excavate overlooked practices, practitioners, and patients, all of which we will see recurring in later chapters when we turn to the Wound Man's own history. But perhaps most relevant of all to understanding the Wound Man's intellectual and aesthetic texture is the way these bloodletting figures reveal an innovative sense of diagrammatic praxis that was alive and well among their makers, visual qualities that bring us back full circle to the broad, busy histories of the late medieval diagram at large.

Fundamentally, across this corpus of phlebotomical figures we find makers struggling with a question of clarity. Consider this point in relation once more to the Wrocław figure contrastingly cataloged by Friedrich and Göber. Its page design is exceedingly complicated. The bulk of its bloodletting information is restrained within a pair of lined text-columns to either side of the figure, but for reasons not entirely clear, twenty-one of the page's labels—a group with no obvious internal consistency—have broken free. Some hover in circular bubbles clustered at the figure's head, feet, and flanks, while other notes pertaining to medicinal cupping have become unanchored even further afield, floating alone at multiple orientations in the spaces immediately above and below the figure's hands and shoulders. Such a sense of informational confusion is in fact incredibly commonplace in these bloodletting figures. Textual phrases and linking lines crisscross back and forth, snaking perplexingly in and out of each other like complex linear puzzles, often with further complementary snippets of information strewn seemingly at random around the page.[115] Some figures are so claustrophobically swamped with words that their details can barely even be seen, while others are placed so far away on the page from their corresponding text that their linking lines converge closely enough on the surface of the body as to appear one atop the other, rendering them all but useless in differentiating important points of practice.[116] In several bloodletting figures, even labels themselves beget more labels, with the names of veins leading via lines to further distinctions, the figures effectively becoming the first in several stages of a branched stemmatic analysis that is particularly exhausting on the eyes.[117]

This clutter was a real problem for the users of these books. Given that their contents demanded the removal of significant amounts of blood from a patient, confusion in absorbing their details was not merely inconvenient for the practitioner but potentially life-threatening for those in their care. Thus, it is not surprising that we find a significant tranche of medieval authors and image-makers developing novel and increasingly subtle diagrammatic approaches to these figures and their information.

German artisans appear to have led the way in this effort, perhaps because of the sheer quantity of figures circulating within their orbit. From the

1420s, bloodletting books produced in the region and written in both Latin and Mittelhochdeutsch began to include figural diagrams that experimented with different modes of annotation, many of which were accompanied by short explanations to clarify how their new systems worked. One Nuremberg book put it as follows:

> *Nun merck das dise her nach geschribne figur weiset vnd leret wi man igliche aderen lassen sol vnd warczu es nucz vnd gut ist das vindestu an ider aderen sunderlichen vnd wo du wilt lassen das such nach der czal als das dise nach gemalte figur aus weist.*
>
> Now note that the following figure indicates and instructs how one should let each vein, and beside each you will also find the use that it serves; and [to find] where you want to bleed it, search for the number on this figure drawn below.[118]

At least ten German manuscripts survive that interrelate text and image on precisely these grounds. Gone are chaotic blocks of text. Instead, the figure's linking red lines lead to a neat key of numbers that in turn correspond to numerated paragraphs of bloodletting instructions on the pages immediately preceding or following the figure (fig. 1.23). Not only did this innovation allow for a much more extensive and detailed textual discussion of the subject than could be afforded by the previous method of miniaturized gobbets, but the placement of this numerated key itself became an arena for aesthetic play. Some rest comfortably on the page around the figure, others curve decoratively into a halo around the head, and yet more sit at the page's edge, forming a neat, numerated border from which hang canopies of red line.[119]

An even greater quantity of manuscripts survive that use a letter-key instead of numbers to form the same correspondence between figure and extended text, an innovation once again first found in the German-speaking world.[120] These examples still vary in quality. Compare, for instance, an impressive figure now in Kassel, whose delicate and extremely expressive features sit within an alternating red-blue mandorla, with a much more basic version now in Frankfurt am Main, where a simpler body sits inside two straight lines of blocky, bold, red letters (fig. 1.24).[121] Yet even the clunkiest keyed figure shepherds its information far more clearly for the user than earlier prototypes did. In fact, these innovative fifteenth-century German phlebotomical manuscripts underline a distinct shift in visual strategy from Europe's first bloodletting figures. Rather than a mere herald, whose streaky bloodlines simply alerted readers to the presence of a bloodletting treatise somewhere nearby, by the end of the period schematic bodies could provide the dominant organizing principle for a piece of phlebotomical writing, the emphasis between text and figure wholly reversed.

Taken together, it is plain to see that these diverse figures—not only this cadre of bloodletting forebears but also medical images of many stripes, stretching back past Erhard Knab to the beginning of the period—have to date been underestimated in all their many aspects, perhaps none more so than in the sheer ambition of their uses. They elaborated, decorated, clarified, and

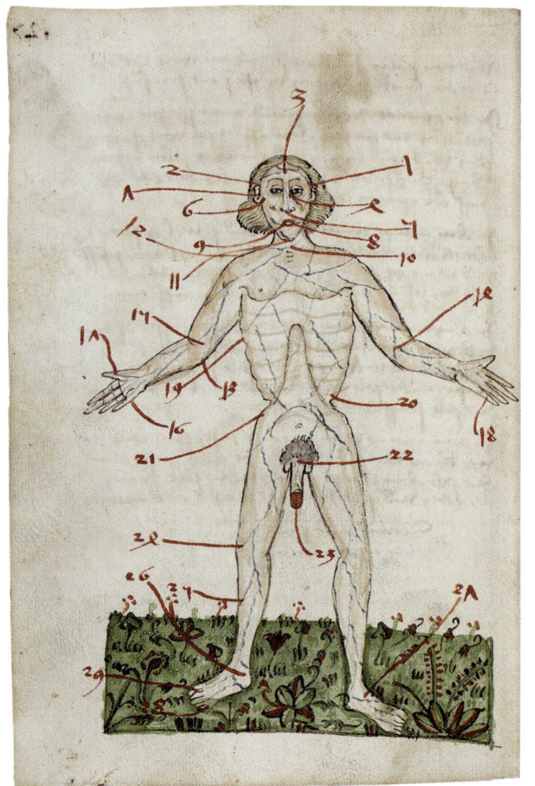

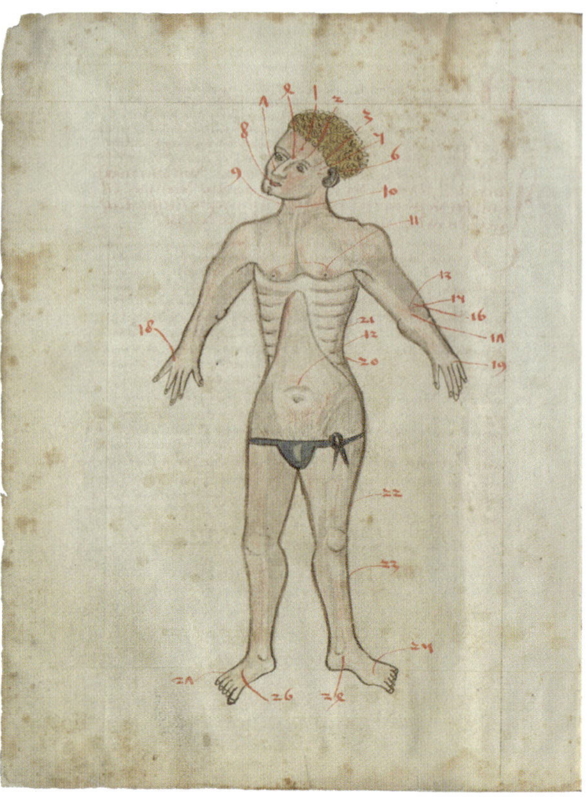

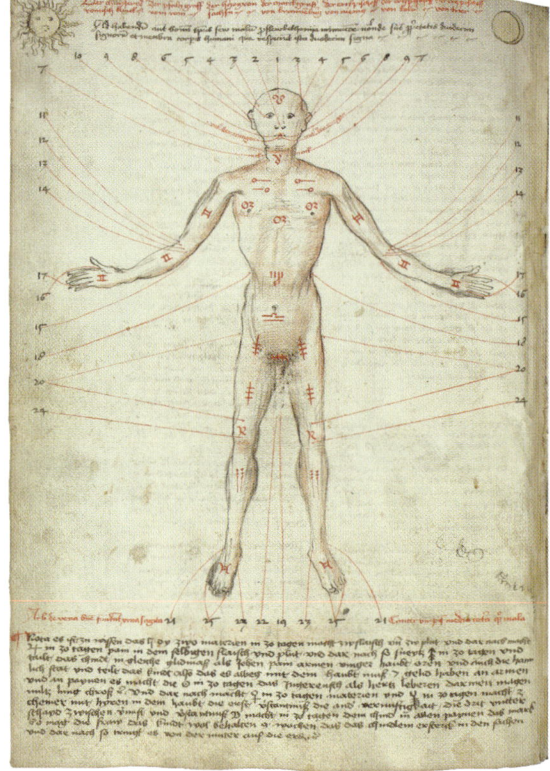

Fig. 1.23. Bloodletting figures with number keys. *(In clockwise order)*: Bloodletting figure, 15th century, Bavaria. Ink and paint on paper, 21 x 14 cm. Vatican City, Biblioteca Apostolica Vaticana, MS Pal. Lat. 1452, fol. 127v. Bloodletting figure, 15th century, Germany. Ink and paint on paper, 28 x 21 cm. Berlin, Staatsbibliothek, Mgq 2021, fol. 181v. Bloodletting figure, 1442, Germany. Ink and paint on paper, 39 x 29 cm. Leipzig, Universitätsbibliothek, MS 1483, fol. 31v.

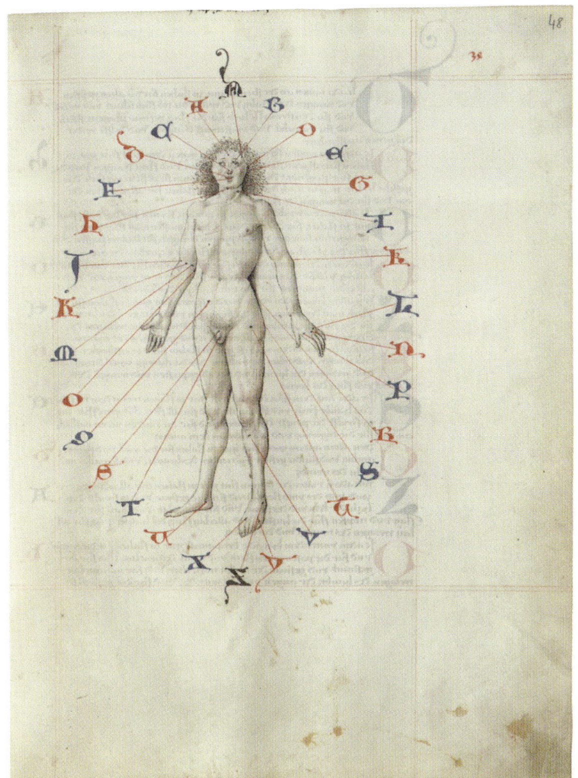

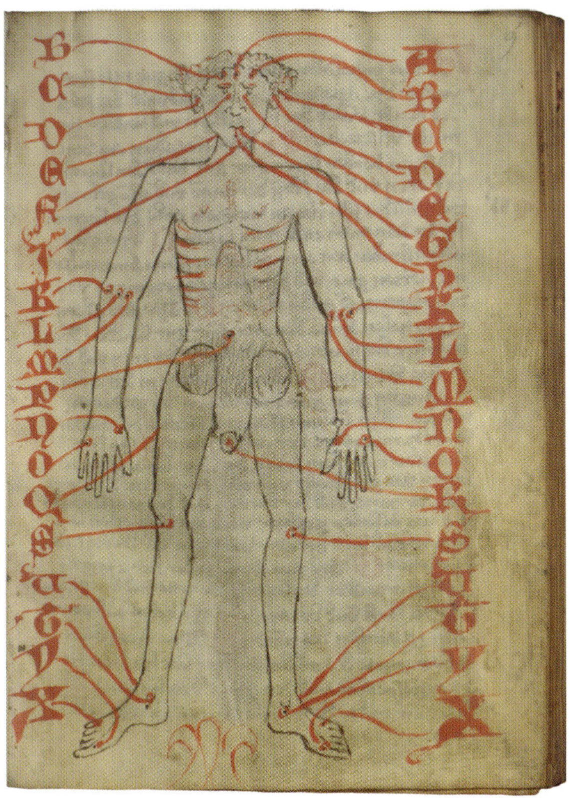

Fig. 1.24. Bloodletting figures with letter-keys. *Left:* Bloodletting figure, c. 1445, Germany. Ink and paint on parchment, 37 x 28 cm. Kassel, Universitätsbibliothek, 2° MS Astron. 1, fol. 48r. *Right:* Bloodletting figure, 15th century, possibly Mainz. Ink on parchment, 18 x 13 cm. Frankfurt am Main, Universitätsbibliothek, MS Barth. 160, fol. 9r.

activated medicine for whole communities of healers. This was the medico-visual world from which the Wound Man would spring, one where medieval makers mined the relationship between image and information with precision to transform their diagrammatic figures into inventive and impressive carriers of knowledge.

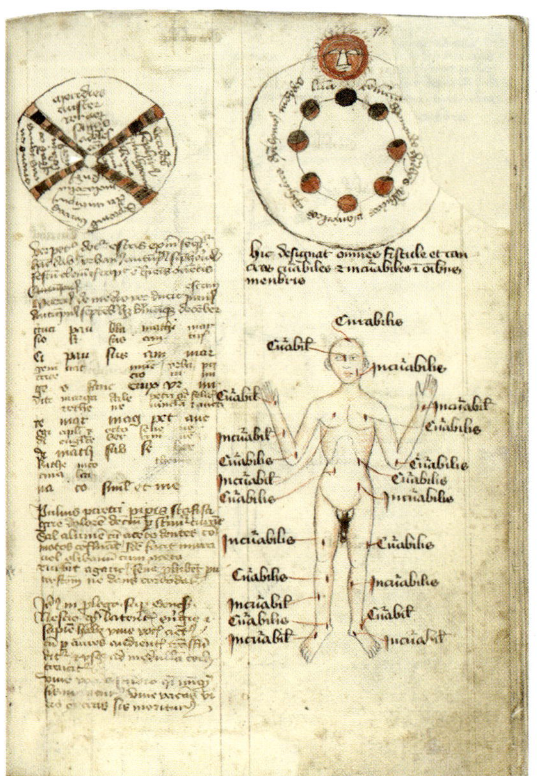

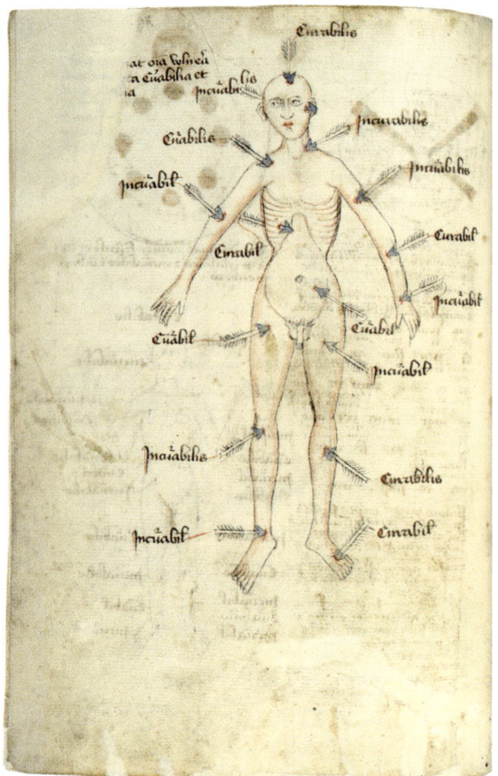

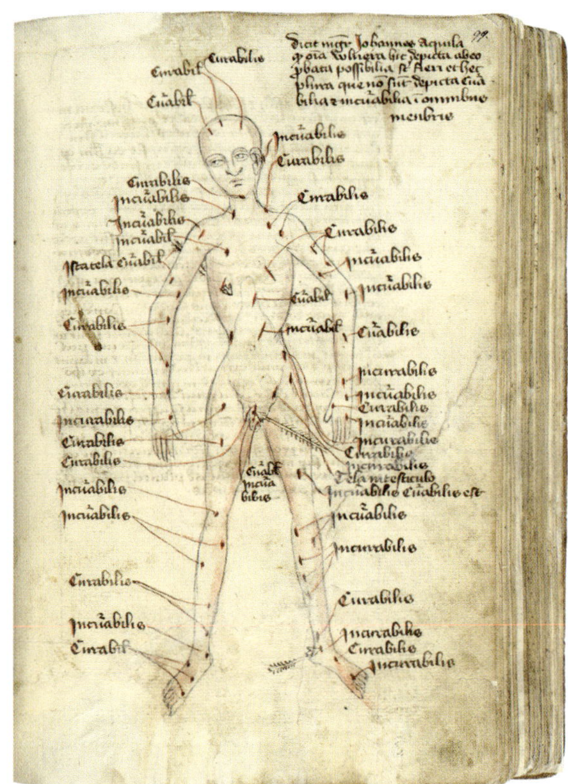

Fig. 2.1. Proto-Wound Men, c. 1399, Bohemia. Ink and paint on paper, 30 x 19 cm (each folio). Prague, Lobkowicz Collection, MS VI Fc 29, 97–99.

CHAPTER TWO

Medicine: Wound Mechanics

Pictured across a pair of folios in a Bohemian manuscript made in the year 1399, three male figures stand naked, bald, and covered in wounds, although to judge by their faces the men seem entirely unperturbed (fig. 2.1).[1] Holding a steady and unflinching gaze, each looks impassively out to their right as if nothing at all was particularly the matter. But their bodies tell a different story. From head to toe, the surface of each figure's skin is blanketed with a regular network of weapons and slit-marks, worrying punctures leaking black and red that give the impression of men fit to burst, each a dense body teetering on the verge of evacuating itself entirely of its blood.

These three remarkable figures are found in a manuscript now in the Lobkowicz Collection in Prague, and they represent the earliest images currently known from the diagrammatic world of late medieval Europe that plot wounds, their effects, and their treatment. These are the first Wound Men, the beginning of the figure's story and its intimate connection to procedures and practices of healing. Such medical functioning was central to the figure's appearance as part of a vivid suite of images recurring throughout medical manuscripts made in Central Europe over the course of the fifteenth century, books that extended the rich figural epistemics explored in the last chapter even further into the sphere of illness and injury. And, as we shall see, the Wound Man in turn marked these manuscripts out as unusual, the product of a complex new wound mechanics that marshaled together a tricky array of healing theory, practical technique, pharmaceutical knowledge, and inventive image-craft.

The Lobkowicz manuscript—indeed, many of the early books in which we find the Wound Man first depicted—is of a type largely referred to by today's scholars as medical "miscellanies," a moniker that reflects their wide assortment of contents drawn from different parts of the late medieval healthscape. This term, however, also conveys an incorrect sense of piecemeal eccentricity, masking the fact that these books were deliberate and structured accumulations, their writings neither miscellaneous nor chosen at random but instead often carefully selected, complementary combinations of healing practice and medical knowledge.[2] In the case of the Lobkowicz book, its multiple texts unfold one onto the other to encompass a substantive and encyclopedic survey of the premodern body, discussing its anatomical systems, good dietary regimen, humoral balance, and herbal medicine. A colophon to one treatise conveniently provides a potential date for the volume's creation, noting its completion on February 12, 1399, during the papacy of Boniface IX, while the work's visual coherence is principally created through a shared pictorial program bunched together in its central section.[3] Among these pages, a number of healing practices are singled out through high-quality diagrammatic images, seemingly completed by the same artist. Five elegant and colorful figures offer schematic outlines of the body's key anatomical systems—veins, arteries, bones, nerves, and muscles—a visual scheme whose earliest iterations appear in southern Germany and England.[4] Several further pages are dedicated to images outlining cautery, the strategic burning of the body with heated irons to balance the humors, in which small figures appear covered with large round spots to indicate points of treatment. And sandwiched in between this anatomy and humoral medicine are the three male figures diagramming the healing of wounds.

The first of these wounded men appears immediately after a broad discussion of medical treatments and their cosmic counterparts. Standing beneath a diagram of the winds and another of the stages of the sun and moon's orbit around the earth, an inscription accompanying the man notes: "*Hic designat omnes fistule et cancres curabiles et incurabiles in omnibus menbris*" (This depicts all fistulas and cancers, curable and incurable, in all members). The figure itself is simplistic but has delicate touches, its outline and features drawn in thin, careful line and accentuated with a light wash. Twenty-two points are marked on the body in black as if they were inch-wide cuts. As well as tiny highlights of red ink, longer red lines flow from these diseased wounds leading to one of two abbreviated and particularly blunt terms: *curabilis* (curable) or *incurabilis* (incurable). On the same folio's verso, a second, significantly larger figure turns up the pressure, this time standing beneath a damaged inscription that likely once read: "*[Hic desig]nat omnia vulnera [sagittis fa]cta curabilia et [incurabili]a*" (This depicts all wounds made by arrows, curable and incurable).[5] Instead of abstract lines alone, this man's sixteen wounds are linked to the same two diagnostic terms by the actual arrows of their making. Most are barely lodged into the figure, their fat shafts protruding from small bleeding wounds, but two have penetrated straight through him, one to the right of his chest puncturing his lung (curable) and another that has passed straight through his head (incurable, unsurprisingly). Finally, across the gutter a third figure combines the visual strategies of his two fellows to showcase yet more wounds, a daunting fifty-eight in total: three are marked by arrows to the chest, groin, and ankle, while the rest are shown simply as red-black slits in the skin. Once more, the diagnoses are binary, curable or incurable, although one curiously notes, "*Ista tela curabilis*" (These darts are curable), another warns of "*Tela in testiculo*" (Darts in the testicle), and a third confusingly states, "*Incurabilis curabilis est*" (Curable and incurable). A legend above this figure also offers the best historical anchor we have for this unusual trio:

> *Dicit magister Johannes Aquila quod omnia vulnera hic depicta ab eo probata possibilia sunt fieri et hec plura que non sunt depicta curabilia et incurabilia in omnibus menbris.*

> Master Johannes Aquila says that all the wounds depicted here, approved by him, are possible to be caused, and also more that have not been depicted, curable and incurable in all members.

A handful of Johannes Aquilae can be found in medieval medical works as the possible source of this advice, the most likely a physician writing at the beginning of the thirteenth century who authored a rhymed bloodletting treatise that survives in a manuscript now in Paris.[6] But even if this is the same Aquila, we do not know whether his wound healing ever constituted more than is shown by these indicatory figures, or indeed whether these men are in fact elaborations on his surgical ideas by later practitioners. Still, these three wounded men reflect what by 1399 was an extensive corpus of medical theory and practice on the healing of wounds. They represent the technical foundations of the Wound Man's image, a medical arena crucial to both his curative function and his gruesome form.

Wounds and the Discontinuous Body

Wounds and their treatment played a significant role in medieval European medicine on a number of levels. In practical terms, wound healing was primarily the domain of surgeons and related hands-on healers, authorities mostly trained in artisanal workshop settings and regulated by a variety of local guild structures.[7] These specialists were well aware of the significant risks associated with invasive procedures, especially those requiring any form of access deep into the bodily interior, and so by the early Middle Ages their training and expertise largely focused on the body's surface. Such surgeons developed significant skill in the healing of ulcers, abscesses, and hernias; they knew how to undertake more specialist operations on particular body parts, for instance, the couching of cataracts or the treatment of fistulas; and in the contexts of both everyday accident and strategic warfare, they also innovated a range of techniques for repairing the bodily surface when it was wounded through injury.

From a theoretical standpoint, understanding wounds was also highly important. Wounds were framed as particularly troublesome intrusions into notions of the continuous body, a foundational concept of corporal unity inherited by medieval Europeans from the writings of Galen and his Arabic commentators. This idea was increasingly encountered through the later Middle Ages as European surgical writers of the twelfth and thirteenth centuries continued to intellectualize their craft and develop a general concept of "the wound" to which they applied overarching curative precepts.[8] The healthy body, as they saw it, was a connected one. Its balanced humors were constantly in flow, and thus a wound represented not only an obvious rupture to the body's surface integrity but a threat to more fundamental forms of biological continuity at work beneath the skin. The swelling that naturally accompanied surface wounds—now understood to be part of the body's immune response as healing cells are transported to the affected area—was seen by premodern thinkers as further evidence of a disrupted bodily flow and a dangerous pooling of humors, something to be avoided at all costs.[9] The term they often used to describe such humoral trauma was *solutio continuitatis* (dissolution of continuity), an idea innovated in particular by the Persian thinker Ibn Sīnā, who also gave European practitioners and writers a sweeping taxonomic spectrum of wounds, ranging in their Latin translation from a simple *incisio* to the more complicated *scissura*, *separatio*, *amplificatio*, *fissura*, *perforatio*, and *ruptura*, among others.[10]

Attending to wounds therefore involved mastering various elements of care, both practical and theoretical, outside and inside the body. Such ideas grew so extensive that at the beginning of the fourteenth century the French surgical author Henri de Mondeville, writing in his canonical treatise the *Chirurgie* (Surgery), thought it expedient to break wound healing down into eight stages: extraction, attending to bleeding, medicating, bandaging, phlebotomy, diet, guarding against infection, and obtaining "*des belles cicatrices*" (beautiful scars).[11] Understanding the gist of these stages is useful for understanding wound practice as a whole. Mondeville's term "extraction," for example, refers to the wound being cleaned and cleared, a process found at the beginning of virtually all medieval wound-healing advice. This would normally have been done by washing the affected area with vinegar and wine, often watered down, although whether a given wound could be fully cleared of bodily detritus seems to have depended on the courage of the healer.[12] A much replicated fifteenth-century treatment for a wound in the head written by an anonymous author in Middle English offers two possibilities: if the wound was found to still contain pieces of the skull, then the pieces should ideally be removed to promote successful healing, but "*ȝef þou dar noȝgh serch ȝe wond*" (if you dare not search the wound)—and why one might or might not dare is left unspoken—the text instead encourages applying a plaster made from ground herbs to steadily draw detritus out from the wound.[13]

Dressing wounds in this way was among the most valued of surgical interventions and built on a long history of discussing pharmaceuticals thought particularly pertinent to the task. A number of recipes survive that outline the production of styptics, medicines normally applied in powdered form and intended to staunch a wound's bleeding. Several recent recreative trials propose to have either confirmed or countermanded the levels of efficacy claimed by medieval healers for their recipes, although to judge this historic medicine by modern standards is to entirely misunderstand both its internal complexity and its cultural specificity.[14] In a move typical of medieval pharmacology's interest in so-called sympathetic healing—wherein certain drugs' material similarities to their intended purpose dictated their clinical qualities—antihemorrhagics were often formed of conspicuously red things: copper ore and dark red wine; the stone hematite, also known as iron oxide, a medieval staple in the production of red dyes and paints; and a tree sap so red that it was given the name *sanguinem draconis* (dragon's blood). The delicate strength of a spider's web was similarly thought an ideal model for the powerful beauty of healing and on occasion was discussed as a viable dressing to reduce swelling around a wound.[15] And in an even more poetic turn, myrrh was thought a particularly good wound salve based on the understanding that it was produced by trees that themselves had been wounded, harvested as a crystallized resin sap from torchwoods whose bark had been broken or slashed.[16] More hard-edged treatments could also be mobilized. Some advocated for the application of caustic substances to burn away dead flesh around a wound, whose presence was thought to lead to further infection. These treatments ranged from gently corrosive herbs and oils to stronger materials such as animal bile, lye, or even arsenic. The presence of pus in a wound also drew keen attention from healers, although this was a more nuanced point of theoretical and practical debate than dead skin. One camp of surgical writers argued that suppuration improved the chance of healing and should be encouraged, while others were insistent that all wounds should be dried out as quickly as possible using various medicaments, before which the healing process could not begin in earnest.[17] All agreed, as a last resort, that a wound hemorrhaging uncontrollably could be staunched by cautery, with thin heated irons applied strategically to seal up bleeding vessels.

Following the stabilization of a wound, a decision then had to be made as to whether the surgeon should encourage closure on its own accord or by suturing the wound themselves. If direct intervention was deemed unnecessary, perhaps because the cut was a particularly clean one, then incarnative medicines to promote the generation of new flesh might be applied, for instance, a paste recommended by the thirteenth-century surgeon Teodorico Borgognoni in his *Cyrurgia* (Surgery) that was made with palm bark, vegetable leaves, ground nutmeg, flour dust, and barley.[18] Some authors argued that such medicines should avoid ingredients that might soften the wound rather than desiccate it, instead recommending the application of gums and mixtures bound in egg white to the skin's surface.[19] Vinegar, a painful but effective astringent that could pull the skin of the wound tighter together, was also thought to help the process, while nonadhesive substances such as animal grease or honey were deemed particularly effective in protecting an open wound, as they would not affix themselves to the skin and cause further damage during redressing or bandaging. Noninvasive treatment of this sort was clearly understood to be effective even in particularly drastic circumstances. Take an episode from the Italian surgeon Lanfranco da Milano's thirteenth-century *Chirurgia magna* (Great Surgery):

> *Et ego vidi hominem septuagenum, et ipsum curavi, qui fuit vulneratus cum telo in ancha, et transivit per carnem anchae per longitudinem unius pedis, sed non tetigit aliquod nervum, quod scivi pro certo propter carentiam doloris, tenui apertum vulnus cum parva et curta tenta, ut viderem si in crastino doloret et praecepi ipsum quiescere, mane autem nullum inveni dolorem nec inflationem. Tunc abieci illam tentulam, et permisi vulnus claudi, et iterum praecepi ipsum quiescere alia die, et in tertia die omnino sanus fuit.*
>
> I saw and cared for a seventy-year-old man who was wounded in the thigh with a spear that passed by the length of a foot through the flesh

> of the thigh, but it didn't hit a nerve, which I knew for certain because of the lack of pain. I kept the wound open with a small, short wick to see whether it would be sore the next day, and instructed him to rest, but in the morning, I found no pain or swelling. Then I took out that little wick and allowed the wound to be closed, and again ordered him to rest another day, and on the third day he was entirely well.[20]

Surgical treatises outlined a broad range of practical techniques to be followed in treating larger or more disruptive wounds that required suturing. Different sorts of sutures called for different sorts of instruments. More delicate operations on the head or face required a thinner, semicircular needle threaded with waxed thread or a thick strand of hair from an ox, a horse, or—if strong enough—a human. By far the most comprehensive source for surgical technique in the period was produced by the tenth-century Hispanic surgeon Abū'l Qāsim al-Zahrāwī, whose *Kitāb al-Taṣrīf* (traditionally translated as his Method of Medicine) was gradually introduced into the Latin world from the middle of the twelfth century onward.[21] He describes four principal types of closure dependent on the size and circumstances of the injury, all of which reveal the intense materiality of wound work. One calls for a series of unthreaded needles to be used as fibulae pinning the wound's edges together, before passing thread around them in repeated figure-of-eight movements and drawing the whole apparatus up tight; another, known today as a purse-string suture, uses a curved needle and is described elliptically by al-Zahrāwī's translators as completed "in the manner of sewing up bags in which goods are packed"; a third, adapted from Galen, who in turn borrowed it from Roman furriers, involves passing a needle along the thick edge of the skin to run in a subcuticular line along the wound, leaving minimal scarring; and a final simple running stitch, the most commonly employed of al-Zahrāwī's techniques, is used to close the skin in even sections "in the manner of a shoemaker."[22]

Various instruments are recommended for this work, from needles of multiple sizes and shapes to different materials for suturing, including wool, silk, linen, animal gut, ants' teeth, and gold or silver wire, the last being thought particularly appropriate for dentistry. This stitching, the stuff of Mondeville's *belles cicatrices*, really mattered. In a legal case recorded from fourteenth-century London, the surgeon John Le Spicer was found guilty of malpractice when attempting to cure a wound on his patient's face, not because the patient died—he was alive and well enough to sue Le Spicer—but because the surgeon had rendered the wound into an impossibly ugly form, what the verdict refers to as an "incurable" scar.[23] We are reminded here of the laconic terms surrounding the three Lobkowicz Wound Men. Perhaps their unelaborated diagnostic judgments of either curable or incurable functioned less as negative markers of surgery's ineffectiveness than as a shorthand warning, advocating that surgeons avoid patients whose sorry fate was already sealed, lest they be blamed for a botched job.[24]

Just as important as technical mastery of wound healing was the ability to control the patient during such procedures. Advice again captured in Teodorico's *Cyrurgia* suggests boiling a sponge in opiates and letting it dry in the sun, to be rehydrated and applied to the nostrils of a patient whenever the surgeon needed to be sure that they were drowsy during procedures; another sponge soaked in vinegar was recommended for waking them.[25] Across surgical sources we commonly find the prescription of such opiates, mostly poppy, henbane, and mandrake, although these techniques would have given patients only limited relief from significant pain.[26] Bedside manner was thus relied upon for putting the patient in appropriately calm and receptive spirits. Lists of positive attributes in a good surgeon, much replicated in the introductions to contemporary treatises, always emphasize the importance of speaking courteously and cleverly to the sick. Gui de Chauliac, one of the last and most enduringly successful of France's medieval academic surgeons, even advised in his fourteenth-century *Inventarium* (Inventory) that a surgeon keep the patient from seeing certain instruments being used for their treatment, since caustics, cautery irons, and knives all had the capacity to spook nonmedics. Chauliac also advises instructing a hemorrhaging patient to shut their eyes and that the surgeon should tell them the bleeding is beneficial in some way, even if this was not strictly true.[27] Calming a patient was not only for their own good. Consider the account of the twelfth-century military writer Usāmah ibn Munqidh, who observed an operation undergone by his father to close a lance wound in his hand. Usāmah records the surgeon's weary frustration at being constantly interrupted in his work:

> Zayd the surgeon was dressing his wound.... My father said, "Zayd, take this pebble from the wound." The surgeon did not reply. He said again, "Don't you see this pebble? Won't you remove it from the wound?" Annoyed by his insistence, the surgeon said, "Where is the pebble? This is the end of a nerve that has been cut." In reality it was white, as though it were one of the pebbles of the Euphrates.[28]

As well as managing a patient's personality, medieval surgeons were also heavily invested in managing other aspects of postoperative wound care. For theorists, the most discussed aspect of aftercare was diet. Some recommended restraint from heavy meals, while others encouraged the consumption of particular foodstuffs thought to refresh the generation of blood, especially meat and wine. On a practical level, however, aftercare mostly involved the application of regular dressings to the wound, and in particular complex and precise systems of bandaging to encourage the healing of sutures and set bones. Like stitching a wound, bandaging was a particularly valuable professional moment. A patient's neat and clean appearance after surgery could serve as a skilled surgeon's calling card, so much so that the fifteenth-century German military surgeon Heinrich von Pfolsprundt titled his entire surgical work the *Buch der Bündth-Ertznei* (Book of Bandage-Healing).[29] Few specifics of these bandaging techniques are preserved for us in writing, but we get something of their sense in an assorted book of medical, religious, and magical texts written in Greek around the year 1440 by a little-known practitioner named John of Aron.[30] The parchment of the manuscript is scuffed and stained, suggesting frequent consultation, but one opening nonetheless clearly preserves a series of faces and bodies, all wrapped in different

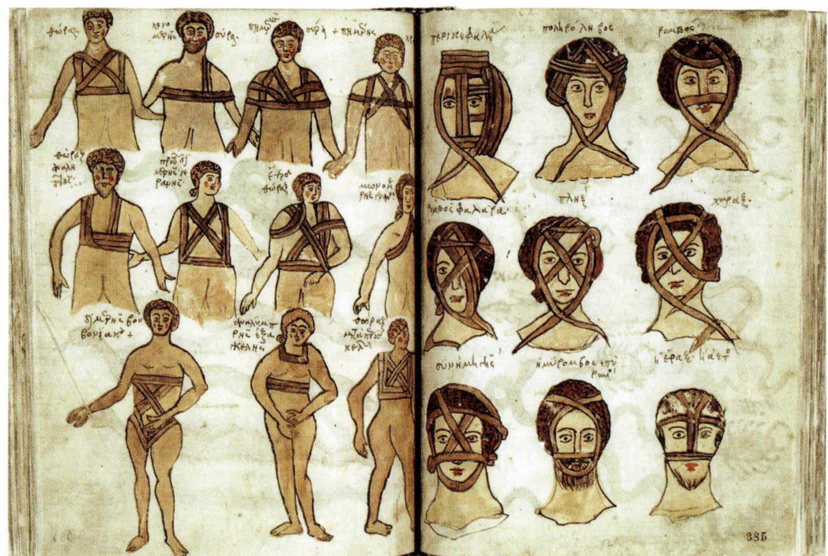

Fig. 2.2. Figures demonstrating bandaging of the body and head, c. 1430–50, Constantinople. Ink and paint on paper, 30 x 22 cm. Bologna, Biblioteca Universitaria, MS Greci 3632, fols. 384v–385r.

snaking webs of brown bandage (fig. 2.2). Their different forms, designed to secure damaged bones and their associated wounds, are each named by shape and style—"Περικεφαλαία" (Around the head, like a helmet), "Πληξ" (Entangled, around the face), "Ρομβός" (Rhombus-shaped)—their intricate designs intimating sophisticated and aesthetically attuned procedures.

Treating wounds in the later European Middle Ages was thus a layered and busy process. Its tenets were open to significant debate and refinement throughout the period. Even holistic understandings of wound healing's very nature could give surgical writers a space to distinguish themselves against their peers. In addition to his eightfold wound process, Mondeville outlines three key approaches to the healing of wounds, all of which were hotly contested. These range from the highly invasive—enlarging wounds to allow for the application of dressings—to dispensing with any actual surgical manipulation and relying only on the consumption of easily digestible meats, eggs, and bread to help cuts heal.[31] Yet regardless of which route a particular surgeon might choose to follow, it is clear that the well trained among them were capable of significant acts of healing. While, in the largely nonliterate craft of surgery, only a small percentage of practitioners had access to a treatise like Mondeville's—or those of Teodorico, al-Zahrāwī, or Pfolsprundt—increasing quantities of archaeological and paleopathological evidence clarify that the wound-healing practices recorded by these scholarly authors were nonetheless well known and widespread.[32] At medieval burials across Europe, skeletons have been excavated complete with circular plates of copper or lead wrapped neatly around damaged bones.[33] Elsewhere, large trauma depressions or the telltale diamond-shaped holes of metal arrowheads have been found puncturing the skulls of skeletons, suggesting head injuries sustained in the course of both daily life and combat. But several of these same skulls also preserve scratch marks on the scalp made during the surgical clearance of their head wounds, as well as signs of bone regrowth that prove the patient lived well beyond the procedure.[34] Such evidence consistently shows that medieval populations were much-healed people, their bodies preserving a large number of old wounds from past injuries that many had no doubt survived through the help of an experienced surgeon.[35]

Disease and the *Dreibilderserie*

Throughout the European Middle Ages, writing about wound healing provided an opportunity for surgical thinkers not only to concretize the specifics of their craft but also to innovate in its literary shape. The wide variety of forms taken by this medicine helped develop an impressively diverse array of material and writerly formats. The earliest medieval wound writings, for instance, are short and fragmentary, surviving embedded within larger treatises produced near the major healing hubs of central and northern Italy and the monastic centers of England, France, and Germany.[36] Others, made later in the period, appear either as part of the far denser and more coherent medical compendia that were foundational to Europe's burgeoning university medicine or in smaller manuscripts focused specifically on elucidating wound theory and practice. Both forms were often calligraphically beautiful treatises that aimed to bring the profession into greater intellectual and social regard.[37] Some wound advice even survives in formats more reflective of medieval religious and superstitious communities, with instructions for the making of pithy wound charms to be recited by a healer or scrawled on small pieces of parchment that could be worn or ingested by a patient, a tradition particularly potent in German-speaking lands.[38] The Wound Man can thus be seen as one of the most unusual outcomes in a long line of surgical literary reformulations, for we find the figure closely allied with a specific group of surgical books whose structure and contents once again aimed to take large swaths of well-established medical knowledge and rework it in innovative ways.

To modern scholars, books in this group have become known as *Dreibilderserie* manuscripts—literally, manuscripts of the "Three-Picture Series"—a term first coined by the historian of medicine Karl Sudhoff in the early twentieth century to describe their shared strategies of medical communication.[39] They are preserved today in at least twenty manuscripts made in southern Germany and Bohemia at various points throughout the fifteenth century, and their creation was clearly a medical project of some importance.[40] To judge by elements of these books' contents and terminology, they probably started being produced within the orbit of the University of Prague or perhaps the busy surgical circles of southern Germany, conceived as a rough-and-ready suite covering several key areas of essential interest to medical students and experienced practitioners alike.[41] As their modern threefold name suggests, each example normally contained a triangulated set of core elements: first, a work addressing internal humoral medicine; second, a work addressing issues of women's health, specifically theories and practices of gynecology and obstetrics; and third, a work focusing exclusively on the healing of wounds. To define these books by their written contents alone, however—as we do with virtually all other medical works of the period—is to miss the point. This group was governed not by a rigorously maintained series of set texts replicated line by line on their busy pages, but instead by a consistent trio of images around which changeable medical writings of various backgrounds were made to coalesce.

The internal logic of these *Dreibilderserie* manuscripts is best understood by taking their eponymous three images in turn. These figures are all molded in what we have already identified as a common yet complicated medieval diagrammatic mode. They appear in individual *Dreibilderserie* manuscripts in various orders, but most often the simplest of the trio leads the group: the so-called *Krankheitsmann*, or "Disease Man," a figure that heralded a turn toward the pathologies of humoral medicine.[42] Take one such figure from a particularly petite *Dreibilderserie* book now in Heidelberg, a bilingual German-Latin work from the middle of the fifteenth century (fig. 2.3).[43] Here the Disease Man is singled out for particular prominence through codicological emphasis, occupying the full length of a fifteen-centimeter parchment insert at the book's opening that unfolds to twice the size of its other small paper pages. He strikes a pose consistent across the group, one that is surely borrowed from contemporary bloodletting figures of the sort discussed in the previous chapter, his legs wide apart, arms bent, and naked except for a small pair of blue drawstring underpants. For a small drawing made only in largely uncolored line, its detailing is still subtle, from the rosy coloring at his concave chest to his tiny, vaguely comical individuated teeth. This sketched body, though, jostles for attention with a far bolder flock of textual elements, words that flank the figure from all angles listing different types of disease.

If we were to flip through the pages of text immediately following this figure, we would discover that these terms in fact function as catchwords linking this body with individuated diseases whose nature and potential cures are elaborated in alphabetical paragraphs of Latin across the next eight folios. In keeping with the flexible ethos of the *Dreibilderserie* group as a whole, the specifics of the textual medicine accompanying the Disease Man vary from manuscript to manuscript. Each book draws on different sources for its curative contents, from the Pseudo-Hippocratic *De morbis* (On Diseases) to Bernard de Gordon's *Lilium medicinae* (Lily of Medicine), as well as ideas borrowed from various other Classical and medieval compilers.[44] Yet when set around the Disease Man, the catchwords' disposition comes together to follow a visual logic rather than a textual one, all localizing illness on the figure's body. The fan of terms spreading out in a corona around his head, for instance, relay diseases of the face and mind.[45] These include some that would present obviously to a patient or medic: *catharrus* (catarrh), *tinitus aurium* (tinnitus of the ears), *obtalmia* (inflammation of the eye), *allopicia* and *casus capillorum* (two forms of hair loss), and *thetanus* (lockjaw). Others, chronic or psychological, might have needed more professional diagnosis: *emigranea* (migraine), *melancholia* and *mania* (both considered malfunctions of the brain), *epilencia* (a disease related to epilepsy), *vertigo* (a dizziness or confusion of balance), *litargia* (a pathological lethargy), and *stupor mentis* (a full-body catatonic state).

This semicorporeal structuring continues to the left and right of the Disease Man. Problems of the abdomen's internal organs run from top to bottom as the list descends, beginning with *arteriaca* (rheuma of the windpipe)

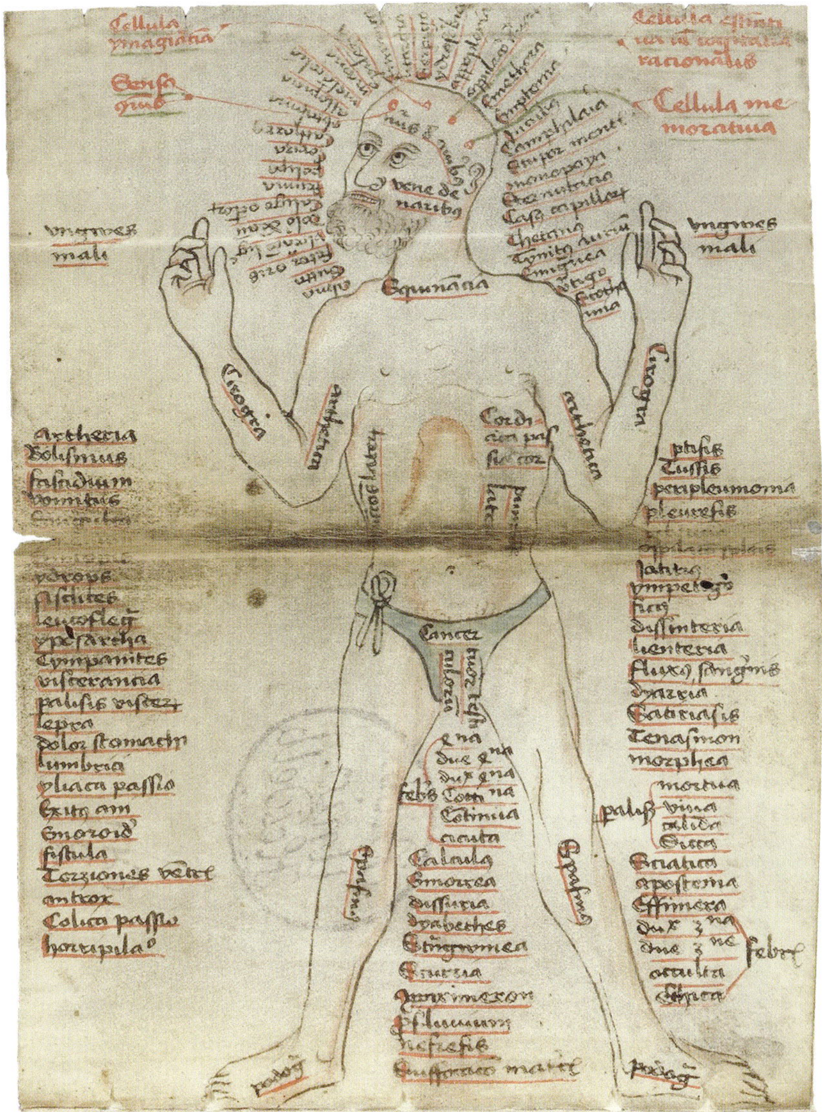

Fig. 2.3. Disease Man, c. 1450–70, southern Germany. Ink and paint on parchment, 20 x 15 cm (unfolded). Heidelberg, Universitätsbibliothek, Cpg 644, inserted as fol. 1.

and *ptisis* (an ulcer of the lung) before moving downward through conditions such as *ictericia* (jaundice), *lumbrici* (long intestinal worms), and both *lienteria* and *diarria* (two irritations of the bowel). A list between the legs takes up this external morbid baton, running vertically from *tumor testiculorum* (tumor in the testicles) down through various urinary disorders—*calculus* (urinary stones) and *strangiurea* (painful urination)—to *nefresis* (a sharp pain associated with kidney stones) and, in an unusually gendered twist to which we will return, *suffocatio matricis* (suffocation of the womb), a gynecological trope inherited from Classical medicine that considered the womb to wander dangerously around the body.[46]

Finally, a small group of terms are reserved for placement atop the Disease Man's body, or perhaps within it. *Squinancia* (quinsy, a swelling in the throat) sits in place at the bottom of the neck; *punctiones lateris* (a pricking sensation in the side) runs down his flanks like a chill; his hands preserve *ungues mali* (bad nails), a growth of dense nail-like tissue; and his feet display *podagra* (a specifically podiatric form of gout). Looking even more deeply into the body, sprouting from the figure's forehead we find listed the so-called cells of the brain responsible, in the medieval view, for the processing of rational thought: the *sensus communis* (common sense), *ymaginativa* (imagination), *estimativa* (estimation), and *memorativa* (memory).[47]

The presence of this semi-anatomical sectioning of the brain reminds us that the Disease Man is playing out a tension familiar to medieval medico-diagrammatic images, his body flipping between the individuality of a patient and the universality of sickness. We are presented with a single, highly tangible man, yet he is exposed to a fantastically impossible multitude of potential technical ills. As a result, artists of different *Dreibilderserie* manuscripts could choose to situate their Disease Men at radically different ends of the diagrammatic spectrum. Some conceived of him as an utterly viable body, a real person whom they playfully set into evocative space—standing on a grass-tufted mound, on the steps of a small tiled building, or simply on a color-wash floor—all the while with his captions hovering over the top of his solid body like a transparent film (fig. 2.4).[48] Meanwhile, other Disease Men are more schematic than human: in manuscripts now in Paris, Berlin, and Prague, his linear body floats abstractedly on the page, the artist highlighting different elements of the brain marked out on the scalp, like a surveyor plotting tracts of land (fig. 2.5), while in another book the figure is even deconstructed down into discrete bodily units spread across four folios, their status as a coherent, continuous man almost entirely undetectable (fig. 2.6).[49]

Twin motors thus power the Disease Man. The insistent presence of medical catchwords emphasizes this picture's technical credentials, reminding the reader that the image functioned as a humanoid marshal organizing the accumulated texts that follow. Yet there is never any doubt that aesthetics takes the reins in these manuscripts' makeup. While its accompanying cures are changeable, the Disease Man's image provides the constant across the humoral medicine of the group. Moreover, his visualized form had its own range of useful purposes. Thumbing through the book, his large body would have caught the reader's eye far more effectively than a mere contents list, assuring them quickly that a particular cure could be found within. Likewise, the ordered mapping of disease about his physical form could serve a mnemonic function for readers keen to memorize the contents of his body and thus the contents of the treatise. Still, it is hard to know exactly how these Disease Men were received or for whom they were specifically intended. Few *Dreibilderserie* manuscripts have reached us with clear enough internal evidence or collecting provenance to link them to particular medieval individuals with much certainty. We might sensibly assume that their visual diversity and handsome images point to patrons who could afford the expense of a relatively accomplished artist. The regular incorporation within *Dreibilderserie* manuscripts of other forms of parallel calendrical and medical materials—bloodletting figures, urine tables, Zodiac Men—indicates that these books were also geared toward medical professionals, or at least toward nonspecialists invested in the impressive learning represented by the healing arts.

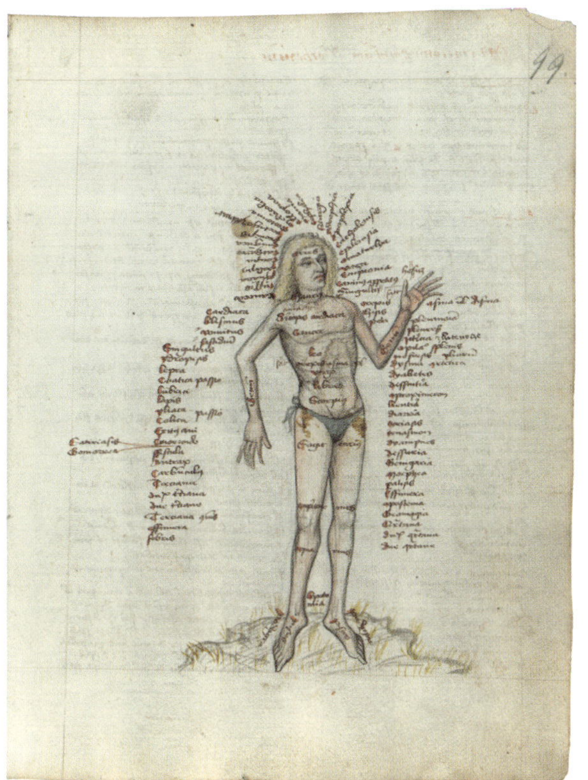

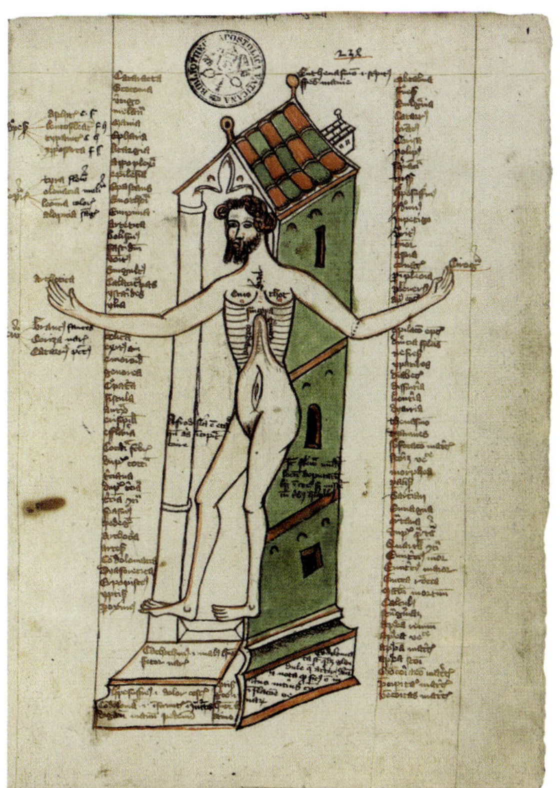

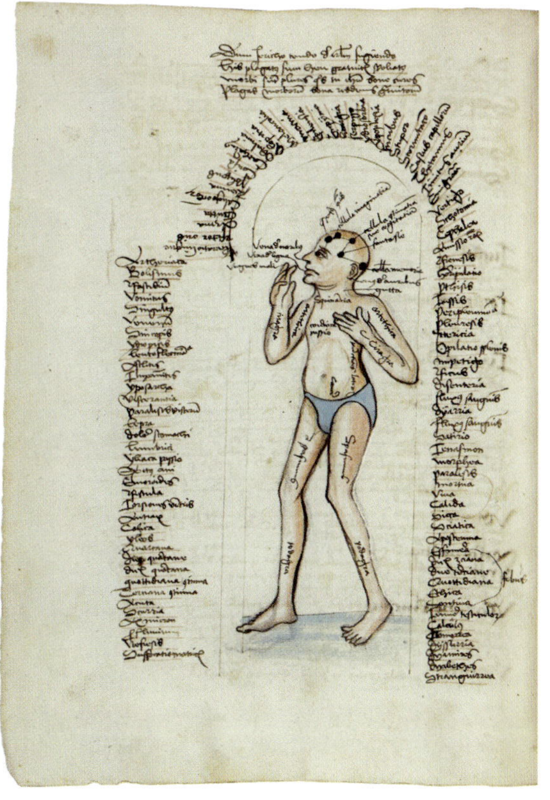

Fig. 2.4. Disease Men placed into semi-realistic settings. *(In clockwise order)*: Disease Man, 15th century, Bohemia. Ink and paint on paper, 28 x 21 cm. Prague, Královská kanonie premonstrátů na Strahově, Strahovská knihovna, MS DC III 3, 99. Disease Man, 15th century, southern Germany. Ink and paint on paper, 29 x 21 cm. Vatican City, Biblioteca Apostolica Vaticana, MS Pal. Lat. 1293, fol. 1r. Disease Man, late 15th century, Germany. Ink and paint on paper, 29 x 20 cm. Vatican City, Biblioteca Apostolica Vaticana, MS Pal. Lat. 1325, fol. 346v.

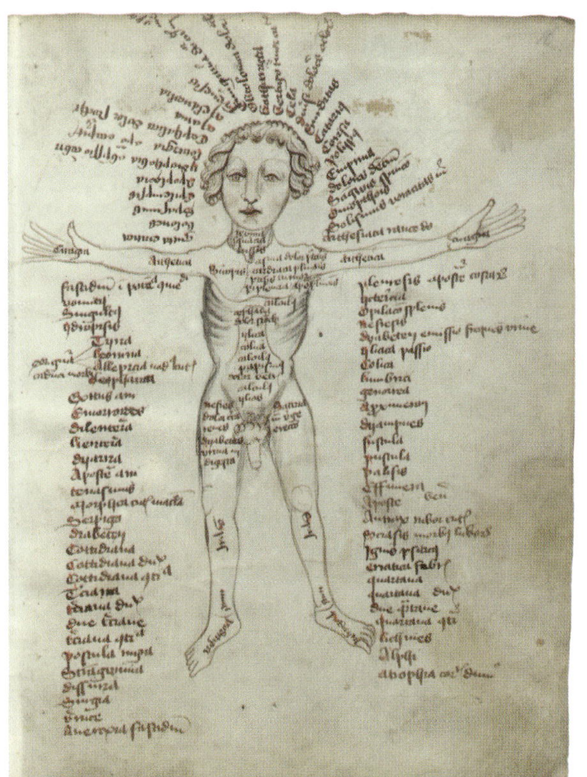

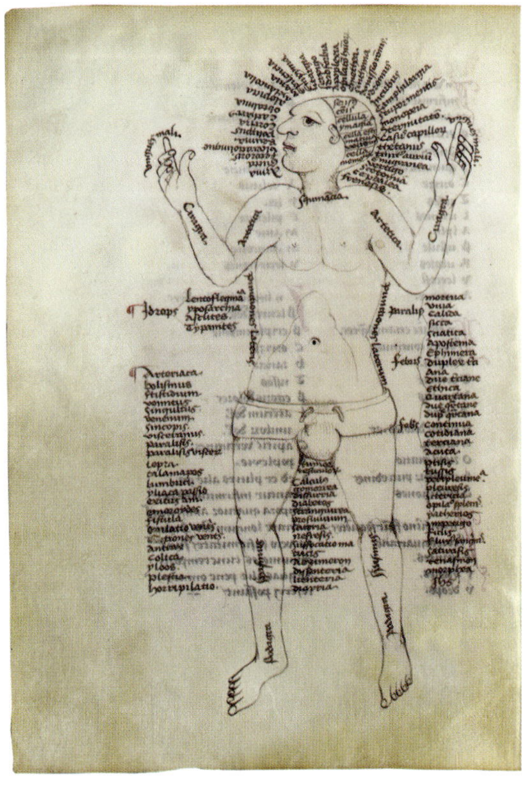

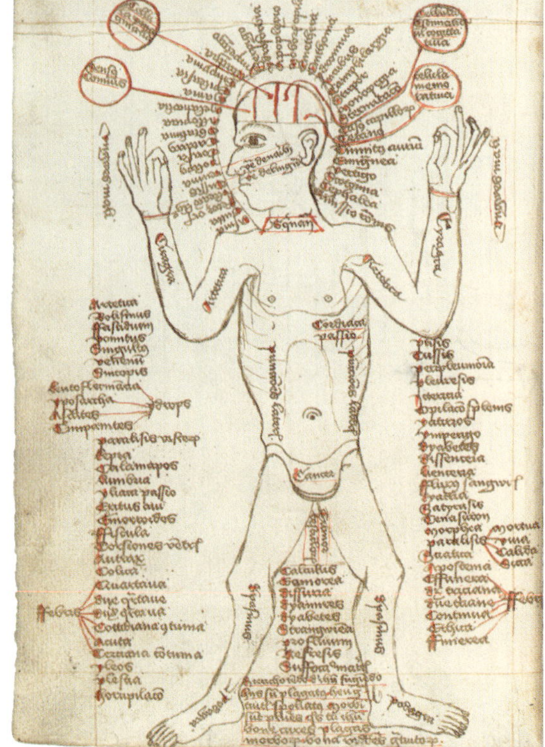

Fig. 2.5. Disease Men with catchword crowns. *(In clockwise order)*: Disease Man, 15th century, Germany. Ink and paint on parchment, 22 x 18 cm. Berlin, Staatsbibliothek, Mlq 275, fol. 16r. Disease Man, after 1417, France. Ink on parchment, 20 x 14 cm. Paris, Bibliothèque nationale de France, MS Latin 11229, fol. 37v. Disease Man, c. 1433–50, Silesia. Ink on paper, 21 x 15 cm. Prague, Národní knihovna České republiky, MS XIX C 49, fol. 176v.

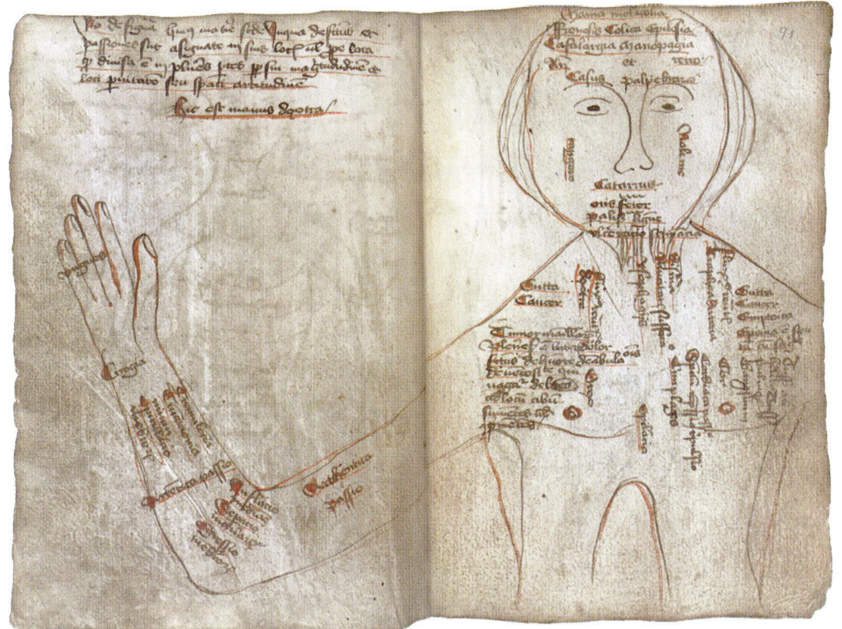

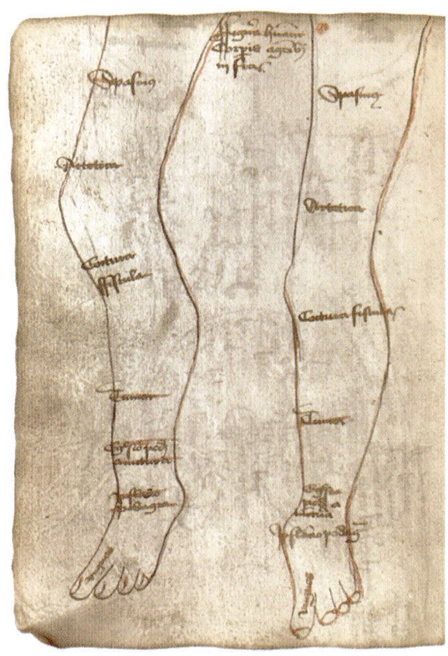

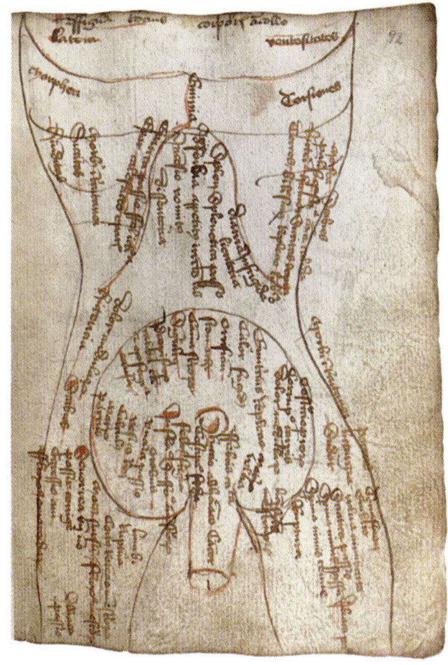

Fig. 2.6. Multiple parts of a divided Disease Man, 15th century, Bohemia. Ink on paper, 21 x 15 cm (each folio). Los Angeles, UCLA, Louise M. Darling Biomedical Library, MS Benjamin 10, fols. 90v–92r.

At the very least, an image found striding across the lower margins of a much earlier German medical manuscript, probably made in Bamberg at some point in the late twelfth century, suggests that an audience for similar figures had existed for some time (fig. 2.7).[50] Depicting a man overwritten with medical terms, it appears beneath the opening paragraph of a short treatise entitled *Tractatus de scemate humano* (Treatise on the Human Figure), a work that draws on much earlier anatomical writings of the fourth-century Roman medic Helvius Vindicianus to outline bodily taxonomies running from head to toe.[51] This medicine is picked up topographically in

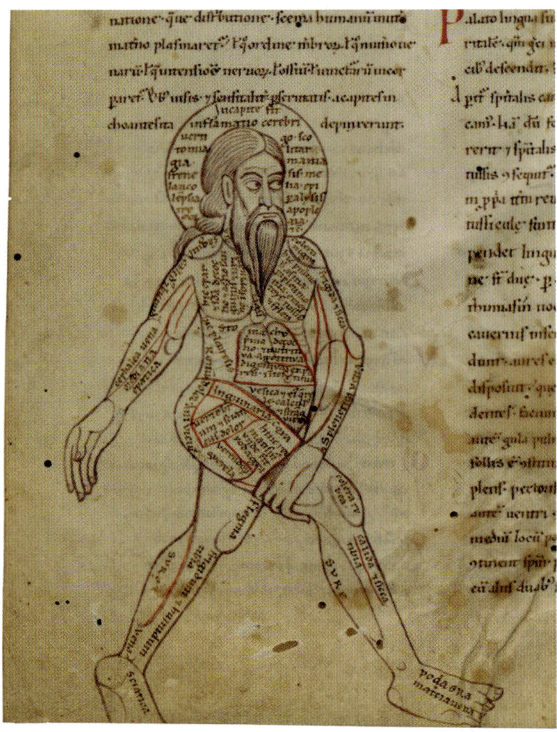

Fig. 2.7. Proto-Disease Man, late 12th century, Germany. Ink on parchment, 29 x 19 cm. Bamberg, Staatsbibliothek, Msc. Med. 6, fol. 142v.

the man's form, his skin divided with a delicate hatch of black and red lines within which the names of veins, organs, and diseases are inscribed onto his body, from *mania* and *epilepsia* around the head down to *pleuresis* over the lungs and *podagra* at the feet. This early Bamberg figure is a historical outlier: nothing like him appears again until the fifteenth-century Disease Men of the *Dreibilderserie*. Yet his presence nonetheless appears to confirm that mapping humoral illness onto bodies had long been embedded in German medical communication, reasoning, and display, proving a keen awareness of how effective and striking it could be to entangle diseases and figures on the page.

Visualizing Women

As well as a historical precedent for figuring disease, this early Bamberg manuscript also inadvertently draws our attention to the second medical arena marshaled by the images of the late medieval *Dreibilderserie*. Overleaf from its striding inscribed male figure, after discussions of the lungs, stomach, and bladder, Vindicianus's anatomical text draws its top-to-tail tour of the body to a close, but not before addressing the morphological specifics of one final organ: the womb. After describing its unique structure—*fragilis* and *mollissima* (fragile and soft)—it summarizes its roles in conception and gives a brief commentary on Hippocratic Aphorism number 5:51, concerning the appearance of the uterus during birth. Yet despite constituting around one-fifth of the entirety of Vindicianus's text, no image accompanies these uterine descriptions. Instead, the Bamberg book leaves its bearded male figure to stand as the sole visualization of a medicalized body, regardless of the obvious fact that he maps pathologies to which both men and women were equally susceptible.

In this decision, the Bamberg book was enacting a misogynistic distinction typical of medical writing in Europe throughout the Middle Ages and beyond. Not that the specifics of women's healthcare were excluded from discussion. On the contrary, several types of text—often anonymously authored, circulating under titles such as *De passionibus mulierum* (On the Diseases of Women) or simply *Genecia* (from the Greek for "women's affairs")—elaborated a broad range of issues pertaining to women's health, with the goal of providing concrete care.[52] But from the thirteenth century, contemporaneous with the birth of the European university movement and its accompanying formalization of academic knowledge, a number of writings began to appear that reframed gynecological ideas for a growing audience of male theoreticians and practitioners. These works often held titles referring to *Secreta mulierum* (Secrets of Women), a double-edged phrase intimating that they would reveal women's inner, anatomical secrets to the reader, but that in fact belied their true intention to guard women's medicine within a male academic elite, a "secret" kept from women themselves. This thinking was central to a broader political shift toward male dominance within medieval European learned medicine, effecting what Monica Green has dubbed the "making masculine" of women's health.[53]

Within this medical world—innovated, recorded, and institutionalized by men—there was no doubt that the male body was the normative one. Humorally speaking, for instance, men were described in theoretical texts as having a warm temperament as opposed to women's natural but inferior coolness, meaning that all medical ideas resulting from this biased central tenet only further compounded women's secondary status, from issues of appropriate diet to questions of practical treatment to the framing of physiologies unique to women, such as menstruation. Again, this is not to suggest that medieval women had no access to effective healthcare. Toward the end of the period, we find a number of healers who were well versed in the practical treatment of women, as well as evidence that women themselves occasionally practiced as surgeons and apothecaries, and that in Germany the first midwifery care institutionalized at a civic level was provided.[54] But their weighting within medicine's fundamentals still governed much of women's healing and confined them to a secondary status that had significant medico-social consequences.

This was as much the case in the realm of imagery and visualization as it was in textual medicine and actual practice. As we saw in the previous chapter, whether plotting anatomy, phlebotomy, or other practical treatments, virtually all medical images found in the medieval European tradition are entirely grounded in male bodily prototypes. Only a scattering of images survive that show women practitioners at work: one depicts a woman administering humoral cupping, while a handful of others illustrate scenes of pregnancy or birth, with post-parturient mothers attended by women birthing experts.[55] These, however, are rare exceptions, highly naturalistic scenes evoking specific everyday spaces. Among more diagrammatic images, only

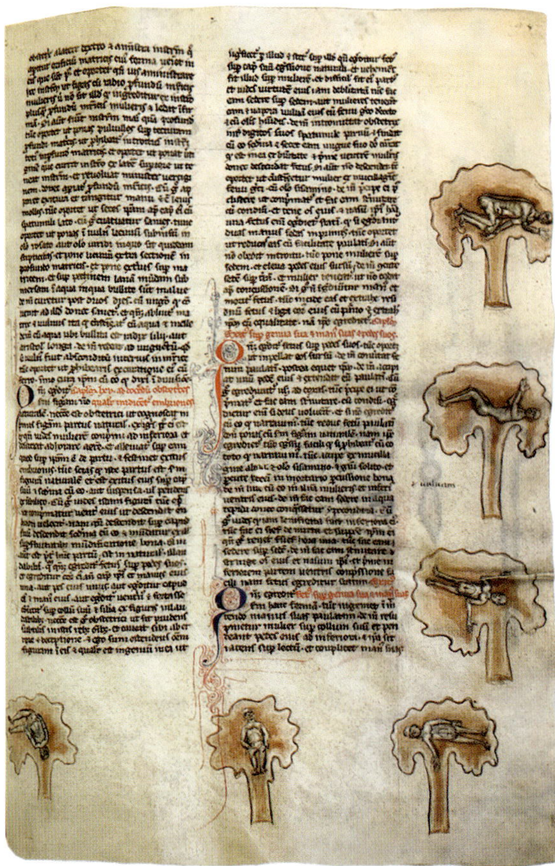

Fig. 2.8. Marginal images showing fetal malpresentations, 14th century, Italy. Ink and paint on parchment. Venice, Biblioteca Nazionale Marciana, MS Lat. Zan. 320 (=1937), fol. 98r.

a handful of traditions that address women's medicine are known to have developed before the fifteenth century. The best-preserved is a scheme stemming from the obstetrical writings of a sixth-century Tunisian scholar named Muscio, who visualized a number of different fetal malpresentations that would have required urgent correction to save the life of both mother and child (fig. 2.8).[56] Yet even this series, aimed in its original Late Antique context at an audience of midwives, was by the thirteenth century being co-opted into an increasingly masculinized academic medicine. Put bluntly, more images of surgical instruments survive in medieval medical books than diagrams elucidating women's bodies.

This may well have been the visual vacuum that authors and artists of fifteenth-century *Dreibilderserie* manuscripts were hoping to address, for they present us with the very first systematic visualization of the full female form to be found in European medicine. This figure, the second of the *Dreibilderserie*'s three core elements, has been dubbed the *schwangere Krankheitsfrau*, or "Pregnant Disease Woman," and in a modern extension of medieval gender biases, she has either gone entirely uncommented on or simply been considered the Disease Man's female equivalent.[57] There are certainly parallels between these two *Dreibilderserie* disease images. The two figures often strike the same froglike pose, their legs and arms outstretched as if they have just flung their bodies open for investigation by the reader, and like the Disease Man, the Disease Woman embodies a clear concern for the topographical mapping of disease through plotted pathologies found listed around her body. Several Disease Women even match the Disease Man directly, with blocks of text beside her head noting nasal polyps and pleural pus, lethargy and tongue ulcers, while her shoulders read as arthritic and her feet carry inscriptive gout. Also similar is the manner in which the Disease Woman gathers together a changeable group of texts, drawing into the *Dreibilderserie* a collection of practically oriented cures variably culled from canonical works of medieval gynecology, including, among others, elements of the *Trotula* ensemble, the Salernitan *De aegritudinum curatione* (On the Treatment of Diseases), the *Viaticum* of Constantinus Africanus, and the so-called *Problemata Aristotelis* (Problems of Aristotle).[58] Collected together, these works take on an encyclopedic yet rather scattered quality typical of the *Dreibilderserie*'s textual medicine, jumping tangentially from topic to topic while overall emphasizing the practical dimensions of the gynecological field, from issues relating to menstruation and diseases of the breasts to conception and contraception, as well as childbirth and its various complications.

However, to conclude that the Disease Woman merely mirrors the Disease Man's labels and textual relations is to overlook the fact that her body is a significantly more sophisticated image, showcasing a far more substantive interest in various interconnected elements of medical knowledge. Take a *Dreibilderserie* Disease Woman from a manuscript now in Copenhagen, pictured alongside other diagrams at the top of a large parchment sheet (fig. 2.9).[59] She is a careful, linear rendering, depicted in thin black ink with light color washes and deep-set eyes. Once more, the figure's surface is thoroughly inscriptive, replete with diseased terms from head to toe. But unlike the Disease Man, her figure's inner anatomy has been paid conspicuous attention. From chin to groin, the front of the body has vanished away to reveal an array of intricately labeled innards. At the neck, two parallel tubes descend to meet two bundles of organs: to the right one meets the heart, picked out in red, while to the left we follow the esophagus down past a lightly shaded gall bladder into a small round stomach, flanked by a curving liver. A network of overlapping passageways sprouts beneath, symbolizing the intestines and colon, while further connections snake out to the right to incorporate an ovate womb containing a fetus—labeled *embrio*—staring out as if looking through a bodily porthole.

These organs all bear additional internal catchwords and strips of texts that continue the *Dreibilderserie*'s general concern for internal disease. Conditions relating to over- and undereating, worms, and constipation have migrated from the Disease Man's external lists to the Disease Woman's inside, crammed one atop the other close to their corporeally appropriate spot. Within her heart we read of *sincopis* (fainting) and *cardia passio* (cardiac arrest), the lower part of her colon displays kidney stones and hemorrhoids, and a long band of terms heading toward her womb begins with the label *suffocatio*, the same uterine suffocation that *Dreibilderserie* authors mapped among the Disease Man's ills. Here, however, the Disease Woman's engagement with anatomy is at once taxonomic and descriptive. All of her organs are presented bearing technical Latin names—*cor*, *stomaci*, *splen*, *renes*, *matrix*,

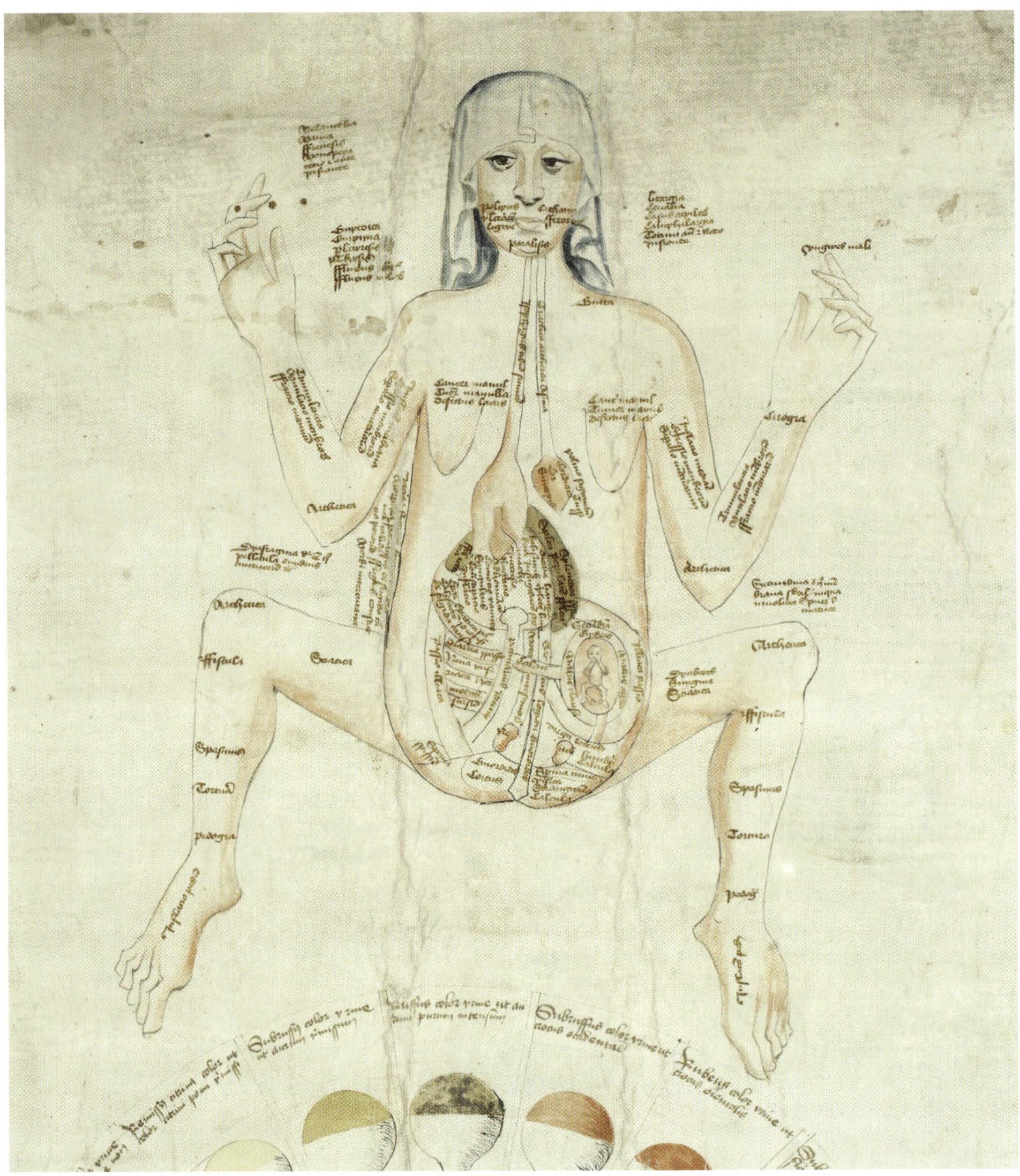

Fig. 2.9. Disease Woman, 15th century, Germany. Ink and paint on parchment, 75 x 55 cm (whole folio). Copenhagen, Kongelige Bibliothek, NKS 84 b 2°, fol. 4r.

and so on—but across the Disease Woman corpus the figure also bears short elaborations that convey to the reader the actual function of some anatomical elements alongside their form (fig. 2.10). The figure in a *Dreibilderserie* manuscript now in the Vatican tells us that the "*dyafragma dividens*" (diaphragm is dividing) the upper and lower chest; another manuscript, now in London, speaks among many other labels of the "*ysophagus cibum sumens*" (esophagus receiving food); and a third, probably made in Regensburg, confirms below her left thigh that the placenta "*est quedam pellicula in qua involuitur puer in matrice*" (is a certain film in which the child is wrapped in the womb).[60]

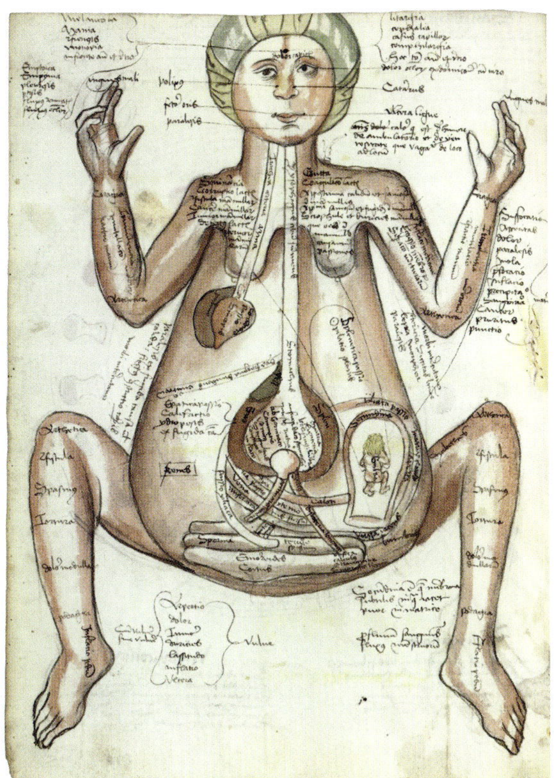

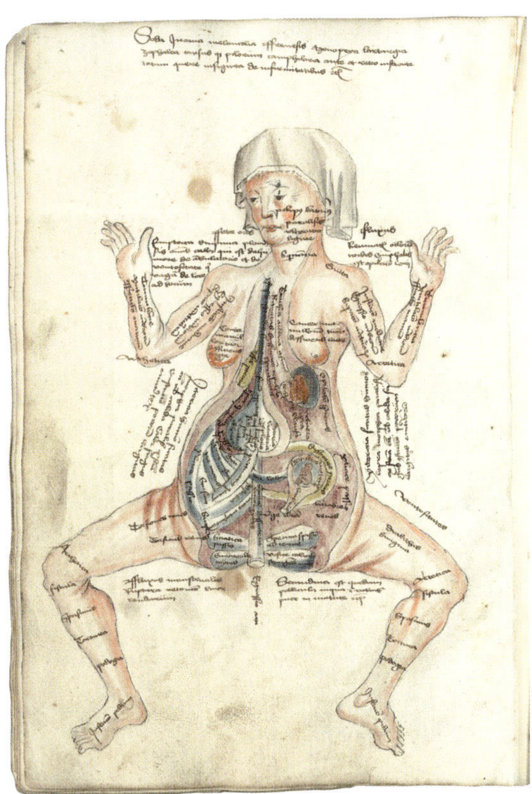

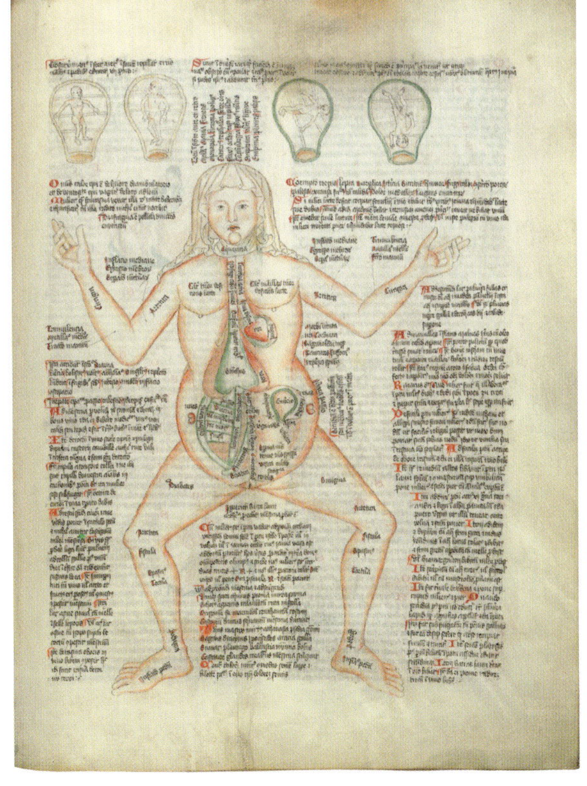

Fig. 2.10. Disease Women. *(In clockwise order)*: Disease Woman, late 15th century, Germany. Ink and paint on paper, 29 x 20 cm. Vatican City, Biblioteca Apostolica Vaticana, MS Pal. Lat. 1325, fol. 349v. Disease Woman, c. 1485, possibly Regensburg. Ink and paint on paper, 31 x 20 cm. Munich, Bayerische Staatsbibliothek, Cgm 597, fol. 259v. Disease Woman, c. 1420–30, possibly Thuringia. Ink and paint on parchment, 40 x 30 cm. London, Wellcome Library, MS 49, fol. 38r.

Katharine Park has suggested that, in contemporary Italian contexts, medico-visual engagement drew highly sexed boundaries through ideas of interiority and exteriority: men's bodies were associated with familiar truths and were used to depict the typical outside of the body, while women's bodies offered answers to complex questions of the anatomical interior and thus were constantly being opened up in imagery.[61] The Germanic-Bohemian Disease Woman, however, seems to combine these ideas rather than separate them out, enabling an understanding of both surface sicknesses and anatomical knowledge in union. Such engagements were clearly prized. In at least five fifteenth-century manuscripts, the Disease Woman was extracted from her *Dreibilderserie* fellows as the series' sole visual representative and included without any form of male counterpart, quite the opposite of the Bamberg manuscript from several centuries earlier.

Another element of the Disease Woman's exterior suggests that we should take seriously her contextual as well as physiological details. Without exception, rather than being shown fully naked, the Disease Woman is presented to us with her head covered. Her hair is restrained within a veil, depicted in one case as a short garment but most often as a long covering that stretches down behind her shoulders and on occasion wraps under her chin to frame her face. As multifaceted social markers, we might read such a veil in a number of ways. Most immediately, it brings to mind contemporary moralizing around female dress, especially in relation to religion, sinfulness, and vanity. Whereas plain veils were considered appropriate for women when visiting church, extravagant headwear could flirt with mistrust and scandal.[62] The latter idea was expressed, for instance, in the sermons of the thirteenth-century Franciscan preacher Berthold of Regensburg, whose writings continued to be popular throughout Germany into the period of the *Dreibilderserie* books. Veils, he stated, especially those garnished with ribbons or bells, were a lightning rod for female vanity, "*ein tuochelach, da iuwer der tiuvel aller meiste mite vahet*" (a cloth with which the devil catches most of you [women]).[63]

A number of images similar to the Disease Woman make clear that such titillation could certainly be courted within contemporary medical manuscripts. Diagrams found in two separate astro-medical handbooks from fifteenth-century Germany both render popular medical tropes not through prototypical male bodies but through deliberately sexually charged female forms. The first, found in a book written in the late 1470s and 1480s, begun by one Brother Wilhelm de Rang at the Benedictine Abbey of Saints Ulrich und Afra in Augsburg, reworks its Disease Man into a seminaked woman.[64] With her cheeks flushed red, she fixes the monastic male reader with a coquettish smile, her modesty barely covered by a small, falling sheet that she holds to her chest with one hand and tugs down with the other, incongruously surrounded by the same diseased catchwords as the male *Dreibilderserie* figure. Even more explicit is a second figure, from a manuscript likely commissioned around the same time in Ulm by a local patrician patron (fig. 2.11).[65] Here it is the Zodiac Man outlining celestial influence—a figure in all other known cases represented as male—that has been replaced with a provocatively naked woman. She ostensibly maps the cosmological correspon-

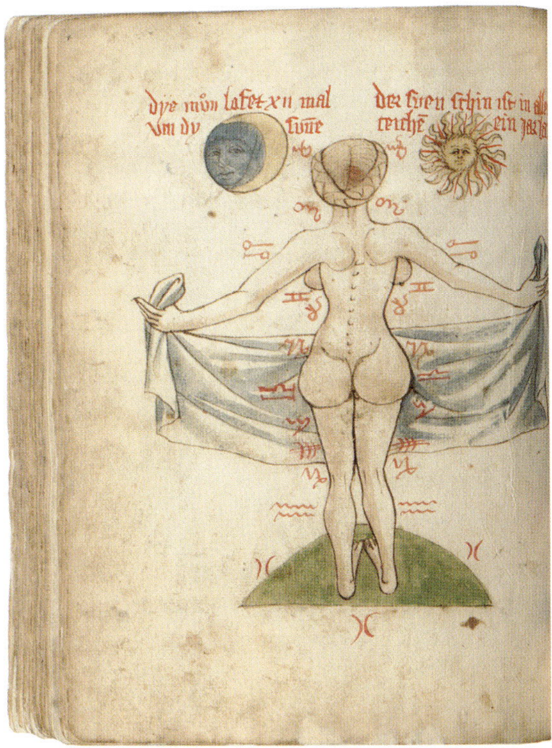

Fig. 2.11. Sexualized Zodiac Woman, c. 1450–75, possibly Ulm. Ink and paint on paper, 28 x 21 cm. Tübingen, Universitätsbibliothek, Md 2, fol. 42v.

dences of the stars onto her body, but in reality she seems concerned with far more earthly matters. Turning away from us, the woman holds up a sheet as if to partly cover her nakedness from the moon and sun, whose smirking partial personifications lurk above her in the sky, but this does little to guard her from the gaze of the reader, who is offered an entirely uncensored view of her behind, where particular care been taken to emphasize her genitals and breasts.

The veiling of the Disease Woman, by contrast, seems an attempt to differentiate her from these potentially sexualized interpretations. After all, the only owners of manuscripts containing Disease Women that we can identify today were men whose religious or medical backgrounds may have kept them particularly alert to the danger of such temptations (fig. 2.12). A Bohemian book owned by a man named Sigismund of St. Mähren, about whom we currently know nothing beyond his name on its inside cover, includes a Disease Woman rather frantically plotted within the lines of an anatomical text.[66] Another example is scrappily sketched in the front of a book owned by one Martin von Geismar, head of the chapter of St. Peter's in Fritzlar.[67] A third appears copied in the notebook of one Jean Gispaden, a peripatetic surgeon based in and around Grenoble.[68] And a fourth has been given a whole page in a university notebook from the 1450s, part of which reproduces notes of several lectures heard at the University of Leipzig by a student named Nicolaus Sturm de Geroltzhoffen, who perhaps also drew the figure.[69] We might also wish to add to this list the deconstructed woman discussed in the

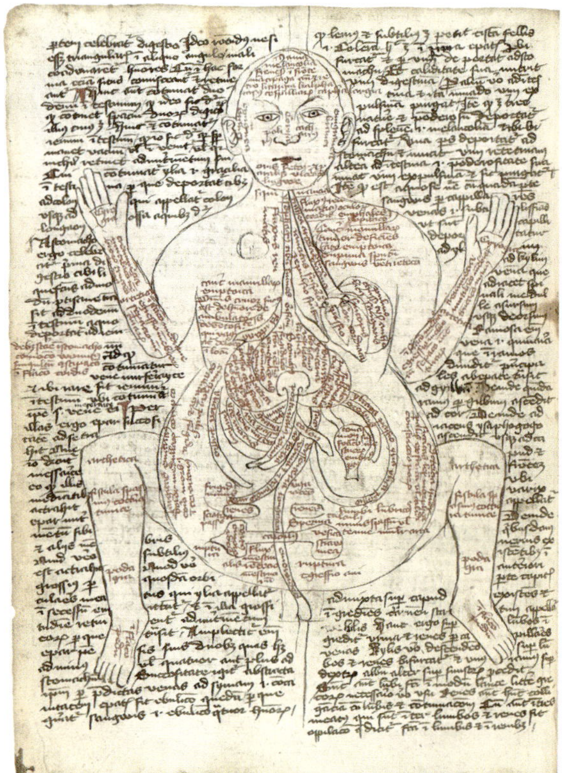

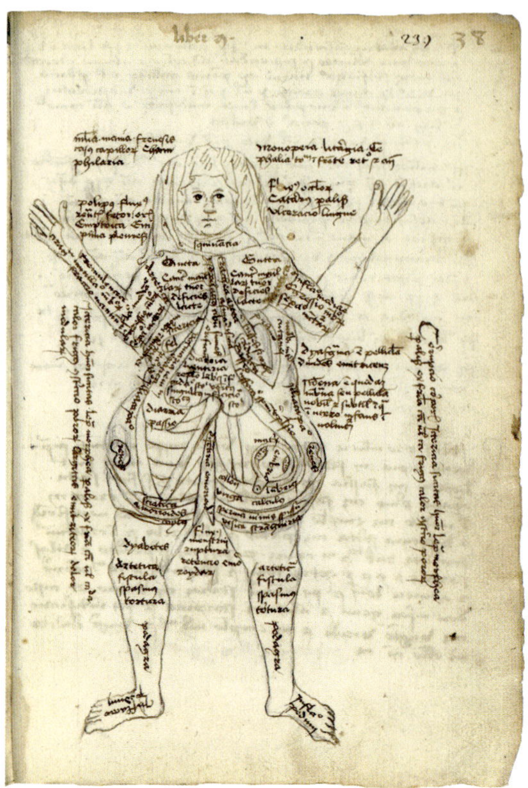

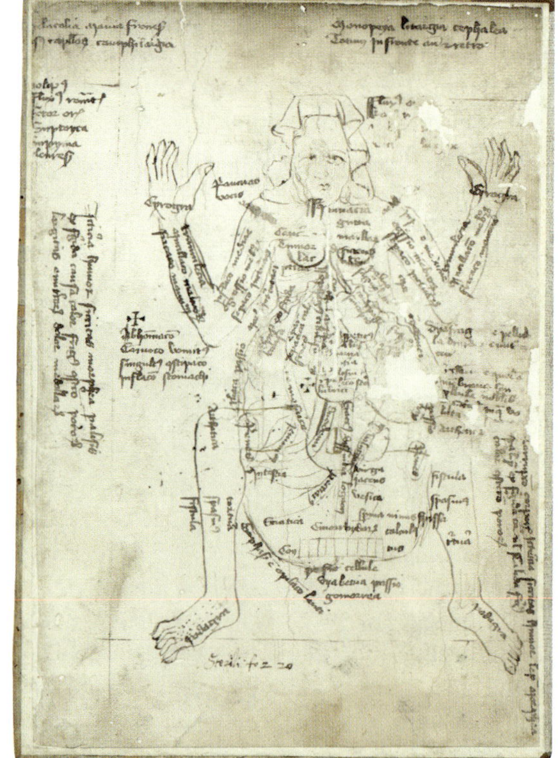

Fig. 2.12. Disease Women in manuscripts owned by men. *(In clockwise order)*: Disease Woman, early 15th century, Bohemia. Ink on paper, 31 x 20 cm. Prague, Národní knihovna České republiky, MS III C 2, fol. 44v. Disease Woman, late 15th century, near Grenoble. Ink on paper, 22 x 15 cm. Paris, Bibliothèque nationale de France, MS Latin 7138, fol. 239r. Disease Woman, c. 1435, Germany. Ink on paper, 29 x 21 cm. Kassel, Universitätsbibliothek, 2° MS Med 7, inside cover.

previous chapter, scribbled by the academic medic Erhard Knab in his 1460s notebook (fig. 1.1).

Clearly, we cannot take this sartorial purification too far. The wimple worn by the Disease Woman is not intended to render her as virginal: she is no nun, or at least not a very chaste one, for she is pregnant. Instead, the wearing of a veil is specified in several contemporary German statutes and sumptuary regulations as a requirement particular to married women in order to differentiate them from their unmarried counterparts, as well as worn by postpartum women during churching ceremonies intended for their ritual purification after recovering from giving birth.[70] The veil's effect thus could well have been to legitimize the Disease Woman's pregnancy within wedlock and other Christian ritual bounds, and it might also have offered more medical reassurance. By this point in the fifteenth century, the physical investigation of women by male practitioners had become a particularly fraught moment of diagnosis and treatment, with taboos forming in some European cultures—especially among higher social classes—against male physicians examining women patients.[71] The Disease Woman's covered head, therefore, could serve to neutralize the medical gaze of its male readers who were turning to *Dreibilderserie* books in order to glean knowledge of women's anatomy and diseases from within her most intimate regions.

Wounds, Words, *Wundarznei*

As well as the Disease Man and Disease Woman, fifteenth-century *Dreibilderserie* books originated a third and final image to steward their tripartite mixed medicine: the Wound Man. Finally we have arrived at the figure in what we might call its quintessential form, or at least its first substantive iteration. A central element of the *Dreibilderserie* series, the Wound Man is known to accompany either one or both of its diseased fellows in at least eight books from the fifteenth century, although new discoveries are surely out there to be made: the latest manuscript containing the figure surfaced on the rare book market as recently as 2023.[72] Yet whether present in examples long known to scholars or only just uncovered, our understanding of its two diseased diagrammatic companions lays good groundwork for appreciating the Wound Man's own underlying mechanics.

One of the most aesthetically impressive of entry points into the *Dreibilderserie* Wound Man is a particularly accomplished version of the figure in a manuscript now in Munich, probably completed around the year 1485 in or near the Bavarian city of Regensburg (fig. 2.13).[73] Standing nearly thirty centimeters high, he is brightly colored and violently rendered, holding a pose now familiar from past figures plotting disease and bloodletting with arms outstretched to either side and naked except for a small pair of blue underpants. The first thing to strike the viewer is a mass of aggressive objects rendered around his body, the most prominent of which are weapons of war. At his uppermost extremity, the tip of a dagger begins to plunge into his forehead; beside it, a short, round-ended club is already making contact, its impact emphasized by a muddy gray bruise forming at his eye; and between them, a stone shaped like a tiny cloud knocks into the side of his temple.

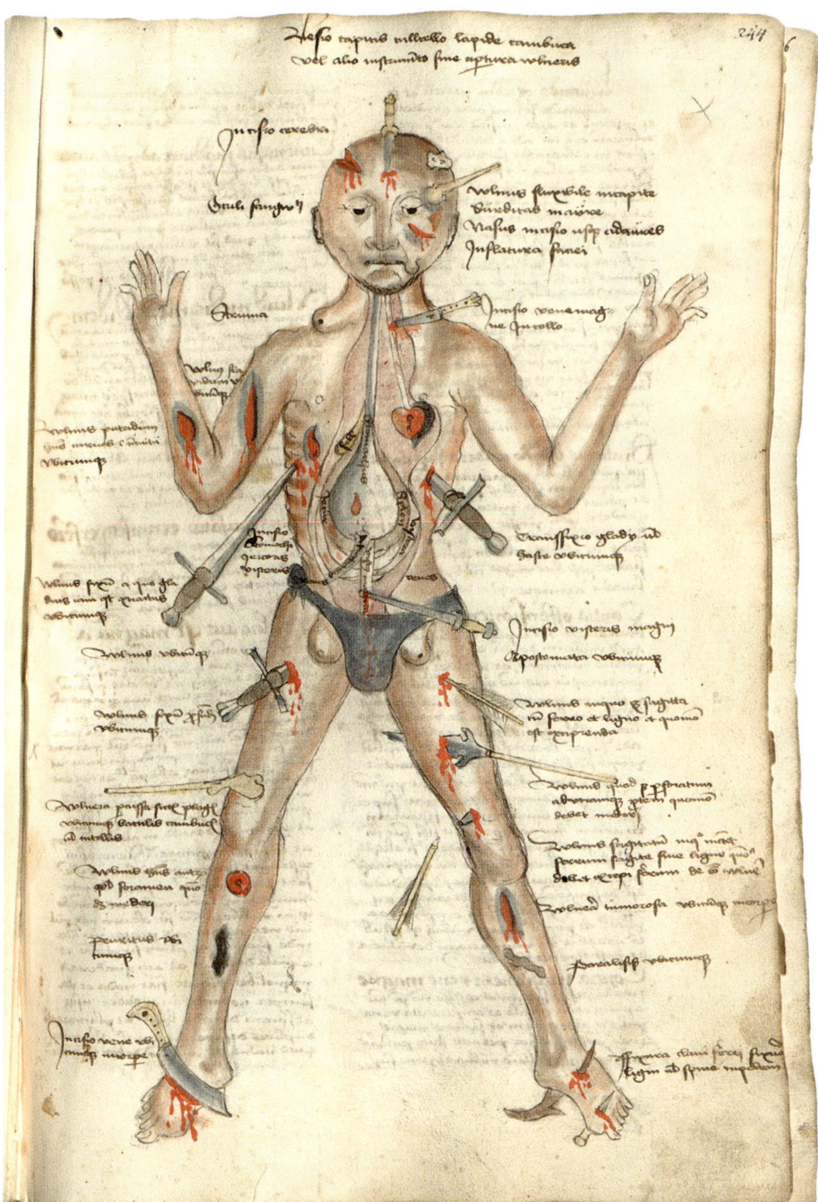

Fig. 2.13. Wound Man, c. 1485, possibly Regensburg. Ink and paint on paper, 31 x 20 cm. Munich, Bayerische Staatsbibliothek, Cgm 597, fol. 244r.

Lower down, his torso and legs sustain even more drastic damage. Four swords draw feathery streams of blood as they perforate his chest, flank, stomach, and thigh, the lowest entering almost to the hilt; a long ranseur has run him through, lancing him with convincing three-dimensionality; and a pair of arrows enter the same leg, one lodged whole between calf and shin and another piercing his thigh, its shaft snapped from the arrowhead.[74] The artist has clearly taken care over these embedded weapons, all delicately illustrated with shaded blades and decorated handles.

Meanwhile, subtle evidence also remains of a different class of injuries, still fresh. Smaller but no less serious, these are markers of more everyday accident. Generalized anonymous wounds pervade the body, a collection of large, bleeding, almond-shaped gashes given depth with further washes of black and gray. Blades slice at the figure's neck and feet, their decorated forms and bolted handles intimating typical kitchen and table knives, perhaps the result of some sort of domestic affray. And two injuries to his left foot seem more unintentional: the sole is pierced with a long, pointed thorn, while an iron nail punctures the foot near the toe, both the result of unfortunate missteps.

Lastly, a third and even subtler patina of injury haunts the Wound Man, indicative of more hidden forms of sickness. Rather than animated by protruding swords or splinters, this is a layer conveyed in worrying, murky marks outside and in. At his left shin, a red circle represents an itchy scab and swelling; a darkened bump to the side of his shaded upper lip indicates a boil; and the figure's neck and groin sport mounds spotted with a pimple-like point, suggestive of abscesses, goiters, or plague buboes. In the same manner as the Disease Woman, between chin and pubis the Wound Man's body switches modes, the naturalism of amassed objects and external features giving way to a schematic outline of his innards. Yet even when granted this unusual view into his transparent torso, we see that all is not well. His major organs—heart, lungs, stomach, gallbladder, and liver—are scarred with light-red blotches.

Importantly, this *Dreibilderserie* Wound Man is not harassed by objects of injury alone. Just as threatening as his accumulated weapons and wounds are the words buzzing around him in all directions. These short phrases serve to both highlight and individuate particular details of the injuries depicted. Some are simple, noting little more than what is shown: "*Incisio cerebri*" (A cut to the brain), "*Oculi sanguinolenti*" (Bloodshot eyes), "*Struma*" (A scrofulous tumor), "*Inflatura faciei*" (Swelling of the face), and so on. Others, by contrast, project a more complicated, abstract, and almost narrative sense of injury or accident:

> *Volnus in quo est sagitta cum ferro et ligno.*
> Wound in which there is an arrow with iron and wood.
>
> *Transfixio gladii vel haste ubicunque.*
> Stabbing by a sword or spear anywhere.
>
> *Volnera tumorosa ubicunque in corpore.*
> Swollen wounds anywhere on the body.

Given the *Dreibilderserie*'s intellectual and curative makeup, it comes as no surprise that these floating phrases formalize connections between the Wound Man's visualized body and the manuscript's textual contents. As with the maladies of both Disease Man and Disease Woman, these topographical captions function as catchwords that link to a longer piece of writing on wound healing that always either preceded or, in most cases, followed the Wound Man. But unlike his *Dreibilderserie* fellows, this text is more consistent than the series' assorted writings on humoral disease or gynecology, a succinct treatise known to modern historians as the *Wundarznei*, or Surgery.[75]

Most likely first compiled around 1400, the *Wundarznei*'s Latin text directly addresses the Wound Man's catalog of trauma injuries, wounds, and other surface issues such as animal bites, rashes, and abscesses, all concerns we would typically associate with the remit of a late medieval surgeon. In the Regensburg manuscript, the text begins on the other side of the same folio as its colorful Wound Man, and from its opening lines it adopts a directness that rarely lets up:

> *Aliquando enim cerebrum penetratur, et aliquando solum cutis offenditur et inflatur cerebrum vulneratum et inficitur. Modo si cerebrum vulneratum erit, tunc videri bene debet, ne ossa essent in vulnere . . .*
>
> Sometimes the brain is penetrated and sometimes only the skin is damaged and the brain becomes swollen and infected. Provided that the brain is wounded, care must be taken that no bone is in the wound . . .

Considering the breadth of medical interventions it covers across only roughly forty-four paragraphs, this familiar yet unrelenting tone feels justified. We read of pierced entrails and broken necks, bloodshot eyes and swollen lips, decaying flesh and arrow wounds, spider bites, stomach cramps, pimples, warts, rheumatism, and much more.[76] Each of these cures is generally granted its own paragraph within the *Wundarznei*, and their explication follows a similar formula. Initially, the issue at hand is named and introduced, using either the "Against . . ." phrasing—"*Contra incisionem cerebri*" (Against a cut to the brain), "*Contra tumorem et ulcerosa labia*" (Against swelling and ulcerous lips)—or by outlining a scenario of serious urgency, such as an animal attack or a patient falling from a height. Thereafter, the text turns to a brief set of practical procedures for treating the problem, for instance, directions on how to clean and stitch a wound or for making up compound medicines for application or ingestion. Entries are typically rounded out by a brief comment on aftercare, either recommending that the patient be monitored for specific signs or that certain prescriptions be repeated at particular times. Many also close with the casual assurance that a certain salve is particularly effective, that a rash will soon abate, or that a patient will no doubt return to good health.

As a historical document in its own right, the *Wundarznei* provides perhaps the best evidence for contextualizing the socio-medical background of the *Dreibilderserie* Wound Man by firmly associating it with the lands triangulated between what we would today call southeastern Germany, southwestern Poland, and Czechia. The inclusion of many botanical plants with Germanic names, as well as regular use of the adjective *bohemice* (Bohemian), suggests a specifically Bavarian or Czech origin for the text, a fact confirmed by the few scant details we do have of these manuscripts' provenance: one was probably written in Silesia, and two others circulated in Regensburg by at least the early sixteenth century.[77] Close analyses by Gundolf Keil and, more recently, by Erltraud Auer and Bernhard Schnell have also shown the treatise's significant debt to an earlier German medical work, the widely distributed *Arzneibuch* (Book of Surgery) of the Würzburg author Ortolf von Baierland, probably written at some point in the 1290s.[78] Ortolf's particular skill in crafting his *Arzneibuch*, an expansive German-language encyclopedia, was to synthesize into the vernacular multiple learned Latin sources—al-Rāzī, Isaac Judaeus, Gilles de Corbeil, Gilbertus Anglicus, the Hippocratic Aphorisms—to form a book of seven parts ordered by area of interest: general medical principles, uroscopy, pulse diagnosis, Hippocratic medicine, bloodletting, disease from head to toe, and wound treatment. Such was the popularity of this seminal work that it became the most copied vernacular medical text of the German Middle Ages, surviving as a complete treatise in over sixty manuscripts and as a cluster of fragmentary parts in more than one hundred books.[79] The *Wundarznei* can, in some senses, be considered among these partial copies, as it borrows either indirectly or directly from at least seventeen chapters of the *Arzneibuch*'s final section on wound surgery.[80]

As well as shortening Ortolf's detailed formulations, simplifying his theoretical content, and often breaking ideas down into multiple smaller entries, the author of the *Wundarznei* also made the intriguing and unusual decision to de-vernacularize the text, moving away from the *Arzneibuch*'s original German to write in Latin. Why precisely this linguistic shift was enacted is unclear. It seems at least somewhat likely that the Latin language was believed to offer a form of aggrandizing authority to this new text. Were the work a product of the newly founded University of Prague—as has been suggested for the entire *Dreibilderserie* corpus—then this would make particular sense, especially as the *Wundarznei* author removes all of the *Arzneibuch*'s regular references to previous learned masters and instead focuses attention squarely on their own command of the materials. Or perhaps, more straightforwardly, Latin simply provided consistency between the *Wundarznei* and the writings marshaled by the Disease Man and Disease Woman, lending textual coherence to *Dreibilderserie* books as a whole. Whatever the reason, linguistic innovation exists in these manuscripts well beyond Latin. One *Dreibilderserie* book wedges a recipe in Old Czech into its Latin *Wundarznei* prescriptions, suggesting a scribe at ease with both languages, while another is written entirely in Czech—complete with a "curable-incurable" proto-Wound Man—and a third from around 1420 includes a *Wundarznei* written in Mittelhochdeutsch.[81] As Gundolf Keil notes, this latter example is a rare case of yoyo-ing medical re-vernacularization, the *Wundarznei*'s Latin translated back into the original German of its *Arzneibuch* source to create a particularly chatty Thuringian version of the text.[82]

Questions of language inevitably spill over into questions of authorship and use, and here the *Wundarznei* again helps shed useful light on the Wound Man's context. In both the regimented structure of its Latin original and the German edition's familiarity of tone, the text brings to mind the emergent fifteenth-century genre of the "How-To" Book, practical treatises designed for professionals in which expertise dwelled not just in the author's reading or thinking but in their doing.[83] The *Wundarznei*'s author refers to their own firsthand experience regularly. We are told often that a remedy can be trusted because it is *probatum* or *vorsucht ist*—meaning that it has been tested by the author—while elsewhere advice on recipe-making or the surgical craft is clearly informed by the author's own professional history. The opening of the Thuringian example begins with an entry detailing several concoctions for killing flies, which feels rather a contrary starting point for a surgical treatise until we consider that this is likely less reflective of general worries about bugs than a concern for cleaning a room of potential pests before treatment. Elsewhere, the author's advice cautions the reader to "watch out for" particular signs in the patient, that certain wounds are particularly "hard to heal," and that certain salves are "particularly extraordinary." A cure for penetrative lacerations even emphasizes elements of good bedside manner, making clear the author's familiarity with typical patient behavior:

> *Wo einer durch stochen wirt mit einem swerte oder spise Deme gib warmen win oder bier mit veistikeit von einer slange zetrincken daz er is nyt wisse daz em dor ab nyt grwße wen wuste er is er trunck sin nicht.*
>
> When a man has been stuck with a sword or spear, give him warm wine or beer to drink with snake fat in it. But don't let him know it, or he'll be horrified. If he knew it, he wouldn't drink it.

We might further contextualize the *Wundarznei* author's practical milieu through connections made throughout to parallel professions in the vicinity of surgery, especially those associated with making books. One entry recommends packing a wound that will not stop bleeding with "*abegeschabte perment daz die permenter abschaben*" (parchment shavings that parchment-makers shave). Another, in the original Latin, refers to *concham*, a type of shell "*in qua colores illuminantium libros reservantur*" (in which the colors for illuminating books are kept).

As for the Wound Man-*Wundarznei* ensemble's specific readership, evidence is harder to come by. Repeated mention in the text of instructions simply to "sew up" wounds or "let blood" from named veins seems to take for granted a reader with basic skills in surgical practice. Yet when compared with other more extensive or learned surgical writings of the period, contemporary expert terminology is in fact largely absent, by contrast suggesting a less experienced user. Only a single mention is made of a specialist surgical instrument—a "falcon," used for extracting arrows—and the bragging, commercialized tendency of contemporary surgical authors to recall successful treatments of particularly well-connected persons is entirely elided.[84] Instead, the direct, easy language of the project feels tailored more toward a capable, literate nonspecialist. Such a reader could have been drawn from the same upper-class urban elites or broad civic audiences that owned contemporary treatises containing bloodletting figures of the sort discussed in the previous chapter. Or these books could also have been catering to more religious audiences whose concern for healing knowledge is well documented, with at least two surviving examples linked to monastic institutions.[85] Evidence of artistic quality only further suggests that the ensemble engaged a

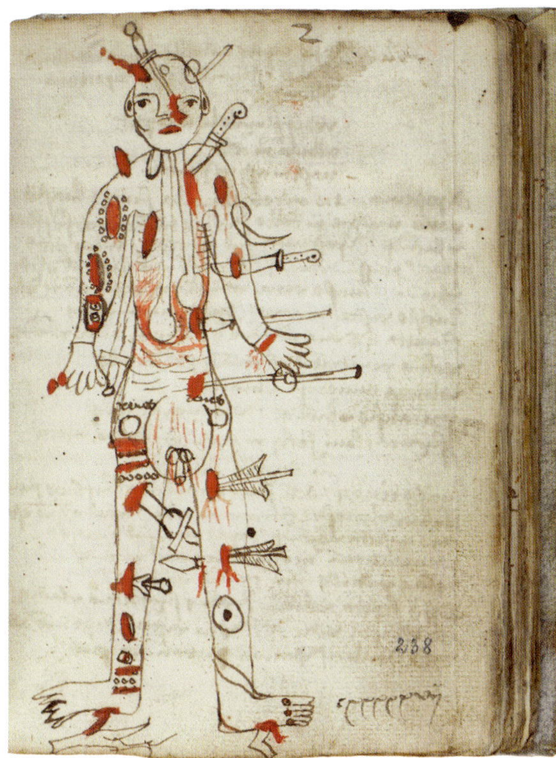

Fig. 2.14. Wound Man, c. 1477–83, Bavaria. Ink on paper, 15 x 10 cm. Solothurn, Zentralbibliothek, Cod. S 474, fol. 238r.

broad spectrum of readers, ranging as they do from luxuriously penned and illustrated editions down to examples such as a Bavarian manuscript now in Solothurn, complete with a hasty, much-abbreviated *Wundarznei* and charmingly scrappy Wound Man (fig. 2.14).[86]

Despite these cloudy specifics, we can still glean certain further concrete detail from the *Wundarznei*'s contents themselves. It is clear, for example, that its author should be considered as much an apothecary as a surgeon. Several surviving *Dreibilderserie* books run seamlessly from Wound Man to *Wundarznei* through to another text, a short *Antidotar* or pharmacopeia listing around fifty recipes to aid in curing the figure's various ills.[87] Among copious concoctions, we read of syrups that help with wound healing, ointments to combat paralysis, salves for burns or improving gums, and one cure for gout ambitiously titled *Gratia Dei* (The grace of God). Yet even if we restrict ourselves to the forty-four entries of the *Wundarznei* alone, we find over one hundred individual ingredients mentioned by name. Again, to the modern reader, certain of these trigger something of a category disturbance. We do not expect to find cat's dung applied to remove a splinter or to be told that applying crushed Spanish fly beetles improves the quality of one's fingernails. But setting the medical efficacy of these cures against twenty-first-century scientific criteria is far less relevant than the clear fact that they were thought impressive enough at the time to record and pass on.

Even more important are the resource networks that these ingredients animate. Many recipes use as their base the ordinary contents of an everyday larder—honey, oils, vinegar, salt, wine—supplemented by the produce of a kitchen garden, such as celery, chicory, onion, cabbage, quince, horseradish, and pumpkin.[88] Animal products, especially egg white and milk, are also often called for, and no inhabitant of the farmyard is spared for its grease, including geese, oxen, goats, rams, and sheep. These are complemented by products from nondomesticated fauna—mussel shells, stag marrow, snake fat, beaver gall—as well as a wide range of cultured or foraged flora that together constitute the vast majority of ingredients listed. Ranging from aloes and yarrows to brassicas and rues, the roots and full plants of around fifty different species are mentioned in the *Wundarznei*'s recipes, to be used either fresh or dried. Many of them could have been cross-referenced with contemporary herbals for a reader interested in their individual healing qualities.[89] Another category of ingredient looks beyond forest and field to again suggest an audience for the Wound Man-*Wundarznei* that was closely connected to parallel artisanal networks. The mention of a pair of pre-prepared compound medicines—*apostolicon*, or "apostle's plaster" (a salve often made from wax, pitch, and vinegar), and *theriacum*, or theriac (an almost mythically efficacious panacea for which various recipes circulated)—implies that the reader would have either known how to make these or had easy access to a local apothecary where they might be purchased.[90]

In fact, for a healer working in southern Germany or Bohemia, these and several of the *Wundarznei*'s other ingredients may well have been imports of significant expense. Probably the most extensive recipe of the entire text is a salve recommended for trauma wounds in which the skin has not been broken but significant bruising and swelling have still been sustained. After mixing together fleawort, yarrow, zinc sulphate, sage, cinquefoil, and wintergreen, the herbs are then boiled with fat from a gelded pig and sweetened with two pounds of sugar, an ingredient that at this point in the fifteenth century would have either originated in European cane fields in Sicily, Cyprus, or western Spain or been imported from more distant Asian markets.[91] As if this expensive product were not enough, the final stage of the recipe calls for these sweetened herbs to be pressed into a paste alongside a quartet of even more far-flung ingredients: myrrh, frankincense, Arabian millet, and mastic.[92] Here, the *Wundarznei* is surely drawing on a common conflation of both exoticism and expense with medical efficaciousness, what Paul Freedman has called the nonexistent medieval boundary between wellness and luxury.[93]

In this and all its many rich material aspects, the *Wundarznei* confirms our building sense of the Wound Man as an image closely connected to multiple strands of medieval medical logic at once. Through its cornucopia of ingredients, this text interlaced the figure with paramedical traditions of apothecaryship, transforming the Wound Man into the locus of a heady international mix of *materia medica*. And at the same time, it distilled complex notions from contemporary medicine into a neatly synthesized and accessible form for communication to several potential communities of healers and artisans, drawing an array of intellectual sources and practical methods alike into the orbit of the Wound Man's body.

“Look to the Man”

If the *Wundarznei*’s curative specifics help us to contextualize the *Dreibilderserie* Wound Man, how precisely did the Wound Man in turn link back to the *Wundarznei*? It might be easy to assume that the figure simply acted as an empty table of contents, an image pointing ever outside itself and toward the substantial medical detail of its accompanying text. But the structural entanglements of Wound Man and cure are in fact far more sophisticated. This is the image’s crucial surgical armature, a matter not of mere signaling but of careful codependence with the written word.

The makers of *Dreibilderserie* manuscripts were themselves keen to emphasize that the Wound Man was more than just the *Wundarznei*’s index. We see this most clearly in a passage from the text that is often boldly underlined in surviving books. On the surface it seems to offer uncomplicated phlebotomical advice, informing the reader of different bloodletting points on the body that could encourage particular types of wound healing. At the end of this phlebotomical material, however, the *Wundarznei* changes tack by stating that the practitioner’s actions in their bloodletting should be governed not only by well-known phlebotomical techniques but also by a short poetic verse.[94] Mostly recorded in Latin—even in the German *Wundarznei*, where it is followed by a vernacular gloss—and in different manuscripts variously labeled *versum*, *versus*, or *metra*, it reads:

> *Hec sunt pensanda medico curare volenti:*
> *Ars, etas, virtus, regio, complexio, forma,*
> *Mos et sinthonia, commixtio, tempus et aer.*
>
> *Daz ist zo vil gesprochen: der arczt, der arczenne wil, der zal an sehen den menschen: noch kunste, noch dem alter, noch kraft, noch der stat, complexion vnd gestalt, noch sitten der gewonheit, noch zu gefelle des siechtvms, noch vormisschunge, noch der zitt, noch der lufft.*
>
> It is often said, the doctor who wants [to practice] medicine should look to the man: the art, the age, the strength, the region, complexion and form, their habits, the disease, the gender, time and air.[95]

On the one hand, this is a straightforward recitation of the so-called Classical “non-naturals,” climactic and lifestyle variables that had long been understood to affect the health of men and women, here expressed in language drawn from a widely circulated twelfth-century medical poem, the *Regimen sanitatis Salernitanum* (Salernitan Health Regime).[96] Yet on the other, the verse’s direct exhortation that the reader should “*an sehen den menschen*” (look to the man)—in Latin versions reference is made to “*homine*” (a man)—explicitly draws our attention to the male figure that this text was universally plotted alongside. The Wound Man himself becomes the man to whom we should look for guidance in giving good health, with the German *Wundarznei* on several occasions even going so far as to directly name its patient as “*der wunte man*” (the wounded man).

This is just one of many playful parallels between Wound Man and *Wundarznei* that we find at work in *Dreibilderserie* books. We see another, for instance, in the structure of the *Wundarznei*'s healing text. Its individuated paragraphs can themselves be read as something of an abstracted body, maintaining an anthropomorphic sequence that runs from cures of the head down to cures of the feet. Such corporeal topography was in part an import from contemporary medicine. The sixth chapter of Ortolf's *Arzneibuch*, which lists general cures for a variety of diseases, adopts the same head-to-toe formatting, as did many medical texts of the time that often proudly state their contents as being listed "*a capite ad calcem*" (from head to heel).[97] But we have also already seen in the previous chapter that the figuring of texts into bodies had a broader, rich heritage as a structural trope among nonmedical works circulating during the later Middle Ages, a scholarly preoccupation that relied on the creative interface of word and image. We might think back to the diagrammatic bodies of Hugh de Fouilloy, Alfonso X's *Libro*, and Thomasin von Zerclêre. Or indeed, we could look to any number of figurative literary products from across the medieval world that utilized similar head-to-toe formatting, from the Song of Solomon to Classical Arabic love poetry to the well-documented insistence by grammarian Geoffrey of Vinsauf in his thirteenth-century *Poetria nova* that ideal descriptions of visual beauty should follow a keen order: as he states, "*a summo capitis descendat splendor ad ipsam radicem*" (let the brightness descend from the top of the head to the very root).[98] By presenting the *Dreibilderserie* reader with an anthropomorphic list of medical cures laid out like a body, as well as the visualization of those same cures as an actual standing figure, the distinction between bodily texts and textual bodies was encouraged to blur.

Images of the Wound Man were themselves constructed with a keen awareness that the figure's graphic body could in turn inventively shape medical writing. This is the case in one of the aesthetically simpler Wound Men to survive from the fifteenth century, found in a Paris *Dreibilderserie* manuscript whose accompanying disease fellows we have already met (fig. 2.15). Sketched out in uncomplicated line and with only minimal shading and color to enunciate his wounds, the image is hardly a virtuoso work of draftsmanship. Yet compare the way that the text circulating around even this straightforward figure has been co-opted into its injurious scheme, a constructional blurring of body and words. Set against the same manuscript's Disease Man and Disease Woman, whose labeling falls in straightforward horizontal lines and regimented columns around them, this Wound Man's textual anchors instead zip to and fro at diagonal angles, deliberately mimicking the instruments that thrust painfully into his sides, even to the point of spinning 180 degrees around the figure, demanding that the disoriented viewer rotate their book in order to read them. It is the structural logic of the image that dominates here, rather than that of the text.

Meanwhile, in more complex Wound Men we get an even stronger sense of the figure's equal footing alongside the *Wundarznei* as an image inhabiting the role almost of a humanoid book. Take one unusually large Wound Man from a manuscript now in London's Wellcome Library (fig. 2.16). This is among the most impressive of all versions of the figure to survive, not only

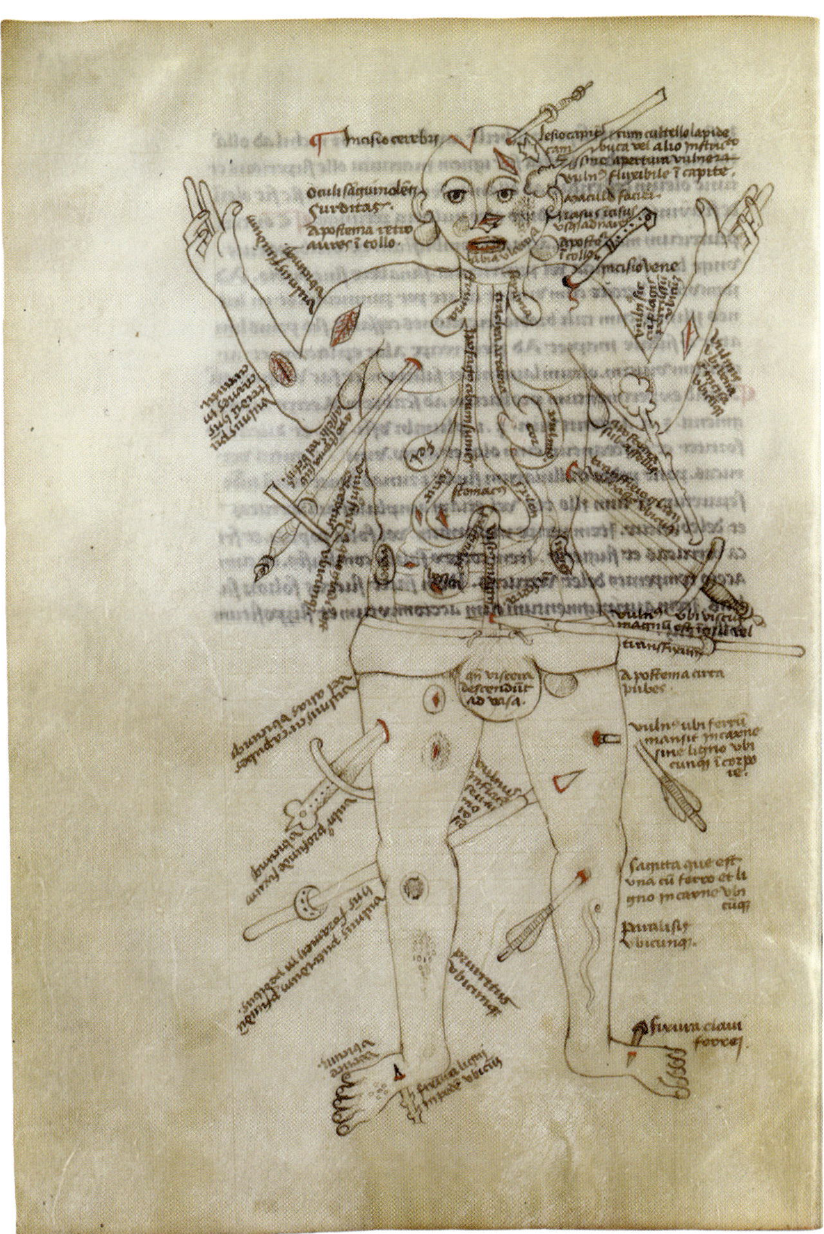

Fig. 2.15. Wound Man, after 1417, France. Ink on parchment, 20 x 14 cm. Paris, Bibliothèque nationale de France, MS Latin 11229, fol. 36v.

for the image's delicate artistry but also for its extremely elaborate detail. The sheer volume of imagery on display is impressive, from increasingly detailed weapons and wounds to a novel menagerie of animal agents, including among other foes a spider crawling up his thigh, a giant yellow bee poised to sting at his elbow, and a camouflaged miniature toad and snakelike worm at work amid his green entrails. Perhaps reflecting this host of fearful critters newly dotted about his body, the curative words surrounding this figure also perform their own type of novel abundance. Rather than chunks of text hovering in the rough vicinity of their respective injuries, each of the image's descriptive catchwords has been vastly reduced and itemized with a

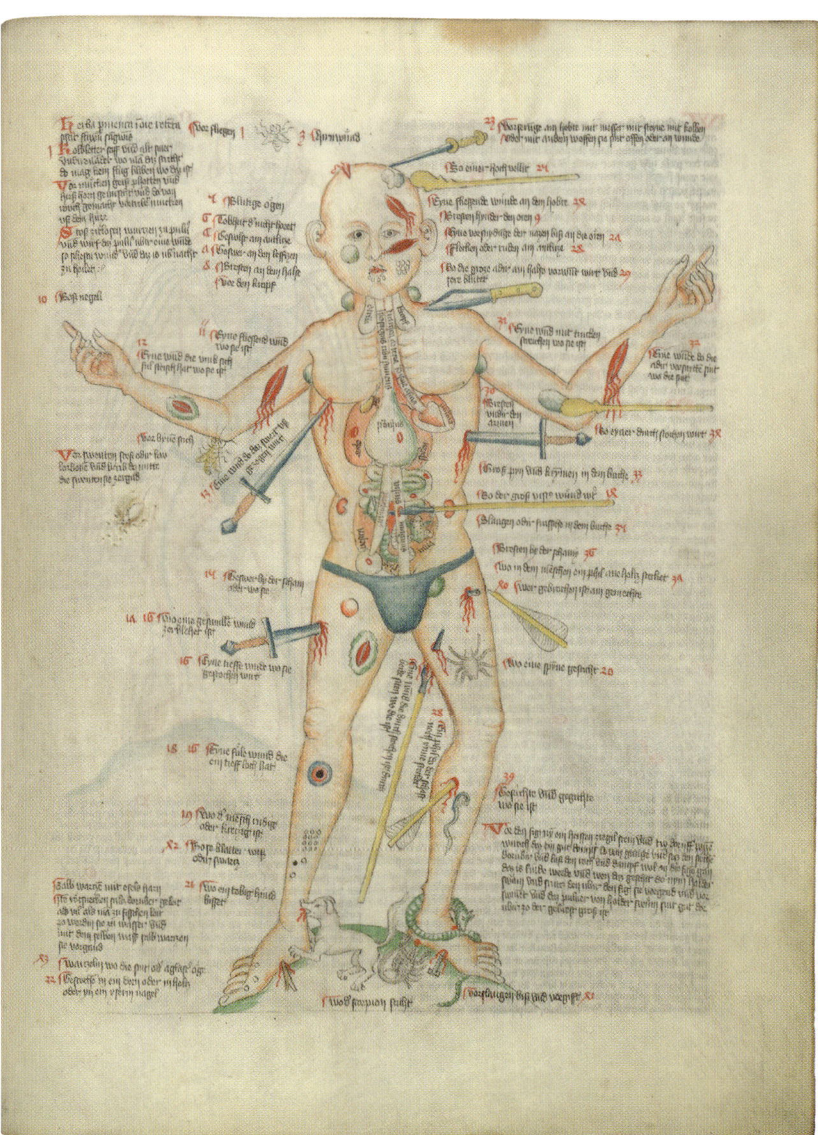

Fig. 2.16. Wound Man, c. 1420–30, possibly Thuringia. Ink and paint on parchment, 40 x 30 cm. London, Wellcome Library, MS 49, fol. 35r.

small red number, linking the Wound Man's debilitating visualizations with a numbered paragraph of the manuscript's *Wundarznei*, reproduced on the preceding folio, in which further elaborations of cures and procedures are to be found. For example, one legend written along the large spear piercing the figure's left side and penetrating into its stomach reads: "*So der gross viscus wund wirt 14*" (If the large intestine is injured 14). This directs the reader to the *Wundarznei*'s fourteenth item, which contains a recipe for the making and application of a styptic, an antihemorrhagic agent in the form of a red powder designed to staunch the bleeding of the wound in question:

> 14. *Item wirt der groze darm oder der magen oder gederme alzo saltu daz heilen. Du salt is zu nehen mit einem subtil fadem und salt doruf schutten rot puluer. Daz selb puluer ist zu allen wunden gut und daz beste. Daz mach alzo*

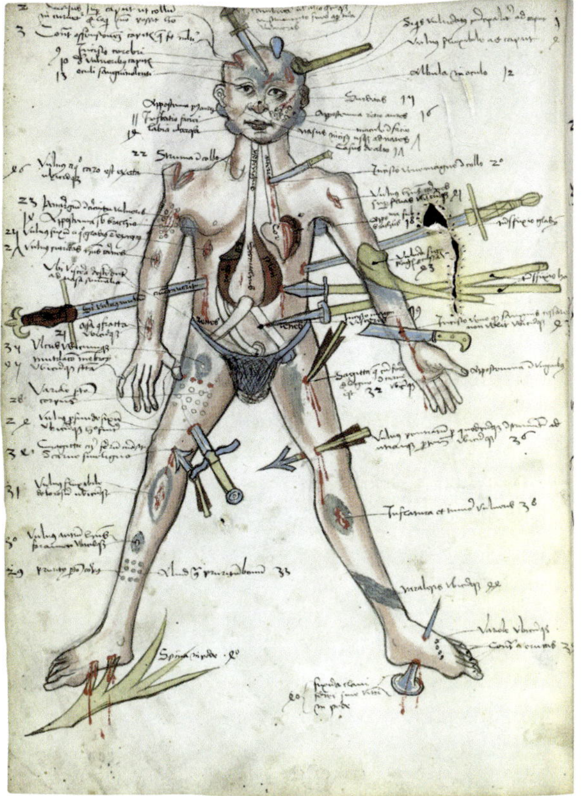

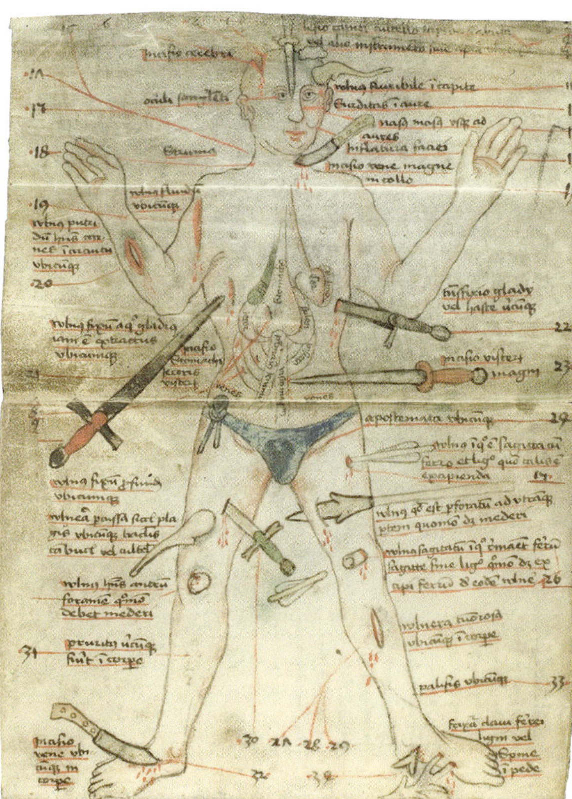

Fig. 2.17. Wound Men with number keys. *Left:* Wound Man, late 15th century, Germany. Ink and paint on paper, 29 x 20 cm. Vatican City, Biblioteca Apostolica Vaticana, MS Pal. Lat. 1325, fol. 360v. *Right:* Wound Man, c. 1450–70, southern Germany. Ink and paint on parchment, 20 x 15 cm (unfolded). Heidelberg, Universitätsbibliothek, Cpg 644, inserted as fol. 78.

Nym swartz win daz uf daz aller rotest si und blutstein i loth muscate und wiß wiroch itzlichs i lod Gummi arabicum iii lod sanguinem draconis und mumie itzlichs i loth Daz zerstoß aller zesammen und mach doruß puluer und behalt das ze notem.

14. Item: If the large intestine [is injured] or the stomach or the entrails, you can heal it thus. Sew it together with a fine thread and sprinkle red powder on it. The same powder is good for all wounds and is the best. It can be made thus. Take black wine that is the very reddest and 1 lot of hematite, 1 lot each of nutmeg and white frankincense, 3 lots of gum arabic, 1 lot each of *sanguinem draconis* [dragon's blood] and mummy. Pound that all together, make a powder out of it, and keep it as needed.

This numerated system not only entangles Wound Man and *Wundarznei* even more directly but also acknowledges the flexible relationship between the two. The placement of one catchphrase—"*Eyne fule wund die ein tieff loch hat*" (An infected wound that has a deep opening)—alongside two numbers, sixteen and eighteen, suggests that both passages might be useful as cures. As a counterpoint, two entries in the corresponding *Wundarznei* are both numbered forty-two, clarifying that either could be used to expedite the removal of the correspondingly numbered pimples that appear overleaf at the figure's shin. This same technique of numbering is used for many fifteenth-century *Dreibilderserie* Wound Men (fig. 2.17).[99] And although their specific details sometimes differ—some covering richly colored figures with webs of delicate black numbers, others opting for fat lines that unsubtly underline the figure's textual surrounds—the fact that such keys survive alongside so many examples confirms that contemporaries considered numeration a particularly valuable visual strategy for connecting wounds and words.[100]

In fact, so thoroughly texted are some surviving Wound Men that we even find substantial blocks of writing in their surrounds that do not defer to the *Wundarznei* at all. These are entirely unique paratextual elaborations containing wholly worked-out treatments to cure the maladies they sit beside, presented exclusively as part of the Wound Man's visualized form.[101] Such cures contain advice for warding off gnats and flies, recipes for pastes to remove tumors, and in one case a particularly long description of a procedure for removing warts:

> *Vor den figen nym ein heissen ziegil stein und tw doruff wizen wiroch daz ein gut dampf do von gange und setz den siechen dorubir und laß den roch und dampf wol an die figen gan daz is linde werde und wen daz geschit so nym halder swam und sturtz den ubir den figen sie vorgent und vorswinnet und daz puluer von holder swum sint gut dorubir zo der gebrest groß ist.*
>
> For warts take a hot brick and put white frankincense on it until a lot of steam comes off, and set the sick man over it and let the smoke and the steam cover the warts until they soften, and when that happens, take fungus from an elder tree and press it over the warts. They'll go away and disappear, and the powder from elder fungus is good if the blemish is large.[102]

While some of these additional chunks of healing text were appended to *Dreibilderserie* figures at their point of creation, others appear to have been added subsequently by later generations of healers. One Wound Man, currently in a private collection in London, is relatively plain in its design, the figure and his weapons rendered only in simple outline (fig. 2.18).[103] Perhaps this is why a later medieval user of the book felt comfortable covering his lower-left side with a block of text summarizing the figure's injuries, weapons, and illnesses, the Wound Man once more transformed into a body to be read.

An especially elaborate Wound Man surviving today in a manuscript in Copenhagen takes this imbrication of text and image to its logical extremes. The figure is exceptional even among his fantastically bruised and battered fifteenth-century fellows, appearing at the center of a single enormous sheet of parchment measuring seventy-five by fifty-five centimeters (fig. 2.19).[104] In some ways he remains typical of the series, his broken body presented unashamedly to us in a fixed stare, pierced by weapons and replete with accidental injuries and signs of illness. Several aesthetic details are particularly fine here. A gray wash enunciates his chin, indicating a weathered five-o'clock shadow. At his shoulder and to the side of his head, slices taken out of his body peel away, modeled in the same convincing three dimensions as his totally severed right thumb. And a deep wound in his arm affords us a view of a snapped radius, plotted out in dark ink beneath his skin. Even more

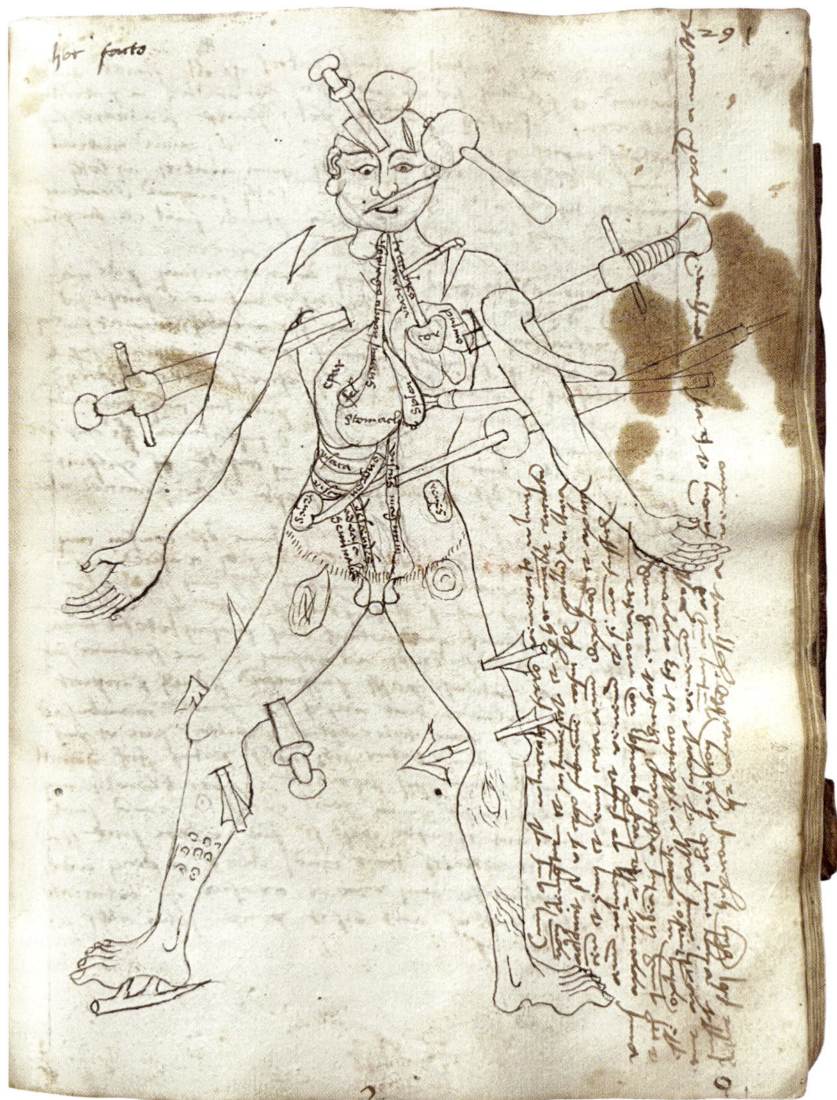

Fig. 2.18. Wound Man, late 15th century, Bohemia. Ink on paper, 21 x 15 cm. London, Sokol Books, no shelf mark ["Medicine"], fol. 291r.

extraordinary than the figure's detailing, though, is its overall setting on the page. Orbiting around this Wound Man is yet another novel presentation of the *Wundarznei*, here not reproduced overleaf as a continuous text or keyed with individual numbers but instead broken up into its constituent paragraphs, each of which appears inside one of forty-three red, compass-drawn circles. Evolving the figure's complex explanatory strategies once again, corresponding sections of curative text are linked to limbs and wounds, rashes and apostemes, by a chaotic network of thin red lines that surround the figure, weaving between bubbles to find their correspondent bodily spot. The result is manic and confusing, with lines that overlap so much that they appear to have even stumped the scribe or artist who plotted them, as evidenced by various corrections that linger on the page as blurry shadows. A later hand has tried to make sense of this discombobulated text by labeling several of the circles alphabetically from A to Z in a light pen, but it is not immediately

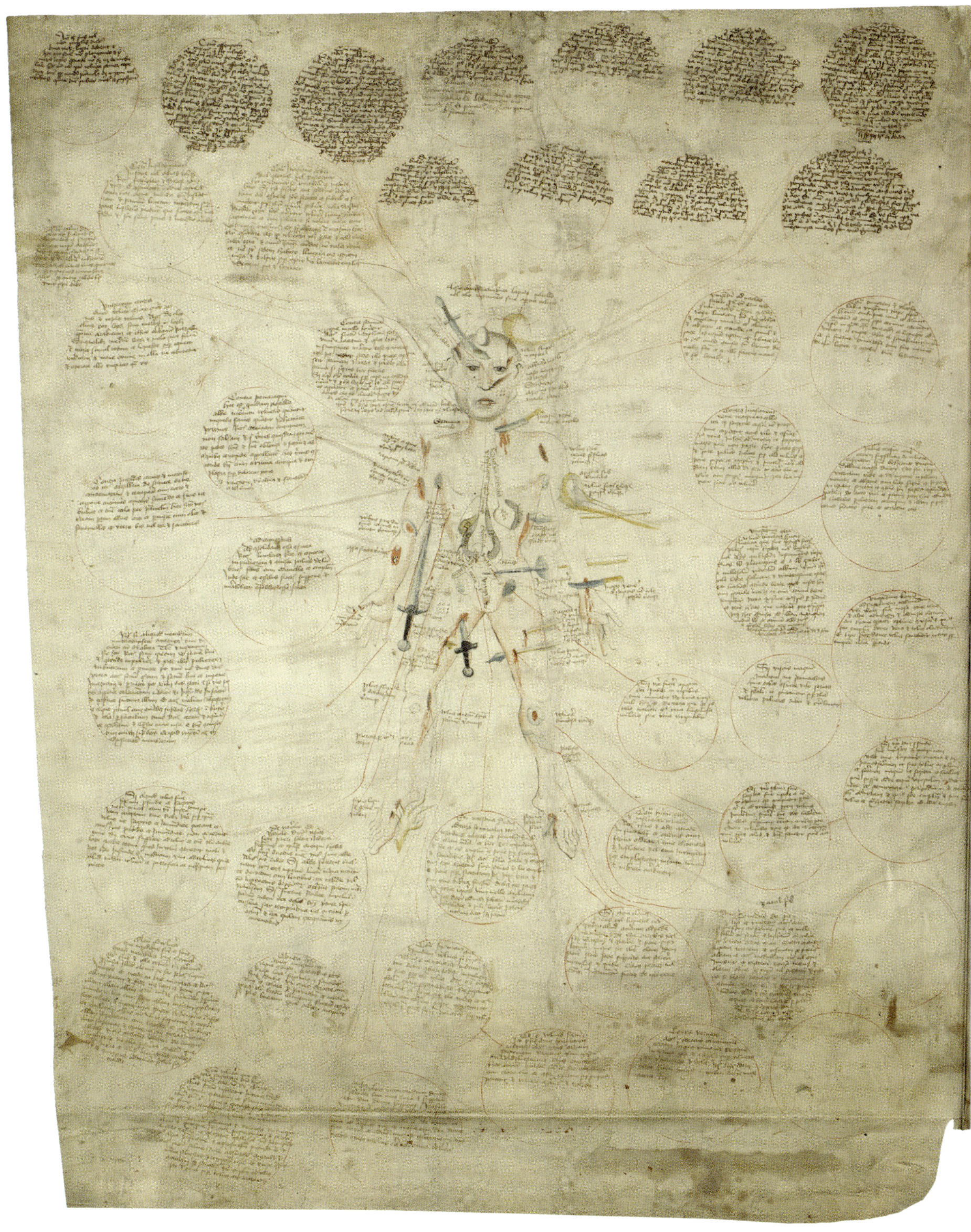

Fig. 2.19. Wound Man, 15th century, Germany. Ink on parchment, 75 x 55 cm. Copenhagen, Kongelige Bibliothek, NKS 84 b 2º, fol. 4v.

apparent what these letters might even correspond to. After all, it is precisely the point of this page that all relevant image and text elements are bound as one in the same space, with no outside referent necessary.

Better than any other *Dreibilderserie* Wound Man, this particularly inventive realization of the figure highlights the shift in diagnostic emphasis that the image was enacting across its entire fifteenth-century corpus. Elsewhere, medical imagery of this sort might easily have been underestimated as an aesthetic bonus, an illustration in the term's most passive sense. But the Copenhagen sheet shows how the Wound Man instead flipped this expected structure, beginning the process of cure not with text but firmly with image. It cannot be read any other way. If a reader tried to begin, say, at the bubble in the folio's upper-left corner, they would find themselves arriving at a cure *in medias res* with advice on aftercare: "*Nota quod prius vulnera singulis diebus bina vice debent ligari*" (Note that wounds first must be bandaged, with two changes every day). Which wounds? The cure actually commences in the bubble immediately to its right, joined to this leftmost circle by a thin red line. It is only by following another line that emerges from this rightmost bubble that we are able to make our way down to the visualization of the relevant wound at the figure's head, although not before speeding past yet another branch of cures for injuries to the brain that sprout off en route as another set of circles. By contrast, when we read from the image outward, this mass of lines and labels makes sense. They unfurl logically as the reader moves from a depicted head wound through to cures for the brain and then those for the skull, before turning finally to issues of postoperative care. The physical structure of the Wound Man's body, always promising to tip over into text, has here finally been fully transformed into a giant anthropomorphic treatise.

This ultimately is the unique nature of the Wound Man's curative mechanics. Emerging as part of the inventive *Dreibilderserie*, its original fifteenth-century iteration acted as a pool of surgical knowledge. On the one hand, it boldly gathered together in a single space an encyclopedic host of contemporary techniques for cutting, suturing, bandaging, administering, setting, and letting. But it also paired these instructions with a canny ability to draw on parallel innovations in visual diagnosis and diagrammatic aesthetics. Although at first appearing to be a pained and pitiless figure, one whose injuries threatened to overwhelm both their victim and the viewer, the Wound Man was in fact one of the period's most sophisticated visual repositories of medical hope, at once enunciating and embodying the many cures he marshaled for the fifteenth-century reader.

CHAPTER THREE

Affect: Wounds in the World

In April 1513, a few miles outside the Alsatian city of Hagenau, a knight named Albrecht von Berwangen was discovered dead. Albrecht had been appointed the previous year to the service of the local count, Philipp III von Hanau-Lichtenberg, but had quickly left amid claims that the nobleman had failed to pay his salary. After an appeal to Emperor Maximilian I, Philipp was compelled to offer the knight 100 guilders in compensation, and it was soon after that Albrecht's body was found in the forest not far from the monastery of Sankt Wolfgang, horribly mutilated.

We know of this affair from several surviving documents now in Heidelberg that record the legal proceedings instigated against Philipp by Albrecht's family through the Imperial Reichskammergericht in Speyer, introduced in a florid notary hand as the "*Endschuldigung unnd Verantwortung Grave philipsen von hanaw*" (Vindication and Justification of Count Philipp von Hanau).[1] Given the damaging financial claims in circulation, Count Philipp was seen as the prime suspect in the murder, and he was called to appear before a Hagenau court. In his testimony, also glossed in the documents, Philipp freely admitted to killing Albrecht, but claimed that he had done so in self-defense after the embittered knight jumped him in the woods. This explanation, however, was deemed unconvincing by prosecutors, at least in part on account of the desecrated state of Albrecht's corpse, whose wounds went far beyond those of an even-handed affray. Found guilty, the count was required to pay an even greater rate of compensation to the family, although he only deigned to do this two years later, in 1515.

Unusually, maybe even uniquely for legal documentation of the time, the pivotal evidence of Albrecht's body was also incorporated into the case's records. It survives in the form of a colorful ink drawing on a single paper sheet, folded into four (fig. 3.1). Lying supine on the ground, the knight is shown dead and violently mistreated. He has been stripped of all his clothes, apart from some white underbriefs and a pair of riding trousers humiliatingly pulled down to his knees. His skin reveals a catalog of heavy bruises and bleeding gashes, while an array of bloody murder weapons lie around him on the floor.

The similarity of the pictured Albrecht to the Wound Man's fantastically injured form gives us pause for thought. By this point in the early sixteenth century, the surgical figure had been in use in the region for over a century, and Albrecht's bleeding wounds, the menacing weapons, and even his similarly styled underpants are at least close enough to suggest that the Hagenau artist—clearly an accomplished painter, presumably well versed in a range of contemporary images—might have been deliberately evoking the Wound Man's well-known woes in their depiction of the stricken knight. More compelling than the visual similarities between the two figures, though, is a key difference. Whereas the wide-eyed Wound Man's weapons always remain lodged in his skin, signaling injuries received recently enough that some hope still remains for speedy intervention and recovery, those surrounding the definably dead Albrecht have been used by attackers long since gone. They are gathered for us in a bloodied pile, as if collected by authorities arriving too late on the scene. This distinction is a pivotal part of the Hagenau image's evidentiary function as a piece of visual legal testimony. The depicted weapons and wounds quantify the knight's suffering, logging the specific cuts and blows that Albrecht sustained during the encounter, each one an individualized affidavit that may have compelled the Hagenau court in its judgment against the count. And at the same time, these forensic details aim to communicate a certain fundamental truth of the event. They argue Albrecht's case: with his sword still sheathed in his right hand, the knight is identified as a victim rather than an aggressor. Taking on the role of important signifiers, these weapons work in consort with the accompanying written account of the trial to convey crucial information about the dead knight, who he was, and what happened to him.

The testimonial qualities of Albrecht's injuries attend to a pressing problem particular to reading occurrences of premodern violence, what the historian Valentin Groebner has called the trap of the *Ungestalt*, literally a deformation or facelessness.[2] Groebner's term specifically describes the flattening tendency often unthinkingly adopted in response to violent images from the historical past, wherein their affective extremes—extreme pain, extreme gore, extreme emotion—can all too easily end up short-circuiting the gap between medieval and modern. Viewed through this ahistorical lens, Groebner argues, such violent images are regularly reduced to generically unnerving things in a manner that anonymizes sufferers and perpetrators alike. Violence itself becomes the subject of the image, rather than the particular bodies that bear it. Unlike with Albrecht, whose corpse is instantly contextualized through name and narrative, the *Ungestalt* presents a real problem in the case of the Wound Man. Already abstracted through the universalizing language of the late medieval diagram, the overwhelming violence on display in the figure draws our focus still further. Hit with its heady technical concoction of potential injury, we never quite stop to ask an obvious yet crucial question: Who actually is this poor soul? And how did he come by such hurt?

To find an answer, we must place the Wound Man back into the broader late medieval and early modern visual ecosystems in which he was conceived. In the previous chapter, we uncovered the surgical potential of the figure, exploring the Wound Man's accompanying *Wundarznei* text to unpack

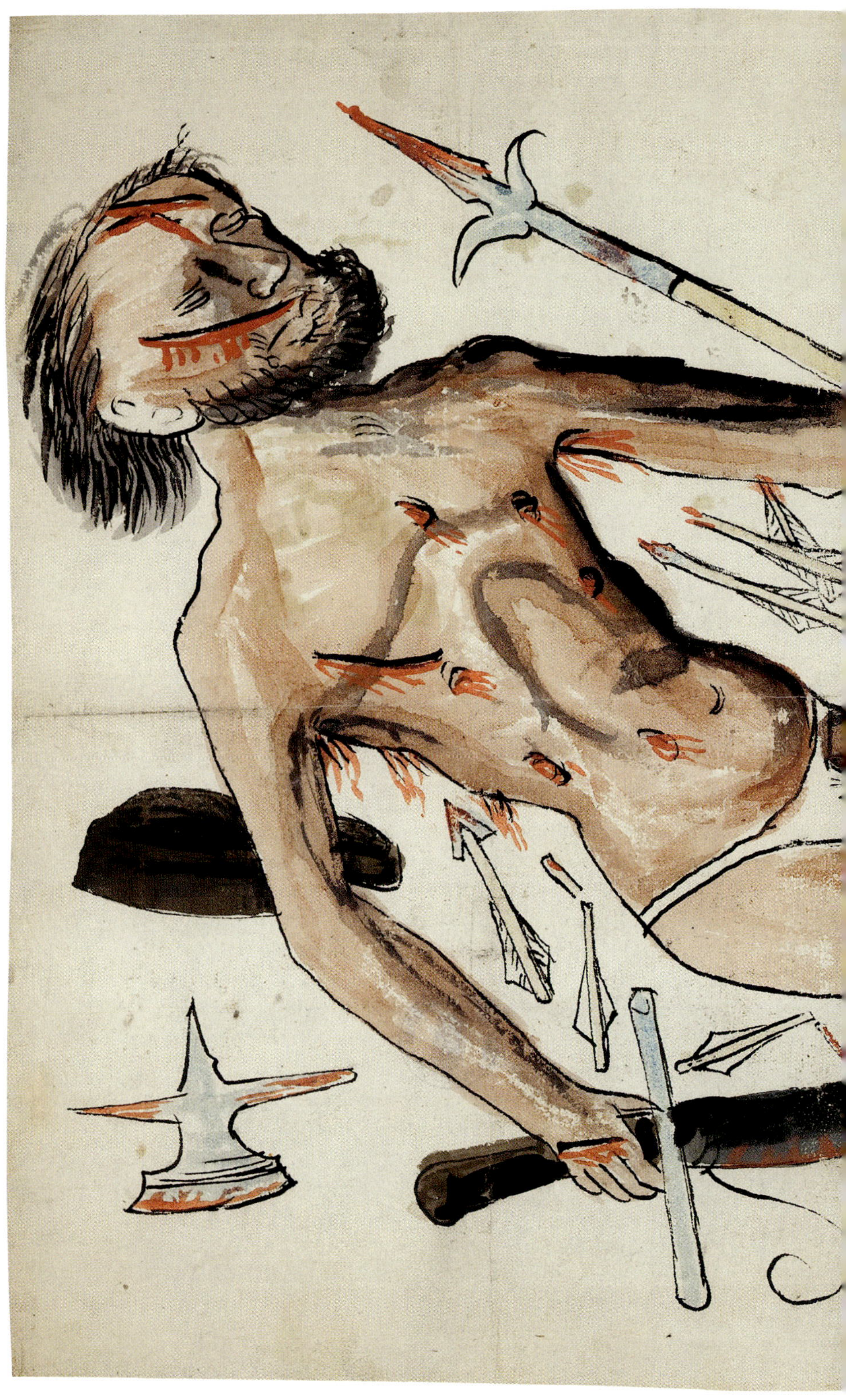

Fig. 3.1. Albrecht von Berwangen discovered dead, 1513, Hagenau. Ink and paint on paper, 33 x 43 cm. Heidelberg, Universitätsbibliothek, Urk. Lehmann 186, fol. supplement 2r.

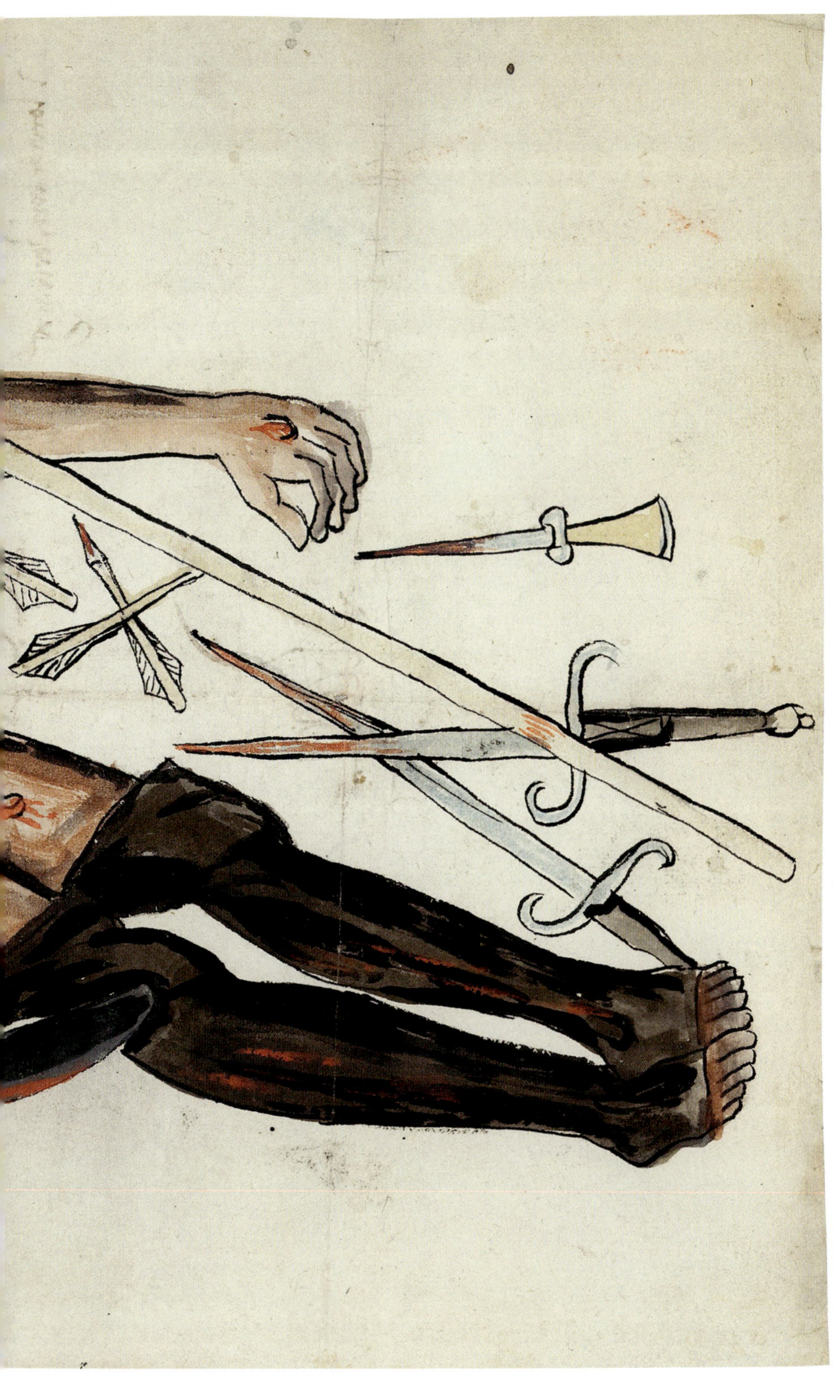

its healing capacities as a medical aid. Yet these medical materials offer us few clues as to the image's more affective valences. By contrast, and as the evidence of Albrecht's body makes only too clear, other corners of contemporary literary and visual culture were full of violent symbolism that makers and readers alike would have brought to the pages of the *Dreibilderserie* books that the Wound Man inhabited. In particular, a range of works from the figure's fifteenth-century homelands of Germany and Bohemia—including epic, spiritual, civic, and superstitious texts—all repeatedly played host to a diverse spectrum of wounded male bodies, the sheer breadth of which opens up a number of new avenues for deepening our understanding of the Wound Man's own form. This chapter looks to forge new connections between the surgical figure and a vibrant range of nonmedical discourses, crafting the beginnings of a wider cultural identity for the Wound Man. Tracing such broad correspondences is inevitably, in part, a speculative history: it foregrounds what viewers might have known rather than what we are certain they saw. Yet in the case of the Wound Man, the value of such readings is firmly concrete. Not only does this contextual material tell us more about what the figure may have meant to contemporary viewers beyond medicine—and what motivated them to replicate the image from the late fourteenth century all the way through to Albrecht von Berwangen's day and beyond—but it also makes clear that the period's ideas of emotion and personhood, of affect and identity, were not distinct from issues of cure. Ultimately, we shall discover that knowing who the Wound Man was in turn helped enhance his healing work.

Written Woundscapes

By the time the family of Albrecht von Berwangen brought successful proceedings against Count Philipp, a powerful secular woundscape had been firmly established across various genres of European literature. From the technical measurements of hardheaded recordkeeping to more symbolic evocations in the narratives of epic prose, the wounded male body was a trope to which medieval and early modern writers regularly returned, and which across its breadth resonates strikingly with the figure of the Wound Man.

Albrecht's own case can itself be seen as part of one branch of this tradition, the culmination of centuries-long developments in legal literature associated with compensation for wounds and wounding. As early as the sixth century, we find enacted across many European societies the enforceable idea that an injured person was entitled to receive proportional restitution for being wounded. This *wergelt* (literally, man-money), as it was normally termed in German-speaking lands, was to take into account both the specifics of the damage done and, more complicatedly, the original capacities and merits of the victim before injury. The result was most often a series of published tariffs, which were particularly extensive in German contexts throughout the medieval and early modern periods. In his examination of Old Frisian tariffs—laws that concretized around the thirteenth century in what is now northern Germany and the Netherlands—Han Nijdam has suggested two principal ways in which wounds were legally conceived in such texts, both of which shed intriguing light on contemporary standards of bodily worth and processes of violence.[3] First, it was acknowledged that different parts of the body required compensation at different levels, an initial quantitative side to the legalese of wounding. The Old Frisian tariffs individuate over 150 bodily locations for injury, running in the same manner as contemporary medical treatises downward from *kop* (head) to *tane* (toe), taking in everything along the way, from the *aghild* (eyelid) and *kanep* (mustache) to the *benete burch* (uterus) and the *knibeltride* (kneecap). Second, in wound law's more qualitative aspect, the specific execution of the injury and its relation to the victim's prior standards of living were also considered. Toward the end of the Middle Ages this evaluation was made by official wound assessors, mostly surgeons, who were dispatched by local authorities and charged with taking context into account to help determine final compensation: they considered, for example, whether the injury was committed in the victim's home, how easy an injury would be to conceal from others, whether a professional would be required to heal the wound, and the degree to which the wound would have a lasting effect on the function of the victim's senses.[4]

The level of detail found in these laws is striking, suggesting a vast array of injuries that civic authorities were familiar with litigating against. Many marry closely with those depicted on the Wound Man's form. For the club injury to his head he would have received a rate of roughly sixteen pennies per inch along the length of the scar, while other open wounds, such as that at his stomach, would have been compensated at eight shillings for the whole, both fines being amplified significantly if the scars healed poorly or became infected.[5] Moreover, by the fourteenth and fifteenth centuries, such wound laws had formalized both financial compensation for injury and, in some cases, a more retaliatory form of punishment, known as *Körperverletzung* (body wounding), which decreed that a guilty individual should themselves be scarred, bruised, bloodied, or otherwise mutilated in direct accordance with their initial crimes, wounding becoming the currency of both perpetrators and victims.[6] Given how widespread this culture of bodily compensation was in German-speaking lands, we can imagine viewers coming across the image of the Wound Man with a sense of legal fright, both for the significant financial compensation he represented and the potential bill of bodily retribution due to whomever had enacted his multiple injuries.

Built into even this most technical and legislative of Germanic wound literature, however, was the fundamental acknowledgment that sustaining violent injury could quickly move beyond the physical ramifications of the body and into more affective territory. As well as *tar* (tears), *lappa* (cut flesh), and *mutha* (wound openings), the Old Frisian tariffs sought to quantify the emotional qualities of wounds, speaking of injured *mod* (feelings), *hast* (anger), and wounds of the *sele* (soul). In a sense, understanding wounds as simultaneously corporeal and heartfelt phenomena followed the teachings of prominent medieval philosophers and theologians, including such esteemed names as Albertus Magnus and Thomas Aquinas, both of whom echoed Aristotle in seeing violence and emotion as inextricably intertwined. True courage, they argued, was both intellectually and physiologically predetermined to realize itself only in genuine moments of violent peril, most notably during extreme personal sickness or in times of war. In the words of a 1435 German translation of Giles of Rome's *De regimine principum* (On the Government of Princes), another Aristotelian offshoot, "*die gewalt irczeigit den man*" (violence reveals the man).[7]

Violence, then, was central to emotional injury, an idea further confirmed by the substantial repertoire of emotionally fraught wound narratives found across parallel spheres of contemporary literature. From the twelfth-century epics of Wolfram von Eschenbach and Gottfried von Straßburg to the fifteenth-century poetry of Oswald von Wolkenstein and the prose of Johannes von Tepl, German-language writing contemporary to the Wound Man was laced with figures made and unmade through particularly brutal means.[8] The texture of this literary violence changed significantly, of course, between different genres and different locales, as well as depending on when across the broad period we look. Nonetheless, key throughout was what Guy Halsall has called violence's "legitimacy": a stark emotional contrast drawn by writers between sanctioned violence, justifiable through legal frameworks like wound tariffs or more chivalric codes of honor, and unsanctioned violence, undertaken by illegitimate actors and expressed in Mittelhochdeutsch through terms like *unmaze*, which suggests a lack of measure or moderation, and *unrehte*, a fundamental unjustness.[9] Freighted with these foundations of just and unjust cause, literal wounds inevitably came to parallel the plight of deeper-set emotional trauma in German romance literature, including festering heartbreak, unsated sexual desire, punishment for social transgression, and revenge.

The specifics of this literary wound symbolism must surely have had some impact on contemporary impressions of the surgical figure, both in a technical and affective sense.[10] For one thing, just as with medieval German wound tariffs, a whole host of the Wound Man's cataloged complaints find popularized precedent within a contemporary courtly literature of violence. The *Wundarznei*'s paragraph 40, for instance, which offers aid to patients whose "*gederme uß gad und gebrochen ist*" (entrails are escaping and ruptured), would have been of particular use to the fated knight Vivianz in the renowned south German author Wolfram von Eschenbach's thirteenth-century epic poem *Willehalm*.[11] Run through with a spear during a tournament joust, Vivianz's stomach is horribly lacerated, but the brave knight battles on regardless, as explained in a particularly graphic stanza:

... daz geweide
uz der tyost ober den sadil hieng.
der helt di banir du gevieng
und gurte daz geweide wider in,
alle ob ime nirgen sin
van dikeyme strite swere:
der iunge lobis bere
vorbaz hurte in den strit.

... his entrails
from the joust hung over the saddle.

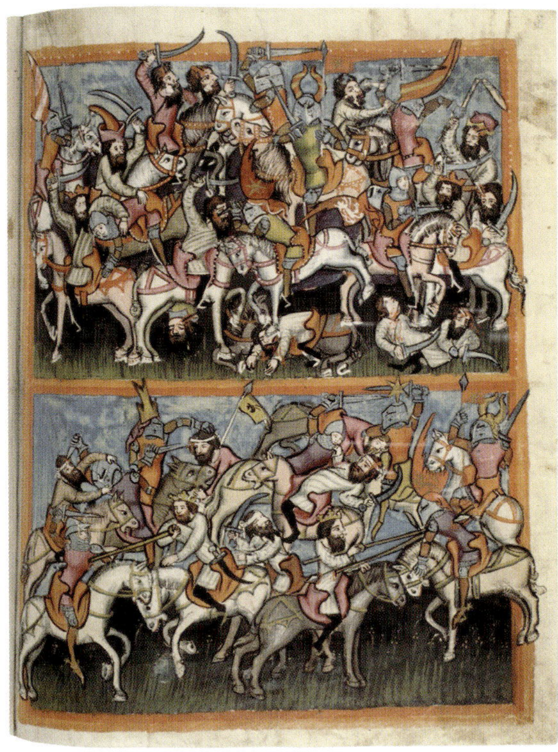

Fig. 3.2. Violent battle scenes from Wolfram von Eschenbach's *Willehalm*, c. 1350–1400, possibly Bavaria. Ink and paint on parchment, 30 x 23 cm. Wolfenbüttel, Herzog August Bibliothek, Cod. Guelf. 30.12 Aug. 2°, fol. 80r.

> The hero grasped his banner
> and stuffed the guts back in,
> all as if nothing had happened to him
> in the fierce contest:
> the praiseworthy youth
> hurtled onward into the fight.[12]

Images that accompany several manuscripts of *Willehalm* further attest to the work's particularly dramatic sense of violence, and Eschenbach ultimately has the injury claim Vivianz's life (fig. 3.2).[13] This was not medical naiveté but a conscious choice by the author, for the knight deliberately sets treatment aside in favor of valiant honor. Later in the same text, by contrast, a similar fate is avoided by the poem's eponymous hero Willehalm, whose wife Gyburc inspects his body for arrow tips—a procedure stressed in the *Wundarznei*'s paragraph 37—and upon their discovery dresses the hero's wounds with vinegar and bean blossoms, just one of several contemporary surgical techniques placed by Eschenbach into the hands of *Willehalm*'s women.[14] We are reminded here of the heavily gendered place of this literary violence: the stuff of specifically masculine fantasies, it is violence meted out by men and received almost exclusively by male bodies.[15]

Beyond simply incurring and curing wounds parallel to those treated in the *Wundarznei*, the affective experiences of these epic figures also trigger a more nuanced series of associations between the Wound Man's medical world and this popular literature. Such an idea flows principally from wounding's formal function within these literary works. Eugene Vance has argued that the cataloging of violent injuries repeatedly present in such texts may have helped form associations between individual characters and discrete narrative events, creating a wound-based mnemonic aid for the performers whose role it was to recite such extensive texts by heart.[16] A similar wound mnemonics has been identified at work in contemporary *lieder*, although in these short, lovelorn songs, memorable wounds tend to be inflicted not by weapons but by sultry glances, the spurning of lovers, or the Venus-like figure of Frau Minne, as neatly summed up in one verse by the anonymous Thuringian poet known as Der Düring:

Ich han leides vil ver wunden,
swunden wunden mir, diu Minne schôz
Do si mich mit blanken armen
warmen, armen leides mich zu ir beslôs.

I have overcome much sorrow,
wounds wasted me, Minne's lap
when she with bare arms
of warm, humble suffering drew me to her.[17]

In terms of narrative too, the dramatic and memorable moment of the wound could also be leveraged by a canny author into a poignant structural tool, at once prophetic and emotive. In siege tales, a warrior's wounds could stand metonymically for weaknesses in the city he was protecting; in Crusader epics, wounded commanders foreshadowed the fate of entire armies; and in military sagas, wounds are spoken of as the "insignia" of combat, ghosts of past chivalric honor fulfilled.[18] We might think as well of the more fantastical side of wounding in such narratives, what Siegfried Christoph has termed the German tradition's particular keenness for "stylized violence."[19] Here, the heroes of such writings could sustain both regular battlefield injuries and absurdly exaggerated ones, a literary equivalent to the Wound Man's own wounded overabundance. Prime among them was the so-called epic blow, a fighting flourish in which a medieval protagonist's swinging sword might not just slash at their opponent but cleave them entirely in two from head to waist (fig. 3.3).[20] Such was the fate of the pagan general Alderot in the poet Der Stricker's renowned epic, *Karl der Grosse*, who received:

... einen slac
dur den helm und dur die hirn scal
und also dur die brust zetal
dur beite satelbogen nider.
daz swert enhabte niht wider,
e im daz ort komen waz
in die erden durch daz graz.

... a blow
through the helmet and through the skull

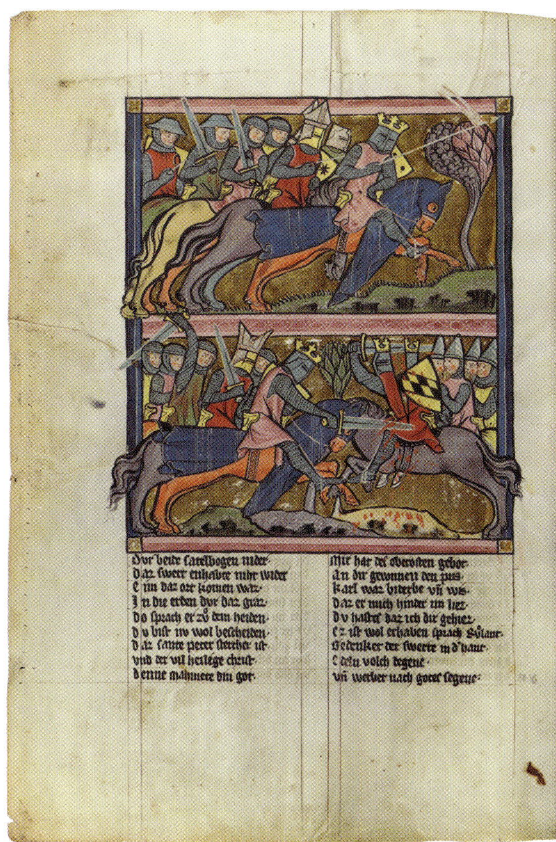

Fig. 3.3. Alderot cut in half by an "Epic Blow" from Der Stricker's *Karl der Grosse*, c. 1300, Zürich. Ink and paint on parchment, 30 x 21 cm. St. Gallen, Kantonsbibliothek, VadSlg MS 302, book II, fol. 35v.

and also through the chest,
through both parts of the saddle.
He did not lift the sword again
before he reached his end
in the earth beneath the sod.[21]

Wounds and the weapons inflicting them functioned as keen symbolic markers in this literary world, thrust intentionally by authors into a narrative even to the point that their presence was made irremovable. One of the genre's most famous deaths is that of Siegfried, crown prince of Xanten, as narrated in the extremely popular twelfth-century epic poem the *Nibelungenlied*.[22] Double-crossed by the vassal Hagen, Siegfried's demise—struck in the back with a spear while bending down to drink—is an archetypal example of an unjust death in chivalric terms. And to underscore Hagen's deceitful knowledge that Siegfried's back was his only vulnerable spot, an area unprotected by his earlier Achilles-like bath in dragon's blood, the text's anonymous author has the spear hold fast in Siegfried's body even as he springs up in retaliation:

Dâ der hêrre Sîvrit ob dem brunnen tranc,
er schôz in durch daz kriuze, daz von der wunden spranc

daz bluot im von dem herzen vaste an Hagenen wât.
sô grôze missewende ein helt nimmêr mêr begât.
Den gêr im gein dem herzen er dô stecken lie.
Alsô grimmeclîchen ze vlühten Hagene nie
gelief noch in der werlde vor deheinem man.
Dô sich der hêrre Sîvrit der grôzen wunden versan
Der herre tobelîchen von dem brunnen spranc.
im ragete von dem herzen ein gêrstange lanc.

As Siegfried drank from the fountain,
he speared him through the mark, so that from the wound sprang
the blood from his heart right onto Hagen's clothes.
No hero has done such a great misdeed since.
He left the spear stuck through the heart.
And Hagan fled with such wild rage
as he had never before run from any man.
When Siegfried became conscious of the great wound,
he leaped madly up from the fountain.
A long spear-shaft was sticking out from his heart.[23]

It was not uncommon to find epic heroes wandering the pages of literary classics beset by just such dramatic weapons or bearing such exaggerated wounds. Take another contemporary scene written by perhaps the most-read medieval poet to write in Mittelhochdeutsch, Hartmann von Aue, in his epic work *Erec*.[24] An adaptation of the earlier French trouvère Chrétien de Troyes's romance tale *Erec et Enide*, Aue's *Erec* was among the first German works to be set in the mythic world of the Arthurian court and follows the eponymous knight Erec as he tries to regain his chivalric honor after neglecting gallant pursuits in favor of his beautiful wife Enite. In one later section of the work—after doing battle with a pair of giants, no less—Erec loses so much blood that he collapses, and a devious local lord, Count Oringles, takes the opportunity to transport the hero's body to his court in the castle of Limors and ply his own advances on Enite. When Oringles strikes her over dinner for not returning his advances, her cries are so powerful that they raise the unconscious Erec, who promptly storms the hall to defend his wife. A crowd of onlookers, fleeing the scene in intense fear of Erec's wrath, finds sympathy from the work's narrator:

nu sprecht, wo ein toter man,
mit plůtigen wunden,
gerůet in gewůnden,
Haubt und hennde,
fuesse an ein gebende,
mit einem Schwerte also bar,
auf ein ungewarnte schar . . .
wer ich gewesen darbeÿ,
ich hette geflohen, wie kuene ich sey.

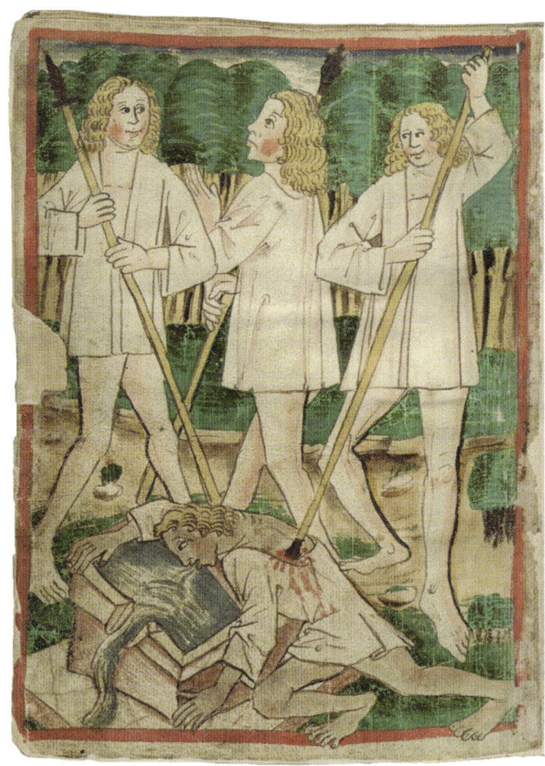

Fig. 3.4. Siegfried lanced in the back in a scene from the *Nibelungenlied* from the so-called *Wiener Heldenbuch* of the Nuremberger Lienhart Scheubel, c. 1480–90, Bavaria or Austria. Ink and paint on paper, 21 x 15 cm. Vienna, Österreichische Nationalbibliothek, Cod. 15478, fol. 291v.

tell me, if a dead man
with bloody wounds,
laid out for burial,
head and hands
and feet in bandages,
was running with sword drawn
on an unsuspecting crowd . . .
had I been there,
I would have fled, however bold I am.[25]

We cannot, of course, say for sure whether a fifteenth-century German reader coming across this account of the wounded yet wandering Erec—or indeed the pin-cushion Siegfried, half-slashed Alderot, or disemboweled Vivianz—would for certain have seen parallels between their evocative narratives and the equally bloody image of the Wound Man. But the pictorial repertoire of wounding and weaponry that accompanied these evocative literary classics suggests that this sort of comparative thinking was at least possible. A fifteenth-century copy of the *Nibelungenlied*, similar in date and likely also in location to the circulating south German *Dreibilderserie* manuscripts that bore the Wound Man, mobilizes Siegfried's dramatic lancing as a frontispiece to the entire Nibelung narrative: the image depicts the very moment that the deadly weapon is driven into the hero's back and is the only illustration from the story to be found in the entire manuscript (fig. 3.4).[26] Likewise,

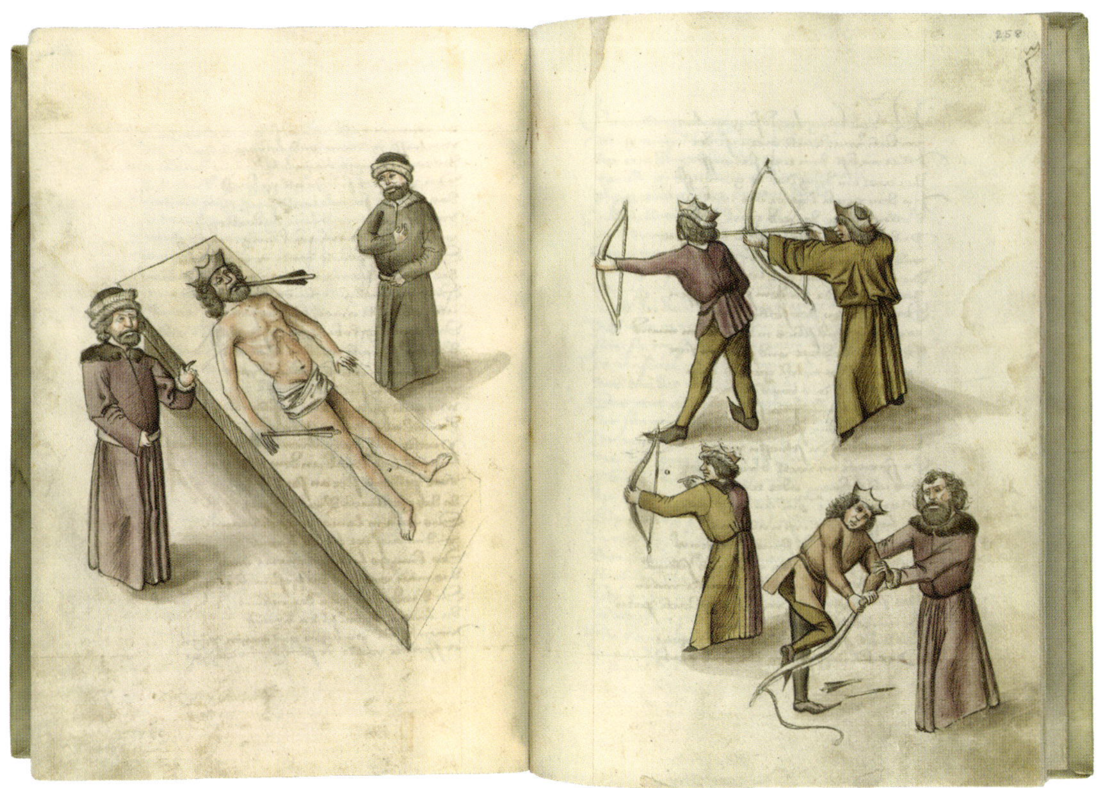

Fig. 3.5. King shot with arrows by his sons from Hugo von Trimberg's *Der Renner*, 1475–1500, possibly Tyrol. Ink and paint on paper, 29 x 21 cm (each folio). New York, Morgan Library & Museum, MS M.763, fols. 257v–258r.

the makers of multiple other contemporary manuscripts took the time to single out instances of particularly gory violence for visualization. Several versions of Hugo von Trimberg's moral compendium *Der Renner* (The Runner) revel in realizing the age-old didactic scene of a king whose sons compete for succession in an archery contest, presenting him riddled with their arrows (fig. 3.5).[27] Meanwhile, at the base of a book decorated around 1445 in the workshop of the popular Hagenau illustrator Diebold Lauber—an inhabitant of the same city that only seventy years later would play backdrop to Albrecht von Berwangen's graphic demise—we find depicted a moment from Wolfram von Eschenbach's *Parzival*, in which the Arthurian stalwart Sir Gawain has survived attack from the swords and spears of the so-called Perilous Bed and is receiving treatment for a series of profusely bleeding wounds (fig. 3.6).[28]

All these heroes are presented on the page in the same abundantly graphic mode as the Wound Man, and we must remember too that for his part the Wound Man was just as intermingled with these wounded romance champions as their images were with him. After all, none of these individual epic characters sport anything as dramatic as the fantastical agglomeration of violent wounds borne by the surgical figure. Viewers might just as easily have been prompted to connect the dots in the other direction, seeing his overwhelming, almost otherworldly injuries as intimating a backstory worthy of contemporary literature, the beginnings of a chivalric personhood emerging for the Wound Man.

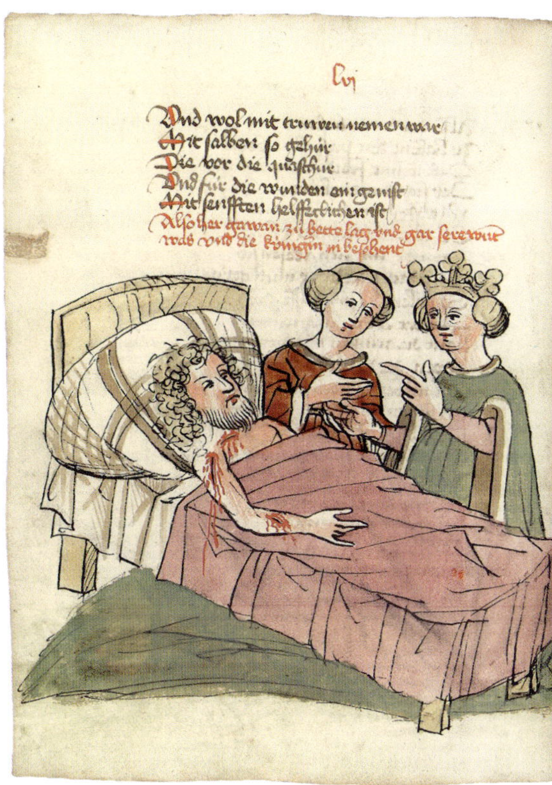

Fig. 3.6. Gawain's wounds being treated in a scene from Wolfram von Eschenbach's *Parzival*, 1443–46, Hagenau. Ink and paint on paper, 28 x 20 cm. Heidelberg, Universitätsbibliothek, Cpg 339, vol. II, fol. 425v.

Wounds as Experience and Technique

Experience, as well as fantasy, could help forge connections across this increasingly expansive fifteenth-century literary woundscape. For as well as the epics of classic romance literature, contemporary German audiences were also being treated to flashy and supposedly authentic accounts of the battlefield through a new literary genre: the military autobiography. Emerging in earnest for the first time in the 1440s and 1450s, these were works published by a generation of landed fighter-writers, such as Ulrich von Hutten, Georg von Frundsberg, and Götz von Berlichingen, all of whom claimed to be reflecting on long careers in the military.[29] Clearly the veracity of these texts as firm historical sources fluctuates, with some seeming to be reliable personal accounts and others inevitably gross exaggerations born of hindsight. But as Jörg Rogge has shown, it was particularly through describing moments of wounded peril that these early war writers developed their texts from mere adventure transcripts into records of more impassioned experience, emotion and injury once again collapsing together in the Wound Man's immediate cultural milieu.[30]

Such violence served two principal narrative functions in these new autobiographical accounts. The meting out and sustaining of wounds courted empathy for their protagonists, who emotively describe their fight for survival amid smashing lances, flying arrows, and sword gashes, while at the same time violent situations offered perfect proof to the reader of these soldiers' hardheaded valor and military mettle. Emblematic of this twin tendency is an account completed at some point after 1467 by a German knight named Jörg von Ehingen, who, after failing to find juicy enough wars in France and Spain, traveled in 1415 to the North African city of Ceuta to fight for the Portuguese.[31] There, he was selected to contend in a duel against a champion chosen from the opposing Berber Muslim army. He gleefully recounts the affair in his autobiography, which is worth quoting at length for both its exciting pace and its florid violence:

> *[Er] rant gar ernstlich gegen mir här und schrai mich an. Allso ließ och gegen im her gonn, hett min spieß uff mein schenkel, und als ich gar nach zů im kam warff ich den spieß inn daß gerüst, und rant im uff sin schilt und wie wol er mich mitt sin spieß in ain flankart oder bantzer ermel ranntt gewan ich im doch von min treffen ain sollichen schwanck ab daß roß und man zůr erden fiellen. Aber sin speiß hieng mir im dem ring harnisch . . . Der häd war mechtiger starck. Er riß sich von mir und kamen allso bäd mitt den lÿben uffrecht und doch kniend nebend ain ander. Stieß ich in mitt mier lincken hand von mir das ich mitt mein schwert ain stich uff in herhollen möcht, alß och geschah. Dan im stoß mit der lincken hand kam er mitt dem lÿb so wÿtt von mir daß ich im ain stich im sin angesicht gab und wie woll ich den stich nitt gar volkůmenlich gehaben möcht verwůntten daß er hinder sich schwangtt und ettwaß geblentt ward. Allso gab ich im erst ain rechten stich im sin angesicht und stach in uff die erden nider und trang allso uff in und stach im den halß ab. Allso stand ich uff nam sin schwert und tratt zů meinem pferdt.*

> [He] ran at me with intent, uttering a cry. So I also went toward him, with my lance at my thigh, and as I approached him, I couched it and thrust it at his shield, and although he thrust his lance into my flank or armguard, my thrust caused him to topple so far that horse and man fell to the ground. But his lance hung in my chainmail. . . . The heathen was enormously strong. He tore himself from me, and we both ended up with our bodies upright but kneeling next to each other. I pushed him away from me with my left hand so that I could strike at him with my sword, which worked out, for the shove with the left hand pushed his body far enough from me that I struck a blow to his face that, although I couldn't make it with full force, wounded him so that he rocked backward and was partially blinded. So I gave him a proper blow to his face and cut him down to the ground, threw myself upon him, and cut his throat. After which I stood up, took his sword, and returned to my horse.[32]

Despite having a lance wedged Wound Man–like in his side, Jörg comes away victorious, and his hyperbolic narrative goes on to claim that following his success the entire Berber army withdrew fearfully and ceded the town, earning the brave knight a full bowl of Portuguese guilders in the process.

However fanciful an outcome, it is the graphic violence of the tale that seems to have lent Jörg's account its authenticity in the eyes of his contemporaries, as we see repeatedly across the new genre. Injury evidenced an author's military fortitude and moral firmness, whether as a result of enemy action or because of more accidental suffering during the dangerous pursuit of war. The fifteenth-century Swiss nobleman Ludwig von Diesbach, for instance, chronicles a moment of what he calls "*grosser schad*" (great injury) while on campaign in Picardy, when the knight's own lance penetrated an artery in his thigh during an encounter with an unpredictable horse.[33] Luckily, with the careful attention of a German *Scherer* (barber-surgeon) he survived the wound, although Ludwig is silent on whether this medic turned to a *Dreibilderserie* book as a curative aid. The *Wundarznei*'s paragraph 34 on the healing of spear wounds would surely have helped, as would many surviving Wound Men who illustrate a similar spear running directly through their left thigh. All Ludwig mentions is the result of his surgeon's successful work, boasting that the injury's only long-term effect was the loss of two lengths from his long-jump personal best.

Although their pages drip with descriptive flair, the new genre of the first-hand military account did not circulate with images that matched their keen investment in wounds.[34] A strong visual correlative, however, can be found in another body of German manuscripts. Emerging at exactly the same time, these books were associated not with military campaigns but with military training, sometimes referred to by contemporaries as addressing the *Kunst des Fechtens* (The Art of Fighting). This was a corpus of military manuscripts that grew to prominence among both high- and low-brow audiences across the fourteenth and fifteenth centuries.[35] And although not always illustrated, nearly fifty German *Fechtbücher* (fight-books) survive that reproduce imagery remarkably similar to the tales of contemporary fighter-writers, their pictures both cataloging and elucidating practical knowledge associated with many different types of martial arts. They include images of disciplines across what Eric Burkart has called a broad "culture of fighting": fencing with swords, daggers, poleaxes, maces, and spiked shields, unarmed wrestling, fighting from horseback, and even crossbow-work, all staged across show fights, legally sanctioned judicial duels, and self-defense during what the manuals term fighting *in ernste*—in the Italian, *d'amore*—namely, genuine, life-threatening combat.[36]

The best-preserved works of this corpus are once more precisely contemporaneous, both chronologically and geographically, with the *Dreibilderserie* Wound Man, most notably a *Fechtbuch* text likely to have been completed in Bavaria at some point in the late 1440s by the Swabian master of arms Hans Talhoffer.[37] One manuscript of Talhoffer's work, now in Copenhagen, shows just how detailed and lavish editions of this work could be. Produced in 1459, seemingly for the master himself, the manuscript names both its scribe, one Michel Rotwyler, and its artist, Clauss Pflieger, who together realized more than 180 painted visualizations of different fighting scenarios (fig. 3.7).[38] Each image is shown in landscape orientation and tightly executed by Pflieger in fine strokes and graded washes of color. Most present two figures, although some show three or four, all caught in the cut and thrust of combat, while above them short descriptions or snippets of advice are offered, often coded for the exclusive knowledge of fighting professionals: "*Daß halß würgen*" (The throat-choke), "*Lern kolben*" (Learn maces), "*Hie macht er ain end stuck*" (Here he makes an end-play), "*Mit dem schwert fur den Slag mit dem spieß*" (With the sword, counter the blow with the spear), and so on.[39]

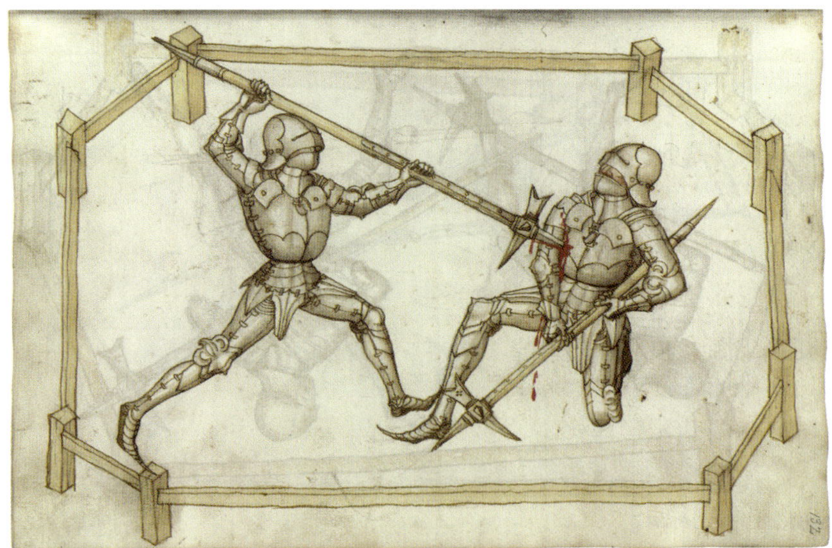

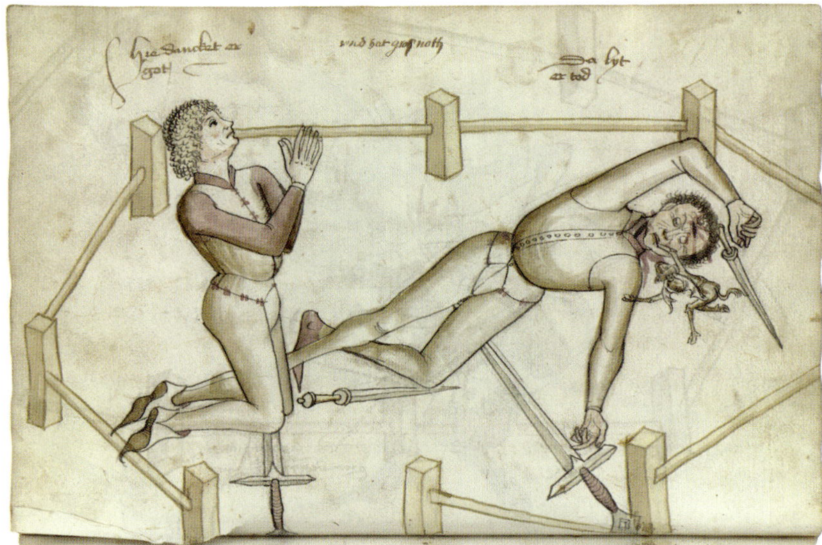

Fig. 3.7. Scenes of combat from Hans Talhoffer's *Fechtbuch*, 1459, Bavaria. Ink and paint on paper, 30 x 21 cm. Copenhagen, Kongelige Bibliothek, Thott 290, 2°, fols. 134v, 93v.

These brief notes offer few specifics to the reader, and instead the majority of practical information on fighting style or equipment is conveyed by the deliberate poses and relative placement of the painted figures. Indeed, as Rachel Kellett has observed, in their structured portrayal of firsthand violence, such *Fechtbücher* were not only elucidating fighterly technique but also tapping into the same long-standing traditions of chivalrous combat as the contemporary German epics explored earlier, a constant among both genres' symbolic vocabulary.[40] These images, for example, convey a wide range of details attesting to more subtle military comportment. In one vignette we glimpse something of the fighter's social world, sitting in the corner of a ring before a tournament bout attended by his squire, while in another we learn of combatants whose stylized clothes and dark skin reveal both the obvious internationalism and the complex racial politics of a fighting life.

Meanwhile, one of the closing images of the Copenhagen Talhoffer book even shows us something of a fighter's moral compass in a scene explaining how to win graciously. The victor of a fight is depicted kneeling on his sword before the bleeding body of his dead opponent—looking not unlike the wounded Gawain or murdered Albrecht von Berwangen—while above this fighter, whose hands are clasped and head is cast upward to heaven, a caption rhymes: "*Hie dancket er got, Da lyt er tod*" (Here he thanks God, There he lies dead).[41]

Close connections abound between the Wound Man and this technical-visual culture of combat, not least because we know that their audiences were in many cases one and the same. *Fechtbücher* were often owned by medical men. Nicholas Pol, for instance, the personal doctor of Holy Roman Emperors Maximilian and Ferdinand, recorded his name in the back of a *Fechtbuch* from his library in the year 1494.[42] Moreover, their contents were not exclusively fighterly. While more aggressive materials certainly tended to dominate, *Fechtbücher* often also incorporated writings geared specifically toward matters of health. Returning once more to the Copenhagen manuscript, we find the master's fighting treatise presented in the book alongside a text extolling the healing properties of bathing, another offering brief anatomical discussion of different body parts, a third dispensing advice on astromedicine in relation to the seven planets, and a bilingual Hebrew-German poem on the health of the body in relation to God.[43] Even Talhoffer's writing itself prescribes certain forms of diet and exercise to focus the health of fighters during training.[44]

From a literary perspective too it makes sense that medicine might have been on the minds of the authors and artists who made these *Fechtbücher*. There is, after all, a close structural kinship between the two genres. Consider the similarities of form between these two passages, one a section on long-sword technique covering *abschniden* (cuts) from the *Fechtbuch* of the fifteenth-century fencing master Sigmund ain Ringeck, and the other a paragraph on combat wounds from a German-language *Wundarznei* accompanying a *Dreibilderserie* Wound Man:

> *Item den schnidt trÿb also. Wenn dir ainer an dz schwert bindt gegen diner lincken sÿtten und schlecht umb vom schwert mitt der zwerche oder sunst dir zuo der rechten sÿtten. So spring mitt dem lincken fůß uß dem haw uff sin rechte sÿttenn und fall im mitt der langen schniden oben uber baÿde arm. Das trÿb zů baiden sÿttenn.*
>
> Item, make the cut as follows. When [someone strikes] you a [blow] on the sword binding against your left side and slides round from the sword, crossways or otherwise, to your right side: jump with the left foot away from the blow to his right side and strike him with the long cut from above over both arms. Do this on both sides.[45]
>
> *Item zo eynem daz hobt vorsert wirt mit kolben mit steinen mit messeren ader wo mitte is geschit Alzo das ein we ist daz er wenet syne synne vorlieren oder ioch vorlurt und ist doch die serde uf getan sunder sußt geknotzt und gemorßt*

> *von slegin deme saltu alzo helffen Er sal lazen die hobt oder daz das ungesunde blut uß gang und mach ein plaster uff die wetund stat.*
>
> Item, for one whose head has been wounded with a club, a stone, a knife or whatever. If he is in so much pain that he thinks he will go unconscious or indeed does go unconscious and the wound is open but all compressed and crushed from the blows, you can help him thus. Let the head vein so that the unhealthy blood goes out, and apply a plaster to the painful place.[46]

A gap of around eighty years between the two manuscripts accounts for certain of their linguistic differences, as do their variant south German dialects. Nevertheless, both take advantage of the same literary style, that of newly emerging fifteenth-century "How-To" literature.[47] Aiming at brevity and technical clarity, the two texts share a directness, both conveying ideas in short, digestible nuggets and in the same frank, imperative voice, even using the same staged itemization of successive moments in a duel or operation.

Given these social and structural relations, the visual similarities that appear between these two fifteenth-century southern German genres take on particular potency. Most obviously, the weapons wielded by *Fechtbücher* figures are often identical to those lodged in the body of the Wound Man, drawn from a shared performative arsenal of late medieval and early modern German warfare.[48] Indeed, in some cases the Wound Man and *Fechtbücher* fighters are even identically dressed. One persistent aspect of the surgical figure is his repeated presentation in the same pair of blue underpants, known in Mittelhochdeutsch as *bruoche*, a detail preserved in several fighting treatises as well. Dress historians have concluded that this form of simple brief was, like both *Dreibilderserie* and *Fechtbuch*, a relatively new phenomenon of the fifteenth century, superseding larger short-like or billowing undergarments favored by thirteenth- and fourteenth-century tastes.[49] Made mostly of

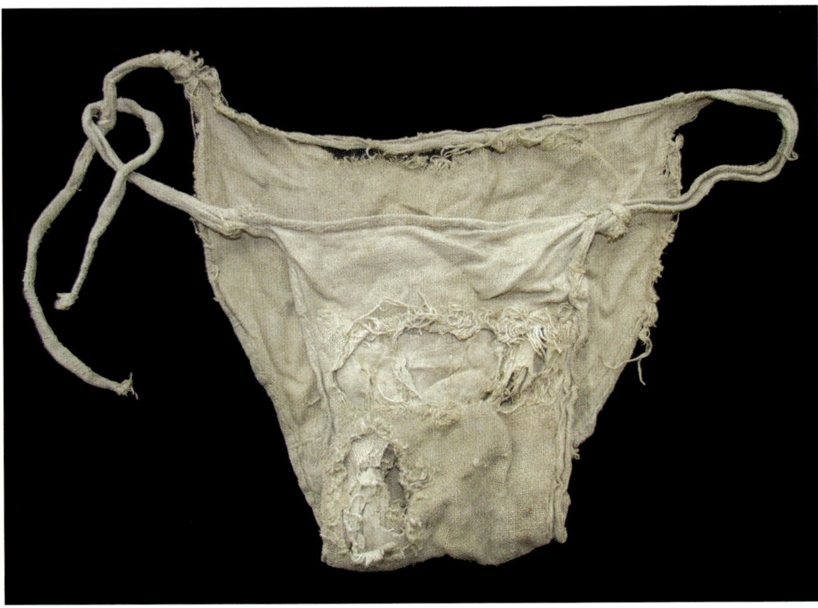

Fig. 3.8. Underpants discovered in excavations at Schloss Lengberg, 15th century, East Tyrol. Linen, width 19 cm (without ties). Innsbruck, Institut für Archäologien.

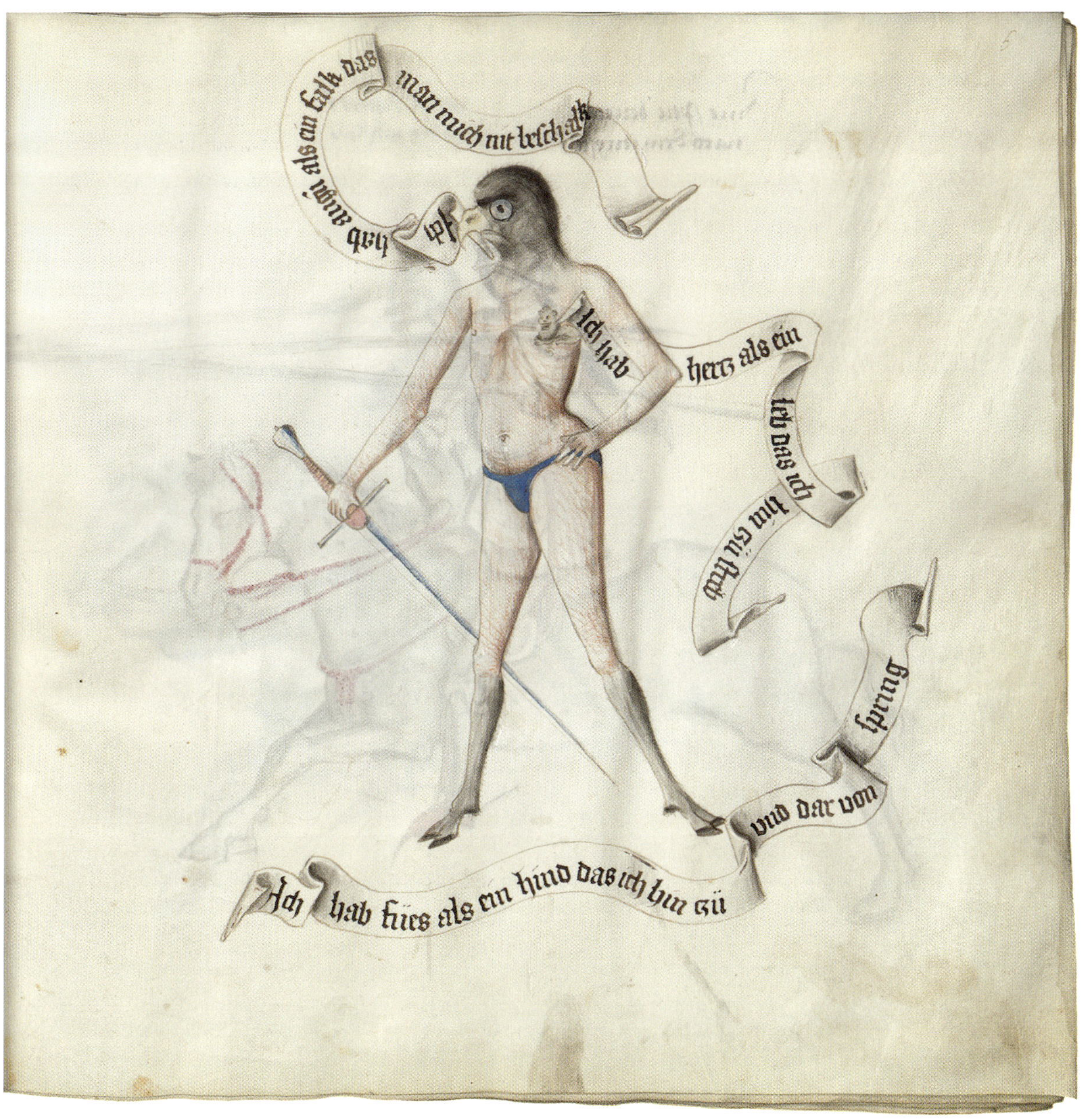

Fig. 3.9. Hybrid figure of an ideal fighter from Paulus Kal's *Fechtbuch*, before 1479, Bavaria. Ink and paint on parchment, 29 x 29 cm. Munich, Bayerische Staatsbibliothek, Cgm 1507, fol. 6r.

highly degradable linen, they are extremely rare survivors, although, conveniently, one of the only pairs to have been preserved was found in southern Germany amid the building rubble used to pack a fifteenth-century vault in Lengberg Castle in the East Tyrol (fig. 3.8).[50] Described elliptically by Elizabeth Coatsworth and Gale Owen-Crocker as "very brief," the garment is indeed skimpy, but even this tatty, disposed-of pair was once valued, as evidenced by three sets of repairs made with linen patches to its central cut of cloth.[51] Their form was clearly a popular choice among fighters, as is made clear in a fifteenth-century *Fechtbuch* by the master Paulus Kal, probably first composed soon after 1460 while Kal was in the service of the Duke of Bavaria-Landshut (fig. 3.9).[52] Fronting one copy of the treatise is an image which presents a hybrid body of Kal's invention, its form clarified in the poetic ditties contained within banderoles of text that swirl about the figure, sword in hand. He claims to be the epitome of an ideal fighter:

Ich hab augen als ein falk das man mich nit beschalk.
Ich hab hercz als ein leb das ich hin czü streb.
Ich hab fües als ein hind das ich hin czü und dar von spring.

I have eyes like a hawk, so you do not overpower me.
I have heart like a lion, so I strive forward.
I have feet like a deer, so I spring forward and back.

Kal's words are gifted monstrous form in the figure. It stands with a large hawk's head, a miniature lion set at its chest, and cervine legs from the knee down, all gathered around a human frame dressed in the very same blue underpants seen on virtually all surviving Wound Men.[53] This comparison only adds further to the sense that, for fifteenth-century contemporaries, *Fechtbücher* figures and surgical Wound Men represented two different ends of a continuous spectrum of practical German literature concerned with bodily injury: the former was responsible for inflicting wounds, the latter for healing them.

In fact, stepping back, this idea of a spectrum of wound-conscious works might also be the most useful way to consider the Wound Man in relation to the entirety of the broad network of German literature we have ranged across so far in this chapter. From legal testimony to poetic fantasy, epic fights to fighting manuals, the catalog of wounded men found in this contextual cultural corpus presents a host of powerful resonances for the surgical figure. Appearing in both the stalwarts of medieval Germanic prose and the most innovative of newly emerging early modern genres, these literary models offer a suite of possible answers to the open question of the Wound Man's personhood. For a fifteenth-century pragmatist, the weapons of war peppered around his body signaled a clear military bent, engendering a view of the Wound Man as fencing model or fighter-writer. For their more romantic counterpart, the overwhelming volume of his injuries—clearly the result of multiple simultaneous encounters condensed into a single moment—signaled the stuff of epic legend, his wounds meted out in the cut-and-thrust of chivalric living. And even if the Wound Man's contemporaries were unaware of or simply uninterested in finding particular parallels for the figure in this cache of literary tropes, such tales and their punchy imagery would nonetheless have furnished readers with a hefty vocabulary of bodily violence through which to frame the figure, a written woundscape into which the Wound Man neatly slotted.

Sacred Wounds

When, in 2013, the fifteenth-century grave of the aristocrat Oswald von Schrofenstein was uncovered in the parish church of Mariä Himmelfahrt in the Tyrolean city of Landeck, researchers found that Oswald had been buried with a 1.24-meter-long sword.[54] Such swords were highly symbolic items to members of the late medieval German elite, and whether this specimen was actually wielded by Oswald on the battlefield or crafted instead just for his interment, the sword's presence was testament to its owner's prowess, evoking violent narratives of the type discussed earlier in a manner that equated swordsmanship with romantic questing and military canny. But the item can also be seen as standing for the close connection of this courtly power with more spiritual concerns. The pommel atop Oswald's sword preserved three neatly etched characters: "IHS," the monogram of Christ. Whether gripping this talisman in battle or burial, Oswald would have been channeling both the superstitious protection of a specific holy name and a far broader, explicitly corporeal healing discourse associated in Christian-majority Europe with the figure of Jesus.

Among the potential conceptual wounded prototypes for the Wound Man, this was surely by some distance the most potent and pervasive alive in contemporary Germany and Bohemia. An integral image across religious life, historians have uncovered references to the corporeality and wounds of Christ in virtually all aspects of fifteenth-century European culture—literary, visual, philosophical, culinary, fraternal, warfaring—to the point that its emblematic qualities feel almost workaday.[55] This enormous breadth, however, should not conceal the pointed currency that religious thinking about bodies held for individual cultural fields, not least among them the medical world of the Wound Man. If we are aiming to insert the Wound Man back into his immediate context, understanding the spiritual aspects of his wounded makeup is key.

It is worth broadening our focus for a moment to consider the wider medico-religious picture of the European Middle Ages. Clearly not all medicine in medieval Europe was practiced by religious Christians, far from it.[56] But it is true that the majority of surviving European medical treatises were produced in Christian contexts, including all surviving *Dreibilderserie* manuscripts containing the Wound Man. Across this large corpus, a multiplicity of medieval holy narratives had created a powerful rhetoric of spiritual healing, evidenced most prominently through metaphors drawn from theological writers of the period who spoke often of different Christological models of cure. Most influentially, the fifth-century church father Augustine of Hippo had in multiple writings painted a complex and enduring picture of Christ as *Christus medicus* (Christ the physician), the Godhead at once inhabiting the figure of the healer and the properties of a drug, while his contemporary, the theologian Saint Jerome of Stridon, introduced similar ideas into the discourse by conceptualizing religious healing as the work of a *spiritualis Hippocrates* (spiritual Hippocrates).[57] By the thirteenth century, this sentiment was being matched in many contemporary confession manuals, mystical writings, preachers' orations, and other types of spiritual guides that spoke of diagnostic sins, holy purgatives, and confession itself as pure medicine. In the words of the fourteenth-century English aristocrat and author Henry of Grosmont, delivered with typical dramatic flourish in his autobiographical Anglo-Norman epic of repentance *Le livre de seyntz medicines* (The Book of Holy Medicines):

Bien semblont mes plaies estre dolerouses qant si envis outre passer me puise.... Tresdouz sires et bon mestres de toutes sciences, ore vous requer qe pour fysisien vous vous moxstres et me deignez a entreprendre en meyn, et me garir de la perillouse enfirmete qest en moy nuyt et iours sanz avoir ent nul alegement.

So painful seem my wounds that I cannot pass over them.... Sweet Lord and good masters of all knowledge, I beg you to be my physician and deign to take me in hand and protect me from the perilous infirmity that night and day rules me without relief.[58]

Medical writers evoked many of the same comparisons as these theological works. Contemporary physicians spoke of Christ as a cure in his own right. The fourteenth-century Genoese physician Galvano da Levanto, for instance, likened the healing effects of wonder drugs and magnetic stones to the compelling cure-all properties of Christ, the *pigmentator celestis* (celestial apothecary).[59] And individual branches of medieval curative professions transformed these metaphors further still to facilitate their own specialisms. For the influential French surgeon Henri de Mondeville, writing at the beginning of the fourteenth century, God was not *Christus medicus* but *Christus cyrurgicus*, not a physician but a tactile surgeon:

Deus ipse fuit cyrurgicus practicus, quando de limo terrae condidit protoplaustrum ... haec enim mirabilia et multa alia consimilia et majora operando cum manibus fecit Deus, quae in divina pagina recitantur.

God himself was a practicing surgeon, when from the slime of the Earth he formed the first man ... these miracles and many other similar and greater ones, which are named on the divine page, God caused by working with his hands.[60]

This sentiment was clearly shared by the artist responsible for the opening images of a contemporary fourteenth-century manuscript made in Picardy and containing the *Chirurgia* (Surgery) of the Italian surgeon Roger Frugardi, which presents a cluster of vignettes that correlated scenes from the life of the Virgin and Christ above with those of a surgeon at work below (fig. 3.10).[61] Similarly, in monastic healing arenas the actual stuff of religious practice could bleed into more medical modes. Eucharistic wafers, the transubstantiated body of Christ, feature as curative medicine in a number of healing treatises, and, as Mary Yearl notes, the rules of their orders commanded monks to offer treatment to the sick, explicitly stating that patients were to be tended to as if they were Christ in person.[62] Such religious comparisons could equally be evoked to the healer's detriment. As Joseph Ziegler has argued, the fourteenth-century sermons of English Dominican friar John Bromyard flipped this medico-religious resemblance, warning that evil might co-opt a sinner's heart in the same way as a physician takes the pulse, a slothful medicine of the devil.[63]

Later medieval Germany was especially engaged in this fruitful back-and-forth between bodily forms of piety and pious forms of bodily care. Re-

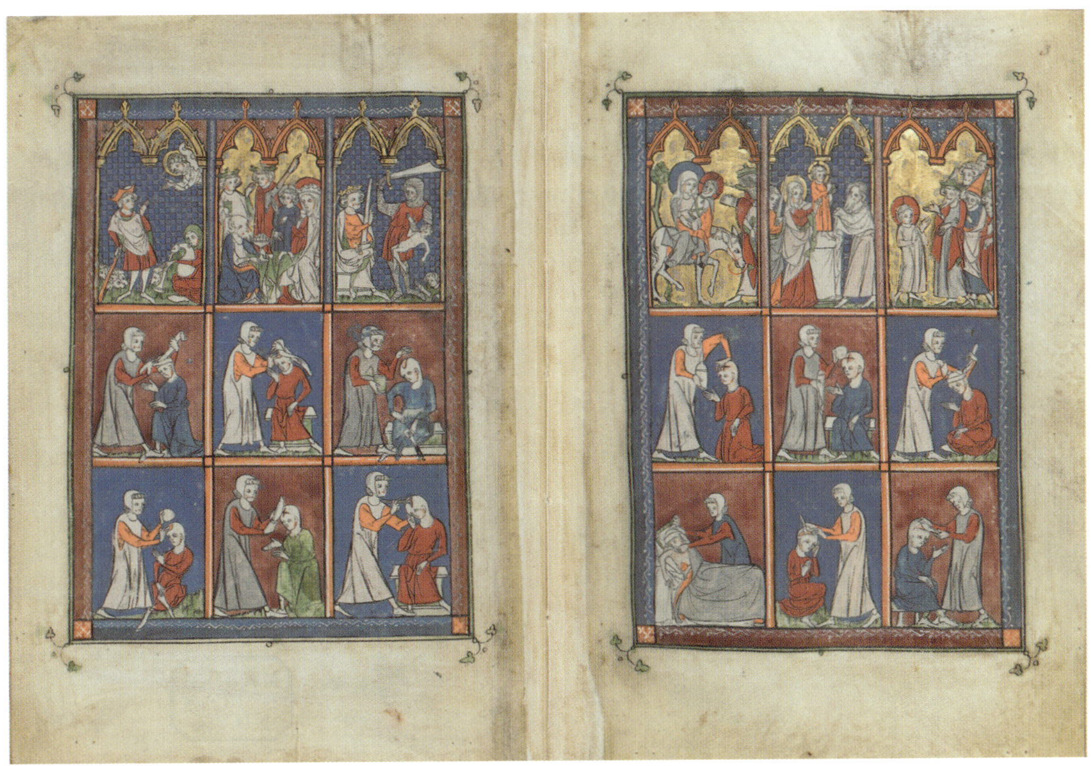

Fig. 3.10. Scenes from the life of Christ paired with surgical operations from Roger Frugardi's *Chirurgia*, c. 1275–1300, France. Ink and paint on parchment, 23 x 16 cm (each folio). London, British Library, Sloane MS 1977, fols. 2v–3r.

ligious invocations in medical texts were common. As early as the 1150s, the famed mystic and medical writer Hildegard of Bingen spoke of embracing the harsh and bitter wounds of Christ, whom she framed as the "*magnus medicus omnium languorum*" (great physician of all diseases).[64] A century and a half later, the opening line of Ortolf von Baierland's *Arzneibuch*—much discussed in the previous chapter—invoked the Solomonic prophecy that "*got hat erczney geschaffen durch ir edelkeit vnd durch ir krafft*" (God made medicine because it is noble and powerful).[65]

As well as mobilizing Christ for supportive metaphor, German healers working in more folkloric traditions invoked this Christian holy presence even more directly in their work. Amuletic charms collected in medical and nonmedical manuscripts alike regularly turned to Christ's Passion for their curative power, especially the tradition of *Wundsegen*, blessings specifically designed to heal a patient's wounds.[66] Surviving examples of these magical excerpts often start with so-called *historiolae*, narrative preambles meant to invoke particular religious personages in the healing process. One popular charm in the case of wounds, the so-called Three Good Brothers Charm, features a *historiola* discussing an injured trio who came across Christ while searching for herbs to heal their wounds, as well as Saint Longinus, whose association with blood and wounding followed logically from his piercing of Christ's side during the Crucifixion.[67] The charm continues by demanding that the wound be anointed with oil or water—another Christological reference—and cleaned with wool before the incantation of specific phrases invoking the wounded Christ and other saints should finally be spoken. Among the oldest such charms is an Althochdeutsch example from around the year 1200 found in a manuscript now in Bamberg, which showcases the typically rhythmic, rhyming quality of their religious healing:

Crist wart hi erden wnt
daz wart da ze himele chunt
iz ne blötete noch ne svar
noch nechein eiter ne bar
taz was ein file göte stunte
heil sis tu wnte.

Christ was wounded here on earth
That then became known in heaven.
It did not bleed or fester
Nor did it bear any pus.
That was a very good hour.
Be cured, wound.[68]

We may recall from the previous chapter that as well as early wound charms, this Bamberg manuscript also contains the earliest version of the *Dreibilderserie* Disease Man, drawing a clear connection between the two traditions (fig. 2.7).[69] Viewed through a religious lens, this medical figure too seems to be drawing on Christian prototypes for aspects of its diagrammatic figuration, his diseased catchwords forming into a circular halo around his head and his heavily bearded form surely borrowed from iconographic models of Christ or Old Testament Prophets.[70]

Although a comparatively niche medical genre, we can see the south German *Dreibilderserie* books as themselves showcasing a similar level of religious inflection. In terms of their contents, laced throughout all three parts of the *Dreibilderserie*—the Disease Man's lists of sickness from head to toe, the Disease Woman's obstetrical treatises, and the Wound Man's *Wundarznei*—we find a host of references that tacitly acknowledge their use by medics working firmly within a Christian setting.[71] When the author of a *Dreibilderserie* text refers to different points in the calendar year, suggesting auspicious times for particular procedures, they invariably work forward or backward from the nearest saint's feast day. A similar logic governs the calendrical timing of gathered ingredients: in a recipe for an unguent against cramps, the *Wundarznei*'s antidotary calls for butter made either in the week before the Nativity of the Blessed Virgin or before the feast of the apostles Philip and James.[72] Occasional liturgical or biblical references likewise appear—again, less for their spiritual content than as practical anchors—for example, in the gynecological section of one *Dreibilderserie* manuscript that cites an unusual discussion of the baptism of hermaphroditic children and invokes Jewish populations in the Book of Exodus as evidence in favor of its advice on fertility.[73]

Even more explicitly, several recipes listed in the *Wundarznei* suggest the medic's direct ability to harness an innate spiritual power of certain ingredients, from cures named *Apostolicon* (Apostle's plaster) and *Gratia Dei*

(The grace of God) to a recipe that "*a solo deo venit*" (comes from God alone) and others rounded out simply with a note that the patient "*sanabitur deo iuuante*" (will be healed by the help of God).[74] The creator of a *Dreibilderserie* manuscript now in Paris made this link even more emphatic when listing the many ills of the treatise's Disease Man, punctuating the final line in the page's lower-right corner with the word *IHS*, the same Christological monogram as on Oswald von Schrofenstein's sword (fig. 2.5).[75] Something similar occurs in a Disease Man from a *Dreibilderserie* manuscript now in Rome, whose sickly form is framed above by a four-line biblical poem that includes the couplet "*Morbi sunt plures quos tu Iesu bone cures*" (Many are the diseases that you, good Jesus, heal) (fig. 2.4).[76] This Disease Man is transformed into Christ himself.

The elaborate nature of the Wound Man's injuries and weapons offered even keener opportunity for contemporary readers to make visual connections between his surgical body and this same Christianized method. Most obviously, this relationship hinged on the image's extreme violence, which accorded with the increasingly elaborate "religiosity of blame and self-reproach"—to use Caroline Walker Bynum's words—that had been amplifying in German-speaking lands since the twelfth century.[77] Late medieval Christian practice in this mold focused on the entangled relationship between pain and piety, a sentiment that took increasingly corporeal and bloody form in both the religious literary and visual imagination. Following an internal spiritual logic, extremes of suffering and salvation were here mediated through the concept of *compassio*, a form of compassion bordering on co-suffering that rendered ever more aggressive depictions of religious violence into ever more effective vehicles for individual devotion.[78] German writers were at the center of this movement, with widely circulated early works by religious authors such as Rupert von Deutz and Elisabeth von Schönau soon joined in the fourteenth century by Ludolf von Sachsen's *Vita Christi* (Life of Christ), Heinrich von Sankt Gallen's *Extendit manum* Passion tract (literally translated as He stretched out his hand), Margarethe Ebner's *Offenbarungen* (Revelations), Marquard von Lindau's German treatise *De anima Christi* (The Soul of Christ), and many others.[79] These writings reworked religious narratives with increasingly grisly determination. By the turn of the fifteenth century, the practice had helped galvanize religious cults centered on Christ's Passion—in particular his "activated" wounds—and stoked antisemitic narratives of the desecration of the host, as well as encouraging the production of increasingly exaggerated and grotesque religious writings.[80]

Among the earliest and best known is a popular anonymous text entitled *Christi Leiden in einer Vision geschaut* (Christ's Passion Shown in a Vision), which purports to be a vision of the Passion recounted by an anonymous nun.[81] It speaks in especially graphic terms, including details such as Christ's heart exploding with blood in "*einen grozen stromigen vlus*" (a great streaming flow) or descriptions of Christ's desecrated corpse at the Deposition as "*swarz und durre, und die wonden ze kenen, und die geleder van eyn geseigen*" (black and dry, and the wounds split open, and the limbs splayed apart).[82] Beyond visionary tracts, contemporary writings of many types contributed to this extreme sentiment. *Fronleichnamsspiele*, or Corpus Christi plays, such as those surviving from the cities of Innsbruck and Eger, brought Christ's acts of suffering to life through procession and performance, with the specific goal that—in the words of one play from 1479, probably written in the southern German town of Künzelsau—"*sein leiden nit werd an euch verlorn*" (his suffering not be lost on you).[83] Biblical events were similarly animated for the compassion of the inner senses through shared song, most notably in the work of contemporary poets such as Oswald von Wolkenstein. One of his fifteenth-century *lieder*, now titled "Im Oberreich" (In Oberland), narrates the Passion with graphic gusto, culminating in a chilling, bloody stanza:

Ein blinder Jude namens Longinus,
der kam mit seinem Speer,
den stieß er in seine heilige Seite.
Blut und Wasser strömten ihm entgegen
bis auf seine Augen.

A blind Jew who was called Longinus
came with a spear,
which he poked into His holy side.
Blood and water gushed toward him
directly into his eyes.[84]

This exaggerated turn toward Christological violence presented itself just as vividly in contemporary visual culture. Walking into a fifteenth-century church or turning the pages of a contemporary religious book, German Christians were more likely to be confronted with doleful images of Christ rendered as a dying corpse than with more uplifting depictions of his triumphant resurrection in heaven. On the one hand, this emphasis was intellectually driven. Image types such as the Man of Sorrows, first emerging in Europe in the thirteenth and fourteenth centuries, focused attention directly on renderings of Christ's injured body by presenting it in iconic fashion, often devoid of tangible time and identifiable space to aid focused devotion.[85] But on the other, the emphasis on violence was unashamedly affective. Christological imagery was pushed to the extreme in much the same manner as the *Christi Leiden* Passion narrative. Consider, for example, the sculpted crucifix likely made for a church in the Bohemian city of Wrocław in the middle of the fourteenth century, a deeply disturbing figure with contorted limbs, a face grimacing in agony, and a body caked in thickly sculpted, three-dimensional streams of blood from head to toe (fig. 3.11). The reception of such graphic works was far from universal in Europe. In a much-discussed case from 1305, the Bishop of London, Ralph Baldock, ordered a German sculptor named Thidemann to swear on the Gospels that he would never again make or trade a *crux horribilis* (terrible cross) like the one he had supplied to the Conyhope Chapel of Saint Mildred's Church, a misshapen crucifix that probably bore a particularly grotesque Germanic Christ and that had been removed under cover of night the previous year amid scandal.[86] Back in Germany, by contrast, sculptures of the type seen in Wrocław were becoming more com-

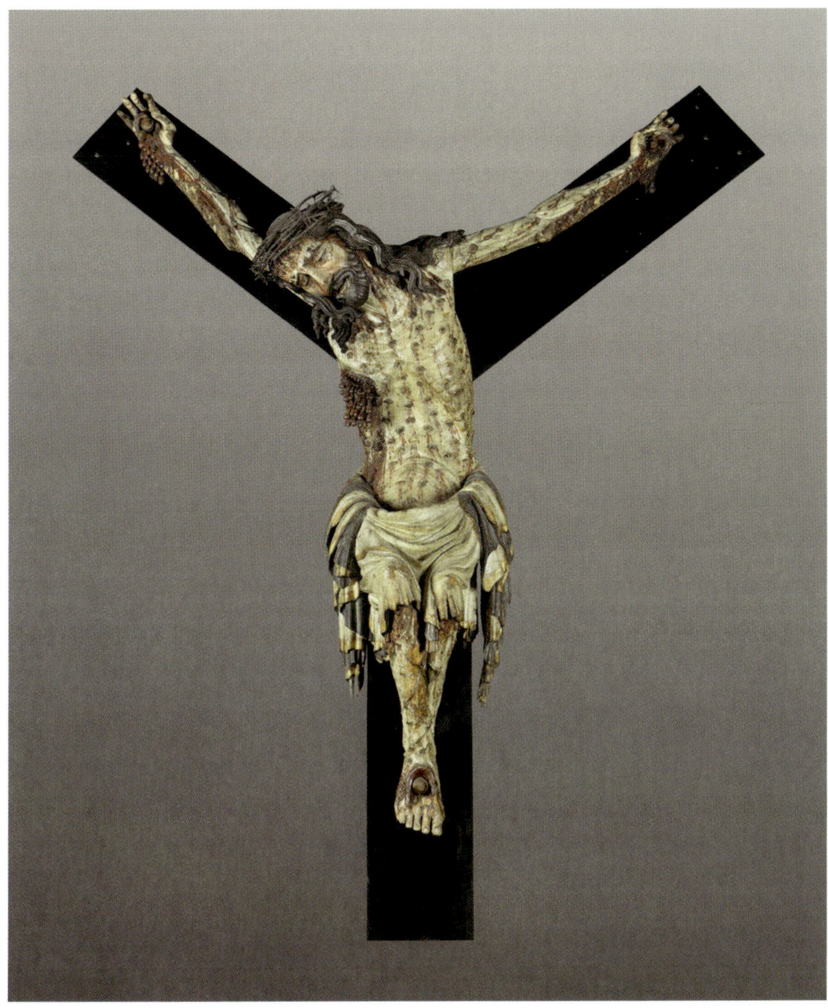

Fig. 3.11. Crucifix, c. 1360, Wrocław. Polychromed wood, 178 x 136 x 44 cm. Warsaw, Muzeum Narodowe, Śr.5. MNW.

mon and their features notably more violent. Recent technical investigation of another fourteenth-century crucifix, today in the Church of Sankt Maria im Kapitol in Cologne, revealed that, a century after the work was first produced, a second paint layer was added to it in the fifteenth century to enhance the bloody red wounds of Christ even further.[87]

Given that medieval medics were so regularly utilizing Christological metaphors to frame their curative practice, it makes sense that the battered body of the Wound Man might itself also court comparison with these contemporaneous and increasingly violent depictions of Christ. Obvious formal parallels can be drawn between their representation of bloodied male bodies in much the same way as we might pair the Wound Man with epic heroes such as Willehalm or Siegfried. In fact, this comparative line of thinking had a rich lineage within contemporary religious works, for instance the popular typology of the *Speculum humanae salvationis* (Mirror of Human Salvation), in which New Testament scenes were prophetically paired with Old Testament and even non-Christian precedents.[88] One surviving copy from the region, made around 1432 in Vienna, juxtaposes a depiction of the wounded

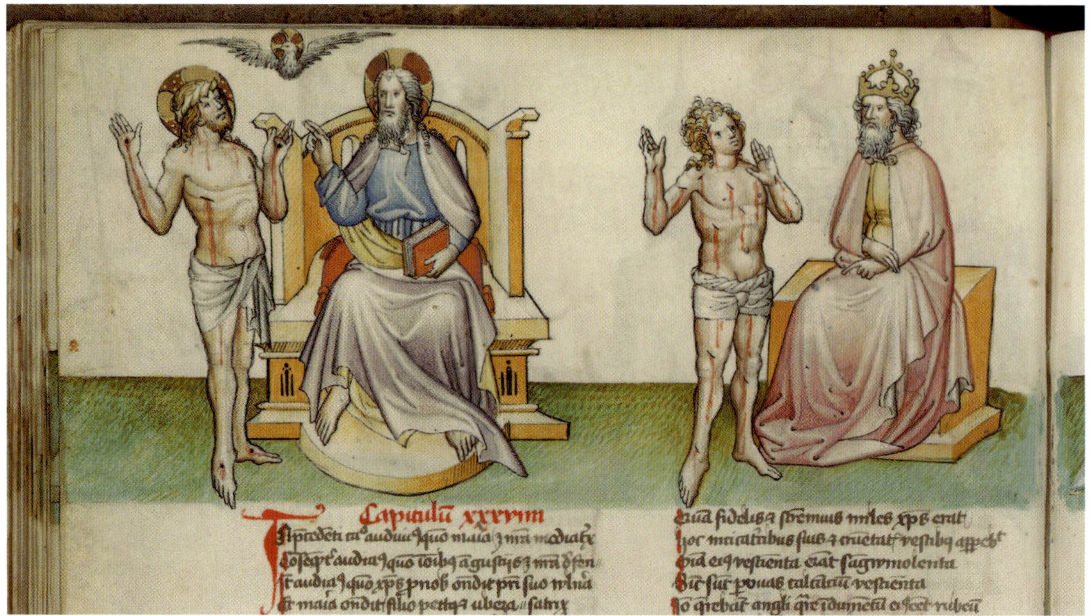

Fig. 3.12. Christ before God paired with the Classical general Antipater before Caesar from the *Speculum humanae salvationis*, 1432, Austria. Ink and paint on parchment, 35 x 26 cm. Madrid, Biblioteca Nacional de España, VITR/25/7, fol. 35v.

Christ interceding with God against an image of the Classical general Antipater baring his wounds to Caesar as a sign of loyalty, both figures adopting the same wide-armed pose to show their scars (fig. 3.12).[89] Were it not for Christ's halo, either could in turn be confused for the Wound Man, who shared with Christ an in-built painful currency: both were seminaked male figures whose wounds—emphasized to the viewer through pose, composition, and sheer number—equated heightened violence with either heightened compassionate potential or heightened surgical skill. The greater the violence wrought upon them, the more impressive each figure appeared within its respective context.

We can push this comparison further. Consider the objects associated with Christ and the Wound Man, the material stuff of two traditions that shared a deep concern for the symbolic potential of wounding things. In the popular motif known as the *Arma Christi*, a flexible and widely employed suite of images that spread throughout European visual culture soon after the Man of Sorrows, Christ's corporeal suffering is conveyed through the instruments of his torture and demise, often without his body present at all.[90] Here the Passion's quotidian tools instead take up the narrative burden of events, an array of miniatures ranging from the whip of the Flagellation to the nails of the Crucifixion to the ladder of the Deposition, all of which mass together in a fragmented ensemble of New Testament moments (fig. 3.13). Functioning effectively as a conglomeration of shorthand pictograms, the *Arma* drew particular attention to the material imagination of the Passion. And in response, late medieval makers rendered these miniature scenes in a variety of media, lending Christ's everyday objects weighted meaning in manuscripts—like the Wound Man, the earliest *Arma Christi* image currently known comes from a book thought to have been illustrated in Prague—as well as in tapestries, paintings, and sculpture on both small and large scales.[91]

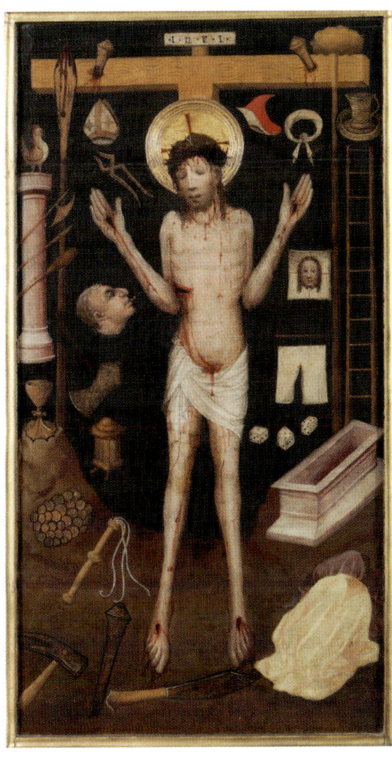

Fig. 3.13. Wounded Christ and the *Arma Christi* on the exterior left panel of the so-called Triptych of the Holy Kinship, c. 1410–40, Cologne. Oil and tempera on oak, 86 x 41 cm. Cologne, Wallraf-Richartz-Museum, WRM 59.

As Bettina Bildhauer has recently argued, paying closer attention to the narratorial qualities of such objects in the medieval German world—what she dubs a "pragmacentric" view—can elevate entirely inert things into far more active protagonists with their own sense of narrative identity.[92] We hear something similar from the twelfth-century theologian Hugh of St. Victor, who observed that it was easy for pain to become passed off on other things, irreversibly entangled with its mediating objects: "*si vulnera et plage non dolerent, quis arma aut tela timeret*" (if wounds and blows did not hurt, who would fear arms or weapons?).[93] Just as with the Wound Man and his *Wundarznei*, the *Arma* come together as a morbid table of contents for Christ's suffering, an act of visual individuation designed in part for mnemonic purposes in much the same way as written Passion accounts could gratuitously list Christ's individual injuries.[94] As such, a particular power of the *Arma Christi* was that it placed the capacity for compassionate suffering even more firmly into the beholder's hands. Through musing on the weapons of the Passion and making narrative sense of their disorder, the viewer held the ability to crucify Christ all over again in their minds, to run events repeatedly backward, forward, or in pieces, as they desired.

This object-based piety was especially popular in Germany, where audiences were regularly asked to objectify emotional pain. German artists tasked with depicting the Virgin's sorrow had for over a century been literalizing the words of Luke's Gospel to show the *Leidensschwert* (sword of grief) repeatedly plunging into Mary's body (fig. 3.14).[95] And we find a similar idea revived and reoriented in yet another related Christological image known as the Sunday Christ, a Sabbatarian missive in which the cause of Christ's

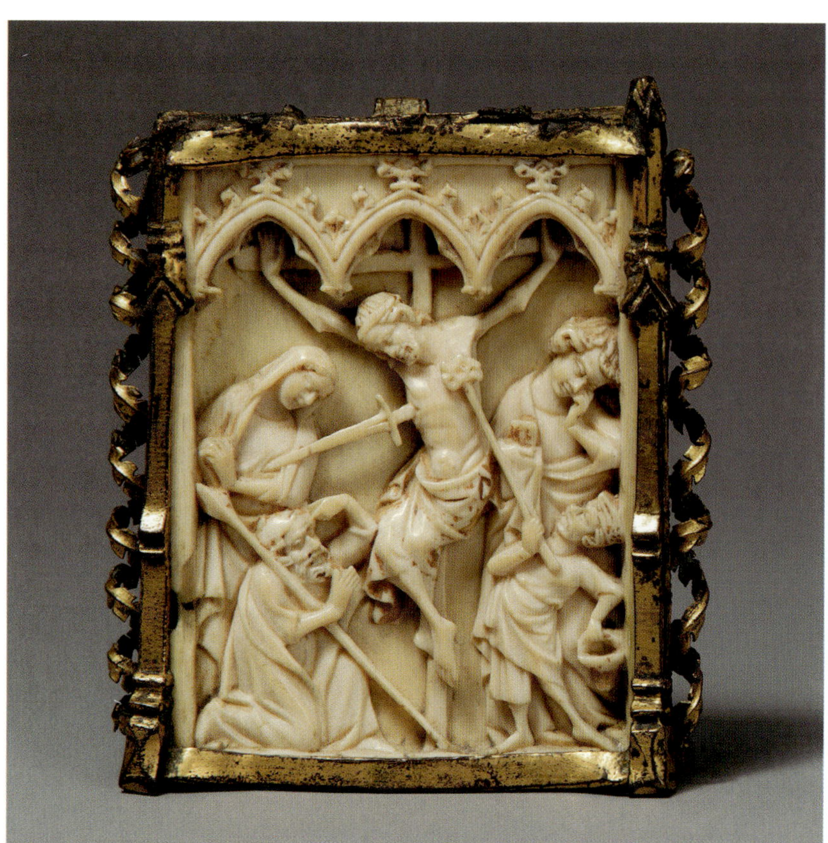

Fig. 3.14. Pax with the Crucifixion, c. 1360–70, southern Germany. Ivory and gilded copper, 10 x 8 x 3 cm. New York, Metropolitan Museum of Art, 1970.324.9.

suffering is the everyday tools of men and women who choose to work on Sunday instead of praying in Church.[96] Among the best preserved of these images—and also probably the earliest, roughly contemporary with the first Wound Men—is a mural completed in or around 1390 on the nave wall of Sogn Gieri Church in the Swiss Alpine town of Rhäzüns (fig. 3.15).[97] Standing like its Christological and medical counterparts with arms raised to either side, this haloed Christ wears only a loincloth, the rest of his body laid bare to reveal dark, dripping wounds. Each injury is linked by a short snaking line to a miniature tool—woodworking saw, wool spindle, rake, hammer, and so on—as if each utensil wielded in vain labor on a Sunday is itself piercing the body of Christ. In some Sunday Christ images, spiritual damage is conveyed by flying arrows or work tools plunged directly into Christ's body, while in others, red lines lead to vignettes of laborers actually at work, harassed by devils for their irreverence. Here we have a religious image utilizing a pictorial device, red linking lines, that had first been popularized in German-speaking lands through medical imagery, both the Wound Man and the widely circulated bloodletting figures of the type discussed in chapter 1.[98] As Achim Timmermann has noted, the Sunday Christ's tools mapped topographically onto logical points of correspondent injury for craftsmen and -women themselves: a slip of the butcher's knife lacerating the wrist, misguided tailor's scissors snipping at the fingertips, a wayward scythe slashing the shin, each one just the sort of accident that the Wound Man was designed

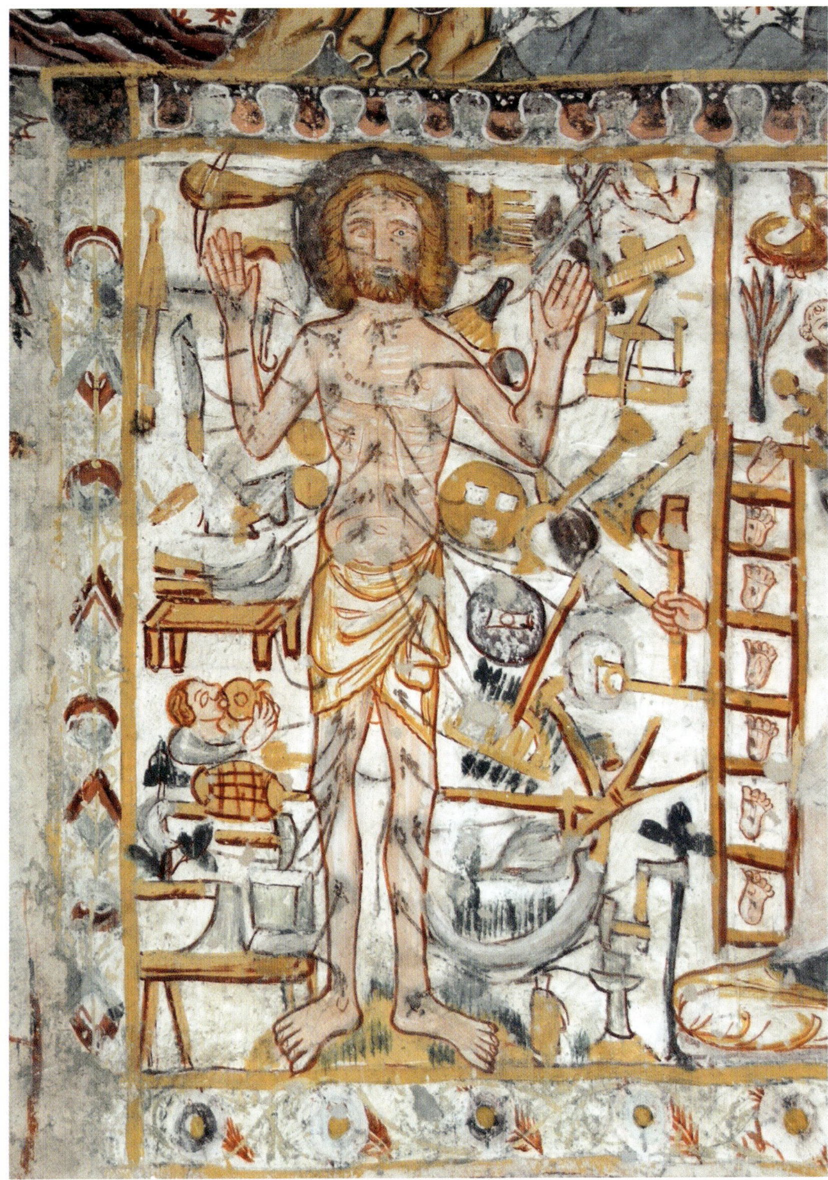

Fig. 3.15. Sunday Christ, c. 1390, Church of Sogn Gieri, Rhäzüns, Switzerland. Paint on plaster, 120 x 95 cm.

to help cure.[99] The effect is a direct correlation of everyday pain with a more expiatory form of religious compassion, all bound together by the framework of diagrammatic medical imagery.

The connection forged by the Sunday Christ between religious violence and more quotidian surgical concerns serves as a reminder that injured holy bodies were of course far more widespread in the period than Christ alone. The first scholarly connection between the Wound Man and contemporary religious practice was in fact not made to Christ at all. Instead, the historian of medicine Karl Sudhoff, in a short 1913 essay, dubbed the figure "*ins Chirurgisch-Groteske verzerrter St. Sebastian*" (Saint Sebastian distorted into something surgically grotesque).[100] This evocation of saintliness is

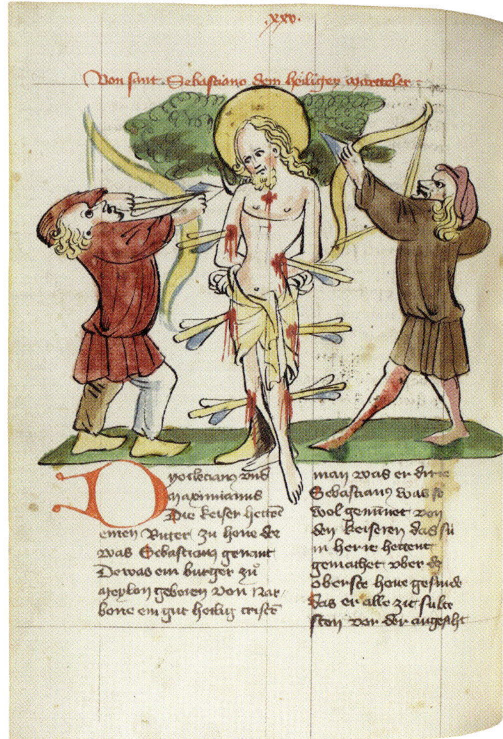

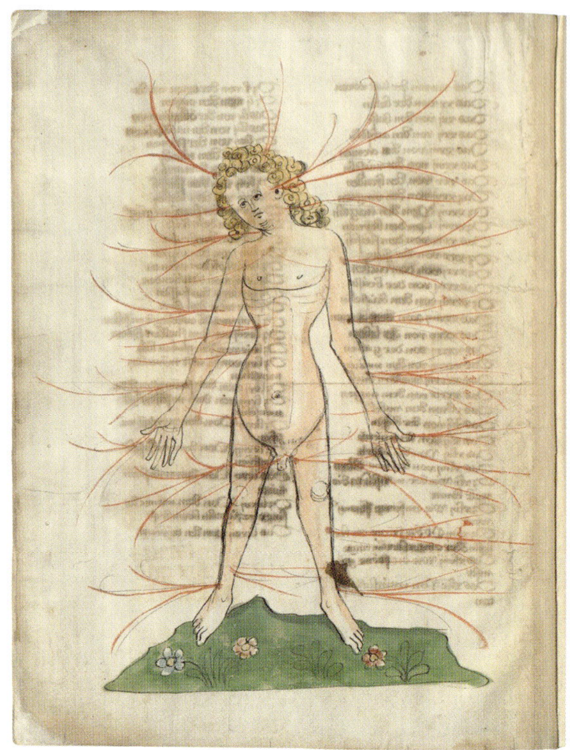

Fig. 3.16. Bloody images from Diebold Lauber's workshop. *Left:* The Martyrdom of Saint Sebastian from the *Elsässische Legenda aurea*, 1435–44, Hagenau. Ink and paint on paper, 27 x 20 cm. Augsburg, Staats- und Stadtbibliothek, 2° Cod 158, fol. 114v. *Right:* Decorative bloodletting figure, c. 1440, Hagenau. Ink and paint on paper, 38 x 28 cm. Frankfurt am Main, Universitätsbibliothek, MS Carm. 1, fol. 2v.

perceptive, for the emphatic violence of late medieval German theology bled just as easily into hagiographies as Passion tracts.

Once more, artists from German-speaking lands working across the material spectrum were particularly well versed in singling out martyrs of the Church through prominent pain, often in an alarmingly decontextualized manner that created what Assaf Pinkus has recently termed a distinct saintly brand of public "visual aggression."[101] In a move that resonated with the proudly borne honor-wounds of romance heroes, medieval theologians such as Bonaventure confirmed that religious martyrs kept their wounds in heaven, a privilege at once taxonomic and glorifying.[102] The graphic image of Sudhoff's Saint Sebastian, for example, which tended to dwell on his torture by archers rather than the final martyred moments of his beheading, was certainly in busy circulation alongside the Wound Man in Germany at the beginning of the fifteenth century, including in some of Europe's earliest printed images, made in the 1410s and 1420s.[103] From the mid-fourteenth century, Sebastian in his graphic torment emerged as a common touchstone of spiritual healing and a particularly important figure in mediating medical and religious worlds. Rolls eaten on his feast day were supposed to ward off plague, and he was often evoked in miraculous accounts of cure, a medico-visual parallel not lost on German artists (fig. 3.16).[104] The Hagenau workshop of Diebold Lauber—the same artists we came across earlier who visualized the wounded exploits of Gawain in Wolfram von Eschenbach's *Parzival*—also produced a series of books containing the so-called *Elsässische Legenda aurea*, the earliest German prose version of Jacobus de Voragine's classic compendium of saints' lives, *The Golden Legend*.[105] Among their pages we find multiple renderings of Sebastian, each vivid in its violence. In what is perhaps the most extensive Lauber *Legenda*, completed around 1440, the saint is shown centrally, bound to a tree, having had arrows fired at him from point-blank range by a pair of caricatured archers, causing thick splurges of blood to run from his body.[106] We are reminded here of another image produced perhaps even in the same year by the Lauber workshop, this one a decorative frontispiece to a copy of the fourteenth-century Bavarian canon Konrad von Megenberg's medical-philosophical *Buch der Natur* (Book of Nature): a bloodletting figure, whose blood spurts outward in all directions with almost comic velocity, tripartite spigots formed from exaggerated lines of red ink.[107] At least for the Lauber workshop, the visualization of wounded, bleeding male bodies in romance epics, medical tomes, and saintly hagiographies all hinged on the same beautifully extravagant violence.

It only takes a brief look through the rest of a hagiographic book such as the Lauber *Legenda* to see that Sudhoff's saintly connection between the Wound Man and Sebastian does not go far enough. Many more of the surgical figure's injuries are paralleled in these images of saintly personnel: the same rock strikes the top of Saint Stephen's head; the same sword plunges into Saint Agnes's neck; the same nails drive through the feet of Saint Felician; Saint Agatha's chest is set about with the same short, sharp dagger; the Evangelist Matthew is beaten with the same clubs; Saint Peter kneels with the same giant cutlass lodged in his head.[108] And as with the compassionate dedication to Christ, so strong was the association of these gruesome attributes with heavenly, martyr-like suffering that they prompted late medieval German followers once more into unusual extremities of devotion. Coming across a striking image in a manuscript from Strasbourg, completed around 1370, one might be forgiven for mistaking its central figure as a strangely dressed saint in mid-torment (fig. 3.17).[109] Stretched long on the page, hands clasped high above its head, the figure's body is beset from all sides: a cross studded with sharp nails and a pair of hanging whips threaten; a snake and toad—the same venomous pests that haunt the Wound Man's stomach—crawl up the figure's legs; a procession of men point up at the figure, thrusting a sponge of vinegar into its face; and above, black devils advance, one poised to drive a carpenter's drill into the figure's cheek. Like the floating torments of the Sunday Christ and *Arma Christi*, these too are symbolic punishments that collapse discrete narrative moments, here not from tales of a saint's murder or Christ's Passion but in the divinely punitive fantasies of the text's author, the fourteenth-century Dominican mystic Heinrich Seuse.[110]

Seuse was one of several contemporary German mystics heavily influenced by the burgeoning theological push and pull of extreme suffering and extreme sanctity, and his religious dedication took particularly corporeal form.[111] This culminated in what was to become an extremely popular semi-autobiographical work conceived by Seuse as a spiritual guide for religious women known as *Das Exemplar*, sometimes referred to in English as *The Life of the Servant*. Channeling tropes shared by other contemporary mystics, such as Mechtild von Magdeburg, Elsbeth von Oye, or Seuse's influential teacher Meister Eckhart, Seuse drew on his own pious life as the

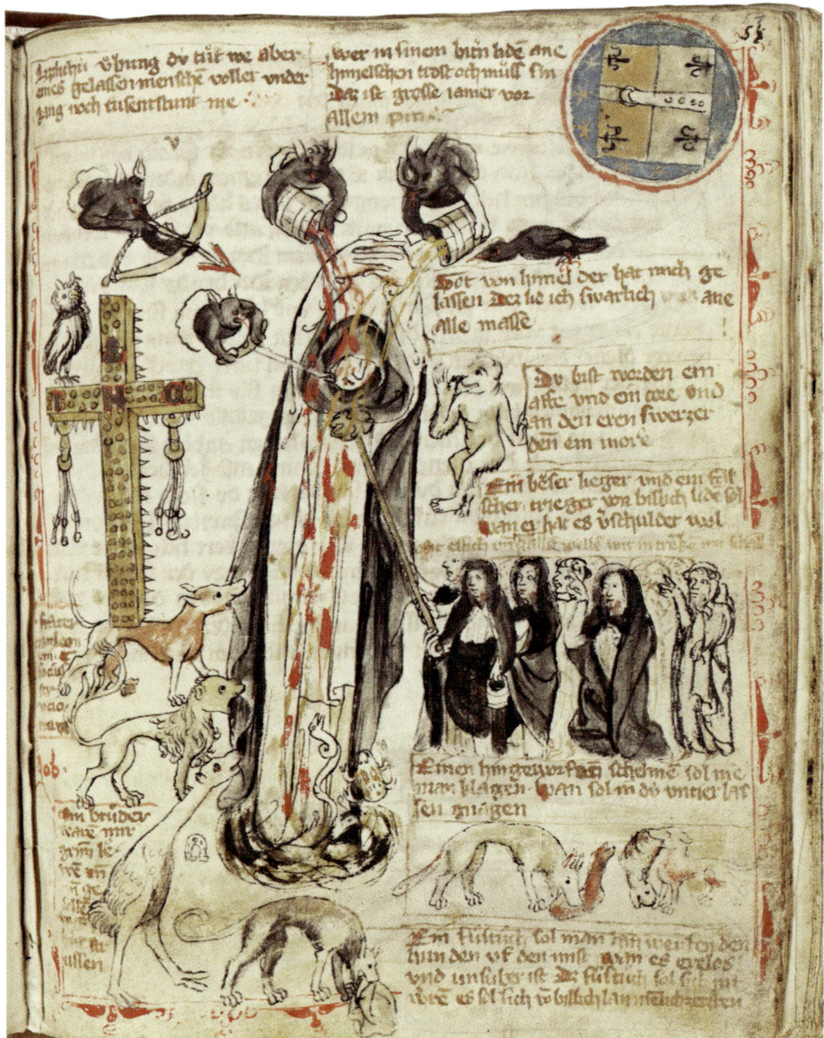

Fig. 3.17. Tormented figure from Heinrich Seuse's *Das Exemplar*, c. 1365–70, Strasbourg. Ink and paint on parchment, 17 x 13 cm. Strasbourg, Bibliothèque nationale et universitaire, MS 2929, fol. 57r.

basis for an elaborate chronicle of mystical visions, emphasizing an *imitatio Christi* that regularly crossed into aggressive self-mortification. A phrase introducing the image on the folio opposite typifies this mystical agenda: "*Diz nagende erbermklich bilde zêget den strengen vndergang etlicher vserwelter gotes frúnden*" (This next pitiful picture shows the harsh downfall of many chosen friends of God). What is being diagrammed for the reader are the text's accumulated torments—shown in much the same way as the Wound Man maps the *Wundarznei*—with multiple tortures made real one atop the other in an overwhelming fantasy of pain.

To pull these religious strands together, we might say that images such as Seuse's worked in consort with a wealth of contemporary religious sources—exaggerated Passion tracts, gruesome crucifixes, bloody martyrdoms—to bring the Wound Man's own injuries, indeed his entire personhood, into contact with a vibrant medieval visual culture of spiritual violence. These texts and images would have been almost unavoidable in the lives of a contemporary reader of the *Dreibilderserie*. Just as much as the valiant, wounded adventurers of contemporary swashbuckling epics, we would be hard-pressed to find a fifteenth-century German who arrived at the Wound Man with absolutely no knowledge of the ideas contained within writings such as the *Christi Leiden* or who had never seen the Man of Sorrows, the *Arma Christi*, the Sunday Christ, or at least some graphic saintly death. The imagery of this violent religious patchwork practiced what the historian of pain Elaine Scarry has eloquently dubbed the "associative" qualities of weapons and wounds, depicted to stand in for violent action and sensation.[112] In the context of Christianized European violence, their association was explicitly aggressive yet salvational, and they in turn imbued the Wound Man with the implicit characteristics of a saintly personage. Descending on the figure en masse, each cut, each blade, helps rebrand the Wound Man's body as a unique medico-religious archive.

Affective Diagnosis and Prognostication

This chapter began with a deceptively simple question: Who is the Wound Man? The words that appear alongside the surgical figure give us few clues. His floating captions present precious little information as to where he sustained his many woes, and the accompanying text of his curative *Wundarznei* is so busy with sharing methods and recipes for urgently tackling his injuries that it never really pauses to tell us how each one came about. As Julie Orlemanski has put it, this is the "melancholy joke" that the Wound Man plays.[113] He seems very much to be someone, his form all too vividly real in front of us on the page, yet at the same time he is somehow nobody concrete at all. This vacuum, however, could quickly be filled. Creative material drawn from a whole range of parallel arenas of Germanic literary culture offered open-minded readers multiple routes for building up a personhood for the figure. They could draw on contemporary cues both secular and spiritual to generate any number of potential contexts within which identities for the Wound Man could grow. But why did this matter? What value did it have for the figure itself that contemporary viewers could so easily project identities onto his deliberately open form?

Contemporary medical thought provides one answer, an idea that hinges on the inverse relationship between anonymity and efficacy. As Peter Murray Jones has shown, by the end of the Middle Ages, concepts of narrative had taken up a central position in European medical writing.[114] In the surgical realm, personalized tales of successful treatment—normally bracketed under the Latin term *narratio*—were presented by literate surgeons with increasing regularity in order to emphasize their exceptional abilities. Boasting of their origination of novel techniques or simply recalling their virtuoso decisions to bring healing to a patient whom fellow medics had given up for dead, they used narratives of cure as both communicative pedagogical tools and upward social strategies. The personalities of these case studies were important. It is no coincidence that such medics gave paramount position to the cure of prominent people, emphasizing their successful treatment of kings, lords, and other well-respected and well-paying clientele. The very authority of a medical text itself was likewise often established through the specifics of the individual testimony it contained in this manner, with so-called *probatur* (witness) statements called upon to attest to the efficacy of particular methods or techniques through real-life stories, a mode we find at work even in the *Wundarznei* that accompanies the *Dreibilderserie* Wound Wan. Moreover, as Eve Salisbury has argued, contemporaries thought that engaging with this type of narrative medicine—that is, both narrations within medical works and nonmedical narratives with healing contents—was a strong enough force to be curative in its own right.[115] Doing so modeled resilience in the face of illness and buoyed the vital spirits of readers to the benefit of their well-being, both mental and physical.

If effective storytelling is thus a crucial part of a medical work's power, the Wound Man certainly tells a good tale. He is after all covered in his own *narratio*, a backstory of objects, each of which a willing reader could track to a range of potentialities. His weapons speak of combat or tournament, his accidental injuries of quotidian work, his wild animals of a rural landscape, his universal diseases of a potential unluckiness courted by all. To put it the other way round, the narrative backdrop of contemporary medicine helps us see that a lack of identity for the Wound Man could have significantly frustrated the figure's curative capacities.

Consider one of the medical notions that dwells at the very heart of the Wound Man's curative matrix: pain. As Esther Cohen has extensively shown, late medieval thinkers of all types considered pain to be highly purposive to humanity, useful morally, theologically, and even historically, just as much as medically.[116] Yet despite its twinned status as both bodily sensation and rationalized emotion, an excess of pain was also understood to fundamentally blunt the human ability to express. Descriptions of pain often fell short. Galen, writing in his *De interioribus* (On Affected Parts), offered what would become a foundational conceptualization of premodern pain, namely that classification was ultimately fruitless given the inevitable shortcomings of expressive language. Pain is always reliant on others to describe, he noted, yet the subjective descriptions of those others—whether patients or fellow medics—were always destined to be extremely difficult to understand.[117] Instead of a quantifiable landscape of pain, medieval thinkers more often framed understanding the pain of others as a highly conditional act, what Anthony Bale has described as premodern pain's close connection to ideas of selfhood.[118] Rather than being determined by the actual gravity of suffering felt, appropriate levels of empathy were instead clarified by the status of the individual in pain and their relationship to those observing. While the pain of the just and the faithful was to be deeply mourned, medieval writings about painful punishment commonly rationalized away the pain of those who deserved to feel it. Criminals who had fallen foul of fifteenth-century legal systems had forgone their right to the compassion of others through social misdeed—what Mitchell Merback has termed a mode of eager "judicial spectatorship" especially common in early modern Germany—while in the religious realm's similar economy of sympathy the painful fires of hell were seen as just reward for spiritual transgression.[119] Knowing this, we understand why it might have been so important for viewers to place the Wound

Man. If a reader did not know who the Wound Man was or how he had come by his pain—to invoke a modern medical parallel, if the reader was unable to take the figure's full case history—how could they know how to respond? Absent a personality, and thus a rationale for his injuries, we can see how the Wound Man's suffering might easily be miscategorized, misdiagnosed, or worst of all, entirely elided.

The Wound Man thus emerges as something of a pictorial empathy machine fueled by multiple associations with contemporary writings, characters, and their associated visual culture. Such empathy had long been understood as a key tool in a healer's arsenal. As early as the 780s, the author of a compendium known as the *Lorscher Arzneibuch* (Lorsch Surgery Book), one of the earliest medical books to survive from German-speaking lands, recognized the fundamental need for medics to feel alongside their patient in order to successfully offer cure. Ideal healers, its text claimed in an echo of the Roman author Cassiodorus, are "*tristes passionibus alienis, de periclitantibus maesti, susceptorum dolore confixi et in alienis calamitatibus maerore proprio semper attoniti*" (saddened by the suffering of others, grieving for those whose lives are in danger, pierced through by the pain of those in their care, and always absorbed in another's calamities, to [their] own grief).[120] By the Wound Man's day, scholastic medics had added to this more complex concepts of *compassio*, often drawn from definitions found in contemporaneous religious and natural philosophical circles, to reorient their empathetic basis toward mechanisms of bodily phenomena.[121] A lack of care was, after all, a central critique of late medieval medics, especially from outside of their field. Francesco Petrarca, among the most vocal of these opponents, spoke in his 1353 *Invective contra medicum* (Invectives against the Doctor) of affective medicine as all but forgotten amid technical debates over cure: "*solebant medici veteres taciti curare, vos perorantes, et altercantes, et conclamantes occiditis*" (ancient physicians used to cure in silence, you [today's physicians] kill while declaiming, arguing, and shouting). It was therefore critical to care about who the Wound Man was. Whether through the varied personnel of contemporary literature or a constellation of religious models, when a tangible identity allowed the reader to empathize with him, his injuries at once became more concrete and, ultimately, more curable.

Crucially, this issue of the Wound Man's pending personality was not something only to be mused upon in the abstract. For some contemporaries, taxonomizing the Wound Man—his pain, his purpose, his personhood—was a matter of real-world consequence, a set of realities for the figure that could be neatly packaged up for export back into the contemporary woundscape from which they came. We see precisely this in a manuscript from the end of the fifteenth century, probably compiled near the southern Franco-German border, which gathers together a wide range of texts on astrology and cosmology.[122] Its primary focus is prognostication, with treatises claiming to aid in the divination of everything from the weather and the course of a sickness through to the personalities and events of an individual's life, all gauged by various extramundane means in the movements of the stars and the semimathematical riddling of numbers. It contains a work authored by the renowned fifteenth-century Alsatian astrologer Johannes Lichtenberger, a geomantic text perhaps by the earlier philosopher Pietro d'Abano, and a group of writings attributed with varying degrees of certainty to the Munich physician Johann Hartlieb, in particular his *Mondwahrsagebuch* (Moon Divination Book), or to use its Latin name, more often cited in other manuscripts, *De mansionibus* (On the Mansions).[123] This text is a lunary, meaning that it contains divinations linked to the moon's course through various so-called celestial mansions, a mantic tradition stretching back to ancient precedents—and in particular developed in early Arabic writings—that used the time of a person's birth to help predict their future.[124] In this German book, it is not only the moon that holds sway over a person's fate but an onomantic formula wherein the letters of a person's Latin baptismal name, as well as the letters of their mother's name, are converted into a numerical total that links them to a tailored prognostication. As the work's opening paragraph explains: "*so mach die rechnung als du wol weist ... wo die recht mansion sey, die im dan zu gehort noch seiner inwendigen natur und auch noch seinen sitten*" (do the calculation as you know ... where the right mansion is, as is proper to him according to his inner nature and also his customs).[125] These divinations were not considered final. Man's *freier wil* (free will), as the text puts it, could well break them. Nonetheless, the work goes on to list the specifics of all twenty-eight mansions in great detail, chopping and changing dramatically over the course of their compressed paragraphs from predictions as to the mansion-dweller's appearance (red under the eyes, gentle face, bad hair, a wonderful head), through to their temperament (lover of all art, a gambler, God-fearing, distant from his brothers), and their lucky or unlucky predispositions (will have three wives, unfortunate around water, excellent in acquiring cattle).

Most prominent among these predictions are divinations on health that note the likelihood of generic diseases appearing and the expected length of the divinee's life, as well as a particular focus on the disposition around their body of various *zeichen*, an interchangeable term that flickers between birthmarks and actual physical wounds that the divinee is likely to one day receive.[126] Conveying these corporeal elements was clearly of particular value to the manuscript's maker, for as well as an opening *rota* to aid in the mapping of name letters onto numbers, each mansion is preceded by the image of a diagrammatic male figure, naked besides a pair of briefs and marked up with neat red slashes that correspond to his bodily fate. These injuries have not been conjured by the author of this divinatory text out of nowhere. Each figure in fact gathers several of the Wound Man's individual painful ills in one spot, his full catalog of woes redistributed across the lunary's twenty-eight figures as objectified portents (fig. 3.18).[127] Mansion-dwellers are shown falling foul of each one of the Wound Man's attributes. One figure, the text informs us, is at risk of being bitten by a dog or other wild animal, shown with a small, bat-eared beast nipping at their ankles. Another is foretold that a stone will be thrown at their head, shown red and round, already lodged above their hairline. Yet more are commanded to avoid swords, clubs, and weapons in general, with the offending items unsheathed from the Wound Man's body and placed into these new images, either clutched nervously in the figures' hands or strewn loose on the ground.

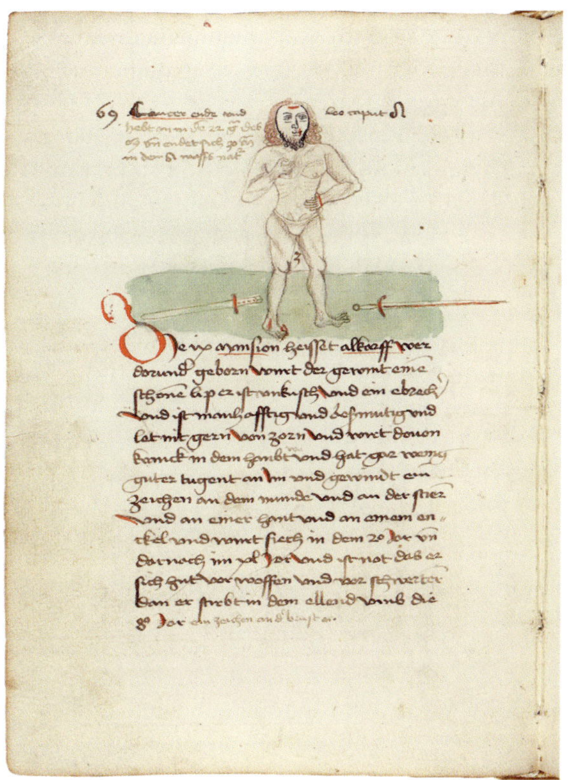

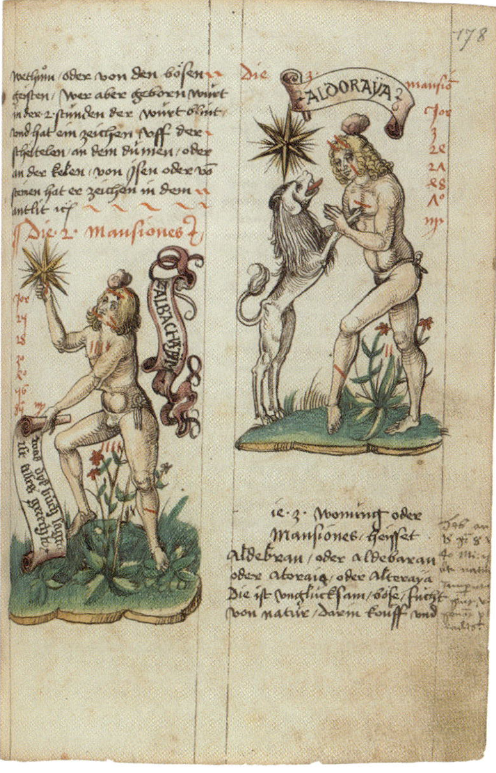

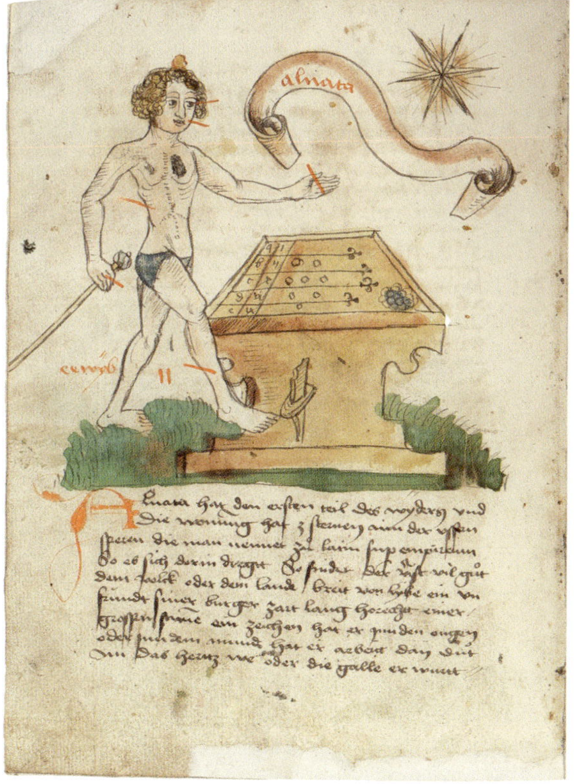

Fig. 3.18. Wound Man as prognosticatory device from Johann Hartlieb's *Mondwahrsagebuch. (In clockwise order)*: Figure of the Ninth Mansion, c. 1490–93, Germany. Ink and paint on paper, 20 x 14 cm. Freiburg im Breisgau, Universitätsbibliothek, Hs. 458, fol. 124v. Figures of the Second and Third Mansions, c. 1490, northern Germany. Ink and paint on paper, 27 x 19 cm. Paris, Bibliothèque nationale de France, MS Allemand 106, fol. 178r. Figure of the First Mansion, c. 1497–1507, Germany. Ink and paint on paper, 20 x 14 cm. Wolfenbüttel, Herzog August Bibliothek, Cod. Guelf. 29.14 Aug. 4°, fol. 10v.

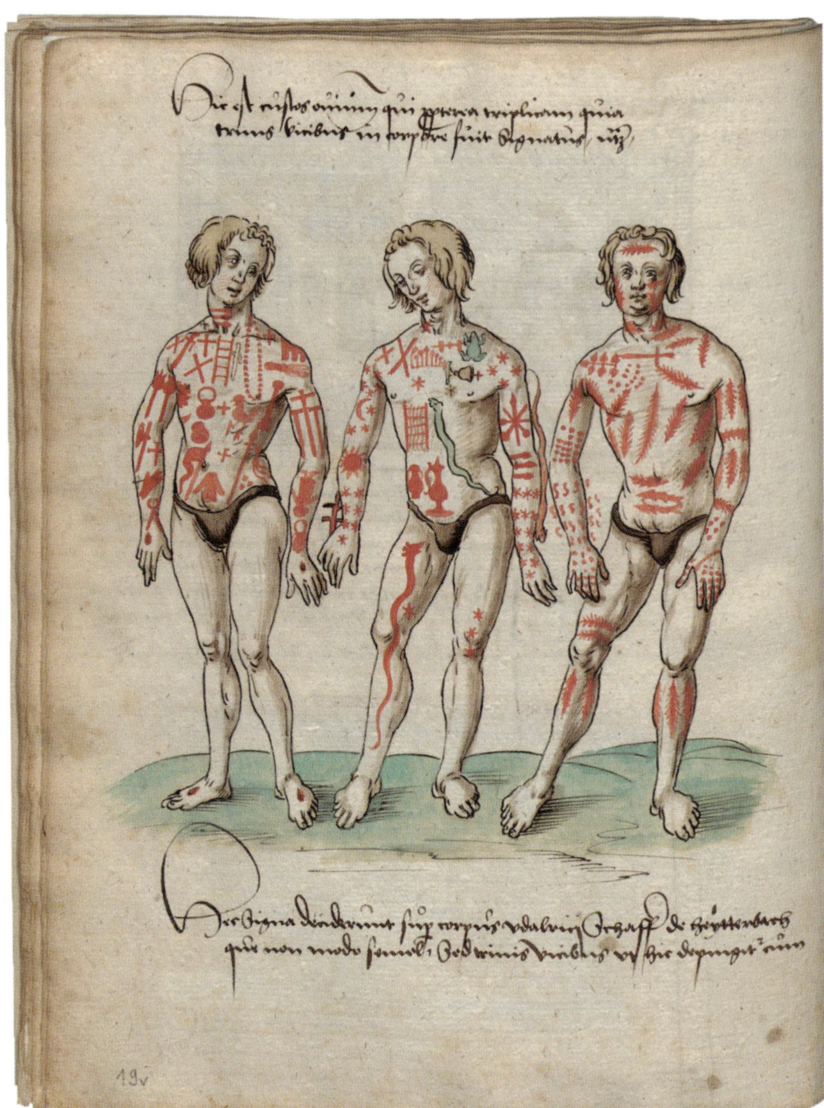

Fig. 3.19. Figures with mysterious marks on their skin from Jakob Mennel's *De signis, portentis atque prodigiis*, 1503, Freiburg im Breisgau. Ink and paint on paper, 30 x 21 cm. Vienna, Österreichische Nationalbibliothek, Cod. 4417*, fol. 19v.

This Franco-German book was not alone. Several other illustrated manuscripts of the same lunary text made in precisely the same period bring even more elaborate, detailed artistry to bear on the same pattern of figures.[128] In one—dated by its scribe, Abraham, to the year 1490—highly detailed Lunar Wound Men pop up throughout with effervescent stars twinkling above their heads, unfurling shaded banderoles bearing the exotic names of their particular mansion. The figures themselves, still slashed with red and wearing blue briefs, play out their fate using an even more elaborate array of the Wound Man's original tools: one named Aldoraya battles off a pouncing white hound at the same moment a rock lodges itself in his skull; another named Almischen traipses his slashed body through a small floating meadow and is bitten by a serpent hiding in the undergrowth; yet another termed Alkraff twists to pull his lover's chest toward him while carrying in his hand a giant threatening arrow. In a third book containing Hartlieb's text, completed in 1497, yet more blue-briefed Wound Men stumble through their cosmic destiny, in one case even shown being bandaged by a surgeon, the connection between the worlds of Wound Man and *Mondwahrsagebuch* made fully concrete.[129]

It was therefore the Wound Man's own openness to the imposition of external personhood—knight, fencer, Christ, saint—that lent his form so well to a book all about predicting personality. No longer merely a bookish diagram, he has here stepped out into the world, the twinned efficacy of his personhood and his healing deliberately entangled. Such an idea was catching. Six years later, when the historian of the Austrian court, Jakob Mennel, came to compose his 1503 *De signis, portentis atque prodigiis* (On Signs, Portents, and Prodigies), a book recording a host of mysterious symbols that had appeared portentously on the skin of several local people that year, we once more find among them many of the surgical figure's wounds, weapons, and attacking animals (fig. 3.19).[130] It is as if anyone could be transformed into the person of the Wound Man, if they were unlucky enough.

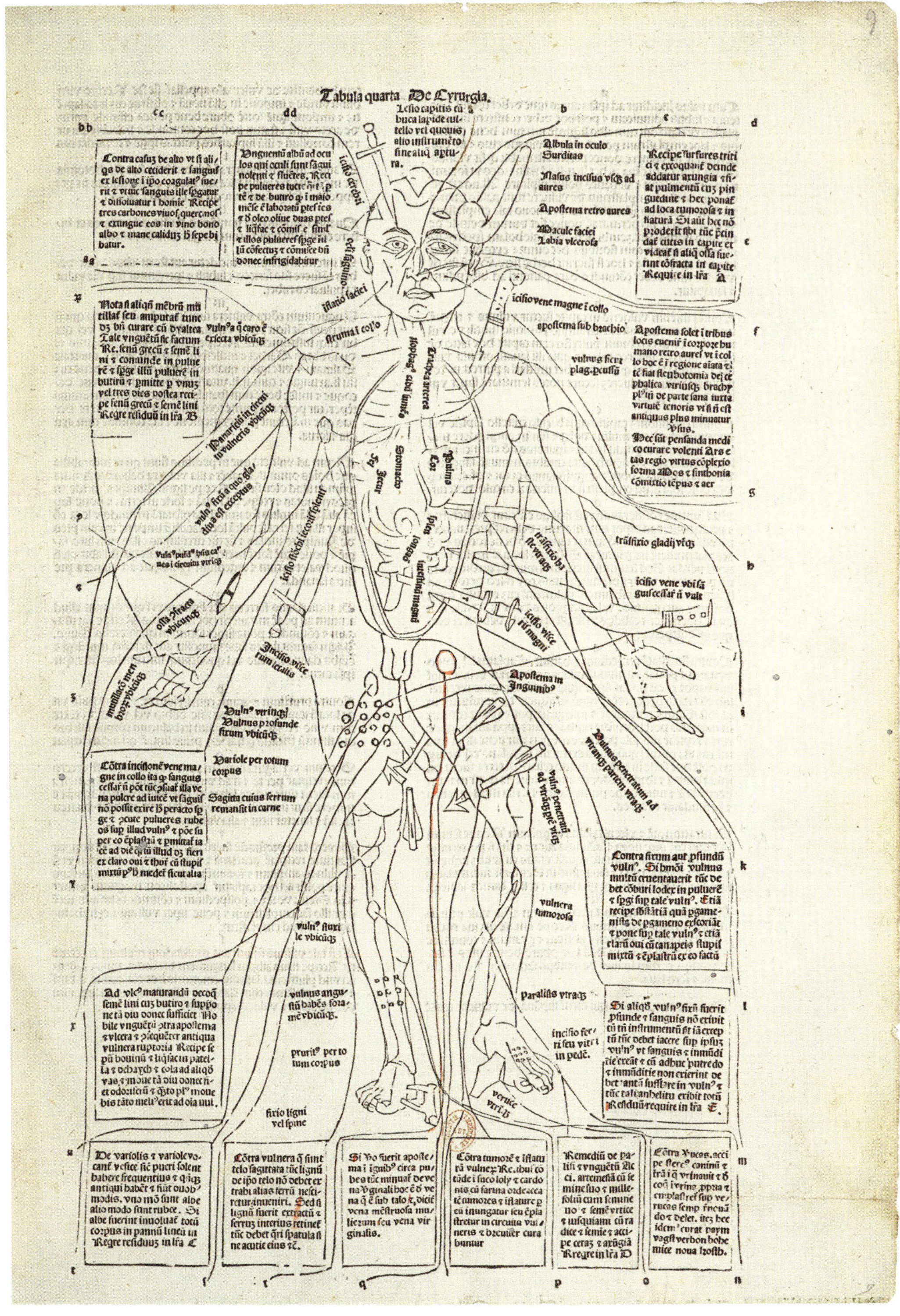

Fig. 4.1. Wound Man from the *Fasciculus medicinae* (Venice: Giovanni and Gregorio de Gregori, 1491). Woodcut with inset metal type, 43 x 31 cm. Paris, Bibliothèque nationale de France, Reserve PET FOL-EB-3, fol. b1r.

CHAPTER FOUR

Into Print: International Intermediality

"Inkunabeln"!—Ein Sport für Bibliographen, so denkt man, so sagt man wohl! Und gewiß geben diese Wiegendrucke den Bibliographen mit die schwersten Nüsse zu knacken!

"Incunables"!—A sport for bibliographers, so one thinks, so one doubtless says! And certainly these earliest prints give bibliographers the hardest nuts to crack!

KARL SUDHOFF, *Deutsche medizinische Inkunabeln*

By this stage in exploring the Wound Man's history, we are well placed to reflect on the unusually multifaceted nature of the figure's evolution across the course of the fifteenth century. This was an image with close connections to many different areas of premodern European culture. Its precursors, as we have seen, lay in a range of dynamic diagrammatic figures, pictures that argued on their own terms through a peculiar yet polyglot visual language. Its own origins lay more specifically in the medical arena, regularly reproduced as part of the inventive *Dreibilderserie* to both visualize and explicate urgent surgical concerns. And, once established, the image grew to embody the multiple resonances developing across different contemporary strands of nonmedical visual and literary culture, from romance poetics to religious piety. So deep are all these contextual ties that it would be easy to typecast the Wound Man as inextricable from its moments of origin, a creature exclusively of the later Middle Ages. But on July 26, 1491, in the printshop of the Venetian brothers Giovanni and Gregorio de Gregori, a version of the Wound Man was produced that was to extend the figure's life into a second impressive wave of action and exchange (fig. 4.1).[1]

A rich tangle of printed lines, body parts, injurious weapons, and curative words, this Wound Man might be less immediately striking than its forebears earlier in the century, less colorful, less gruesomely glamorous. Yet both the origins and consequences of this print are pivotal. This chapter explores these two aspects in turn. First, it develops an understanding of how the medium of press printing—new to Europe in the 1440s and 1450s—dealt with the medical world of the Wound Man, at once suggesting that we expand what we might consider early printed medicine to be, and in so doing that we think through how a figure born of German and Bohemian manuscripts could make its way across the Alps into an Italian printed book. And second, it traces the near-instantaneous passing of the Gregoris' first printed Wound Man into an even busier international circuit of visual exchange, the almost viral spread of the figure both within and, crucially, beyond the medium of the printed book itself.[2]

The story of European print has been told many ways, and as Peter Parshall reminds us, such narratives are all too often characterized by the sheer extravagance of their claims.[3] In the twentieth century, scholars became fascinated by the intensity of print's diffusion, waxing exaggerative as to the all-consuming impact of the so-called Print Revolution on virtually every aspect of fifteenth-century life.[4] This move has since been tempered by more focused approaches, including studies that address the work of particular printers, explore the print networks of specific towns and cities, and, most recently, employ more statistical approaches to the increasingly enormous amounts of incunable information stored in digital repositories.[5] All this work is crucial to understanding the Wound Man's emergence into the print sphere. But tracing the Wound Man through this printed maze—and out the other side—allows us to splice the story of early European print in yet another way: not by its practitioners, geographies, or statistics but by the journey of a single image. It offers a useful case study in how one flexible visual trope might become untethered from a unique medical, cultural, or artistic point and cast instead into an emerging network of thinkers and makers. What the Wound Man affords us is the opportunity to nuance the often-siloed sense of this moment in the history of bibliographic technology, revealing in particular the figure's international and intermedial potential.

Medicine in the Press

How and why did the medical materials of the later Middle Ages, Wound Man included, find their way into Europe's earliest printed books? Even if its all-encompassing influence has at times been overstated, the speed with which printing presses sprang up throughout Europe is nonetheless testament to the close concordance of the continent's artisans, technologists, bibliophiles, entrepreneurial financiers, and—in the case of the Wound Man's story—medical practitioners. Between 1471 and 1480, presses appeared in more than one hundred European towns, with ninety more locations following suit in the 1480s and another fifty founding their first press before the end of the century.[6] As part of this rapid increase, genres of all types were quickly subjected to the press, and medical texts were among some of the earliest to appear on the scene.

This fifteenth-century European printed medicine, however, is an area that to date has been largely overlooked, confined almost exclusively to matters of precedent and convention.[7] Scholars have affirmed that its foundations were closely modeled on those of the continent's manuscript traditions. Unsurprisingly, Classical authorities and their commentaries, the backbone of much medieval medical theory and resultant practice, maintained a key importance in the new medium. Between 1473 and 1481, works by renowned ancient authors such as Galen, Celsus, Serapion, Dioscorides, and the Hippocratic Corpus had all found their way into print, mostly produced in cities within striking distance of important centers of university medicine.[8] This academic market acted as a substantial driver for printed medical texts, a fact confirmed, for instance, by the printing in 1476 of the *Articella*. This extensive and constantly evolving compilatory work, first gathered together in the thirteenth century for widespread use as a medical textbook, was printed no fewer than eighteen times before 1534.[9]

Such long-standing learning was also accompanied in early print by another group of works authored by later medieval European and Arabic writers, again consisting of key texts from the manuscript medical corpus. To take just one fruitful example, consider the medical works printed in Italy in the space of a single decade, the 1470s. This cluster of titles makes clear that medical printing was present in a wide range of flourishing hubs, each of which had been quick to adopt print technologies following their initial European emergence in central Germany. For instance, in Padua, one of the foremost centers of late medieval European medicine, printed editions encompassed a range of works by the late medieval greats: the anatomical writings of the Bolognese master Mondino dei Liuzzi, a tract on bathing by his contemporary Gentile da Foligno, and what was probably the first printed edition of Ibn Sīnā's *Canon*.[10] In Venice, the region's leading powerhouse for printing, publishers oversaw multiple similar works, especially grand collected editions such as Nicholas of Salerno's *Antidotarium* (Antidotary), a medieval pharmacological mainstay, and the more than four-hundred-page collected *Opera* of the eighth-century Arabic author Yūhannā ibn Māsawaiyh, known in the West as Mesue.[11] Meanwhile, during roughly the same years yet more Italian cities premiered the production of yet more diverse medical works: the Latin translation of al-Rāzī's encyclopedic mainstay *Liber ad Almansorem* (Book of al-Mansur) was printed in Milan; the Catalonian master Arnau de Villanova's *De arte cognoscendi venena* (On the Art of Knowledge of Poisons) was printed in Mantua; writings on eye disease by the ocular specialist Benvenuto Grassi were printed in Ferrara; a fifteenth-century treatise on plague attributed to Antonio Cermisone was printed in Naples; and, recognizing the intercultural nature of these texts, a book of regimen attributed to the Hebrew thinker Moses ben Maimon, better known as Maimonides, was printed in Florence.[12]

Medical texts were likewise being sporadically printed beyond the Italian peninsula in this early period. German-speaking lands, with their multiple major print centers and strong tendency toward vernacular works, also generated a substantial amount of incunable medical material, including the first editions of Ortolf von Baierland's *Arzneibuch*—which we first encountered in chapter 2—as well as various bilingual German-Latin books of regimen, the earliest printed vernacular works on pediatrics, and a large number of so-called *Pestblätter*, single-page ephemera offering advice on combating plague.[13] A similar cache of nascent works was becoming available in the Netherlands, most notably some of the earliest editions of the thirteenth-century surgeon Guillermo da Saliceto's *De salute corporis* (On the Health of the Body), printed at some point before 1472.[14] And for their part, French printers, especially those in the popular print center of Lyon, were also mobilizing medicine, originating editions of two further key surgical works written by authorities once local to the city: the late thirteenth-century *Chirurgia* (Surgery) of Lanfranco da Milano and its fourteenth-century counterpart written by the Frenchman Gui de Chauliac.[15]

Although this cavalcade of works from across the continent might seem numerous, the period's boom in printed materials was so substantial that strictly medical books such as these were still very much in the minority. They have been estimated to account for only a little over 3 percent of the total books printed in the fifteenth century, perhaps explaining why their investigation has largely focused on enlivening this corpus via matters of medieval medical heritage.[16] But with such a single-minded view of this material dominating, the strong presence of medicine and its varied practices amid a number of other parallel literary products has gone largely unnoticed. When we keep in mind the field's often porous boundaries, a far more prevalent and expanded sense of early print medicine begins to emerge.

A good example of this phenomenon is the large number of surviving printed almanacs produced in the early decades of the new medium.[17] These single-page prints, which were found first in German contexts and later internationally, quickly emerged among European presses as a popular genre excellently suited to print's emerging markets for cheap, small-scale texts. Almanacs have often been seen as generic compilations of different forms of calendrical knowledge, mostly prognostications distilled from longer treatises by well-known prophetic authors set alongside sporadic predictions based on cosmic and astrological events thought to foreshadow changes in weather, impending environmental disaster, and even political revolt.[18] Yet the astrological concerns of such incunables were also patently medical, utilized in particular for matters of phlebotomical practice and the sharing of appropriate dates for the bleeding of patients to provide relief for a wide range of conditions. Produced in large batches, almanacs were known to circulate individually, to be incorporated into larger-scale practical texts, and also to function publicly, with local authorities often requesting their display on the walls of a city's guildhall to fix appropriate days for bloodletting among local practitioners.[19] Far from a simple refashioning of the academic greats, this was a grassroots proliferation of medico-therapeutic knowledge, and it was a going concern for the very earliest of Europe's printers: the first-known phlebotomical calendar—the so-called *Mainzer Aderlasskalender*, or *Laxierkalender*, which appeared around 1456—was printed using the very same type as Johannes Gutenberg's famed thirty-six-line Bible.[20]

Similar concentrations of subtle medicine can be found in a variety of places. Europe's earliest printed encyclopedias and natural philosophical works—from Aristotle's *De animalibus* (On Animals) to the writings of Pliny the Elder or Hrabanus Maurus—all first produced in the mid-1470s, were compilations that covered many topics relating to human health.[21] Likewise, we might expand our medical net to include more esoteric material appearing in early print that expounded the therapeutic properties of different concoctions, such as cookbooks and treatises on viticulture.[22] Even texts that on the surface seem entirely unrelated to medical topics could nonetheless share valuable healing information. A 1472 booklet on marriage by the Franconian humanist Albertus de Eyb includes sporadic discussion of contemporary gynecological thought, while a 1469 *Vocabularius* (Vocabulary Book) published in the Rhine-side town of Eltville defines enough medical words to make clear that a basic understanding of the field was available to both its creators and its audience.[23] Moreover, as Sabrina Minuzzi notes, the fact that both mainstream medical incunables and these parallel early works were most often published anonymously or pseudonymously surely also conceals the presence of a greater network of medically attuned practitioners and printers than titles alone can convey.[24]

A similar sense of neglect also haunts the early history of visual materials from this period of newly emergent print medicine. In some ways this is more understandable: virtually all the printed works listed in this chapter thus far are unillustrated, and this was not atypical for the majority of European incunables as a whole, their printers' focus more often trained on mastering the complex novel technologies and production lines of movable type and the practicalities of producing a viable book for a volatile market. Increasingly, though, historians of early print are now attuning themselves to the small but important body of images contained within early incunables, both for their technical aspects and their cultural impacts.[25]

It was not in fact long after German presses of the late 1450s began to innovate in woodcut and metalcut printing within their books that images started to slowly surface within the printed medical realm, although, surprisingly, the scholarly narrative of this early visual medicine has to date focused extremely narrowly on only one genre: medicinal herbals (fig. 4.2).[26] This is a story often seen as beginning in October 1475, when the Augsburg printer Johann Bämler kick-started what would become a substantial canon of European botanical printing by publishing an edition of Konrad von Megenberg's seminal *Buch der Natur* (Book of Nature), another work we have already encountered in manuscript form. His book included a handful of full-page woodcuts, two of which present botanical materials discussed in the text for their pharmacological properties, with plants feathered gently into receding layers of a single scene from foreground to background.[27] Megenberg's work was highly successful, reprinted four further times over the following seven years, each time with planted, potted, or uprooted specimens blossoming into carefully allotted spaces alongside descriptions of their natural philosophical and medical properties, their characteristics simply rendered yet clearly individuated: fruit trees standing tall in the background, vines twisting and turning along trellises, the wide leaves of wildflowers hugging flat to the ground. Perhaps inspired by Bämler, at some point between February 1482 and early 1483, the Roman publisher Giovanni Filippo de Lignamine printed an extremely extensive herbal in which each of its more than 130 chapters was afforded a large rectangular print, hand-colored in many editions, showing a particular plant's schematic characteristics.[28] In 1484, the Mainz printer Peter Schöffer published a *Herbarius latinus* (Latin Herbal) in a similar format, its roughly 150 woodcuts each glossed with the given plant's botanical name in German.[29] And similar works soon followed across Europe in Speyer, Leuven, and Paris, as well as two extremely popular expanded

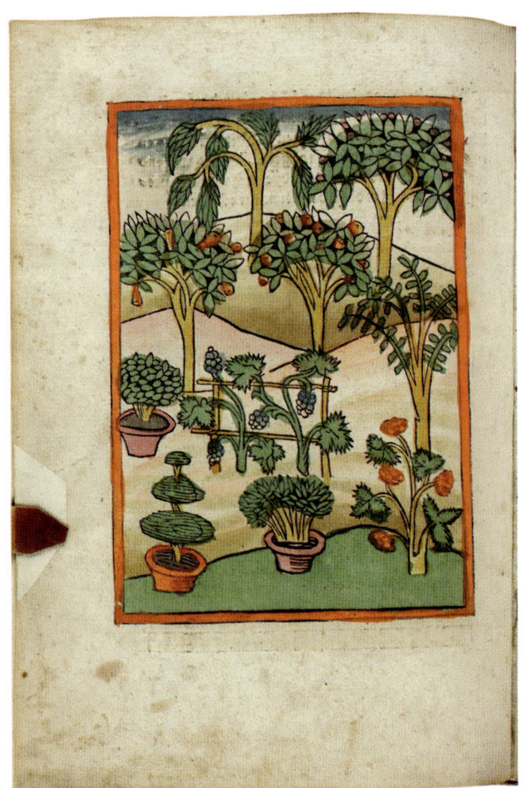

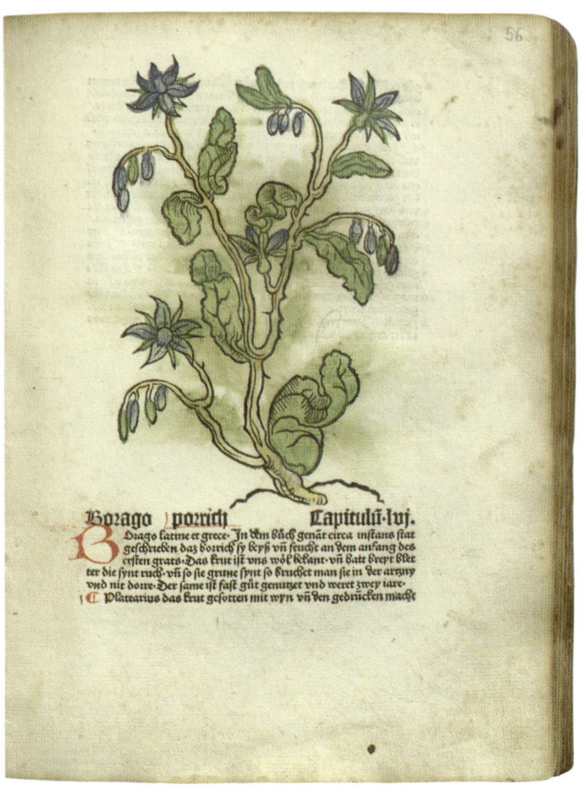

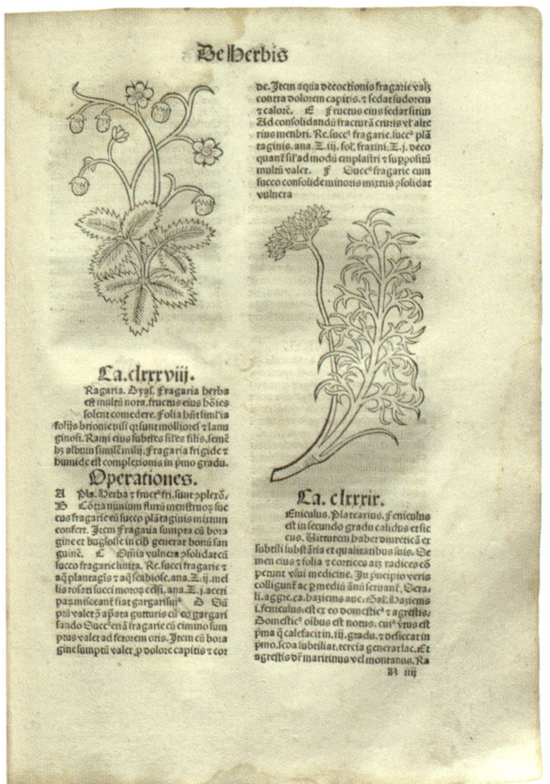

Fig. 4.2. Herbals with increasingly complex imagery. *(In clockwise order)*: Assorted plants from Konrad von Megenberg's *Buch der Natur* (Augsburg: Johann Bämler, 1475). Hand-colored woodcut, 27 x 19 cm. Erlangen, Friedrich-Alexander-Universität, Universitätsbibliothek, H62/CIM.P 21, fol. 183v. Borage from the *Gart der Gesuntheit* (Mainz: Peter Schöffer, 1485). Hand-colored woodcut, 20 x 15 cm. Frankfurt am Main, Universitätsbibliothek, Inc. fol. 131 (Ausst. 135), fol. 56r. Wild strawberry and fennel from the *Hortus sanitatis* (Mainz: Jacob Meydenbach, 1491). Woodcut, 28 x 19 cm. Erlangen, Friedrich-Alexander-Universität, Universitätsbibliothek, H61/2 TREW.G 136, fol. n4r.

editions again printed in Mainz: Schöffer's 1485 *Gart der Gesuntheit* (Garden of Health), prefaced with a grand illustration of medieval intellectuals discussing herbs and featuring nearly twice as many illustrated plants as his earlier *Herbarius*, and the 1491 *Hortus sanitatis* (again, Garden of Health), printed by Jacob Meydenbach, whose illustrations numbered well over one thousand.[30]

Several useful critical ideas have been extracted from this incunable herbal tradition and its equally busy sixteenth-century legacy, shedding light on their novel status as an emergent genre of technical imagery. First, scholars have examined the complex practical, legal, and economic concerns represented by such pictures. Early print entrepreneurs were highly sensitive to the significant costs of their new enterprises, investments that in the extreme were capable of bankrupting their financial backers. Images could serve as rich advertisement for the visual capacities and higher-value markets of the new medium, but equally, if the audience for such expensive volumes was misjudged, they could doom an entire press to failure.[31] Medical printers were clearly happy to gamble, and we know that woodblocks from herbal works regularly passed back and forth between pharmacological printers, sometimes legitimately through sale or inheritance and other times through acts of copying and barefaced plagiarism that prompted attempts at legal recompense.[32] Second, these botanical books have also been explored more art historically as a vehicle by which medical imagery from the rich manuscript traditions of the later Middle Ages found its way into print alongside the texts of early printed medical treatises. We read in Lignamine's introduction to his herbal, for example, that the work was based on a ninth-century manuscript to which he had been granted access in the library of the nearby abbey of Montecassino, and comparison with this original, still surviving at the abbey, proves it was indeed the model for both Lignamine's Pseudo-Apuleian text and its chunky botanical illustrations.[33] And third, these same medical herbals have also been made to play a dominant role in more theoretical discussions of printing aesthetics, especially those around issues of naturalism and the vivacity of images. Partly this has to do with the blurring—sometimes helpful but often not—of aesthetic styles and technical developments, the teleological assumption that a shift away from schematic representations of plants toward a concern with increasingly veristic botanical images was in some way reflective of printing's ineffable technical advancement over time.[34] But more productively, it has also led to the interrogation of such images' epistemic concerns, what Sachiko Kusukawa has termed their claims to "counterfeiting" the forms, media, and knowledge contained within the natural world.[35]

It is important to emphasize, however, that this herbal tradition was hardly the only genre of printed medical illustration to have been produced in fifteenth-century Europe, nor the only form of contemporary medical images to prompt practical, art historical, and epistemic consideration. Take the output of just one prolific early printer, the Nuremberg medic Hans Folz, who published over forty short works in German between around 1479 and 1488, all of his own composition.[36] A barber-surgeon by training and a master of the city, Folz was located at the heart of the medical and artistic networks in which the contemporary *Dreibilderserie* Wound Man continued to circulate. It is assumed that his medical work financially supported what must have been an expensive printing enterprise, and this training certainly had influence over the contents of his writing. Among Folz's more popular works—mostly carnival plays and poetic parodies, often strongly antisemitic—we find many medical products. An early broadside satirizes both the form and language of popular bloodletting calendars, noting that "*die gülden zal ist heür übel geraten pey dem merern teil des folcks*" (the golden hour this year looks bad for most people), mainly because the calendar's prognostications were aimed at "*dausent eyer unnd cccc pratwürst und lxxx pfaffen*" (one thousand eggs and four hundred sausages and eighty priests).[37] Another early piece, *Von einem griechischen Arzt* (The Greek Quack) from 1479, skewers the elaborate recipes of the medical profession in knowing terms:

und wer do sech ein rawch auff gon
von einem feur von schne gemacht
des nem zu ostern vor fasnacht
mit acht lot milcz von zweyn socken
und des gederms von einem rocken
das als sol man zu reyben cleyn
mit zwey lot newes mones scheyn . . .
wer das temperirt es wirt nit arck
doch man es vor am sascz versuch
des nis der siech auf virczehen schuch
gemessen vor der stuben thür.

and when you see smoke rising
from a fire made out of snow,
take of this at Easter before Carnival
with eight measures of spleen from two socks
and the intestines of a frock,
which you should grate very finely
with two lots of new moonlight . . .
whoever mixes this will have no trouble,
but only if one tries it first with some sauce.
The invalid takes this at fourteen feet
measured from the door of the room.[38]

More serious medical texts by Folz also survive, nearly all of which open with half- or full-page woodcuts commissioned from unknown makers to reproduce extant visual traditions of fifteenth-century manuscript medicine. At the beginning of his 1482 *Von der Pestilenz* (On Plague), a versified set of instructions against the disease, an entire page is given over to the image of a doctor lancing a boil in the armpit of a grotesque plague victim, stripped to his underwear and covered in lumpy buboes (fig. 4.3).[39] By the time of his death in 1513, Folz's books had presented readers with an impressively wide

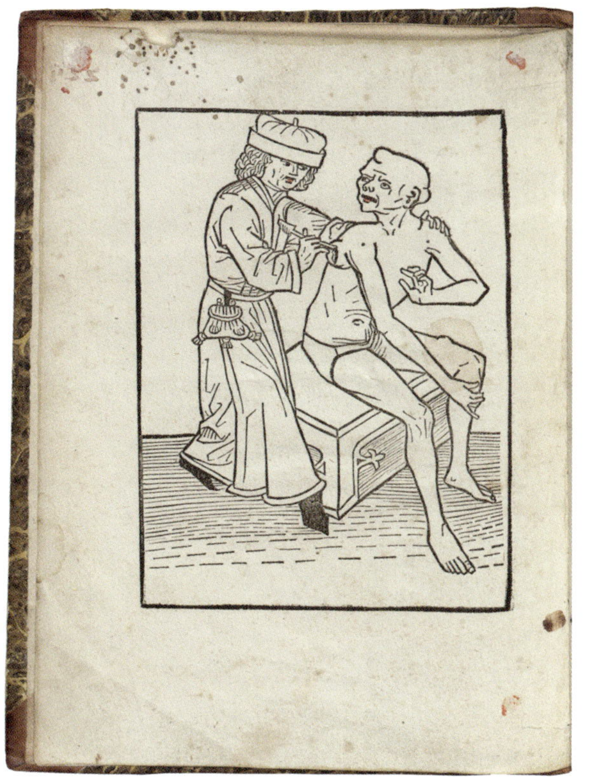

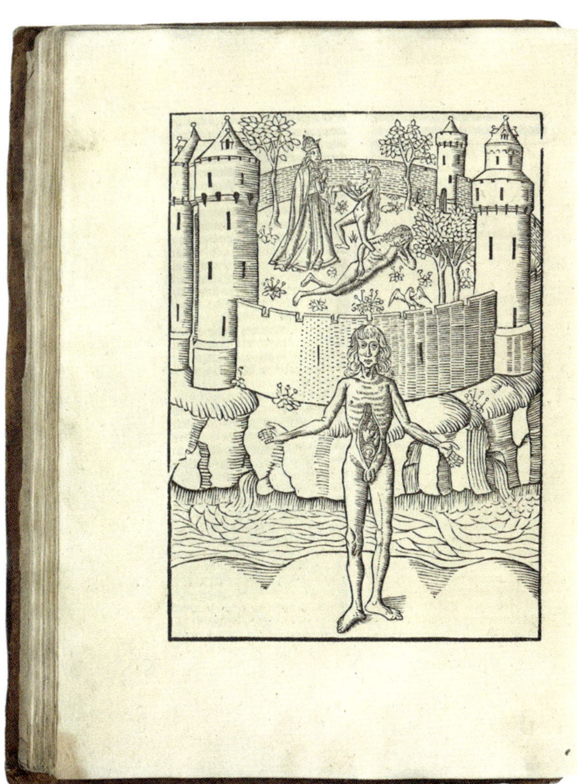

Fig. 4.3. Doctor lancing a patient's bubo from Hans Folz's *Von der Pestilenz* (Nuremberg: Hans Folz, 1482). Woodcut, 18 x 14 cm. Munich, Bayerische Staatsbibliothek, Rar. 185, fol. 1v.

Fig. 4.4. Anatomical figure and the Creation of Eve from Bartholomew the Englishman's *Van den proprieteyten der dinghen* (Haarlem: Jacob Bellaert, 1485). Woodcut, 24 x 17 cm. Valenciennes, Bibliothèque municipale, INC 45, fol. c4v.

range of other well-known medical images in print, from scenes of therapeutic bathing and distillation to portraits of historical physicians in conversation and iconic images of healing personalities such as Saint Sebastian, the last appealing to what by this point was a highly developed marketplace for printed evocations of the saint for curing plague.[40]

Showcasing far more than printed plants, the trajectory of Folz's increasing use of a variety of medical images holds firm for incunables more widely. From the early 1480s, medical readers could find in print a large number of visualizations familiar to them from manuscripts of the previous century, including scenes of physicians examining urine flasks, patients having blood taken from the elbow, chiromantic hand-diagrams covered in portentous symbols, fully realized anatomy scenes showing assembled medics disputing over unpacked cadavers, and even figures standing in front of religious scenes presenting their bisected innards for the reader's own examination (fig. 4.4).[41] But by far the most common element of this evolving printed visual medicine was another import from earlier traditions: diagrammatic human figures, images even more ubiquitous in printed books than the bountiful botany of pharmacological texts. As with their manuscript histories, discussed in chapter 1, such figures once again seem to have undertaken important conceptual groundwork for the Wound Man, affirming the connection between medical knowledge and the schematic use of the human form in the minds of both early printers and their audiences.

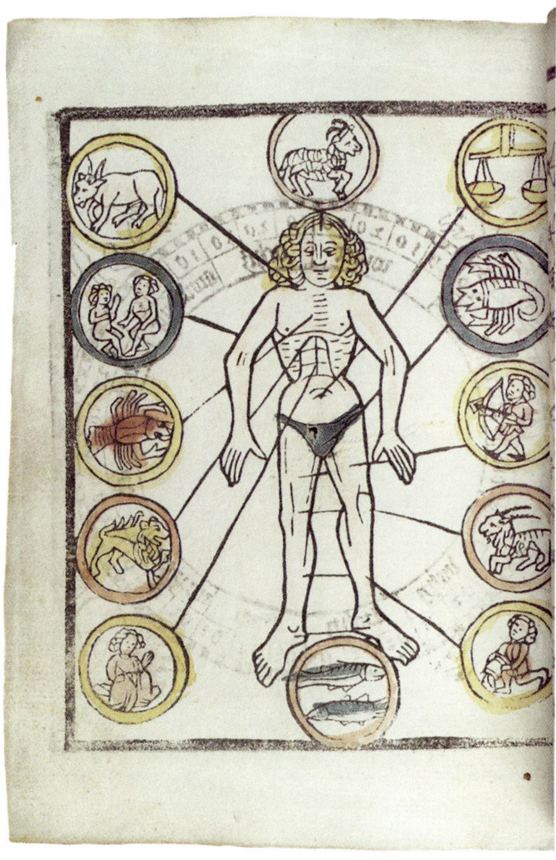

Fig. 4.5. Zodiac Man, c. 1457, central Germany. Hand-colored woodcut, 14 x 10 cm. Wolfenbüttel, Herzog August Bibliothek, Cod. Guelf. 1189 Helmst., fol. 9r.

The first to feature in printed works were bloodletting figures, which appeared initially in the output of German presses that began, from the early 1480s, to produce editions of the so-called *Teutsch Kalender* (German Calendar), a short but influential booklet covering issues of astro-medicine and the fundamental linking of the body and the heavens as a vital arbiter of human health. The earliest such text to survive was produced in 1481 by the Augsburg printer Johann Blaubirer, who looked to capitalize on the marketing potential of this medical subspecialty's all-encompassing remit by producing an initial version of the *Kalender*.[42] His book was itself effectively a print iteration of an earlier medieval genre, the so-called Iatromathematical Housebook, and as Francis Brévart has shown, the 1481 edition was produced directly from a manuscript tradition stretching back to the early 1400s, drawing too on midcentury xylographic printed precedents (fig. 4.5).[43] Blaubirer's text incorporated a range of treatises typical of these pan-disciplinary books, including a yearlong calendar alongside short works on the labors of the months, the signs of the zodiac, the planets, the winds, and other assorted cosmological and medical concerns, almost all of which were accompanied by woodblock illustrations commissioned from a now-anonymous artist. In Blaubirer's 1483 edition of the *Kalender*, this astrological material was joined by another familiar schematic body, a male bloodletting figure, who was also given his own

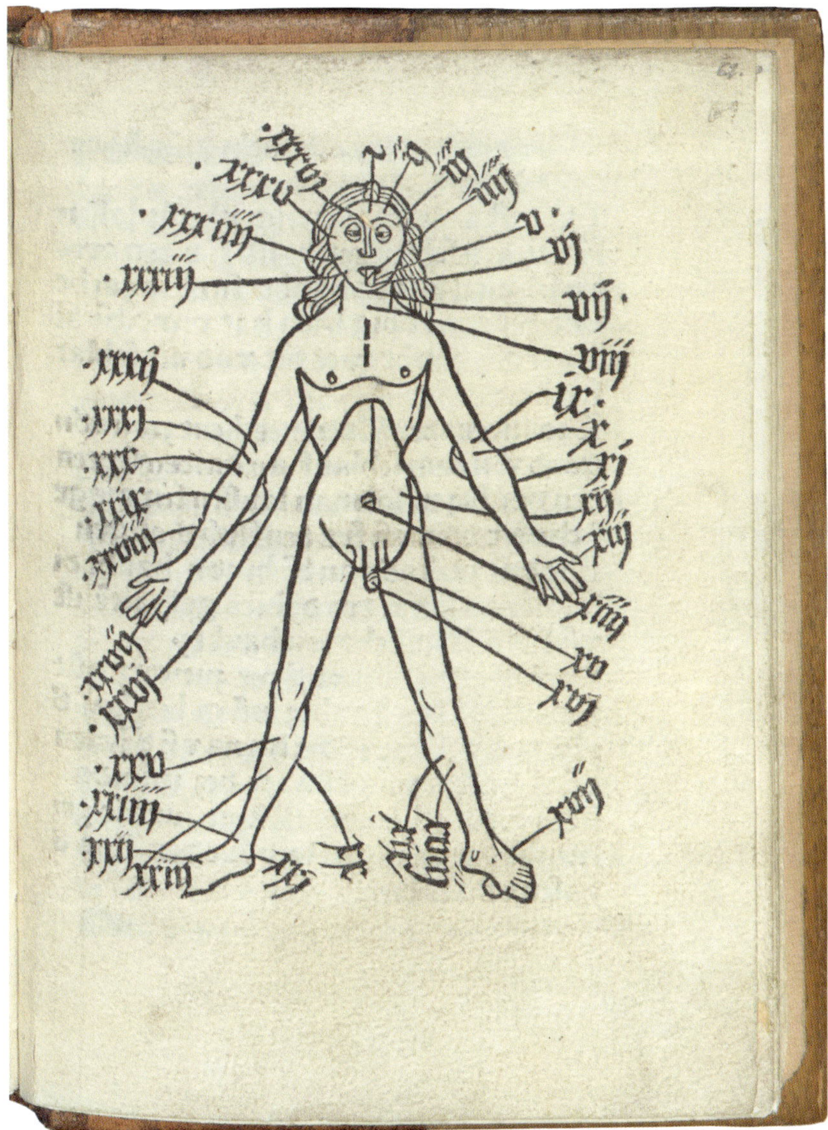

Fig. 4.6. Bloodletting figure from the *Teutsch Kalender* (Augsburg: Johann Blaubirer, 1483). Woodcut, 17 x 13 cm. Augsburg, Staats- und Stadtbibliothek, 4 Ink 162, fol. h8r.

full page toward the back of the book (fig. 4.6).[44] This diagrammatic man adopts the same splayed stance and stuck-out tongue as previous manuscript iterations, while also retaining the crucial technical capacity of earlier versions of the image to link body and text. Each of the figure's bloodletting sites is numbered, keyed in correspondence to particular relevant passages of a bloodletting treatise that follows the image, with thirty-six points emanating elegant lines carved smoothly from the wooden block, snaking their way up to the spiky, xylographic *X*s, *V*s, and *I*s of Roman numerals that explode at the figure's edge like miniature fireworks.

The immense popularity of such bloodletting figures is attested by their repeated presence across the early print landscape. At present, at least thirty-three editions of the *Teutsch Kalender* by multiple printers have been identified

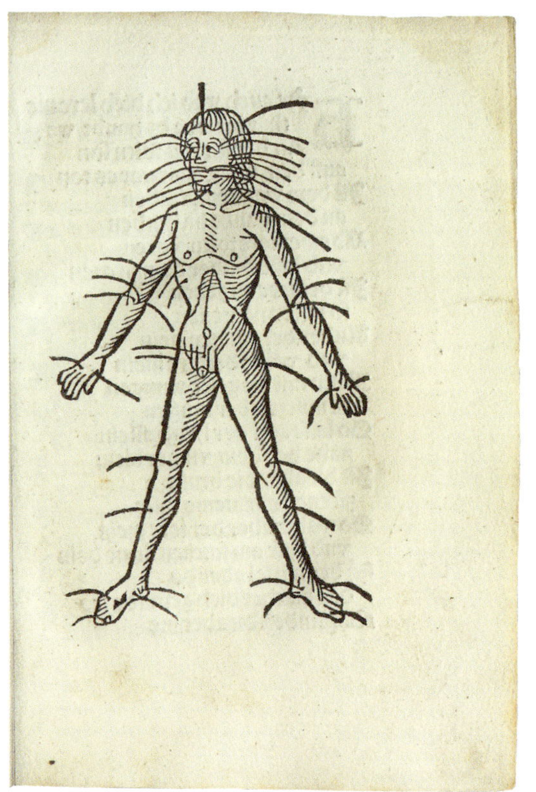

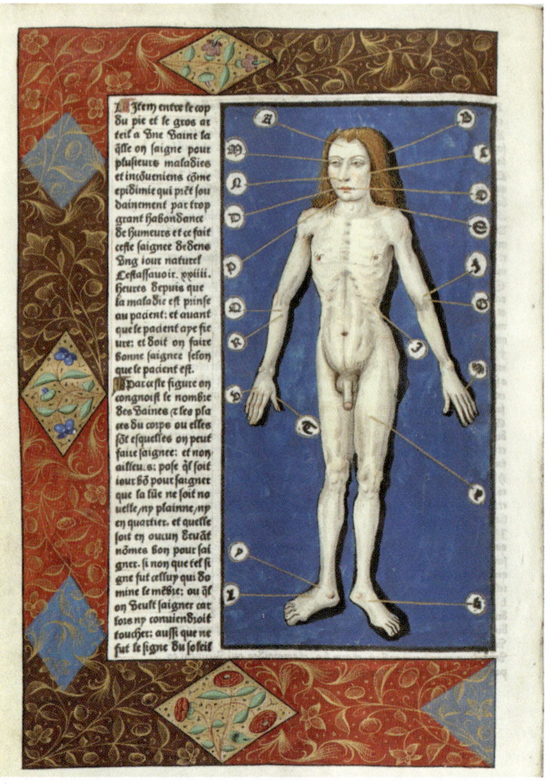

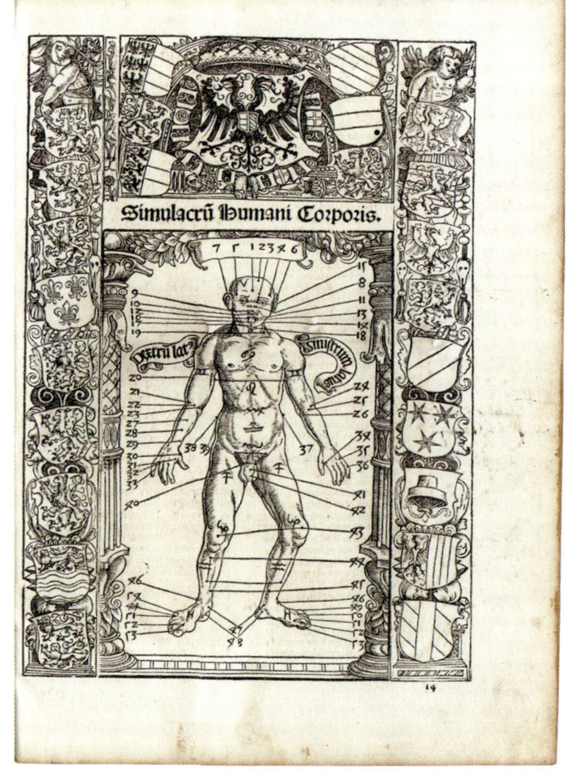

Fig. 4.7. Early printed bloodletting figures. *(In clockwise order)*: Bloodletting figure from Heinrich von Laufenberg's *Versehung des Leibes* (Augsburg: Erhard Ratdolt, 1491). Woodcut, 15 x 10 cm. Wolfenbüttel, Herzog August Bibliothek, 167.9 Poet, fol. l5r. Bloodletting figure from the *Calendrier des bergers* (Paris: Guy Marchant, 1493). Hand-colored woodcut, 25 x 20 cm. Paris, Bibliothèque nationale de France, VELINS-518, fol. h3r. Bloodletting figure from Johannes Stöffler's *Calendarium Romanum magnum* (Oppenheim: Jakob Köbel, 1518). Woodcut, 29 x 20 cm. Zürich, Bibliothek der ETH, Rar 8909, fol. 14r.

between 1481 and 1522, every one of which features increasingly intricate, diagrammed phlebotomical men (fig. 4.7).[45] In 1491, the earliest known French-language printed astro-medical treatise appeared, produced under the title *Calendrier des bergers* (Shepherds' Calendar) by Parisian printer Gui Marchant, affirming such figures' widening appeal in translation.[46] The same year saw an edition of Heinrich von Laufenberg's *Versehung des Leibes* (Care of the Body), a text that came complete with an extravagant and entirely decorative pseudo-bloodletting figure whose cross-hatched body sprouts miniature decorative fountains of blood from punctures in his veins but with no corresponding phlebotomical text.[47] And by the early sixteenth century, the image was appearing in influential scholarly works, for instance in the Tübingen professor Johannes Stöffler's *Calendarium Romanum magnum* (The Great Roman Calendar)—a proposal for reworking the entire European calendar—where it featured in extravagant heraldic surrounds labeled as a "*simulacrum humani corporis*" (simulacrum of the human body), showcasing no fewer than forty-nine bloodletting locations.[48]

Just as these diagrammatic images proliferated, so too did their audience. The fact that such figures survive in both their unadorned original printed form and also in extremely elaborate hand-colored editions, complete with expensive rubrication and decoration, suggests that they would have entered the market at a variety of price points in order to attract a broad potential readership drawn from different parts of the fifteenth-century European social spectrum.[49] Moreover, the eagerness of early printers to usher such figures across boundaries of textual genre suggests an interest in mobilizing their diagrammatic forms as widely as possible for different types of potential readers.

To get a sense of just how fluid this movement could be, we might again look across the work of a single printer, this time the Strasbourg press of Johann Prüss, active from the late 1470s until his death in 1510.[50] Prüss's publishing range was particularly impressive for a printer of this period, spanning nearly 250 editions, from *Schwankromane* (folk tales) to Latin and vernacular editions of Classical writings and multiple religious works and their commentaries—including several gargantuan, multivolume Bibles—as well as grammar books, imperial edicts, travel itineraries, and statute books. A portion of this output encompassed the medical, including a printing in either 1483 or 1484 of his edition of the *Teutsch Kalender* first pioneered by Blaubirer.[51] Prüss significantly developed his version of the work, incorporating into his Strasbourg edition both amended texts and reformulated images. Once again, the only visualization granted a full page all to itself is a diagrammatic figure, and not just a bloodletting image but a hybrid schematic of shared astrological and phlebotomical intent (fig. 4.8). Rather than floating abstractedly on the page, the figure commissioned by Prüss now stands relatively firmly on grassy ground, and instead of individual bloodletting points, he is surrounded on either side by a grid showing the twelve zodiac signs, each linked to its area of general phlebotomical influence by a thin line emanating from a small notch or slit in the figure's body, as if it were let blood snaking out from a wound. Strikingly, the figure is also visually anatomized, his inner organs revealed through an incision from beneath the chin down to

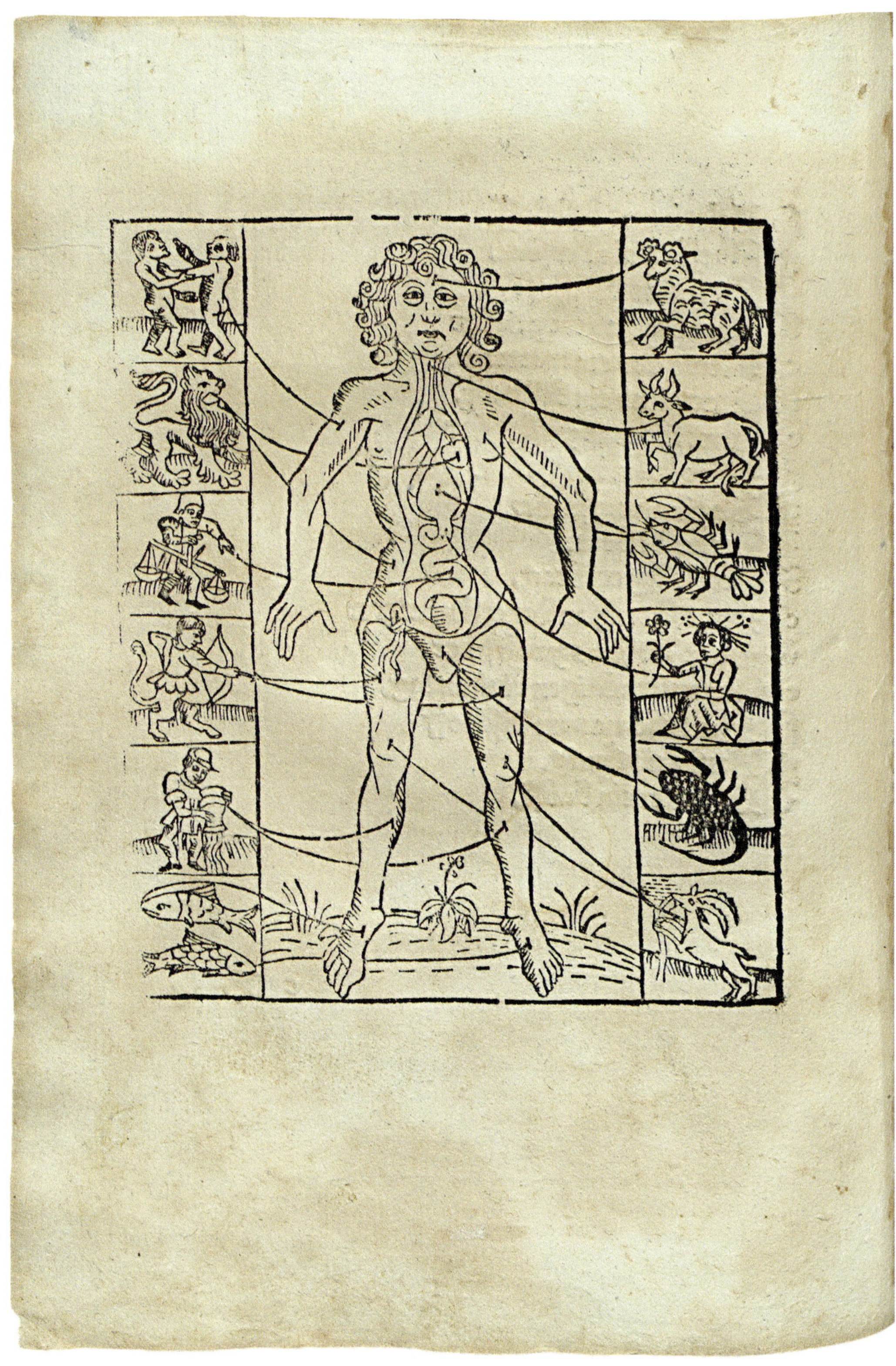

Fig. 4.8. Hybrid bloodletting-zodiac figure from Johann Prüss's *Kalender* (Strasbourg: Johann Prüss, c. 1483). Woodcut, 21 x 15 cm. Gießen, Universitätsbibliothek, Ink S 67065(3), fol. c4v.

the groin, suggesting that its now-anonymous maker was familiar not only with manuscript bloodletting figures but also with the *Dreibilderserie* Wound Man or Disease Woman, whose bodies similarly expose the contents of their torso to the viewer.

This figure was to dance around Prüss's oeuvre for over a decade (fig. 4.9). Within a year of its initial appearance, the image had already begun to spring up in new contexts, appearing as a visual conclusion to the opening calendar section of his 1484 *Martyrologium der Heiligen* (Martyrology of the Saints).[52] This was not an astrological text but a religious martyrology that mapped a full year's worth of feast days, prayers, and other religious practices associated with a local catalog of Christian saints. Yet here Prüss's bloodletting figure is the visual star of the book, which contains only a handful of other tiny astrological visualizations and not even any images of the very saints to whom the work's rituals were designed to appeal.[53] Not satisfied with only reviving his figure in a religious setting, later in the same year Prüss put the woodblock to work yet again, this time in pursuit of audiences with more specifically astrological interests as part of his first attempt at a printed broadside almanac.[54] Prüss clearly saw the image as a fitting way to enliven the page, tucked at the bottom of a long doubled sheet whose calendrical and prognosticatory text is topped with a wide woodcut showing seated holy figures and flanked by a pair of decorative borders, one writhing with playful grotesques and the other inhabited by personifications of the planets.[55] The efficacy of this image in almanac form must have stayed with Prüss, for it appeared several years later, in 1494, in another of the printer's extravagant broadsides where it is presented to the reader in an even more overtly medicalized setting. Here the double page concludes with a cluster of images at its base, small windows showing scenes of bloodletting, cupping, the repair of a dislocation, and the administering of medicaments to an ailing bedbound patient, all set around Prüss's earlier hybrid figure.[56] We even seem to find the figure spilling out from the Prüss workshop and into the work of his competitors. One almanac from around 1490, attributed on the basis of its typography to a Basel printer known only as the Printer of the Form der Copyen, ends abruptly at its base, either a deliberate cut for the page to be reused or perhaps where a second page, now lost, would have taken up the reins.[57] But just before the paper breaks, we see the unmistakable head of Prüss's hybrid woodblock. How is he here? Is this almanac in fact the work of Prüss's press? Or was the woodblock closely copied, sold, stolen? With only this incomplete sheet known to have survived, specific answers are hard to come by. But the back-and-forth of this diagrammatic man makes clear that such imagery remained a central part of an incunable printer's medico-visual arsenal, used to plot ideas onto patients in a way that both enlivened the intellectual value of their works and bolstered their aesthetic appeal to readers.

We can safely say, therefore, that printers of the late fifteenth century had a far greater and more varied range of medical investments than just the floral *materia medica* with which they populated botanical books. In fact, we might briefly return to Johann Bämler's edition of the *Buch der Natur*—the work hoisted as foundational to early print herbals—and note that even this book does not actually open with an image of a plant. Instead, after a short outline

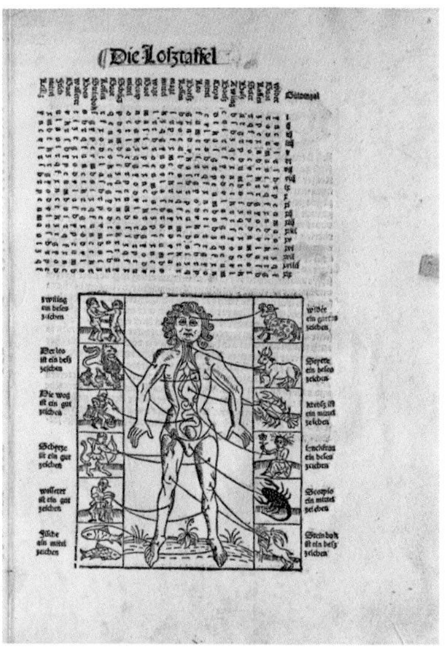

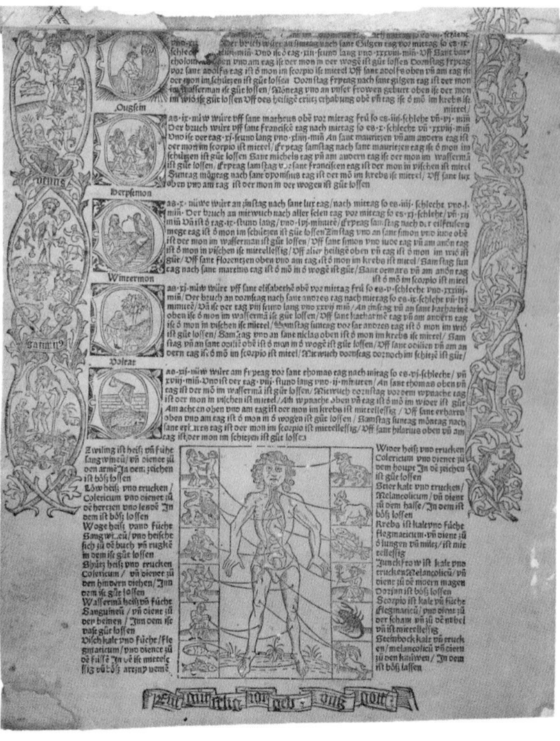

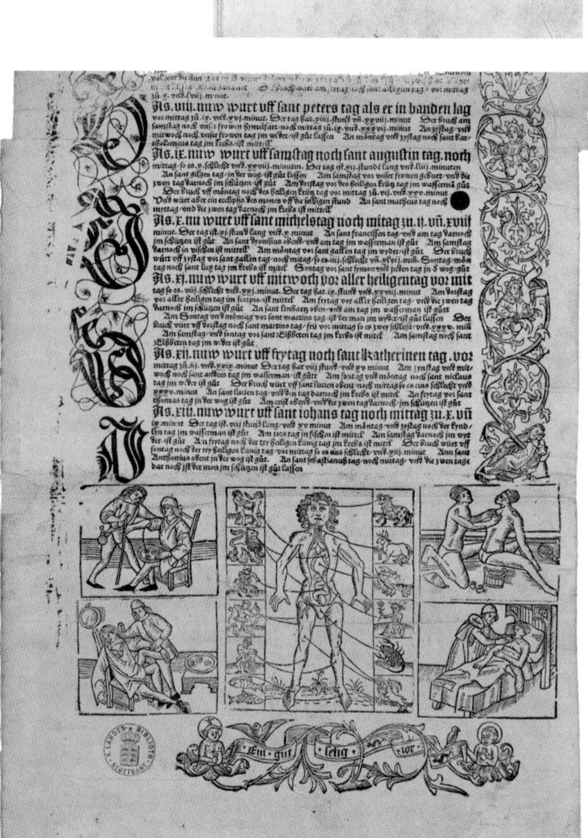

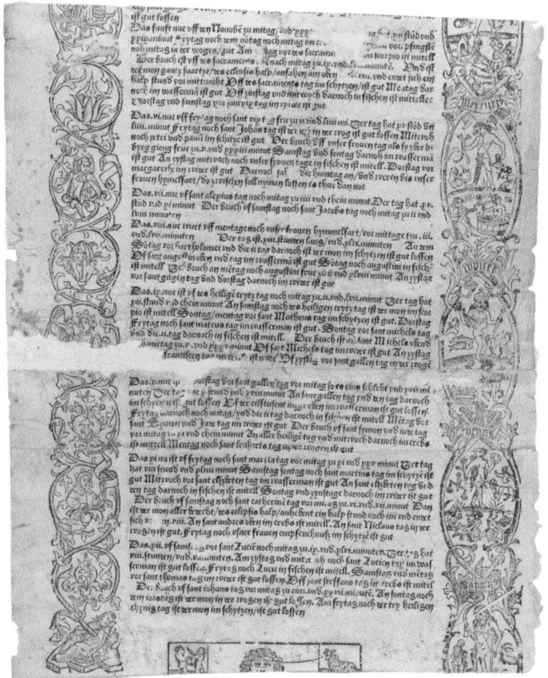

Fig. 4.9. Johan Prüss's hybrid figure reused in multiple works. *(In clockwise order)*: Bloodletting table and figure from the *Martyrologium der Heiligen* (Strasbourg: Johann Prüss, 1484). Woodcut, 29 x 18 cm. Darmstadt, Universitäts- und Landesbibliothek, Inc IV 142, inserted after opening calendar. Hybrid figure from an almanac (Strasbourg: Johann Prüss, c. 1484). Woodcut, 36 x 28 cm (lower sheet). The Hague, Huis van het boek, 039 C 009. Hybrid figure from an almanac (Basel: Printer of the Form der Copyen, c. 1489–90). Woodcut, 32 x 25 cm. Munich, Bayerische Staatsbiblithek, Einbl. Kal. 1490 p. Hybrid figure from an almanac (Strasbourg: Johann Prüss, c. 1494). Woodcut, 37 x 28 cm (lower sheet). Stuttgart, Württembergische Landesbibliothek, Inc.fol.87b.

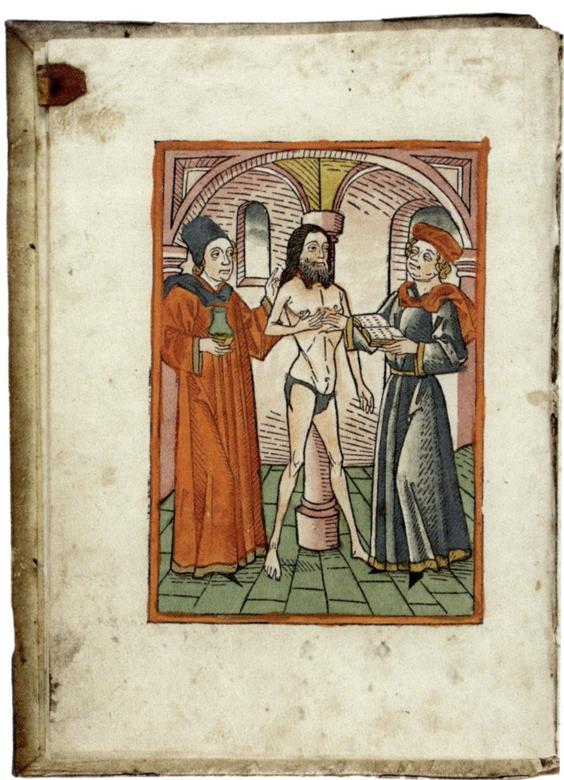

Fig. 4.10. Doctors examining a figure from Konrad von Megenberg's *Buch der Natur* (Augsburg: Johann Bämler, 1475). Hand-colored woodcut, 24 x 19 cm. Erlangen, Friedrich-Alexander-Universität, Universitätsbibliothek, H62/CIM.P 21, fol. 3v.

of its chapters, the beginning of its text proper is heralded to the reader by a full-page woodblock, brightly hand-colored in many versions, depicting a male figure attended by a pair of doctors (fig. 4.10).[58] His generic nature has at times confused catalogers, who have variously described him as a leper being checked over for boils, as a patient being treated by Saints Cosmas and Damian, and even sometimes as the figure of Christ. But in the context of the earliest incunable medical imagery, of which Bämler's *Buch* was a key part, we must surely recognize this figure as responding to more diagrammatic bodies in the model of the Wound Man, blue underwear and all, drawn forth from the late medieval manuscript corpus and forming a central part of the visual repertoire of early medical print.

The *Fasciculus medicinae*

This emerging print market for illustrated medical texts clearly made an impression on one pair of printing entrepreneurs in particular, the brothers Giovanni and Gregorio de Gregori, whose work was to act as the most significant spur to the Wound Man's story since its first appearance in the *Dreibilderserie*. Originally from Forlì, the Gregori brothers began their print careers peripatetically, working their way northward from their hometown through presses in Vicenza and Padua before setting up in the major print center of Venice.[59] Here, first Giovanni and then his younger brother Gregorio were printing together by the early 1480s.

Their output varied during the first decade of their Venetian press. Initially their work was dominated by printings of Classical works, the likes of Cicero, Valerius Maximus, Horace, and Terence, often made in collaboration with other Venetian printing houses.[60] This was supplemented by the occasional contemporary work in Italian, for instance the so-called *Frottola di un Caligaro*, a short folk song about a knight, or the *Storia della battaglia di Campo Morto*, an account of a military victory by Roberto Malatesta in 1482.[61] Following this phase was a period when the brothers focused on legal texts, most likely aimed at the renowned law school of the nearby university at Padua, as was a short subsequent period when they printed academic philosophical works.[62] And medicine too made increasingly significant appearances throughout this period. From the mid-1480s onward, the Gregoris can be linked with a small group of prognostications and bloodletting calendars, and by around 1488 they were producing a number of more explicitly medical works: editions of Guillermo Saliceto's *Chirurgia* (Surgery), Michael Scot's *Liber physiognomiae* (Book of Physiognomy), assorted natural philosophical discussions of the body as part of the writings of Albertus Magnus, and the *Corona florida medicinae* (Flowering Crown of Medicine) of the contemporary Paduan professor of medicine Antonio Gazio.[63] This medical specialism was to gain even greater momentum throughout the 1490s, when they produced editions of well-known medical treatises by Abū Marwān ibn Zuhr, Aristotle, Bernard de Gordon, Ibn Māsawaiyh, and Ibn Sīnā, alongside two editions of the popular *Articella* and the writings of contemporary Venetian army surgeon Alessandro Benedetti.[64]

It was during the early stages of this sustained interest in medical printing that on July 26, 1491, the brothers printed a sixteen-page booklet entitled *Fasciculus medicinae* (Little Bundle of Medicine).[65] This work is often hailed as Europe's first illustrated medical treatise in print, and although the account of incunable medicine provided earlier shows that this was clearly not the case, the pages of the *Fasciculus* are nonetheless replete with a particularly impressive and extensive combination of practical medical texts and intricate medical images.

A brief tour through this often misunderstood booklet makes apparent that we have in fact seen much of its contents before in manuscript form (fig. 4.11). The opening of the work sets out its epistemic stance boldly. Its title, printed at the top of its first folio in red Gothic type, is entirely dwarfed by a full-page circular diagram, alerting the reader to the specifically visual qualities of the medicine to come. This particular schematic is a uroscopic wheel of the type found in Europe from the thirteenth century onward: twenty-one wide-brimmed flasks of urine are arranged in a circle according to their colorific tone and labeled on a spectrum from clear as well water through to a deep, dark black.[66] Acting as partner to a short text beginning on the opposite page elaborating urological diagnosis, this opening sets up the vital intertwining of diagram and text that forms the principal mode of medical explication in the *Fasciculus*. Just two folios later we find another textual-visual combination, labeled "*tabula secunda*" (second table), a set of writings on phlebotomy that opens with a full-page bloodletting figure, naked, muscular, and somewhat exhausted looking. Again, this printed figure harks back

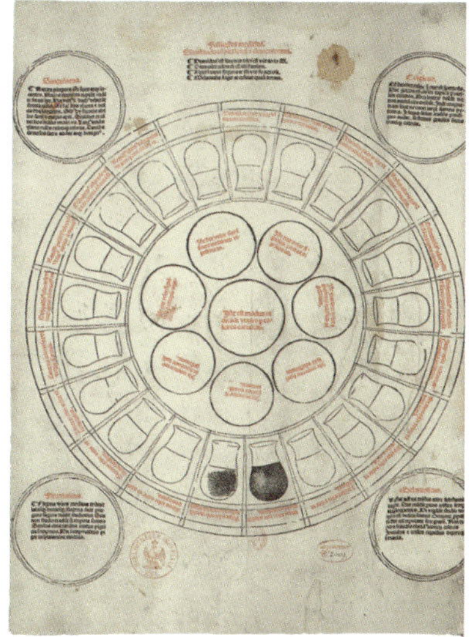

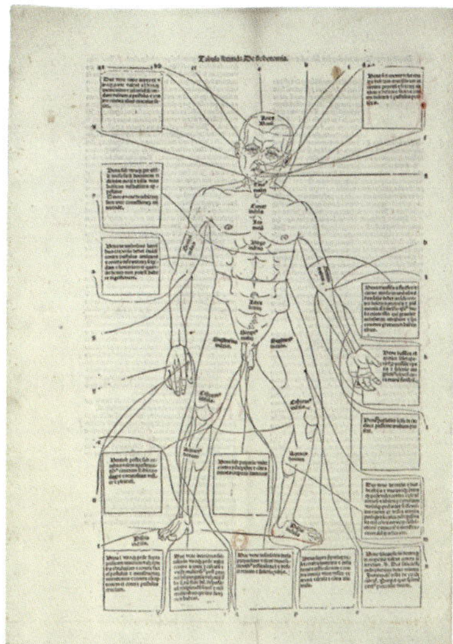

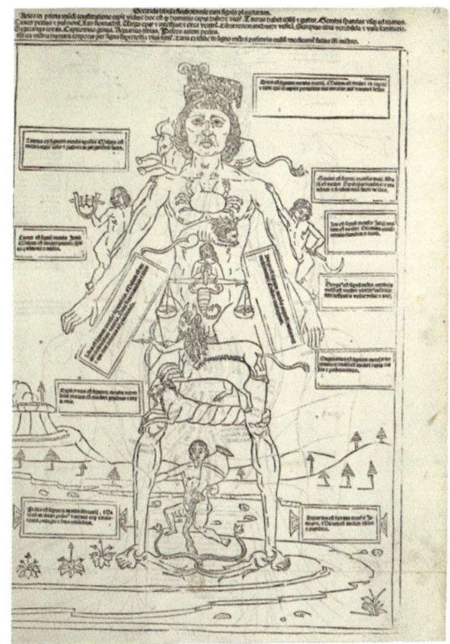

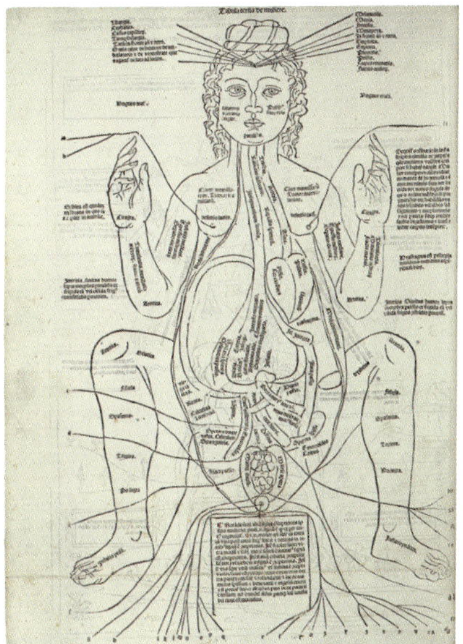

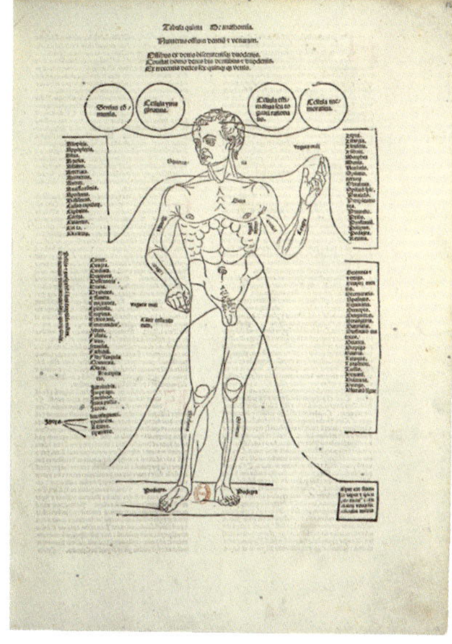

Fig. 4.11. Urine wheel, bloodletting figure, Zodiac Man, Disease Woman, and Disease Man from the *Fasciculus medicinae* (Venice: Giovanni and Gregorio de Gregori, 1491). Woodcuts with inset metal type, 43 x 31 cm (each folio). Paris, Bibliothèque nationale de France, Reserve PET FOL-EB-3, fols. a1v, a2v, a5r, a5v, b4r.

directly to manuscript models by the labeling of his form from head to toe with a key of letters—running from *a* through to *cc*—each of which connects different bloodletting locations on his body to their explanation in individuated paragraphs of a phlebotomical treatise that follows.[67] At the other end of these bloodletting materials, the booklet continues with what it names a "*secunda tabula fleubotomie*" (second phlebotomical table), this one showing a shaggy-haired Zodiac Man standing in a river bend, the playful warping of scale between his body and the landscape lending the image a particularly fantastical air.

Proceeding through the rest of the booklet, we find three further groupings of medical texts, each with its own full-page diagrammatic herald. In fact, these are the three key figures of the fifteenth-century German *Dreibilderserie* tradition: Disease Man, Disease Woman, and Wound Man. The *Fasciculus* turns first to the Disease Woman, depicted with particularly elegant poise despite her overwhelming size on the page and a notably tubular anatomy within. Much like her manuscript precursors, she is marked by a key of lines and letters that match parts of her body to a set of texts that follow on women's medicine and outline various cures to her visualized ills, themselves drawn from earlier models.[68] Second, we are presented with the Wound Man, whose generalizing label—*De cyrurgia* (On surgery)—makes clear the booklet's shift into more hands-on territory (fig. 4.1). As we would expect, his body is covered with its typical array of wounds, buboes, and violently lodged foreign objects, while its lettered key links his multiple ailments to a curative text that follows, the earliest printed edition of the *Dreibilderserie*'s Latin *Wundarznei* and *Antidotar*, which we have also met before. And toward the end of the booklet, the reader finds a carefully posed Disease Man whose upper bubbles of text label the four so-called cells of the brain and whose extensive bracketed rosters to left and right list a range of pathologies, the cures for which are discussed in a text on assorted diseases that follows.[69]

Judging from this delicate concoction of practical texts and active images, we can characterize the Gregoris' *Fasciculus* as effectively a fifteenth-century *Dreibilderserie* manuscript in print, although the matter of the booklet's specific heritage has been drawn somewhat off course by the fixation of many twentieth-century scholars on questions of authorship. The text itself offers a deceptively simple account of its origins in its two brief colophons:

> *Finis fasciculi medicine Iohannis de ketham. Revisus per georgium de monteferrato Artium et medicine doctorem qui insuper apposuit titulum, auctoritates et loca plura.*
>
> *Impressum venetiis per lohannem et Gregorium fratres de forlivio. Anno domini millesimo quadringentesimo nonagesimo primo mensis iulii die xxvi.*
>
> The end of the little bundle of medicine of John of Ketham. Revised by Giorgio dal Monferrato, doctor of arts and medicine, who also added the title, authorities, and further references.
>
> Printed in Venice by the brothers Giovanni and Gregorio of Forlì. In the year of our Lord 1491, the 26th day of the month of July.[70]

The Gregoris are noted as the book's printers, and while the artist or artists responsible for its woodcuts go unmentioned, we do read of one Giorgio dal Monferrato, a doctor who can be located in Venetian sources as early as 1475 and who is listed as the book's editor. Responsible for titling the work and developing its scholarly references to include a number of major medical authorities, Monferrato claimed in a 1496 request for privilege from the Venetian Collegio that he had labored for sixteen years on the text.[71] The identity of the third name mentioned, Iohannes de Ketham, has prompted more extensive debate, stretching back as far as bibliographers of the sixteenth century. To summarize a now well-worn discussion, it was the authoritative voice of medical historian Karl Sudhoff who incorrectly canonized the colophon's Iohannes as one Johannes von Kirchheim, a Viennese university medical professor in the late 1450s and 1460s with a specialty in anatomical demonstration.[72] After much back-and-forth among historians of medicine, this tempting hypothesis has since been rejected, not least because a number of surviving *Dreibilderserie* manuscripts are known to have been made several decades before von Kirchheim's career began, proving that he could not have been the originator or original compiler of the texts or images included in the group. Instead, his name is likely to have been added to the *Fasciculus*'s colophon either with the explicit intention of inflating the price of the book—especially in Germany—through the glamorous draw of a known academic personage or simply in error. Maybe, for instance, Monferrato misread an inscription in one of his sources that was originally intended as a marginal commentary or note of ownership, rather than authorship.[73]

This topsy-turvy historiography now settled, it is the *Fasciculus*'s Wound Man that in fact offers the only small piece of direct evidence we have of the printed work's material provenance. As Tiziana Pesenti has highlighted in her extensive examination of the writings grouped within the *Fasciculus*, toward the end of the work's printed *Wundarznei* we find an editorial note explaining that this surgical text's final five items—paragraphs marked with uppercase letters *A* through *E*—do not appear as part of the diagrammatic key placed about its correspondent printed Wound Man.[74] The paragraphs themselves are garbled to the point almost of nonsense, suggesting that their transposer, perhaps working from a damaged manuscript source in which these snippets of text were largely illegible, felt compelled to include what little information they could make out for accuracy's sake. What exactly this original exemplar might have been, however, remains unclear.[75] If we look to existing *Dreibilderserie* manuscripts as potential models, those now in Paris, London, and the Vatican preserve all six of the same diagrammatic elements found in the *Fasciculus*: the urine wheel, the bloodletting figure, Zodiac Man, Disease Woman, Wound Man, and Disease Man (figs. 2.3–2.18). But none of these elements appear in the same order as the figures in the Gregoris' work, nor are they a precise match for the *Fasciculus*'s textual contents, which draw on slightly different combinations of advice from the medieval medical canon for their healing information. Pesenti posits that the large, rectangular shape of the *Fasciculus*'s paper—an unusual *super-reale* sizing of forty-three by thirty-one centimeters—suggests that the Gregoris were attempting to evoke a particularly large-scale original.[76] Perhaps their model was something more akin to the giant pages of the Copenhagen *Dreibilderserie* folios discussed in chapter 2, whose medico-visual materials sprawl dramatically across enormous parchment sheets via a network of linked text bubbles (fig. 2.19). This would also align with a detail preserved in cure *c* of the treatise accompanying the *Fasciculus* Wound Man, which for a head injury recommends applying a plaster "*ut inferiori circulo docetur*" (as is shown in the circle below).

Given the strong connections between southern Germany and northern Italy in the later fifteenth century, it would not have been hard for such a German or Bohemian *Dreibilderserie* book to make its way to Venice. The city was, after all, a print center whose very foundations rested on an exchange of artisans across the Alps, and whose earliest printing presses were set up almost in their entirety by northern immigrants such as Erhard Ratdolt and Nicolas Jenson.[77] The products of these early presses were themselves also eminently peripatetic things, and material evidence even helps us directly implicate the Gregori brothers in this international network. One copy of their 1483 Venetian edition of Horace's complete works was recently discovered to contain a recycled page from the so-called Fust-Schoeffer *Donatus* inside its intact original binding.[78] This hidden page was a product of one of the very earliest presses in Mainz in the late 1450s, proving that Italian and German early printed materials could be happily compacted together into a single object from a very early date.

The *Fasciculus*'s contents and organization might not have been an idea original to the Gregoris, but their unique treatment of these *Dreibilderserie* medical themes nonetheless marks a significant milestone for printed medicine, both economic and technical. Commercially speaking, the Gregoris' booklet tells us much about the market for medical figures like the Wound Man in the final decade of the fifteenth century. As well as continuing a popular manuscript tradition by then nearly a century old, the *Fasciculus* represents a canny synthesis of two contemporary market strands that we have already seen were emerging at precisely the same time. On the one hand, from the 1470s onward, major European print centers were producing tomes of medical theory aimed at a learned academic audience, and on the other, printed medical imagery itself was gaining in popularity among a non-academic readership, flourishing especially in more commonplace paramedical genres such as broadsheet almanacs. Bridging these two approaches, the Gregoris took aim at a viable middle market, creating a book that presented theoretically sound practical medicine—punched up for the learned reader by Giorgio dal Monferrato, as we read in the colophon—and yet that also still foregrounded a suite of popular, vibrant images as a way of organizing and advertising its abbreviated medical contents.

Moreover, the *Fasciculus*'s images are revealed as even more remarkable when we consider them within the artistic context of Venetian print at this precise moment. As Lillian Armstrong has shown, the beginning of the 1490s was something of a turning point in the city's print culture.[79] During the first two decades of Venetian printing, the 1470s and 1480s, clients with an interest in images—and the budget to afford their comparatively high prices—turned almost exclusively to hand illumination and rubrication to enliven the pages of their texts, most often in the form of colored frontispieces with elaborate personalized details. This was the case for several of the Gregoris' own clientele, whose surviving books showcase a keen awareness of the early printed page as an opportunity for visual spectacle. A pair of Justinianic legal texts printed by the brothers in 1484 and 1485, both in the collection of the Bavarian Benedictine Abbey of Tegernsee, were at some point embellished with twin painted scenes on their opening pages, the first showing the book's presentation to Justinian by two scholars and the second showing a marriage ceremony (fig. 4.12).[80] Another of the Gregoris' books, containing the medical writings of Antonio Gazio, survives embellished with inhabited initials and floral banderoles attributed to Antonio Maria da Vil-

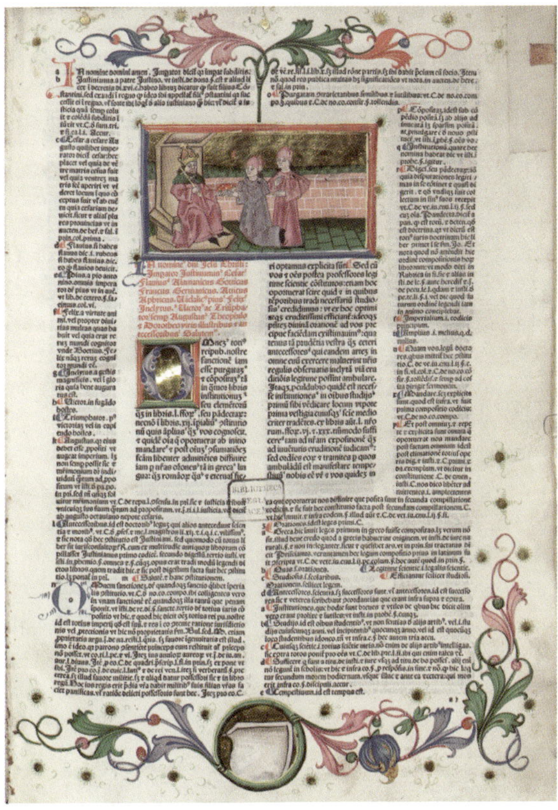

Fig. 4.12. Hand illustration in a printed edition of the *Digestum vetus* (Venice: Giovanni and Gregorio de Gregori, 1484). Ink and paint on paper, 42 x 28 cm. Munich, Bayerische Staatsbibliothek, 2 Inc.c.a. 1453, fol. a2r.

lafora, a prestigious illuminator recorded in the employ of the University of Padua.[81] Villafora even added the arms of the powerful Visconti family, a move that has led some to suggest that the copy was presented to the Dukes of Milan in an unsuccessful attempt by Gazio to gain their patronage.

By contrast, images printed directly alongside such early texts were a far less common feature of nascent Venetian incunables. Only a handful of examples are known from the 1470s and early 1480s, almost all small-scale mathematical or astrological diagrams produced by German printers in the city, especially at Ratdolt's prolific press, the products of which record his collaboration with an artist named Bernardus Maler in the colophon of several books.[82] Only three works linked to the Gregoris from before 1491 include images of any kind, all of which are of contested date and provenance.[83]

By the later 1480s, though, this visual pool was widening among printers in the city to include different forms of printed aesthetic detail: large decorated initials, half- and quarter-page vignettes in religious and secular works alike, and increasingly ornate illustrated frontispieces that aped the dancing figures and abundant vegetal forms of earlier hand-illuminated work, perhaps even designed in the new medium by the very same artists.[84] Clearly the Gregoris were alert to this sea change, and in the summer of 1491 they decided to act, by producing not only the heavily illustrated *Fasciculus* but also—released on the very same day—an edition of Abū al-Saqr al-Qabīsī's *Libellus isagogicus* (known in English as his Introduction into the Art of Astrology), an astrological work whose circular diagrams and illustrated tables were likewise integral to understanding its texts.[85] These works were followed in 1492 by both an edition of Aristotle's *De animalibus*, boasting an elaborate frontispiece complete with a Classicizing frieze and processions of dancing putti, and the very first illustrated printing of Giovanni Boccaccio's *Decameron*, laced throughout with 120 vignettes depicting the text's unfolding narratives.[86] One work printed by the Gregoris even allows us to observe their embrace of printed imagery in real time. Over the course of more than a year, the brothers were at work on a gargantuan edition of the complete works of Boethius printed in two volumes, one in March 1491 and the other in August 1492. The difference between these volumes is striking: the earlier, printed before the *Fasciculus*, is entirely plain, devoid of both decoration and imagery, while the other, printed after the *Fasciculus*, contains page upon page of elaborate diagrams.[87]

The *Fasciculus* thus appeared at a moment of change for the Gregori press, a matter of aesthetics but also innovation. Novel technological thought was put into the book from the very first image, its uroscopic wheel, a diagram that is all about the diagnostic value of color (fig. 4.11). Clearly, the Gregoris could not reproduce the broad colorific spectrum we see in some manuscript versions of the same picture, yet they nonetheless turned to recent advances in two-tone printing to produce the page in red and black, most likely in two pressings using a frisket and quads, adopting a technique still relatively new in Venice.[88] In addition, the brothers set their resident artist—or artists—the tricky task of conveying color where they could through the subtleties of their woodblock carving. At the base of the scheme, we find two flasks labeled with particularly dire terms for black urine specimens, one described as "*ut cornu bene nigrum*" (like very black horn) and the other, of an even deeper tone, "*ut incaustrum*" (like ink). Picking up on this material cue, the maker of the woodblock has varied the depth of the inner spaces of these flasks, making one slightly less shallow and leaving the other entirely ungouged, allowing the block to pick up subtly different levels of ink and reproduce two shades of black to match the two shades of urine.

Even more technically adventurous is the *Fasciculus*'s complex combination of image and text in a single space. This was, we must remember, by far the most significant difficulty presented to any printer who wished to translate the *Dreibilderserie* images into print. In older manuscript models, line-drawn diagrammatic figures and their penetrating textual elements could interweave with ease. Not so in the printed realm. Combinations of text and image that utilized movable type, as opposed to the xylographic texts of carved block books, are known in printed incunables as early as the 1460s, most of them created simply by either printing a woodcut image and metalcut type side by side in a single forme or printing them in turn, one pull after the other. However, for the densely packed images of the *Fasciculus*—and none more concentrated than its Wound Man, whose many labels sit at multiple angles in finely tuned relation to its fragile lines—the Gregoris and their woodcutters instead employed the hybrid technique of insetting pieces of movable metal type as precise plugs into the body of the woodblock (fig. 4.13). This method is evidenced in Germany as early as the 1460s, but its adoption in Venice is only known from the late 1470s, with largely unimpressive results (fig. 4.14).

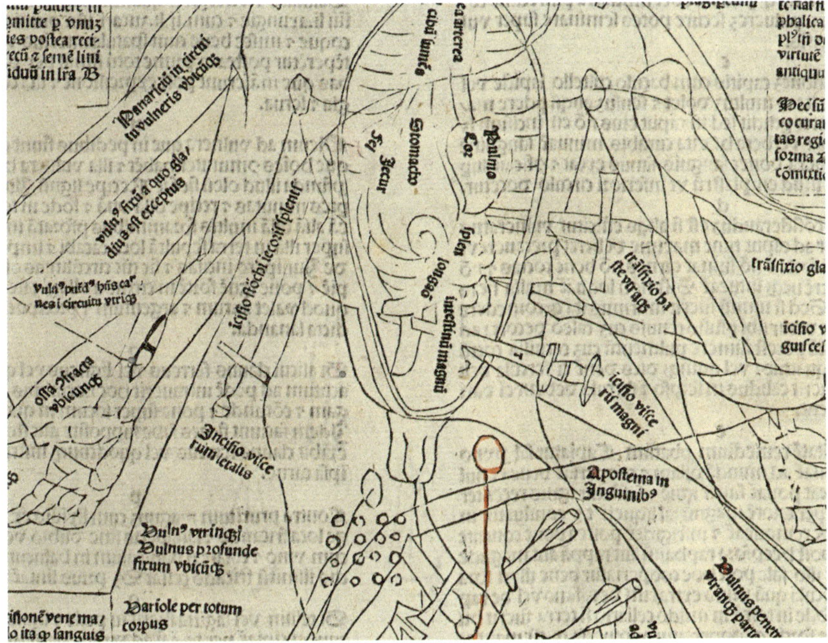

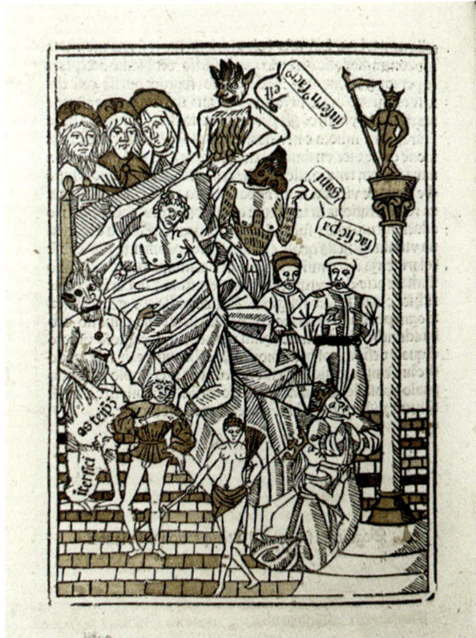

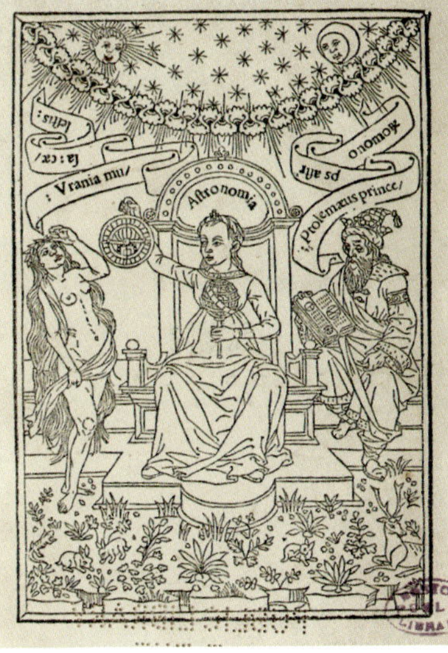

Fig. 4.13. Detail of the *Fasciculus* Wound Man's metal type letter plugs (fig. 4.1).

Fig. 4.14. Venetian incunables with poorly inset text. *Left:* A man on his deathbed from the *Ars moriendi* (Venice: Johannes Clein and Piero Himel, 1490). Hand-colored woodcut with inset metal type, 21 x 14 cm. London, British Library, IA.23743, fol. a3r. *Right:* Astronomia enthroned from Johannes de Sacro Bosco's *Sphaera mundi* (Venice: Bonetus Locatellus, 1490). Woodcut with inset metal type, 21 x 15 cm. Boston Public Library, Q.405.41, fol. a1v.

Observe how clumsily text is set into two works from late 1490, contemporary to the *Fasciculus*, an illustrated *Ars moriendi* printed by Johannes Clein and Piero Himel and an image from Bonetus Locatellus's edition of Johannes Sacrobosco's *Sphaera mundi* (On the Sphere of the World).[89] Clein and Himel's book, the first Venetian attempt at an illustrated edition of this popular manual on death, extracts the detail of its woodcut images in great chunks in order to insert its type, leaving its wording floating in ghostly halos. The opening frontispiece of Locatellus's *Sphera mundi* manages this element somewhat better, although here it is the text that suffers from incorporation: the blank space of a pair of banderoles held by the figures of Urania and Ptolemy makes room for cramped lettering, heavily abbreviated, while above the central personification of Astronomia her name has been inelegantly inserted into a semicircular niche in three distinct, clunky chunks, *Astro-nom-ia*.

Text in the *Fasciculus*'s Wound Man, by contrast, darts smoothly around its companion imagery, its typographic plugs interrupting the integrity of carved lines only infrequently and even then just for a moment, its words instead molded in delicate visual consort with their woodblock.[90] Scholars of incunables have to date tracked the growing reputation of the Gregori brothers through the impressive abundance of their printed type: twenty-five distinct Gothic fonts have been identified in their products, as well as eight Roman, two Italic, two complete Greek sets, and one set of Hebrew lettering. Looking closely at their *Fasciculus*, however, we surely must extend an appreciation of their workshop's technical capacities to image-making as well as typesetting. The cutters and setters of the booklet's figures might still be unknown to us today, but their skill in helping the Gregoris translate a highly complex fifteenth-century manuscript into the new medium of print nonetheless remains remarkable.

Fasiculo, Compendio, Epilogo, Cyrurgie

It would be easy to assume that the Gregoris' 1491 printing of the *Fasciculus medicinae* concretized the Wound Man and his fellow *Dreibilderserie* figures: that through their production of multiple copies of near-identical booklets, these manuscript images became somehow stable. This was not the case.

Even as they first passed into print, these fifteenth-century pictures underwent subtle but detectable aesthetic shifts in comparison to their earlier manuscript form (fig. 4.11). Such revisions are mostly modest, although none are unaffected by the shift in medium. The items of the *Fasciculus* urine wheel, for instance, have grown in number from a typical twenty to twenty-one with the inclusion of an unexplained flask to the upper left. Its bloodletting figure appears more emotive than most manuscript versions, staggering forward toward the viewer with one palm outstretched. The astrological symbols sitting comfortably atop the Zodiac Man's skin have been remodeled, especially the intertwined dolphin-like Pisces, which could have paddled onto the page from the base of one of Venice's more elaborate well-heads. The Disease Woman has undergone both sartorial and anatomical change. Instead of a long flowing wimple, she wears a stylish striped hat, while her uterus has been rearranged from its usual inaccurate position on her left-hand side to a low central position, a shift that brings the organ closer to its realistic site within the human body, but that also radically rearranges the figure's distended outline to fit its innards. For his part, the Wound Man is the figure perhaps least directly affected by the transition into print, with only occasional details of his weapons updated to fit Italian tastes of the 1490s. The Disease Man, on the other hand, is the most significantly revised. Not only have his listed diseases been rearranged from topographical to alphabetical order, but he stands in a striking Classical contrapposto, one arm by his side with his elbow pulled back, the other angled upward with delicately raised hand, his stylistic texture feeling significantly different in print.

How scholars have framed this aesthetic shift has depended largely on their own biases. Tiziana Pesenti sees the reoriented Disease Man as a definitive, Italianate success. The image, she claims, has "abandoned any diagrammatic intent" and no longer has "anything in common with the schematic, flaccid young bald man in blue underpants," who, in her opinion, is an impoverished medieval model.[91] Instead, she conjures abstract connections to renaissance greats for comparison, stating that he bears "the posture, the physiognomy of a nude designed by Mantegna." Others have taken this idea even further, using the figure's bearing as ammunition in increasingly circular and ultimately unnecessary attempts to ascribe the woodblock to assorted grand figures of the Venetian renaissance: Vittore Carpaccio, Gentile Bellini, the so-called Master of the Dolphins.[92] In this view, the appearance of these figures in print marks a moment of arrival and permanence, the *Fasciculus* announcing the *Dreibilderserie* images' transition into a modern mode of specifically fixed address. We could see this chiming with what Lorraine Daston has suggested to be true of early modern epistemic images more broadly: that one of their functions was to build ontological consensus through their printed visual consistency, forming shared "working objects" that enabled increasingly far-flung users to see in scientific union.[93]

Claims for the stability of this particular body of images, however, are a fiction. On February 5, 1494, a little less than three years after their first printing, the Gregoris produced a second edition of the same book.[94] This 1494 "little bundle" was even littler than the 1491 edition, a good bit smaller at thirty-two by twenty-one centimeters. But running at fifty-two folios, its contents had been notably expanded under the guidance of a new editor, the humanist scholar Sebastiano Manilio, with whom the Gregoris had already collaborated on two books in 1492.[95] Most significantly, the entirety of the 1494 edition was translated by Manilio into Italian, and the work was retitled *Fasiculo de medicina in volgare* (Little Bundle of Medicine in the Vernacular).[96] Although Manilio preserved much of the sentiment of the original Latin, maintaining the complexities of its technical language and resisting the editor's urge to add significant passages of commentary or summary, he did instigate the inclusion of two further treatises within the bundle: a short herbal extracted from the writings of Albertus Magnus, entitled *Proprieta de herbe* (Properties of Herbs), and a vernacular translation of Mondino dei Liuzzi's famed anatomical treatise the *Anathomia (Anatomy)*.[97]

To match this enlarged text, the Gregoris also added four new full-page woodblock plates to the *Fasiculo* (fig. 4.15). Spread throughout the book, these supplemental images offered the bundle's hodgepodge of gathered treatises something of a continuous narrative quality. The first of them, a frontispiece showing a humanist at work transcribing a book amid a significant medical library, opens the 1494 edition. As with "Iohannes de Ketham" before him, the precise identity of this figure—labeled "Petrus de Montagnana"—has been the subject of some debate, but it is nonetheless clear that the frontispiece was designed to capture the editorial spirit in which medical books like the *Fasiculo* were being generated.[98] Three figures are also gathered at the foot of Petrus's desk, each holding a wicker-lined urine flask, presumably waiting for the medical professional's diagnosis on these deliveries

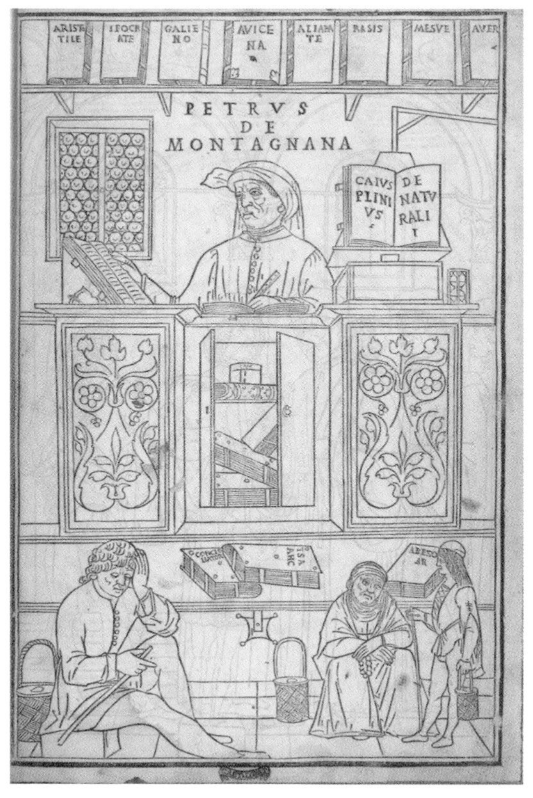
ARISTO TILE
IPOCR ATE
GALIE NO
AVICE NA
RASIS
MESVE
AVER
PETRVS DE MONTAGNANA
CAIVS PLINI VS
DE NATV RALI

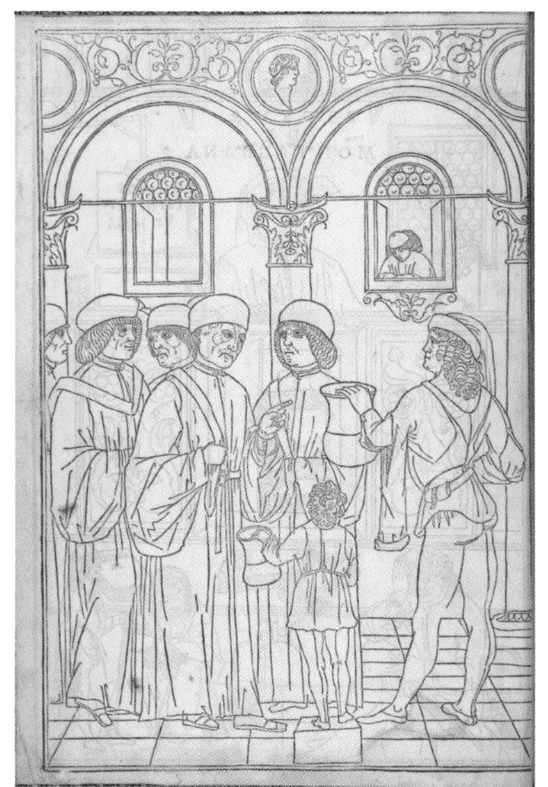

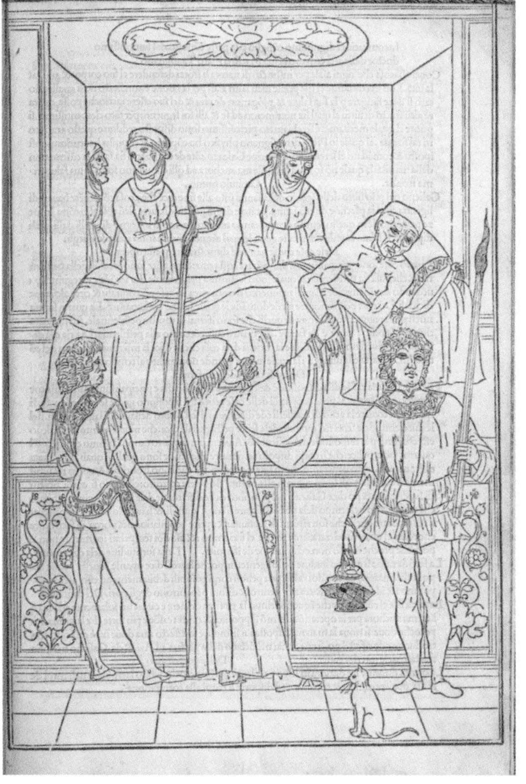

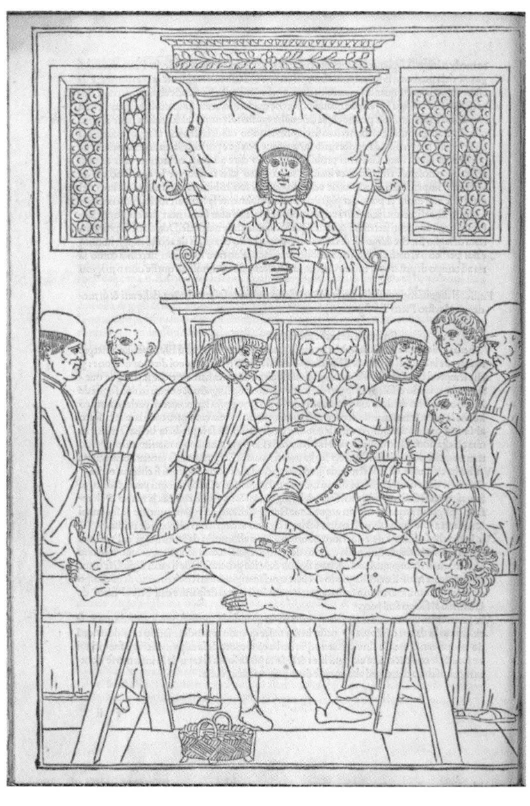

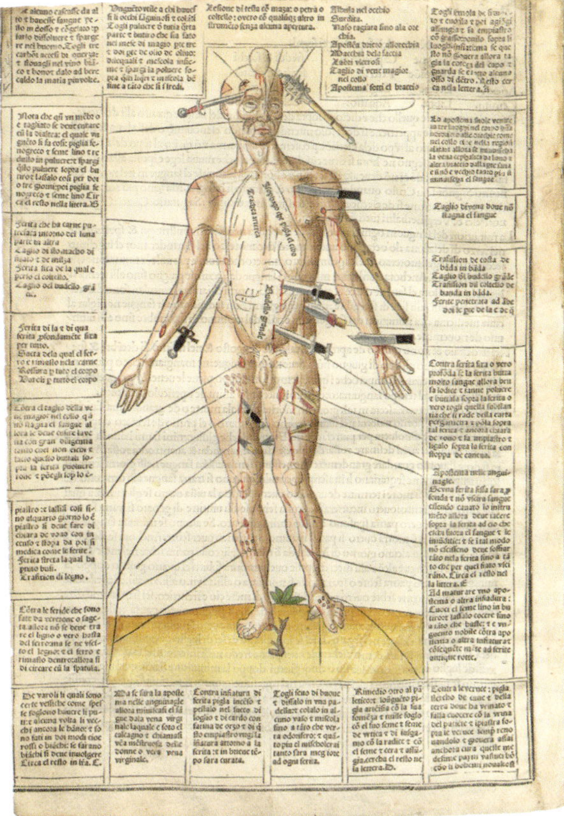

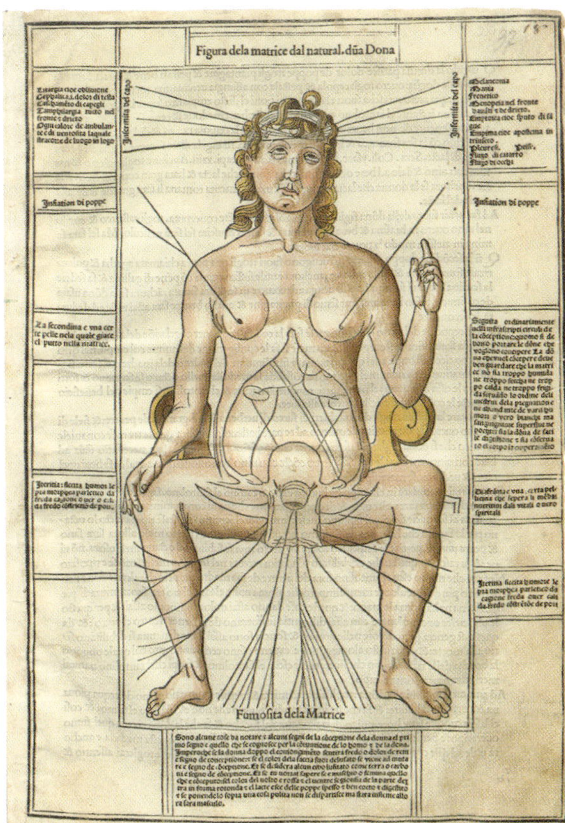

from patients. This touch of real-world, quotidian medicine serves to link the frontispiece with the three other scenes that are newly inserted throughout the book and act, in turn, as prefaces to three of the book's later texts. Its writings on uroscopy are introduced by the scene of a physician in public consultation beneath Corinthian arches as he inspects a large urine flask. A plague treatise is announced by an image of a physician attending a sick man in bed, perhaps the same doctor as in the earlier scenes. And immediately before the newly included text of Mondino's *Anathomia* we find a university anatomy taking place, the scene most likely modeled on the academic dissections that are occasionally attested as having taken place in the medical school of the nearby university at Padua.[99]

As for the six original images of the *Fasciculus*, these appear reordered and revised in the 1494 edition. Some, like the Zodiac Man, Bloodletting Man, and Disease Man, are relatively unchanged. The Disease Man was even printed from the very same woodblock as in 1491.[100] But two figures have undergone what Pesenti calls a radical "metamorphosis" in the shift from *Fasciculus* to *Fasiculo* (fig. 4.16). The Disease Woman has once again been reimagined. Looking exaggeratedly to the sky, she sits with her hair tied back in a grandiose chair whose volute arms are designed to match the curving forms of her now simplified innards, her pubis also dramatically opened and issuing forth a cluster of lines that no longer link to specific paragraphs of

Fig. 4.15 (*opposite*). New narrative scenes from the *Fasiculo de medicina in volgare* (Venice: Giovanni and Gregorio de Gregori, 1494). Woodcuts, 32 x 21 cm. Bethesda, National Library of Medicine, WZ 230 K43fI 1494, fols. a1r, a1v, e2r, f2v.

Fig. 4.16 (*above*). Wound Man and Disease Woman from the *Fasiculo de medicina in volgare* (Venice: Giovanni and Gregorio de Gregori, 1494). Hand-colored woodcuts, 32 x 21 cm. New Haven, Yale University, Harvey Cushing/John Hay Whitney Medical Library, Incunabula +K-17 (Goff), fols. b6v, d1r.

text but rather are relabeled as "*Fumosita dela matrice*" (Fumes of the womb). The 1494 Wound Man too is substantially revised. With his right hip swung outward and his head tilted, he exhibits a rather more elegant sense of poise than was evident in previous iterations, with a slender muscularity delineated through careful lines at his arms and thighs. His presence on the page has likewise been tinkered with. Instead of simply floating in blank space, he is now grounded in the most basic of landscapes—a horizon line and a small sprouting shrub—as well as being surrounded on all sides by a frame of continuous text blocks. The weapons still protruding from his body are far more detailed than those attacking his previous print counterparts. Swords and knives include refined leather grips and decorative pommels, each line of fletch on his three arrows is individuated, and the club pounding the side of his head has been upgraded from a rounded wooden design to a violently spiked, metallic mace. In other elements, though, his details have been strangely stripped back. His internal organs retreat into a fuzz of sparse lines, with the fifty or so catchwords that once surrounded his body and penetrated his abdomen reduced to a mere three, highlighting the "*Isophago che pigla el cibo*" (Esophagus that takes the food), "*Trachea arterea*" (Trachea), and "*Budello grande*" (Large intestine). The snaking linking lines that once wove between his wounded body and the outermost blocks of text are now straight and cursory. Moreover, despite occasional mention of several "*lettre de alphabeto*" (letters of the alphabet) in Manilio's translation of the figure's accompanying *Wundarznei*, the alphabetical key that once linked the Wound Man's ailments with their associated cures has vanished, leaving the reader no clear route for connecting treatments and their visualization.

Just like their manuscript precursors, then, the visual specifics of the *Fasciculus* images were clearly flexible in print. Indeed, the Gregoris made no fewer than five further editions of the booklet, with text and images that fluctuated subtly with every new version. Manilio's editorial work must have proven popular, for the brothers' next edition appeared a mere year and a half later, in 1495, with the entire expanded contents rendered back into Latin, the text blocks surrounding its diagrammatic figures edited once again, and their alphabetical keys resurrected.[101] This seems to suggest a stronger market at work in Venice for the Latin than the vernacular, or at least greater interest in a more detailed work whose diagrammatic images connected clearly to its text. Certainly a frustration with the lack of captioning around the *Fasiculo*'s figures moved at least one reader to annotate their 1495 edition with a full suite of figural catchwords, copied by hand from its 1491 predecessor.[102] This push and pull continued: a pair of editions in 1500 and 1501 stuck to the Latin text and alphabetized key and bulked up the book even more by including a short treatise on disease by al-Rāzī; in 1508, the Gregoris published the Italian text once more, this time keeping the catchwords in the woodblocks—presumably still in place there from the 1501 edition—but offering no corresponding key in the text of its treatises; and in 1514, their last edition, the brothers reverted to the Latin text, including plates from the 1494 book that had survived twenty years of printing remarkably well.[103]

It may well have been this shape-shifting variation that also led the text some way beyond Venice. Sabrina Minuzzi notes that of all surviving Latin editions of the *Fasciculus* and *Fasiculo* printed by the Gregoris before 1500, only 11 percent remain on Italian soil.[104] Even accounting for losses over the centuries and movement in the later rare-book trade, such figures suggest that for all its popularity in Venetian printing circles, the *Fasciculus* was also conceived as a book for export. Just as its *Dreibilderserie* contents showcase the fluidity with which fifteenth-century medical ideas and images could traverse the Alps, its printing on the eve of the sixteenth century was likewise a traveling affair. Inscriptions and annotations still present in the margins of these Venetian books attest to the geographical diversity of their many illustrious owners. At least one copy of the Gregoris' 1495 edition found its way into the library of famed Nuremberg humanist Hartmann Schedel before his death in 1514, bound together with three other medical works, two of which were also printed by the Gregoris.[105] Another copy of their 1500 edition contains a near-contemporaneous note of ownership scribbled by Ulrich Zwingli, the Swiss theologian and reformer.[106] A third, the 1514 edition, is recorded in Denmark by at least the 1530s and noted in the collection of the Bishop of Odense at his manor house on the island of Fyn.[107] In the 1540s, a copy of their 1495 edition was gifted from one Swiss physician, Christoph Klauser, to another, the humanist Conrad Gessner, and a note of the exchange is still preserved on its inside cover.[108] And by the end of the century, another copy of their 1500 edition was to be found in the Ashwellthorpe library of the Englishman Sir Thomas Knyvett, Lord High Sheriff of Norfolk.[109] In fortuitous circularity with Johannes von Kirchheim, the infamous Viennese figure incorrectly once thought to be the *Fasciculus*'s originator, in 1520 we find a later professor of medicine at the University of Vienna named Martin Stainpeis recommending that sections of the booklet be read by all his first- and second-year medical students.[110]

More than merely circulating, however, the move into print helped propel the *Fasciculus*'s diagrammatic figures themselves into an international market (fig. 4.17). On August 15, 1494, only six months after the Gregoris produced their first Italian edition of the *Fasiculo*, the Zaragoza printer Paulus Hurus published his *Compendio de la salud humana* (Compendium of Human Health), effectively a Castilian-language version of the 1491 Latin *Fasciculus*.[111] Hurus, originally a native of Konstanz, had arrived in Zaragoza in 1476, a time when printing shops were still not common on the Iberian Peninsula and were mostly run by immigrant merchants and businessmen, especially Germans.[112] The press he founded there grew to significant renown, fueled in no small part by Hurus's frequent journeys throughout Spain, France, and Germany under the auspices of the Große Ravensburger Handelsgesellschaft, one of the continent's most extensive trading companies. These international mercantile connections allowed him to be present at Europe's increasingly frequent book fairs, through which he brought an influx of foreign printing expertise into Spain alongside both used woodblocks and complete printed books.[113] It is likely that he came into the possession of a copy of the *Fasciculus* at one of these book fairs.

His *Compendio*, one of only a few medical incunables to be printed in Zaragoza, translates much of the Gregoris' original booklet, reproducing—and in some cases in fact correcting—each of its central treatises inherited

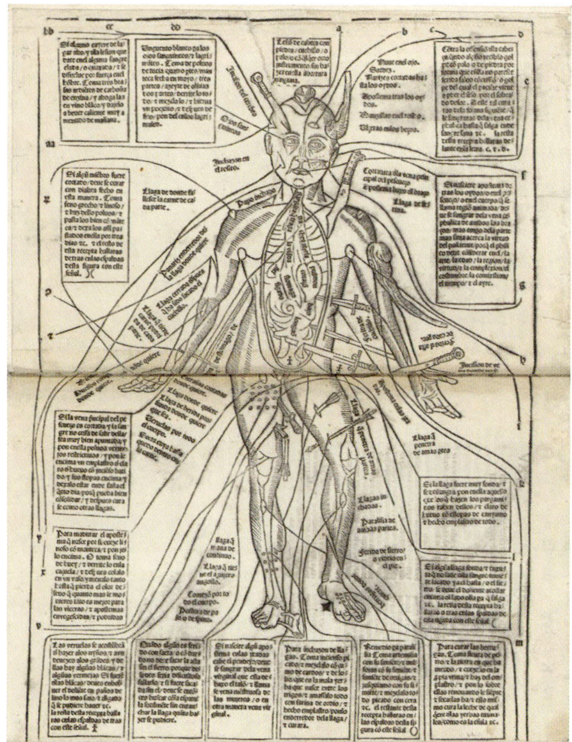

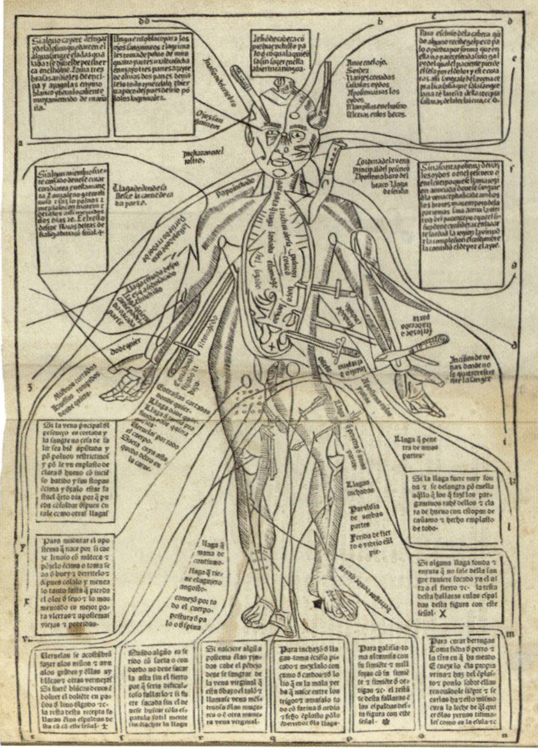

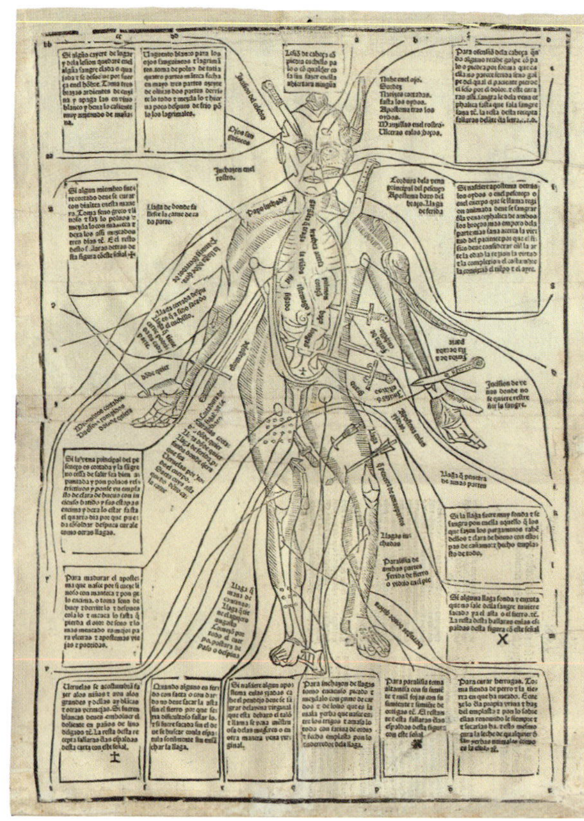

Fig. 4.17. Spanish Wound Men. *(In clockwise order)*: Wound Man from the *Compendio de la salud humana* (Zaragoza: Paulus Hurus, 1494). Woodcut, 39 x 25 cm (unfolded). Madrid, Biblioteca Nacional de España, INC/51, inserted after fol. XXIIII. Wound Man from the *Epilogo en medicina* (Burgos: Juan de Burgos, 1495). Woodcut, 38 x 25 cm (unfolded). San Marino, Huntington Library, 86926, inserted after fol. XXIIII. Wound Man from the *Epilogo en medicina y en cirurgia conveniente ala salud* (Pamplona: Arnaldo Guillen de Brocar, 1495). Woodcut, 38 x 25 cm (unfolded). Madrid, Biblioteca Nacional de España, INC/1335, inserted after fol. XXV.

from the German manuscript tradition, as well as their six accompanying diagrammatic images.[114] These are near-direct copies of the Venetian originals, reworked in woodblocks either by a native Zaragozan cutter or, as has been suggested for other Hurus books, a German artisan who had accompanied the printer in his move from Konstanz.[115] Such a practice was not uncommon, especially at the Hurus press. In 1493, the workshop produced a translation of John of Capua's moralizing treatise the *Directorium humanae vitae* (Guide for Human Life), decorated with extremely close copies—perhaps even prints from the original blocks—of the images that accompanied the text in its first printing in Urach by Conrad Fyner, around a decade earlier, and had already been recycled through editions in the German presses of both Johann Schönsperger and Johann Prüss.[116] The engravings of Hurus's *Compendio* are distinct enough from the *Fasciculus* figures as to clearly be copies rather than imports, yet even as copies they are attentive. Little sets them apart besides the generally sharper angles of the figures' features and the insertion of hatched lines down the sides of objects and bodies to act as shading. The only significant difference in these Zaragoza versions is their dimensions: three of the figures, the Disease Woman, the Bloodletting Man, and the Wound Man, have been doubled in size and inserted horizontally as folded loose leaves, forcing the reader to spin the book ninety degrees in order to take them in.

Why these particular images were selected for expansion is unclear, but their success—and that of the *Compendio* as a whole—was proven a mere ten months later when, in May 1495, the Burgos printer Juan de Burgos produced a second Hispanic edition, complete with both small- and large-scale plates of the six diagrammatic *Fasciculus* figures.[117] This was swiftly followed in October of the same year by yet another printing, the Pamplona printer Arnaldo Guillén de Brocar's version of the *Compendio*—now titled the *Epilogo en medicina y en cirurgia conveniente ala salud* (Epilogue on Medicine and on Surgery Beneficial to Health)—which contained images copied in turn from the Burgos edition.[118] Marginal notes found across all three Spanish editions and collected by the keen eye of Folke Gernert make clear the diversity of these books' readers, including early annotations made by friars, surgeons, and at least one writer working in the circle of the Archbishop of Toledo.[119] Within just fourteen months, the Gregoris' *Fasciculus* Wound Man had been recycled throughout the major print centers of Aragon, Castile, and Navarre, reaching beyond medics and into a broader learned milieu.

These Spanish copies set the tone for further regional engagements with the *Fasciculus* tradition. In northern Europe, for instance, an even more complex situation was emerging (fig. 4.18). As Christian Coppens has carefully deduced, the Gregoris' images must have made their way to the Netherlands by at least 1508, for a close copy of their *Fasiculo* Wound Man appeared that year in a Dutch translation of the surgical works of Gui de Chauliac entitled *Die Cyrurgie van meester Guido de Cauliaco* (The Surgery of Master Gui de Chauliac) and produced by the established printer Henrick Eckert van Homberch.[120] This was followed in 1512 by the up-and-coming printer Claes de Grave's Dutch-language translation of the entire *Fasciculus*, which preserved the original's Latin in title alone.[121] Helpfully, this second Dutch

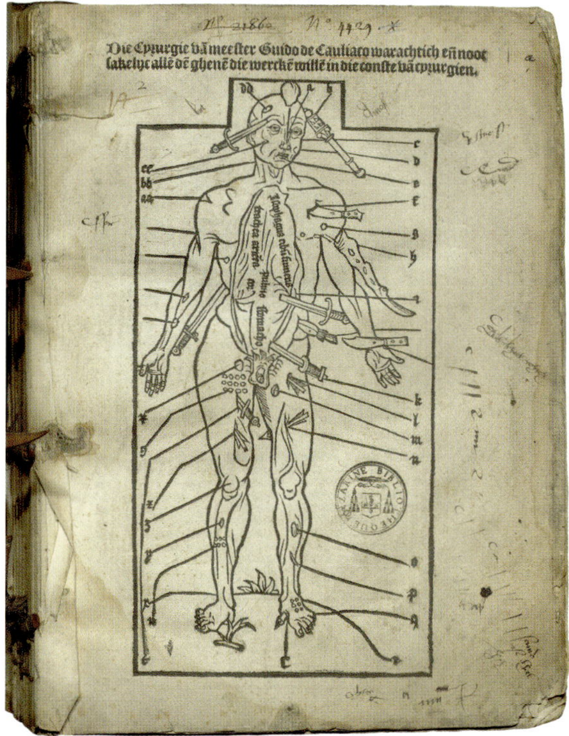

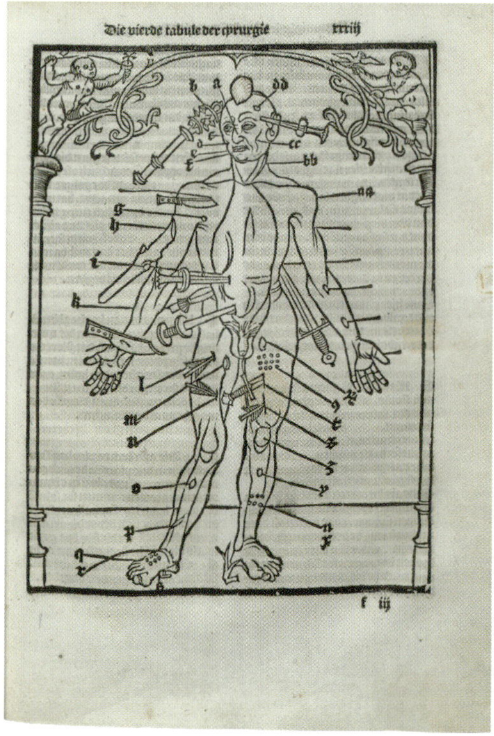

Fig. 4.18. Dutch Wound Men. *Left:* Wound Man from *Die Cyrurgie van meester Guido de Cauliaco* (Antwerp: Henrick Eckert van Homberch, 1508). Woodcut, 29 x 21 cm. Paris, Bibliothèque Mazarine, RES-TD73-13, fol. a1r. *Right:* Wound Man from the *Fasciculus medicine* (Antwerp: Claes de Grave, 1512). Woodcut, 27 x 21 cm. Ritterhude, Milestones of Science Books, #002039, fol. f3r.

work's translator, one Petrus Antonianus, gives a clear citation of his source in the book's introduction, as well as a strong sense of the motivation behind this edition:

> *Hieroneme hebbe ic Petrus Antonianus ter eeren vander generoser stadt van Antwerpen een ten profijte vanden gemeinen volcke, eenen boeck wt den latijne in dye duytsche sprake ghetraeslateert geheeten Fasciculus medicine.*
>
> This is why I, Petrus Antonianus, in honor of the generosity of the city of Antwerp and for the benefit of ordinary people, have taken a book written in Latin and translated it into Dutch, called *Fasciculus medicine*.

The practically orientated contents of the Gregoris' *Fasciculus*, free of theoretical nomenclature and the baggage of medical heritage found in many comparable specialist books, clearly chimed with Antonianus's intention to return medical knowledge to "*gemeinen volcke*" (ordinary people). To this aim, the 1512 work enlarged the Venetian model in its contents, providing Dutch texts that expanded on the themes of the core *Fasciculus* treatises. In visual terms, the Antwerp volume borrowed only loosely from the Venetian editions of the 1490s. Two of the Gregoris' narrative vignettes are included—scenes of the physician visiting a plague patient and receiving urine samples, the latter relegated to the very back of the book—and all six of the diagrammatic *Fasciculus* figures remain. But crammed into the Dutch book's smaller margins, the style of these figures' bodies and borders reflects their doubled geographical allegiances. Italianate putti play in the upper corners of the Wound Man plate and along the armrests of the Disease Woman's ornate seat, while the Zodiac Man's long flowing hair seems much more closely aligned with the astrological figures found in German bloodletting calendars and almanacs like those of Johann Prüss.[122]

In short, the *Fasciculus* and its figures were anything but static. By the turn of the sixteenth century, buoyed by the international popularity of its incunable vehicle, the Wound Man was to be found across Europe in printed books that were just as innovative and changeable as their manuscript forebears in terms of both their medical contents and their aesthetic character. In fact, the *Fasciculus* continued to prove popular for at least a generation. Back in Italy, this time on the opposite side of the peninsula in the Duchy of Milan, the printer Giovanni de Castellione produced his own edition of the Italian *Fasiculo* in 1509, incorporating reversed interpretations of the Gregoris' images from their first Italian edition.[123] At some point around 1513, a brief vogue for sections of the *Fasciculus* and its imagery emerged in Germany, with printers making miniature booklets focusing on either the Disease Woman or the Wound Man.[124] Another Milanese edition appeared in 1516, this one an exact reproduction of Castellione's book, produced by the printer Giovann'Angelo Scinzenzeler.[125] In 1517, the Seville printer Jacob Cromberger reprinted the work yet again in Spanish, part of a broader pattern in the Cromberger press of revival and reissue.[126] By the 1520s, the Gregoris' plates appear to have found their way into the hands of the Arrivabene family of Venetian printers, who produced their own Latin edition in 1522 and another Italian edition in 1523.[127] And in the Netherlands, Claes de Grave was tempted to return to the book for a second Dutch edition released in 1529, a full seventeen years after his first publication of the treatise and its figures.[128] Year after year, the Wound Man and his fellow *Dreibilderserie* images continued to be mobilized as pictorial stalwarts amid the burgeoning market for medical print, their innovative mechanics fine-tuned for mass appeal as a pan-European visual phenomenon.

Flickering Media

As well as highlighting emerging international networks of European print, the reworking of the Wound Man across multiple editions of the *Fasciculus medicinae* offers us a route into understanding the particularly intermedial texture of medical imagery at the end of the fifteenth century and the beginning of the sixteenth.[129] The acknowledgment of the relationship between technologies of the hand and of the machine at this moment in the history of printing is of long standing, stretching back to early modern chroniclers themselves who regularly mentioned the connections between printed texts and earlier manuscripts. But it is only relatively recently that scholars of book history have placed the relationship between these two media under sustained critical pressure. Chiming with the tendency toward overstatement found in pioneering commentators on the so-called Print Revolution, early and mid-twentieth-century writers most often framed the manuscript-incunable relationship as a simple story of progress. Their methods relied upon what Sonja Drimmer has recently dubbed the "prepositional paradigm," an ineluctable sense of technical change in which both texts and images moved unidirectionally from an "old" medium of manuscripts into the "new" medium of the printed book.[130] However, the nuanced work of a significant number of subsequent scholars—including Curt Bühler, Julia Boffey, Donald McKenzie, David McKitterick, Sandra Hindman, and others—has since questioned such an assumed teleology, evoking instead models of interdependence to situate late medieval European manuscripts and early printed books more firmly alongside each other.[131] The case of the Wound Man only confirms such hybridity at work, an image that we can watch flickering excitedly back and forth between manuscript and print.

As early as the 1470s, makers and owners of both medical printed books and manuscripts were beginning to envision their products as sites for media exchange. We have already seen that Europe's earliest incunable users, keen to develop treatises that matched a marketplace well attuned to the value of handcrafted work, commonly called upon book artists to embellish their titles by hand. These intermedial interventions could range from small-scale illuminated initials or minute flurries of rubrication to full-page portraits of historical medics or fully worked-up scenes of treatment. Some even deliberately left blank spaces in and among printed texts for the reader to populate with their own diagrammatic or decorative commentary.[132] However, to think that fifteenth-century intermediality consisted only of skeuomorphic manuscript imports into the finishing of incunables is to overlook important evidence from the opposite side of the corpus. We might just as well approach such hybridity from the perspective of the manuscript, for handmade fifteenth- and sixteenth-century medical books of course continued to be made. In much the same way new printed texts took advantage of older systems of hand-produced imagery, so too did these manuscript-makers take advantage of the cheapness and flexibility to be found in the new print medium.

Most visually exciting among these trends is what we might call medical collage, a technique found in many surviving manuscript books produced by scholars, students, and learned amateurs alike in the era of early print. These are instances in which European medical writers chose simply to dismember the printed works at their disposal—most often segments of inexpensive, single-sheet *Flugblätter*, although sometimes parts of pages from larger print volumes—and glue them into books alongside handwritten texts, annotations, and images, producing a cut-and-paste aesthetic that wore its bibliographical credentials unashamedly.[133] At its most sophisticated, this could result in multimedia medical books whose shared material dependence produced aesthetically fantastic hybrids. Perhaps none is more impressive, in either concept or sheer visual punch, than the pages of a book now in the Národní knihovna in Prague (fig. 4.19).[134] Over 250 folios long, this manuscript contains a collection of around forty texts written by hand in a combination of Old Czech and Latin. Some are only short recipes no longer than a page in length, while others are formal copies of complete treatises with a substantial medieval pedigree, including the so-called *Františkánova kompilace* (Franciscan Compilation), a bilingual Latin-Czech compilation by

Fig. 4.19. Stephanus Plebanus's multimedia manuscript, including a dismembered almanac spread across multiple pages and a print of *The Martyrdom of the Ten Thousand*, c. 1498–1503, Bohemia. Ink and paint on paper with glued paper woodcut and metal-cut inserts, 31 x 21 cm. Prague, Národní knihovna České republiky, MS XVII D 10, fols. 42v, 46r, 242v, 244v.

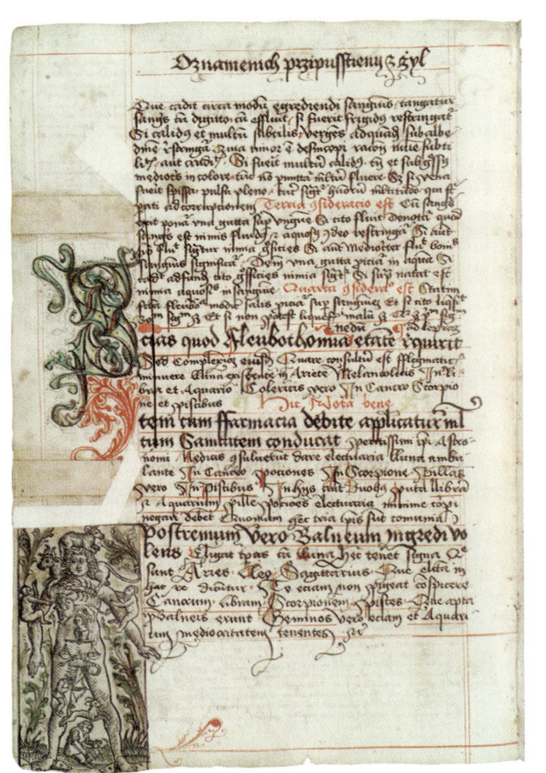

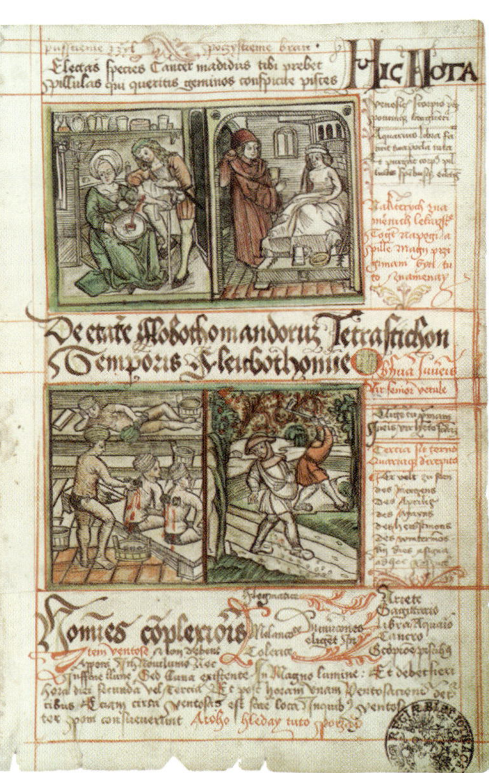

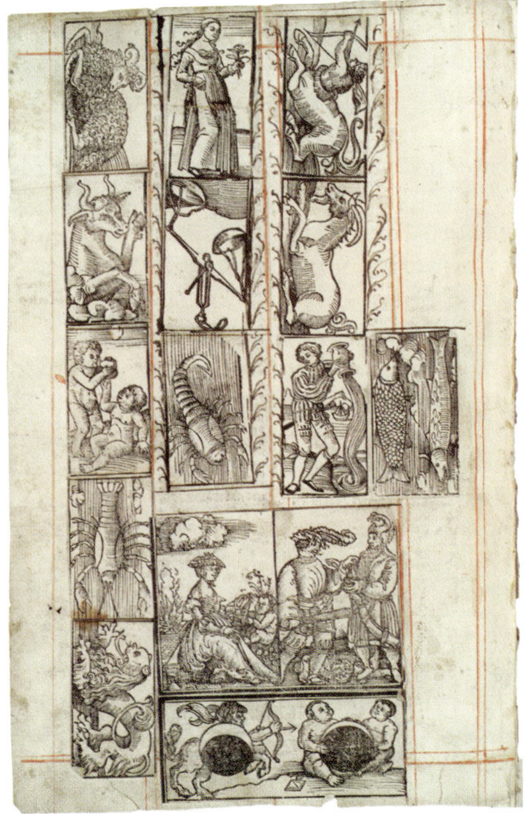

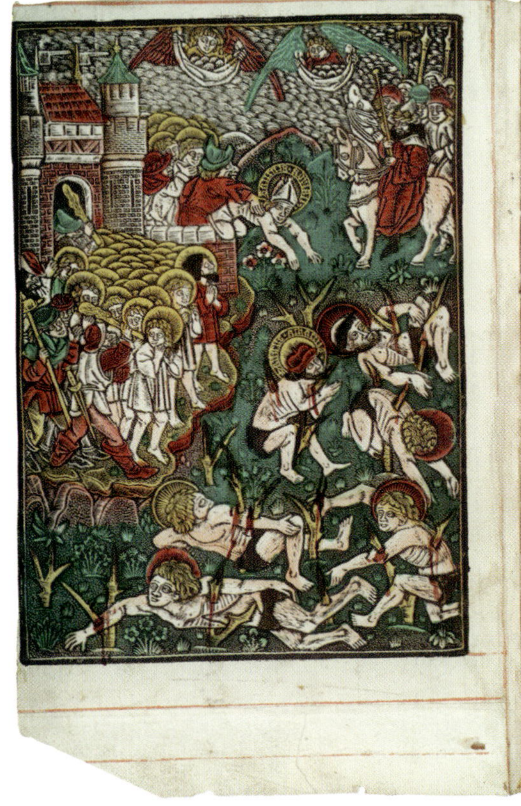

an anonymous Franciscan citing bodily cures that run topographically from head to toe.[135] Three of the book's texts include the name of their scribe as one Stephanus Plebanus and note dates between 1498 and 1503, suggesting that their contents were built up over this period of five years, a fact confirmed by the cumulative nature of the book's imagery as a whole. Although Stephanus's hand is relatively neat, its pages betray a flurry of active, real-time thought. Texts are densely overwritten with notations in all four margins, red rubrics endlessly punctuate mops of black words, floral motifs spill out from grand initials across the gutter, and in certain particularly striking sections Stephanus shifts media in order to amplify the book's creative energy further still, introducing cut-and-paste print elements.

We can track some of these unique printed details back to their published originals. One, a banderole proclaiming "*Ein gut selig new iar*" (A good, blessed new year) that lies pasted beside a handwritten discussion of pleurisy, matches precisely a woodblock being used in the first decade of the century by the Nuremberg printer Hieronymus Höltzel to head a number of single-sheet Czech and German almanacs.[136] Another, a medical broadside on the uses of petroleum pasted into Stephanus's book as its own full page, was originally produced around the year 1500 in the Nuremberg press of Ambrosius Huber.[137] And toward the end of the book we come across multiple such elements running in a frenetic multimedia sequence: first the reader is presented with twelve printed zodiac symbols cut from a dismembered almanac and stuck to the page; then follows a handwritten text on dream divination; then a full-page, pasted, metalcut print of the Martyrdom of the Ten Thousand; then a handwritten Latin indulgence by Pope Alexander V glossed in Italian, German, and Czech; and finally a series of five full-page religious scenes, three of which are pasted xylographic prints—the Five Wounds of Christ, the Mass of Saint Gregory, and Saint Jerome—and two of which are depictions of the *Arma Christi* drawn entirely by hand.[138] Clearly Stephanus was channeling a broad range of written and visual material circulating across the region in both manuscript and printed form and seemingly made little distinction between the two types of media.

As well as these literal acts of print transposition, other manuscript medical works pursued a more subtle style of translation between their pages and the new medium (fig. 4.20). A book now in Basel appears on the surface to be just another of the many astro-medical manuscripts produced in Europe during the later fifteenth century, containing written information on the health landscape of the year across different months and seasons.[139] On closer inspection, however, the contents in fact closely mirror a text already explored in this chapter, the 1484 edition of the *Teutsch Kalender* printed in Strasbourg by Johann Prüss. A note specifically ascribing the book's commission to the Basel councilor Leonard Iselin, as well as the presence throughout of this wealthy family's arms, suggests that it was produced to both abbreviate and elevate the popular printed work in a decorated calligraphic form more fitting for an elite library. As part of this process, the scribe responsible for the manuscript—noted in the work as one Jacob Meiger, or perhaps another unnamed accompanying artist—has also reproduced Prüss's much-utilized hybrid zodiac-bloodletting figure (figs. 4.8 and 4.9). Although not a verbatim

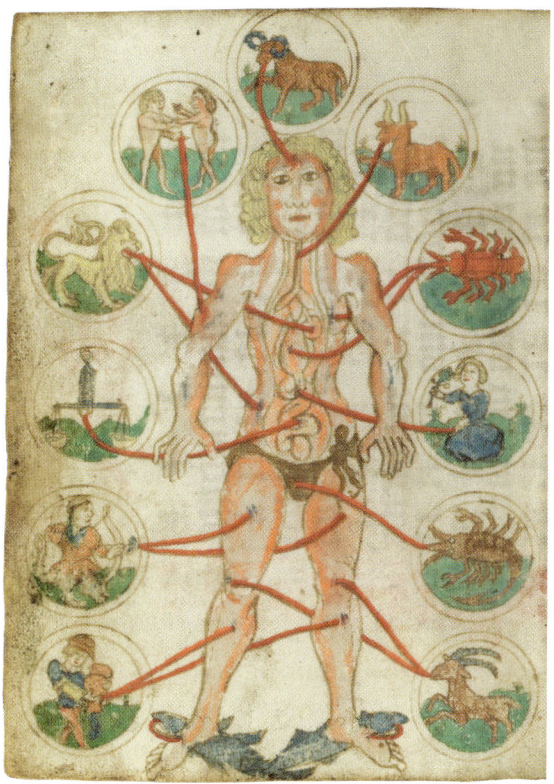

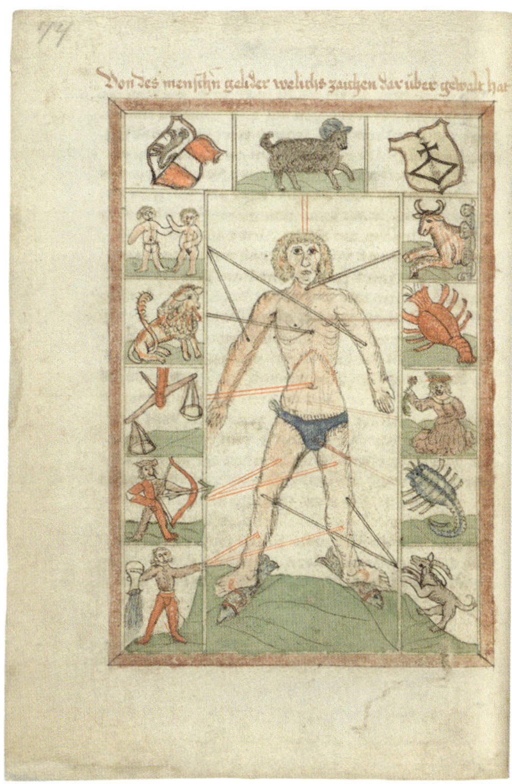

Fig. 4.20. Hand-illustrated copies of Johann Prüss's hybrid figure. *Left:* Hybrid figure, 1490, Basel. Ink and paint on parchment, 10 x 8 cm. Basel, Universitätsbibliothek, O IV 38, fol. 14v. *Right:* Hybrid figure, c. 1518, possibly Salzburg. Ink and paint on paper, 20 x 14 cm. Budapest, Országos Széchényi Könyvtár (Széchényi-Nationalbibliothek), Cod. Germ. 56, fol. 37v.

copy, the Iselin book is entirely indebted to the printed original in both its composition and content, sporting the same flowing hair, the same strangely anatomized innards, and even the same underbriefs as Prüss's almanac figure, tied in a florid knot at the hip. This is an image that flips the accepted teleological narrative of media progression, with print firmly the model for hand-produced work. Moreover, it was one of many. Precisely the same act of faithful reproduction occurs again in another housebook made for an aristocratic Bavarian or Austrian family around 1518, with Prüss's figure once more appearing translated as a colorful freehand drawing, the cheap, disposable print image reworked across media for a new audience.[140]

Given its widespread popularity across Europe, it is unsurprising that we also find the texts and images of the Gregoris' *Fasciculus medicinae* receiving similar intermedial treatment amid what we have already established as their highly international band of users. The simplest form this could take is evidenced in a medical book, now in the library of Trinity College Cambridge, whose handwritten title proclaims itself as *Fasciculus medicine rerum naturalium collectus anno 1507* (Little Bundle of Medicine of Natural Things Collected in the Year 1507).[141] This is a hybrid work in the most literal sense: its initial fifty-four paper folios contain a collection of handwritten medical treatises in Latin and Middle Dutch, while its final twelve comprise a booklet cut wholesale from an early incunable, preserving the opening of Guillermo Saliceto's *De salute corporis* (On the Health of the Body) printed in the Netherlands around 1472.[142] Their combination is particularly useful

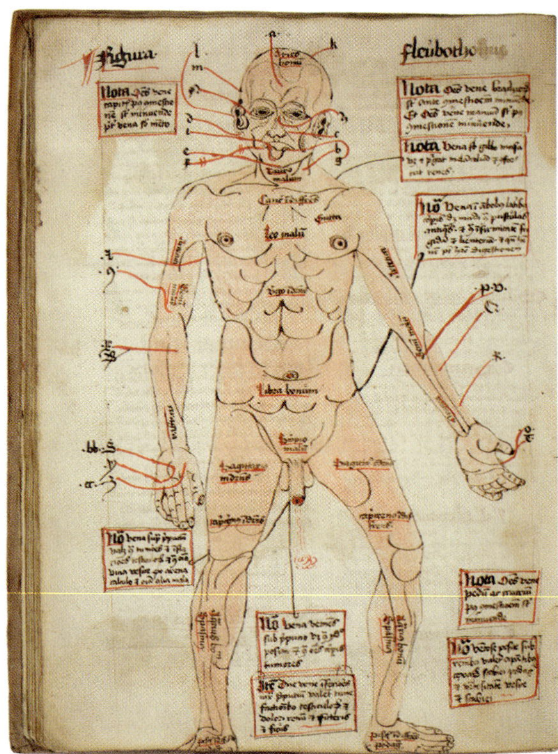

Fig. 4.21. Bloodletting figure copied from the printed *Fasciculus medicinae*, 1507, probably the Netherlands. Ink on paper, 28 x 20 cm. Cambridge, Trinity College, Wren Library, O.9.31, fol. 29v.

for understanding the value of the incunable, a possession prized enough to have been bound alongside the handwritten treatise more than forty years after its printing. And the contents of the book's manuscript elements also speak directly to the influence of print. Two portions of its handwritten text are copied verbatim from the 1491 Latin *Fasciculus*—one reproducing its pair of phlebotomy treatises and the other its treatise on urine—while wedged between them is a full-page drawing of a standing man, instantly recognizable as a duplicate of the *Fasciculus*'s bloodletting figure (fig. 4.21).[143] Colored in an orangey pink and staggering toward the reader in a pose identical to his printed double, its detail suggests a particularly attentive copyist who has engaged with the subtle linearity of the Gregoris' original closely, from the figure's curvaceous receding hairline to the repeated shell-like bulges used by the 1491 woodcutter to delineate the inner edge of his rib cage.[144] This 1507 image is not without its own sense of invention. Some of the information that surrounded the original printed figure has been streamlined, with six of the venous descriptions that once floated rather ambiguously in boxes now moved to the back of the manuscript's accompanying phlebotomical text, and the image's corresponding key has also been extended to incorporate these new descriptors.[145] Nonetheless, we get the sense that for the maker of this book, "using" the *Fasciculus* was not only an invitation to read and absorb its information but also to replicate and reformat it.

Ann Blair has thought through many of the specific reasons why late fifteenth- and early sixteenth-century individuals might have wished to make manuscript copies of printed incunables in this way.[146] These range from practical worries over the long-term durability of paper to the cognitive or spiritual values of copying by hand, as well as more conceptual investments in the look or feel of a decorated manuscript in comparison to the relative sparsity of early print. We know too that hand-copying processes had long played an important role in the exchange and transformation of knowledge and did not simply stop with the advent of the press. Blair cites the case of the prolific fifteenth-century Burgundian book collector Raphael de Marcatellis, whose extensive library was largely constituted of manuscript copies of printed books: forty-eight of the fifty-eight books owned by Marcatellis that still survive were formatted in this manner, most of which were works unavailable in eastern France and that would have been temporarily borrowed from Italian contacts for transcription.[147]

Many *Fasciculus* manuscripts produced from the work's early printed editions preserve a similar investment in the cognitive benefits of copying, showcasing the customization of medical knowledge through addition, excision, and combination. In one Dutch example from around 1500, for instance, three of the Gregoris' texts have been copied as a continuous block alongside a vast array of complementary medical materials.[148] The work's images have been excised: the section simply begins with the Wound Man's accompanying text on surgical cures, copied without its marshaling figure, and where the Disease Man should appear the manuscript instead reproduces his labels alone, affirming its focus on specifically textual medicine. But this scribe's copying is still actively synthetical. Rather than opting for a verbatim transcript of the printed original, they have chosen in their manuscript to mix remedies and recipes on the same topic drawn from different parts of the printed work, a cross-fertilized *Fasciculus* tailored to their particular needs and interests.

A more extreme version of this same idea is found in another surviving manuscript now in Vienna, dated on the basis of its paper watermarks to the 1540s or 1550s (fig. 4.22).[149] At only thirteen folios, this booklet certainly meets the Gregoris' "Little Bundle" on its own terms, its author having opted not for a full *Fasciculus* transcription but rather for swapping and splicing elements of its printed text and images to produce a manuscript with a flavor of the Venetian original yet at the same time almost entirely new. Five of the *Fasciculus* figures are replicated here, although this manuscript's maker, rather than placing them opposite full explanatory treatises, has reproduced only condensed snippets of their counterpart texts in doubled columns framed with decorative arches and floral motifs. The images themselves, shaky yet somehow still hard-edged and precise, have a faltering precision that suggests they are in fact direct tracings of an early Venetian version of the printed work. Even working within these confines, however, their maker has still exercised independent vision. While four of the figures are precisely traced echoes of their incunable counterparts, one appears to be a concoction of this new booklet, a mix-and-match *cadavre exquis* that sets the head of the *Fasciculus* Zodiac Man—complete with askew dimples and ear-length shaggy hair—on top of the unmistakable staggering body of the printed book's bloodletting figure, the combination given away by the presence of rather too many lines at the neck and shoulders.[150]

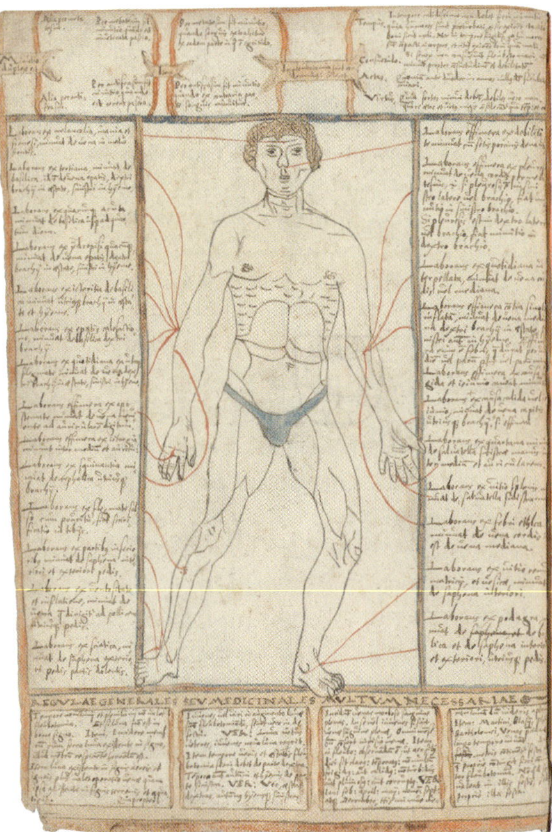

Fig. 4.22. *Cadavre exquis* copied from different parts of the printed *Fasciculus medicinae*, c. 1540–50, Austria or southern Germany. Ink on paper, 33 x 22 cm. Vienna, Österreichische Nationalbibliothek, Cod. 14034, fol. 4v.

Caught up in this inventive replication of the *Fasciculus*, we also find the print Wound Man preserved by hand in several manuscripts from the early 1500s. This was more than just a passive exercise. Like many of their intermedial medical counterparts, the visual innovations and recombinations of these images are deft, at once careful and imaginative enough to make clear that translating the Wound Man from one medium to another was considered a creative act in its own right. On the one hand, we find copyists focused on clarity and faithfulness in their reproduction. Take a manuscript now in Leiden's Universiteitsbibliotheek, which, apart from a single short phlebotomical treatise—written in Dutch, confirming the book's origin in the Netherlands—meticulously duplicates in a neat hand the full text of the Gregoris' first-edition *Fasciculus* (fig. 4.23).[151] It copies the original's diagrammatic figures as well, each occupying a full page and preserving the Gregoris' letter-keys, including a sparse Wound Man that finely reimagines the linear quality of the original's woodblock in shades of black ink.[152]

On the other hand, we find Wound Men translated across media with originality and flair. The most extravagant is a manuscript now in Ljubljana's Semeniška knjižnica, titled on its frontispiece *Ein khleins Püschle von Practickhen* (A Little Bundle of Practice) (fig. 4.24).[153] It contains a detailed and complete translation of the *Fasciculus* into German—something never produced in full in print—with the translator's text bearing such a close

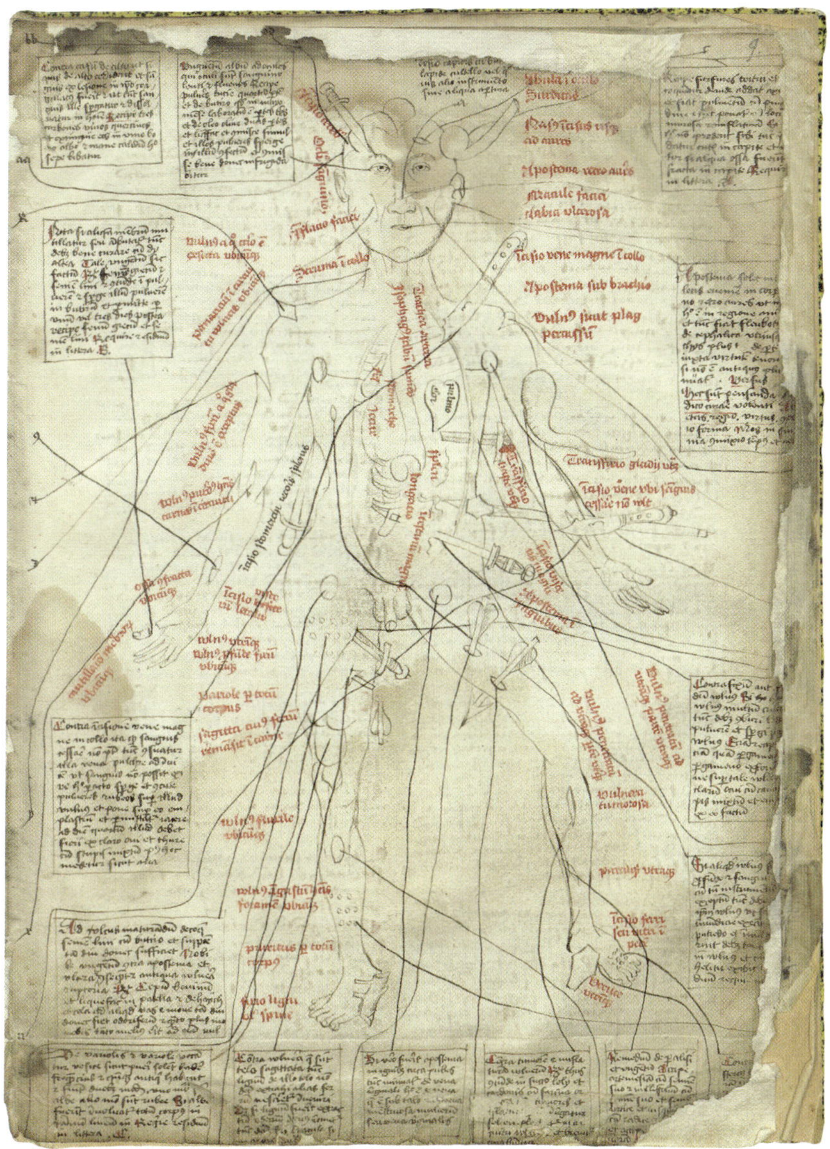

Fig. 4.23. Wound Man copied from the printed *Fasciculus medicinae*, after 1491, the Netherlands. Ink on paper, 29 x 17 cm. Leiden, Universiteitsbibliotheek, MS BPL 1905, fol. 9r.

correspondence to the original that we can tell its exemplar was the final Latin edition of the book to be published in Venice, a 1522 printing by Cesare Arrivabene. At this point in the *Fasciculus*'s history, the booklet had grown to contain eleven different treatises, and this German manuscript diligently translates them all, as well as including remarkably sophisticated copies of nearly all the printed original's woodcuts.[154] Signed in two places with the initials N.P. and in one place dated 1559, they are doubtless the work of an extremely skilled professional artist with a particular sensitivity for the original printed work's twofold mode of woodcut address. The German version marks a clear distinction between narrative and diagrammatic imagery. When reproducing the quotidian scenes of doctors and patients, the artist employs a confident graphic style of hatched shading with only the slightest

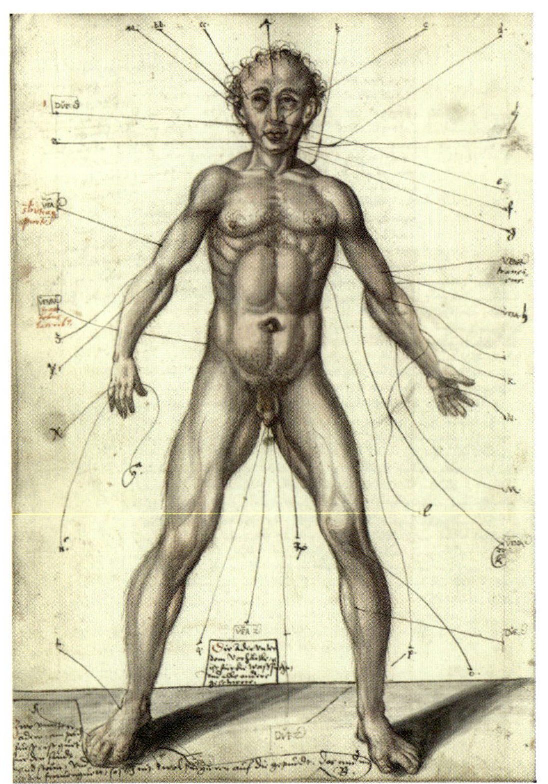

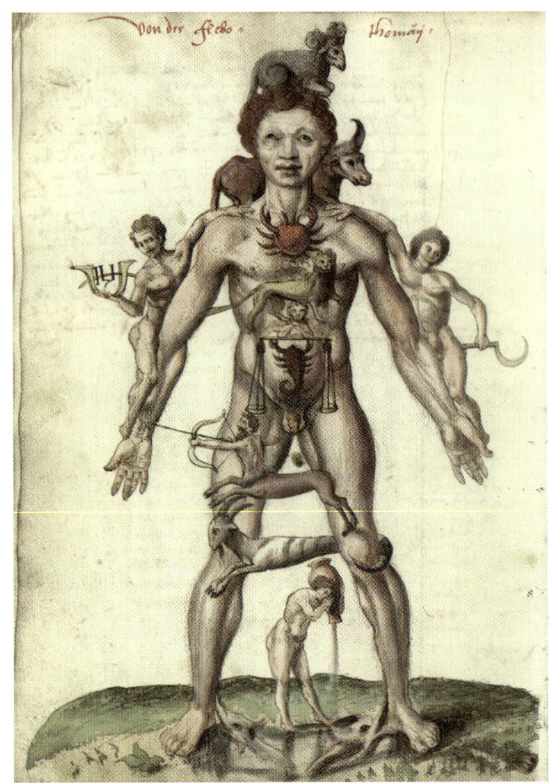

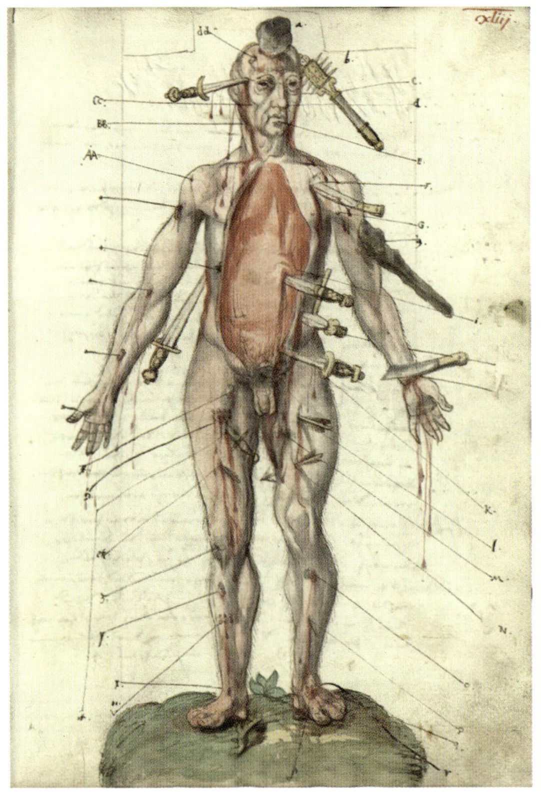

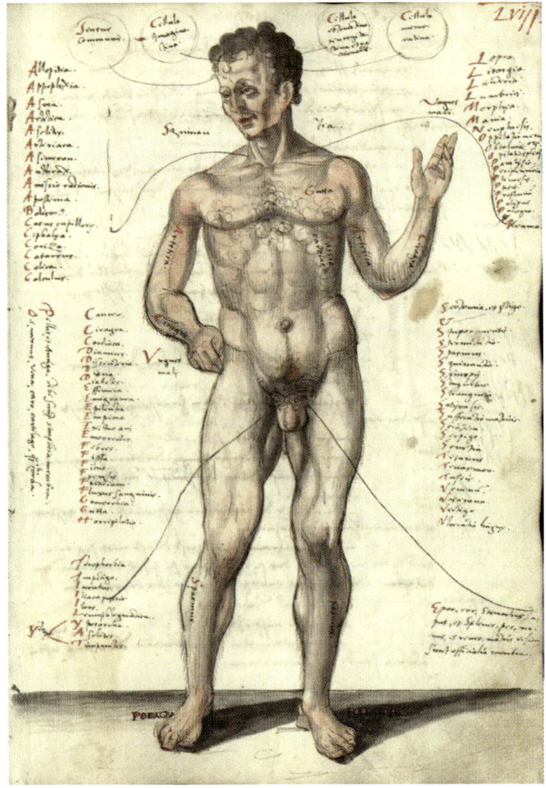

occasional highlights of color, an approach particularly fitting for reinterpreting colorless ink prints. But for the Ljubljana book's cadre of *Dreibilderserie* images and related diagrammatic figures, a much bolder treatment takes over. Flooded with color, their rounded forms leap off the page in a way unimaginable in a printed work. The muscular body of the bloodletting figure is highly detailed, even down to the curly hairs on his chest. The Zodiac Man gazes to the heavens as his body is beset by astrological signs whose acute naturalism only further emphasizes their playful, monstrous qualities. The Disease Man strikes his pose with a smile, casting a realistic shadow behind him on the floor. And each of the Wound Man's outrageous injuries is laboriously individuated through darkened bruising, with streams of blood and subtle gradations of red used to model his fleshy opened chest.[155]

Fig. 4.24. Bloodletting figure, Zodiac Man, Wound Man, and Disease Man copied from the printed *Fasciculus medicinae*, c. 1559, Germany. Ink and paint on paper, 36 x 25 cm. Ljubljana, Semeniška knjižnica, SKLJ Rkp. 2, fols. Vv, XIXv, XLIIIr, LVIIIr.

The story of the Wound Man's emergence in print, we might therefore conclude, was as much an intermedial phenomenon as it was an international one. Passed from German and Bohemian manuscripts into an Italian incunable, then onward into Spanish and Dutch printed editions, and further still into a cross-continental network of hybrid and hand-drawn copies, at each stage in the figure's late fifteenth- and early sixteenth-century life its makers placed a premium on the reproduction of bodies across regions and across formats. That historians have not much cared about this story to date is surely once more a question of disciplinary bias. Virtually all scholars writing on the *Fasciculus* have arrived at the "Little Bundle" from a definably early modern point of view, the beginning of the story of renaissance print rather than a second stage in the life of a medieval group of images. It is perhaps for this same reason that they have also been content to leave the story there. Happy to compartmentalize the *Fasciculus* in its incunable moment, its texts and images are only really spoken of as the starting gun on printed medicine. But if we stick with the Wound Man once more, we will discover that the image's shift into the sixteenth century and beyond holds more in the way of connections than breaks. If the *Fasciculus* formed one point of pivot for the history of the Wound Man, opening it up to new media and new audiences across Europe, then the subsequent early modern history of the image amplified its impact further still as it reached new intellectual and aesthetic networks, both local and global.

CHAPTER FIVE

Image: Wound Man Aesthetics

Thanks to the royalty-free image policies of London's Wellcome Library, the most widely reproduced Wound Man comes from a manuscript currently in its care (fig. 0.1).[1] This figure has graced the front cover of academic books, appeared on album sleeves, and even featured as a prop on a prime-time US television show.[2] It also acts as a useful hinge between the concerns of this chapter and the last.

It is certainly among the most eye-catching versions of the image. Occupying the entirety of a small parchment page, this Wound Man is brought to life through a combination of bold color and intricate line, his skin painted in a thick pastel-pink wash and given depth through an unusual form of scratchy penwork shading particularly evident at his face. As we have by now come to expect, he is beset by the typically overwhelming hallmarks of highly specific injuries and illnesses, many of which are finely detailed in this example: the bulging woodgrain of the rounded club at his left shoulder, the scratched metal blades of various knives slashing his skin, the elegant, decorated hilts of the swords that slide into his body. His wounds are somehow both subtle and elaborate, small in size and yet enunciated with deep black centers or individuated streams of red, flowing downward like bloody petals. So evocative are these tools and their effects that one user—perhaps contemporary, perhaps later—has been moved to stab through the parchment page multiple times with a pin at the figure's knees.

Placing this particular Wound Man historically, however, is tricky. His body is surrounded by a cluster of underlined, abbreviated Latin catchwords that elaborate some of his conditions in a familiar format: *Incisio cerebri* (Incision to the brain), *Inflatio faciei* (Swelling of the face), *Veruce utrique* (Warts on both sides), *Vulnus angustum habens foramen ubicunque* (Narrow wound with an opening in any place), and so on. Yet what sets this Wound Man apart, separating it in fact from every one of the many examples of the image considered in this book so far, is that these limited, floating sentences are the only text found across this entire manuscript that directly relates to the figure and his cure.

Kathleen Scott and Jesús Romero-Barranco have examined the rest of this book's decoration and hand, as well as its use of certain linguistic patterns, and both have soundly concluded that it was produced in southern England around the mid-fifteenth century.[3] Its main sections preserve a pair of anatomical treatises. The first is a Middle English text, forty-eight folios long and ascribed pseudonymously in a Latin incipit to Galen, that lists the internal structure of the body in five chapters, organized from the *soyft brayne* downward. The second is a Middle English translation of the *Anatomia porci* (Anatomy of the Pig), a well-known and much shorter text originally produced in the eleventh or twelfth century that describes the theoretical dissection of a pig, attributed to the Salernitan master Copho.[4] Apart from the occasional illuminated initial, it is only in the manuscript's final pages—a suspiciously separate quire of eight folios—that the book's diagrammatic medical imagery appears. This includes a pair of nude male figures, a pair of skeletons, and a pair of figures with exposed nerves or veins, each duo shown doubled across facing pages from both front and behind, followed in turn by two images drawn from the late medieval *Dreibilderserie* tradition: the Disease Woman and, at the very back of the book, the Wound Man.[5] These figures, separated out from the medical substance of the manuscript's two core treatises, lack any textual elaboration besides the occasional hovering label.

Looking back on the history of the Wound Man, we recognize this as highly unusual. Throughout its fifteenth-century usage, the figure helped marshal surgical knowledge through its close relationship with an integral accompanying treatise, the so-called *Wundarznei*, which listed procedures and recipes to combat the ills illustrated about his body. Both figure and text needed to be present for the user to successfully cross-reference a depicted injury with its correlative cure and vice versa. Appearing alone in this Wellcome manuscript, the medical mechanics of the image simply fail. What then was the purpose of this isolated Wound Man, tucked away at the very back of the book?

We are helped in answering this question by attending to this figure's visual particularities. These bear a striking resemblance not to its fifteenth-century manuscript fellows but to the earliest known printed version of the figure, produced in Venice in 1491 as part of the *Fasciculus medicinae*, the assorted medical booklet discussed at length in the previous chapter (fig. 4.1). Like its incunable counterpart, the Wellcome Wound Man holds a tight pose, with muscular arms drawn down and palms outstretched toward the viewer. The two images boast the same square jawlines, hairless heads, open-eyed stares, and rounded chins, they share twin transparent stomachs, and the cuspular detailing of their knees matches line for line. The loose, fuzzy shapes of their internal organs are likewise extremely similar—something no manuscript Wound Men share so closely—and they even bear identical murderous instrumentation. Swords, spears, daggers, and clubs attack their bodies at precisely the same locations, they bleed from the same cuts, and they share sores of the same shape, orientation, and size.

These similarities prompted early observers to argue that this Wellcome Wound Man formed the prototype for the printed Venetian figure, although from our earlier exploration of the *Fasciculus* and its history, we know this cannot have been the case with this textless image.[6] We also know that the

1491 book and its subsequent editions generated a flurry of intermedial copying, with hand-written and hand-illustrated versions of the printed work surviving in a spread of sixteenth-century manuscripts now in Cambridge, Vienna, Leiden, Ljubljana, and elsewhere (figs. 4.21–4.24). The Wellcome figure must thus have come about through the same process of visual rephrasing from print to manuscript and is in fact explicitly confirmed as a copy by the presence of certain peculiar elements lost in translation. The top of the head of the printed 1491 *Fasciculus* Wound Man, for example, depicts a stone lodged inside a circular wound or bruise—plainly identified as such with the label "*Lesio capitis cum lapide*" (Lesion of the head [made] with a stone)—yet the flattening and saturation of this detail in print seems to have produced some confusion for the Wellcome artist. With little regard for the original text, or perhaps limited ability to understand its Latin labels, they have instead merged their version of the stone with its accompanying lesion to produce a uniform gray patch, maybe intended as an ill-fitting hat or metal helmet to emphasize the general warfaring ethos of the battered figure.

This Wound Man and the entire independent quire of figures at the back of the Wellcome manuscript were therefore produced at some point after the printed *Fasciculus* was first published in 1491. It may well have been very soon after. Sonja Drimmer has drawn attention to a scientific manuscript compendium completed in London in 1490 that illustrated the astrological text of Ptolemy's *Almagest,* with personifications of star signs and planets copied directly from the woodcuts of another Venetian printed book, the Roman author Hyginus's *Poetica astronomica* published by the German printer Erhard Ratdolt in 1482, 1485, and 1488.[7] As little as two years could have transpired between the Venetian printing and the English copy. Evidence from the contemporary English medical scene likewise corroborates that Italian printed medical books were circulating in the country soon after publication. Vivian Nutton has noted that Garret Godfrey, for instance, an early sixteenth-century bookseller in Cambridge, could arrange for shipments of recently printed material from both Lyon and Venice to cross the Channel at speed.[8] A tantalizingly unfinished note on the Wellcome manuscript's final page opposite the Wound Man reads, "This is . . . ," likely the beginning of a colophon formulation familiar to English readers around 1500: "This is a book belonging to . . . ." Beyond this fragment, though, we cannot be sure who precisely commissioned the copying of this booklet as a luxurious flourish to the earlier medical work.

This Wellcome example highlights a final crucial aspect of the Wound Man and its history. We have seen that the figure was originally born of a medieval surgical text and was subsequently popularized through printed medical books across the European continent. But the elaborate paintings at the back of this otherwise quite normal English manuscript suggest that by the turn of the sixteenth century there was something more about the Wound Man that appealed to readers. As a striking picture, it could be reproduced in its own right without any real accompanying medicine. In the previous chapter, we saw the Wound Man become detached from a particular medium, moving from manuscript to print and back again. This chapter extends that logic by tracing the drifting of the figure away from its diagrammatic origins altogether and showing how it emerged as a representative of the medical field in a far more aesthetic sense. Relieved of its duties as a mediator of specific medical cures, the Wound Man was granted yet another life: an extensive, independent existence that from the turn of the sixteenth century went on to unfold for some three hundred years around the world. In short, this chapter charts the Wound Man's evolution into an untethered artistic image.

The Wound Man as Medical Title Page

The Wellcome's English Wound Man is in fact one of several surviving late fifteenth-century works to evidence the beginnings of a new, specifically aesthetic direction for the figure. Foremost among them in terms of both innovation and influence is a figure that appears on the title page of a book from 1497 produced by the Strasbourg printer Johann Grüninger, the so-called *Buch der Cirurgia* (Book of Surgery) of the surgeon Hieronymus Brunschwig (fig. 5.1). Brunschwig and Grüninger's collaboration is a sizable treatise formed of eight chapters that cover the treatment of many different kinds of surgical trauma.[9] And in a number of ways its canny coupling of advice on wound healing with novel print technology is a highly appropriate vehicle for the very first version of the Wound Man to be printed north of the Alps.

As we might imagine for a region that a century earlier gave rise to the diagrammatic *Dreibilderserie* manuscript tradition and its practically oriented cures, German-speaking centers such as Strasbourg had continued to emphasize hands-on healing as the fifteenth century progressed. Medical practitioners in the region exhibited less of a concern for the highly scholastic forms of medical writing popular in some other parts of Europe, and the subject was rarely a substantive focus of German academic life, certainly less so than in the university cities of France and Italy. The vast majority of healers in the region instead learned their craft in more practical environs, trained through apprenticeship amid a wide-reaching network of masters and guilds.[10] Born around 1450, Hieronymus Brunschwig received this typical German training through the local Strasbourg guild of barbers and bathmasters. After working as both a surgeon and an apothecary in a number of nearby regions across the southern Holy Roman Empire, he returned to the city and began channeling his wealth of practical experience into a number of publications on pharmacology, anatomy, distillation, and surgery.[11]

For these texts, Brunschwig opted to write in his native Alsatian dialect, following in the footsteps of earlier German-language medical authors, such as the influential fourteenth-century surgeon Ortolf von Baierland and the fifteenth-century knight-physician Heinrich von Pfolsprundt. This decision opened up Brunschwig's work to a much wider variety of non-Latinate readers, his *Cirurgia* being the earliest known surgical treatise from the region to be printed in the vernacular. The book's aspirations to broad appeal can also be gleaned from its contents. While Brunschwig writes with a keen awareness of medicine's more academic facets, evident in his citation of multiple Classical authors and a liberal sprinkling of traditional theoretical dictums, he more often favors explanations of medicine as a manual craft. Among

Dis ist das buch der Ci/
rurgia. Hantwirch
ung der wund artzny von
Hyerõimo brũschwig

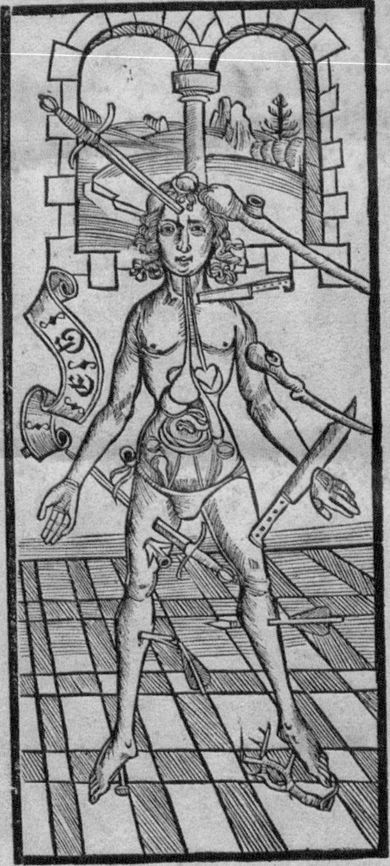

Liber hic editus Argentorati, per Joannem
Grüningerum, anno 1497. rarus; ac Typographiæ
incunabulis adnumerandus.

Fig. 5.1. Title page of Hieronymus Brunschwig's *Buch der Cirurgia* (Strasbourg: Johann Grüninger, 1497). Woodcut, 28 x 20 cm. Munich, Bayerische Staatsbibliothek, 2 Inc.c.a. 3452, title page.

other things, he informs the reader of the different roles and capacities of an ideal surgeon, the different types of wounds and their cures in head-to-toe format, the ways in which injuries can be sustained through different kinds of accidents, and the most effective pharmaceutical recipes for curing different types of ailments. It was this highly practical focus, coupled with learned expertise and expressed in accessible language, that quickly made the text a best seller upon its publication by Grüninger in July 1497. The *Cirurgia* would circulate widely among a substantial audience of medical professionals and learned laypeople alike.[12]

Returning to the book's title page, we find Brunschwig's clever positioning of his medical expertise neatly proclaimed in a short phrase at the top of the page stressing the experiential nature of his surgical skill: "*Dis ist das buch der Cirurgia, hantwirchung der wund artzny von Hyeronimo Brunschwig*" (This is the book of surgery, handiwork of surgery by Hieronymus Brunschwig). This sentiment is echoed too by the particularly thin woodblock of the Wound Man standing beneath these words. Stretching precisely as wide as the author's name and rendered in a long rectangular frame with a thick black border, this figure has little in common with any of the printed Wound Men in contemporaneous circulation around 1497. He has neither the poised muscularity of his Venetian counterpart in the 1491 *Fasciculus medicinae* nor the rounded features of subsequent Italian and Spanish editions of the same book produced in 1494 and 1495 (figs 4.1 and 4.16–4.17). Instead, and fittingly for the book's contents, this woodblock draws on a more local lineage, echoing many of the same features as earlier German *Dreibilderserie* manuscript versions of the figure: he wears the same recognizable skimpy briefs, is impaled by similarly rendered weapons, and presents the same schematic internal anatomy through his strangely transparent stomach.

What is more, Brunschwig's Wound Man has been newly narrativized. Unlike its predecessors, who all stare blankly out at the reader from an equally blank parchment or paper background, the figure of the *Cirurgia*'s title page has been placed firmly in an everyday interior. This is emphatically not a Wound Man presented for its original diagrammatic purpose. No number or letter-key is present linking his injuries to specific cures, and the figure's floating descriptive catchwords have entirely disappeared. The figure is instead alarmingly present, standing in the middle of a checkered tile floor and framed by a double archway giving on to an Alsatian landscape of hills and trees. It is as if we have just turned a corner and stumbled across the Wound Man standing right in front of us, a creature no longer of the neutral picture plane but of the reader's own space.

The relocation of this Wound Man into a semi-realistic setting stems in part from the technical advances in woodblock printing on display in the *Cirurgia*. As a highly active printer on the Strasbourg scene, Grüninger would have been well aware of a woodcut's potential power within the region's burgeoning incunable market. His press produced more illustrated volumes than any other Strasbourg printer of the period, including various editions of Sebastian Brant's *Narrenschiff* (Ship of Fools), several Bibles with woodblock images, an illustrated edition of Hieronymus Baldung's *Aphorismi* (Aphorisms), another chronicling the life of Saint Ursula, and a number of early illustrated political broadsides.[13] This visual engagement extended to his medical works as well, producing a pair of busily illustrated herbals in 1487 and 1489, as well as a Book of Hours in 1494 that included a bloodletting figure among its calendrical materials.[14] The *Cirurgia* also benefited from this visual expertise. It boasted nearly fifty large-scale images placed throughout the book, most stretching the full height of the page and punctuating Brunschwig's writing with a range of medical scenarios that would have been well known to readers. Familiar scenes are populated by familiar characters—an apothecary in his shop, sick men lying in their beds, a surgeon kneeling to begin work on a patient—and importantly, the images included both contemporary medical professionals and, as Tillmann Taape has shown, the figure of the so-called *gestreiffelten leyen* (striped layman), the stereotype of a highly fashionable yet capable layman inserted to flatter the book's ideal nonmedical reader.[15]

More curious, however, is the fact that only around half of the *Cirurgia*'s images were printed from complete woodblocks. The rest follow a complex modular composition produced by chopping and changing different combinations of half-sized blocks that could be paired to produce a range of seemingly unified single images. This technique was new to the Grüninger press. First used only months earlier in November 1496 in a heavily illustrated edition of Terence's *Comedies*, thin blocks depicting individual characters were rearranged page by page, depending on the casting of a particular scene.[16] This visual practice served a similar function in the *Cirurgia*, but with two groups of more clinical personnel: roughly half of the half-blocks are dedicated to tight gatherings of healers, and the remainder depict different individual patients, allowing Grüninger to stage multiple types of novel surgical scenarios in deceptively continuous interiors.[17] One such half-block portrays a group of three particularly busy practitioners gesturing in almost frantic dialogue, a trio who appear multiple times throughout the book paired with at least four other half-blocks to conjure up four separate vignettes (fig. 5.2). In one image, they point to a patient dressed in a cloak and seated by a door. In another, their fingers gesture across a room that has morphed relatively convincingly into an apothecary's shop, complete with a young assistant grinding ingredients. In a third, they have been transported to a room flanked by shelves of medicine jars, where they attend to a different seated patient. And in several further scenes, the gestures of these same doctors are redirected to a half-block Wound Man, the very same figure used for the book's title page. This is what accounts for the particularly long, thin dimensions of the *Cirurgia*'s opening Wound Man and explains why the figure itself is placed into such realistic space. Doing so allowed the image to be neatly slotted into a multitude of printed realities later on in the book. No longer a surgical diagram but a portrait, this Wound Man comes alive to stalk the stone halls of contemporary healing spaces and to be examined by several different groups of medical professionals.

A question still remains as to why the Wound Man was selected by Grüninger for the book's title page. Given their interchangeable nature, any of the book's half-blocks depicting troubled patients or capable healers would have been an appropriate choice for elevation to the *Cirurgia*'s first folio.

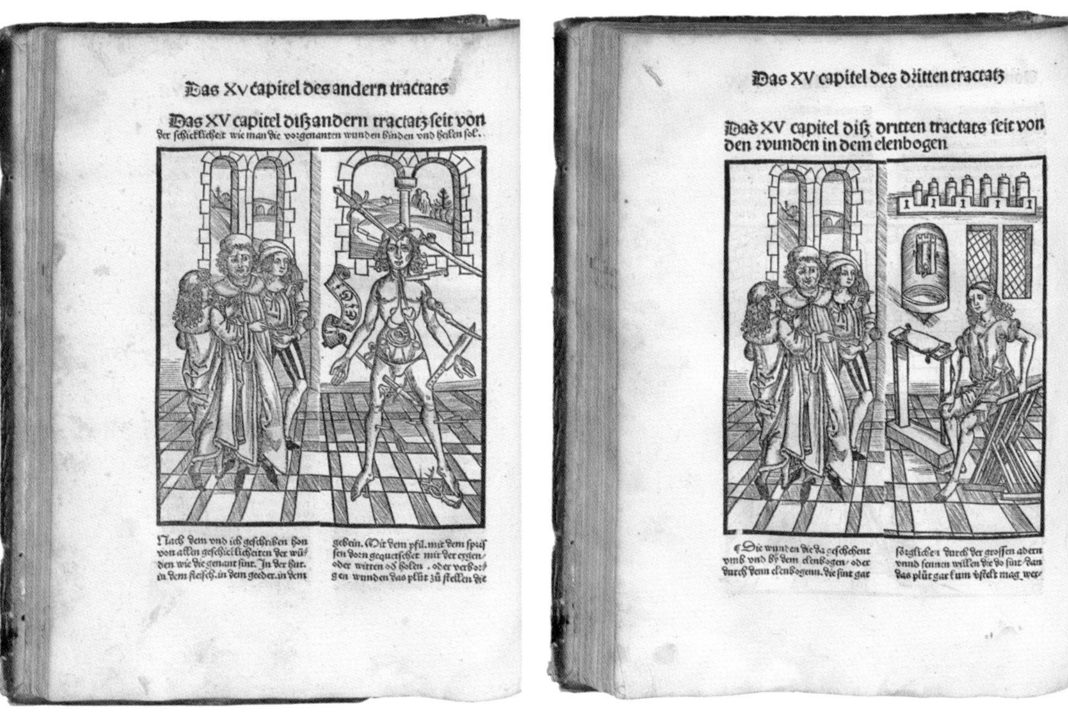

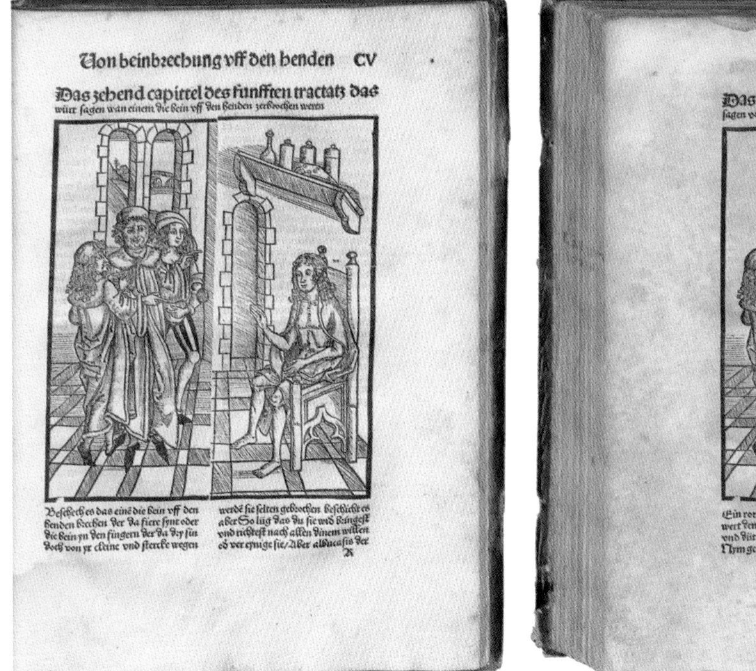

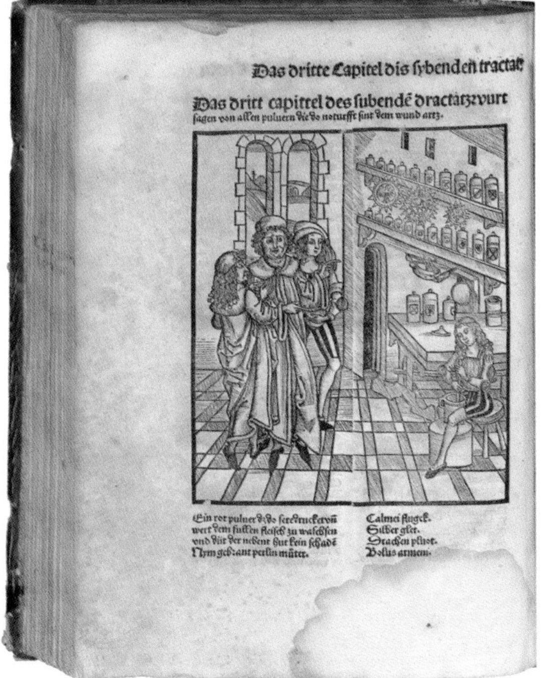

Fig. 5.2. Scenes made by combining a half-block depicting three doctors with various patients and the Wound Man, from Hieronymus Brunschwig's *Buch der Cirurgia* (Strasbourg: Johann Grüninger, 1497). Woodcuts, 28 x 20 cm. Munich, Bayerische Staatsbibliothek, 2 Inc.c.a. 3452, fols. XXXVIIv, LXVv, CVr, CXXIIv.

So why choose the Wound Man? Consider Brunschwig's work more closely in its immediate artistic context. At this point in time, the very concept of a title page was still a relatively new, flexible phenomenon in European printed books. As Ursula Rautenberg and Margaret Smith have both shown, these bibliographic spaces were still highly varied in the late fifteenth century.[18] Some incunable works were titled only with text—fulfilling the need for quick identification of a book—while others gradually introduced front-page images of various types in the hope of appealing to different potential audiences. We might read the choice of the Wound Man as a smart piece of marketing on the part of Grüninger and Brunschwig. Certainly, if such title pages were born of a competition for attention, late fifteenth-century Germany was producing a significant roster of ever more remarkable printed bodies against which Grüninger's Wound Man would have been compared. Images of graphic male subjects—often religiously oriented scenes of Saint Sebastian, Christ in agony, or the Seven Deadly Sins—had been circulating for decades in Germany as woodblock broadsides. But by the 1490s they were being joined by representations of even more extreme bodies, especially those ostensibly linked to real-world medical events.

In late 1495, a short printed pamphlet authored by Sebastian Brant and entitled *Von der wunderbaren Geburt des Kindes bei Worms* (On the Wondrous Birth of the Child near Worms) began to circulate throughout the region as a broadsheet. In Strasbourg, it was reworked into Latin and produced as a folio booklet by the printer Johann Prüss, whom we met in the previous chapter printing astro-medical almanacs.[19] In the volume, Brant framed the recent birth of conjoined twins in the town of Bürstadt as a religious portent reflecting the abnormality of contemporary politics, especially the recently concluded political diet held in the city of Worms, only seven kilometers from the site of the twins' birth. Prüss's Strasbourg booklet reproduced Brant's extended satirical and prognosticatory poem over six short pages, and the volume as a whole was fronted by a woodcut title page: a halved composition—fittingly for its doubled subject matter—presenting the reader with a condensed view of the city of Worms on the right and on the left an image of the twins themselves, alive and well despite being dramatically fused at the forehead. Elsewhere, even more explicitly medicalized images were being similarly mobilized for dramatic printed effect. Around 1496, a young Albrecht Dürer is likely to have provided the central woodcut for another broadside produced in Nuremberg by the printer Hans Mair, depicting a syphilitic man surrounded by verses narrating an astrological dream of the Dutch doctor Theodorus Ulsenius, who had been brought to Nuremberg in the hope that he could provide a cure for the disease (fig. 5.3).[20] Dressed as a *Landsknecht*, one of the Teutonic foot soldiers thought responsible for spreading syphilis northward through Switzerland and Germany, the man stands with arms outstretched, almost as if he were a mournful Christ—or perhaps a figural medical diagram—with his bright red, hand-painted robe raised at the thigh to teasingly reveal sore-stricken skin.

These were the figures with which Grüninger's Wound Man was competing. Brant's politicization of conjoined twins or Dürer's sickly soldier may have come with far inferior medical pedigrees, but they caught the reader's

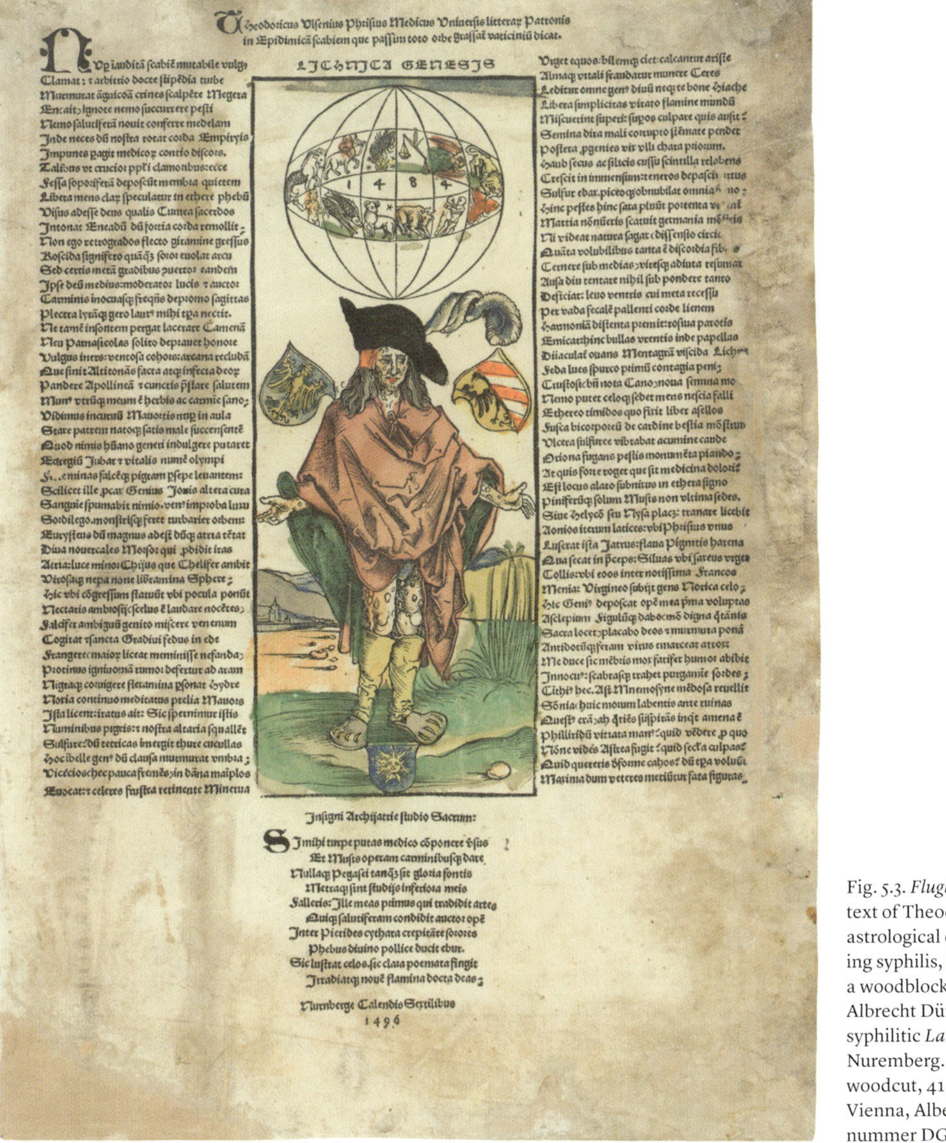

Fig. 5.3. *Flugblatt* with the text of Theodorus Ulsenius's astrological dream discussing syphilis, illustrated with a woodblock attributed to Albrecht Dürer depicting a syphilitic *Landsknecht*, 1496, Nuremberg. Hand-colored woodcut, 41 x 28 cm. Vienna, Albertina, Inventarnummer DG1930/210.

eye in a busy marketplace. Given this backdrop, it was likely the Wound Man's strikingly graphic nature that made Grüninger and Brunschwig so keen to co-opt it for the *Cirurgia*'s title page. Their figure was set up as an aesthetic lure, although happily it was one that nonetheless also functioned as an appropriate meditative entry point into Brunschwig's surgical world. What more vivid a medical symbol could one wish for when proudly launching the first printed German-language surgical work onto the market? The image's potential for sensation was at least clear to the unknown artist responsible for the half-block, who chose it as a space to prominently display their initials, E.G., in a floating banderole to the figure's right: the very first Wound Man to be signed as an artwork.[21]

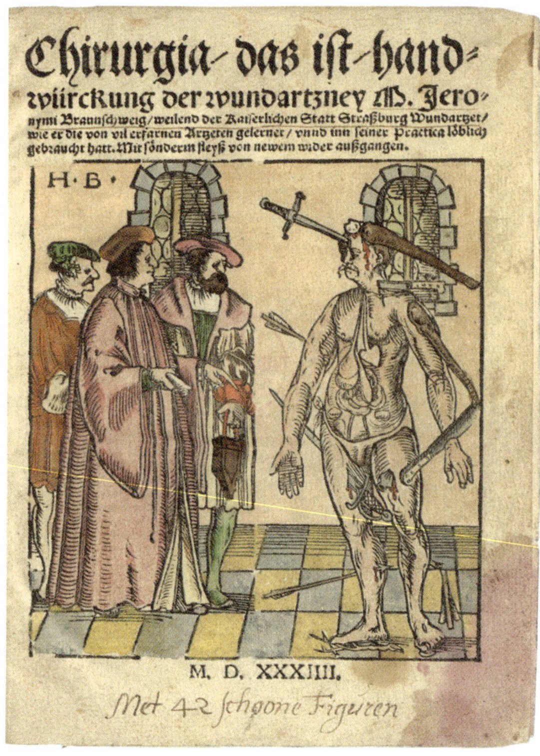

Fig. 5.4. Title page of Hieronymus Brunschwig's *Buch der Cirurgia* (Augsburg: Alexander Weißenhorn, 1534). Hand-colored woodcut, 20 x 15 cm. Berlin, Staatsbibliothek, Jg 3486, title page.

Another testament to the immediate success of both the *Cirurgia* and its Wound Man was their regular reprinting. Less than five months after Grüninger's edition first premiered in Strasbourg, a near-identical version was published in Augsburg by the printer Johann Schönsperger, who reproduced the full text of Brunschwig's surgical treatises alongside almost exact copies of Grüninger's modular woodcuts, missing only the occasional details of their complex changeable plugs. In 1513, Grüninger himself reprinted the work, this time including Brunschwig's short treatise on anatomy, while a few years later the first of what would grow to be several translations of the work appeared: in 1518 the Rostock printer Ludwig Dietz produced a version in Low German; in 1525 an English edition emerged from the London press of Peter Treveris; and in 1535 the book was translated into Dutch for publication in Utrecht by Jan Berntsz.[22] Back in Germany, a 1534 edition produced by the Augsburg printer Alexander Weißenhorn furnished the work with a new complete set of modular woodcuts, including a reworked Wound Man—this time a far more muscular, mustachioed presence—who is once again elevated to the work's title page, shown turning to face a trio of medics in three-quarter pose (fig. 5.4).[23]

The continued presence of Brunschwig's popular book helped drive the production of further illustrated medical works in German presses. These ranged in style and form, from the bizarre rectangular diagrammatic torsos of Johannes Peyligk's 1499 *Compendium philosophiae naturalis* (Compendium of Natural Philosophy) or Magnus Hundt's 1501 *Antropologium de hominis dignitate* (Anthropology: On the Dignity of Man), to the philosophical anatomies of sweeping textbooks like Gregor Reisch's 1503 *Margarita philo-*

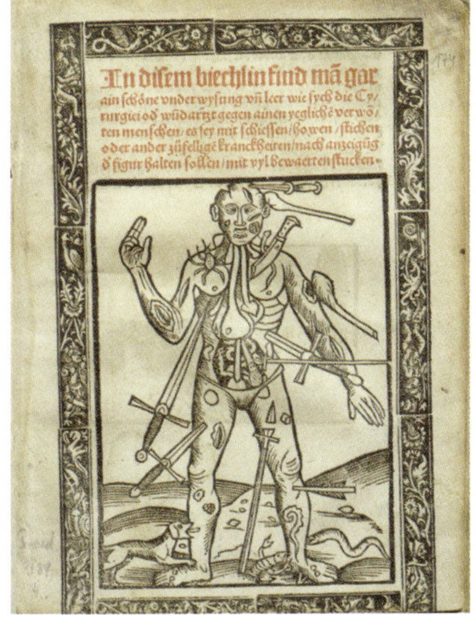

In disem biechlin find mā gar ain schöne vnderwysung vñ leer wie sych die Cyrurgici od' wūdartzt gegen ainen yeglichē verwōten menschen/ es sey mit schiessen/ howen/ stichen oder ander zůfellige kranckhaiten/ nach anzaigūg d' figur halten sollen/ mit vyl bewaerten stucken.

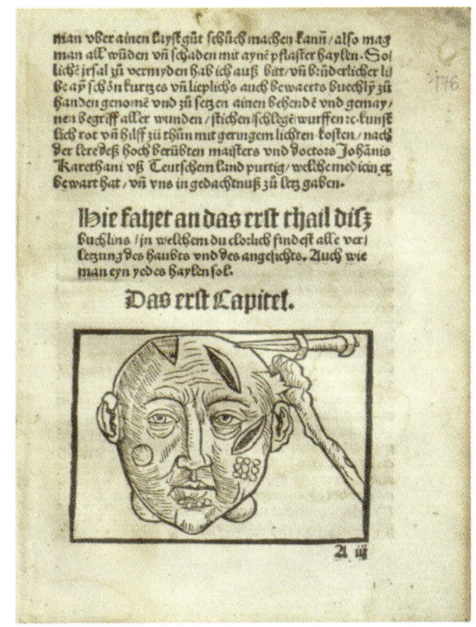

Hie fahet an das erst thail disz büchlins / jn welchem du clorlich findest alle verletzung des haubts vnd des angesichts. Auch wie man eyn yedes haylen sol.

Das erst Capitel.

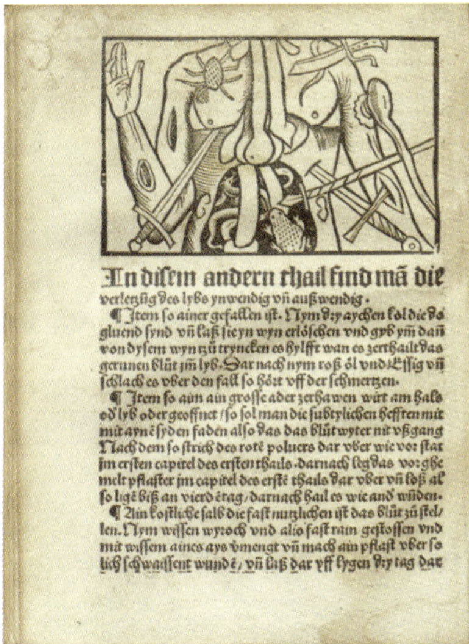

In disem andern thail find mā die verletzūg des lybs ynwendig vñ außwendig.

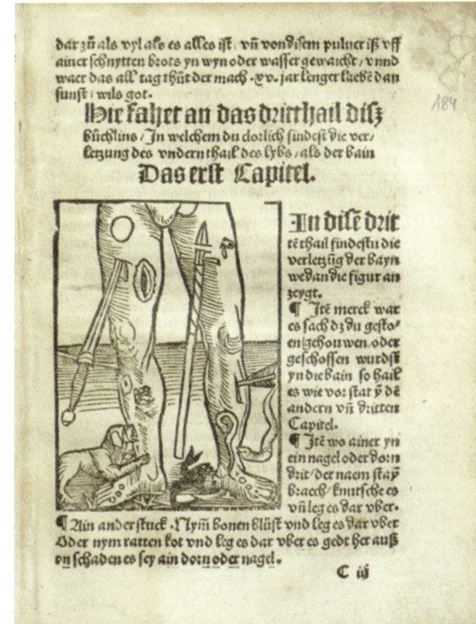

Hie fahet an das dritthail disz büchlins / In welchem du clorlich findest die verletzung des vndern thail des lybs / als der bain

Das erst Capitel.

Fig. 5.5. Title page and amputated close-ups of the Wound Man from a surgical *Biechlin* (Cologne: Arnd von Aich, c. 1515). Woodcuts, 19 x 14 cm. Frankfurt am Main, Goethe Universität, Universitätsbibliothek, rebound as part of incunable sammelband Ausst. 253, Nr. 4, fols. 174r, 176r, 179v, 184r.

sophica (Pearl of Philosophy) or scenes of everyday cure in vernacular medical mainstays like Lorenz Freis's 1518 *Spiegel der Artzney* (Mirror of Surgery), a work that was also printed by Grüninger in Strasbourg and that reused several woodcuts from his earlier editions of Brunschwig.[24]

But more specifically, Brunschwig's work also kick-started a broader and more regular German engagement with the figure of the Wound Man as an aesthetic rather than technical image. Most likely inspired by Grüninger's second reprint of the *Cirurgia*, at least three publishers working between 1513 and 1516 in Basel, Cologne, and Augsburg—Pamphilus Gengenbach, Arnd von Aich, and Hans Froschauer—produced a series of short *Biechlin* (booklets) on surgery that claimed to be vernacular condensations of the *Fasciculus medicinae*.[25] Although they bear only a limited likeness to the Venetian book, their images all follow a consistent format (fig. 5.5). First, the reader is presented with the Wound Man's scarred and scabby head, beset with weapons yet floating entirely disembodied against a blank background. A second image focuses on the torso, relishing the details of the figure's transparent chest and the animals crawling inside its stomach. And a third shows the Wound Man from the waist down against a loosely sketched landscape, making the presence of yet more attacking animals particularly lucid. None of these figures contains any sort of key that links them diagrammatically to particular passages of text. Instead, they take on the role of chapter headings, guiding the reader respectively to medicine concerning the head, abdomen, and lower appendages, once more providing a visual hook around which a fifteenth-century reader could conceptualize cures. All three printers also fronted their work with a full figure of the Wound Man who stands starkly on their title pages, again placed into realistic space, this time a field before low rolling hills. Unlike Brunschwig's *Cirurgia*, whose opening so proudly affirms the name and skills of the surgeon, these shorter booklets offer no comparable hint as to their authorship. They simply start by intoning a shared mantra that "*In disem biechlin find man gar ain schöne underwysung und leer wie sich die Cyrurgici oder wundartz gegen ainen yeglichen verwundten menschen ... nach anzegung der figur halten sollen*" (In this booklet one finds fine instruction and teaching on how the *Cyrurgici* or surgeons should treat any wounded person as shown by the figure). Yet hanging this bold claim above the image of the Wound Man—who points knowingly up to the phrase with his right hand—almost has the effect of attributing the entire work to the figure himself. The picture is at once a diagrammatic instructor and at the same time some sort of strange patient-herald, bedecked with his trademark wounds, weapons, animals, and underwear.

Poetry and Personality

This growing parade of German medical books featuring the Wound Man had a major impact on one Strasbourg artisan in particular, the printer Johann Schott, who in 1517 turned his press's attention away from the largely Latin, humanist works for which he was well known to publish its first-ever book in the vernacular, the surgeon Hans von Gersdorff's *Feldtbuch der Wundtartzney* (Fieldbook of Wound Surgery).[26] Like Brunschwig, with whom he was roughly contemporary, Gersdorff was a Strasbourg medic whose writings channeled an explicitly hands-on surgical training that was largely undertaken, if we are to believe the *Feldtbuch*'s brief autobiographical comments, on the battlefields of the Burgundian Wars.[27] A practically oriented text, the *Feldtbuch* was aimed at a broad audience of specialists and nonspecialists alike, and while Gersdorff refers to himself in the book's opening as merely a *zusamen läßer* (compiler), this simplification is far from the case. His work is novel and extensive, spread over four chapters that address a vast array of key tenets in contemporary surgical practice, moving from bedside comportment and treatment narratives of past patients to anatomical breakdowns of the body and a subject-specific Latin-German glossary. In particular, he elaborates two areas of specialty: a short chapter concerning the diagnosis and treatment of leprosy, and a very long second chapter, which takes up the majority of the book, in which he addresses traumatology, namely the treatment of fractures, dislocations, and wounds.

Recognizing the growing market for visualized vernacular medicine, Schott matched Gersdorff's substantive body of cures and techniques with a handsome volume, printing the text as a thick quarto book illustrated with twenty-eight full- or half-page woodblocks whose subjects reflect the *Feldtbuch*'s wide-ranging influences. The work opens with a double portrait of the healing saints Cosmas and Damian, the first of a string of religious references that run through the treatise, picked up in further images of Saint Anthony and of Job as a leper, as well as Gersdorff's dedication of the book to God and the Virgin Mary in aid of what he calls "*christlichen menschen,*" good Christians in need of cure. Other images are more procedural, responding to particular treatments that Gersdorff advances in his text: crooked arms and legs appear locked in metallic, armorlike vices for slow manipulation; surgical instruments are presented in detail with decorated ends, as well as the floating hands of the surgeon; and a surprisingly calm head of a patient is shown pushed flat against the table as a large corkscrew trepan begins to drill into the side of his skull. These blocks also present their medical elements in an increasingly intimate way, from the skyward glance of a restrained soldier undergoing the extraction of a bullet or arrowhead in the middle of the battlefield to a portrait of the author himself frowning in concentration at his desk, his pen guided by an angel visiting at his side.

To visually announce the beginning of Gersdorff's key second surgical chapter on wounds, Schott did not turn to the latent power of religious imagery or the technical persuasion of fancy instruments. Instead, no doubt influenced by the model of Brunschwig's *Cirurgia* and the rich visual ecosystem it had already prompted in Germany, the printer chose to front the book's surgical specialisms with a full-page Wound Man (fig. 5.6).[28] Some elements of this 1517 figure feel familiar when we look back at the genre as a whole. Looking out wearily at the reader, he is nearly naked, pierced by foreign bodies at all the usual points, the club and stone at his head, the spear in his side, the thorn in his foot, and so on. Yet certain subtle changes to the figure's makeup also indicate a continued move away from the Wound Man's diagrammatic origins and toward certain new realities of early modern life. Not only have the image's traditional sketched-out anatomical elements disappeared from this figure's stomach—his organs now firmly covered beneath a fully realized muscular abdomen—but the *Feldtbuch* Wound Man is also the first to bear the burden of a new kind of warfare. Two large circular pieces of shot the size of cannonballs smash into his shin and wrist with such explosive force that the skin violently fans out in all directions, miniature explosions that stand as testament to the ravages of developing military technologies with which contemporary surgeons were increasingly being confronted.[29]

Another key element adds to the sense of this Wound Man as an independent artwork with an increasingly tangible contemporary presence: for the first time in the figure's history, this Wound Man speaks. Printed above the woodcut is a short, four-line rhyming verse, written in the first person:

Wie wol ich bin voll streich und stich,
Zermorrscht, verwundet iamerlich,

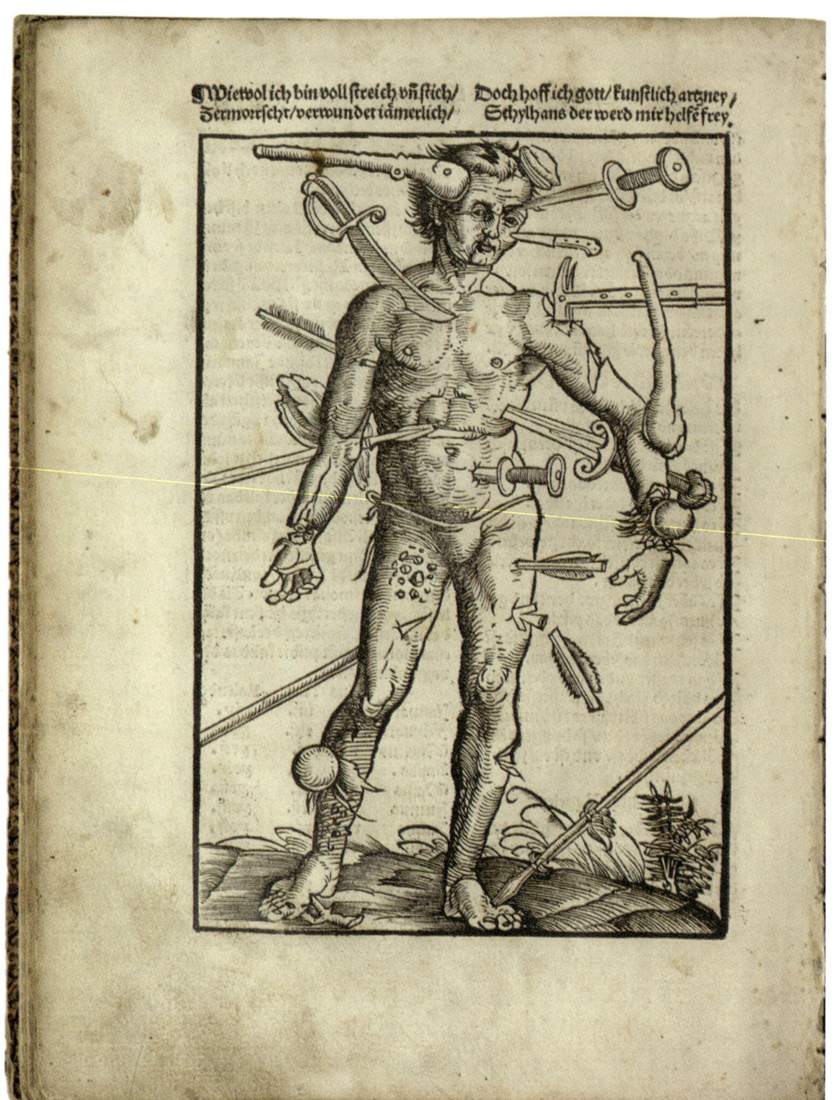

Fig. 5.6. Wound Man with poem from Hans von Gersdorff's *Feldtbuch der Wundtartzney* (Strasbourg: Johann Schott, 1517). Woodcut, 29 x 21 cm. Erlangen, Friedrich-Alexander-Universität, Universitätsbibliothek, H61/2 TREW.F 389, fol. XVIIIv.

Doch hoff ich gott, kunstlich artzney,
Schylhans der werd mir helfen frey.

Though I am full of strokes and blows,
Broken, pitifully wounded,
Still I hope to God, the artful surgeon,
Schylhans will help me freely.

Through this ditty, the figure emphasizes the violent nature of his own wounds in more affective terms than usual. As well as being graphically rendered in the woodcut, we learn straight from the Wound Man's mouth that his injuries are piteous, that he is *zermorrscht* (broken or crushed, both literally and emotionally), and that he hopes for salvation in the form of surgical intervention. The *Schylhans* mentioned in the verse's final line refers to Gersdorff himself, employing a nickname that the surgeon uses repeatedly throughout the *Feldtbuch*, and it is through his art that the Wound Man openly appeals to be released from his pain.

In some ways, this poem recalls earlier verses already associated with the figure and his healing. Think, for instance, of the mnemonic found in the fifteenth-century *Wundarznei* discussed in chapter 2, whose similar four-line structure reminded readers to "*an sehen den menschen*" (look to the man) when listing the different versified ills affecting the human body. It appears reminiscent too of the figure's carefully poised personhood as discussed in chapter 3, which allowed the Wound Man to remain constantly open to different individuated readings from literary epics and religious scripture. The *Feldtbuch*'s poetic exhortation, however, operates on a somewhat different register. Rather than giving advice to the surgical reader or offering an abstracted intimation of the figure's identity, this Wound Man's direct appeal to the surgeon—and to God—brings him vividly into the human realm as an image of a patient in need.

In this new poetic framing, Schott's figure may have been taking its lead less from Wound Men past and more from other items circulating in contemporary sixteenth-century German material culture. The precedent for bookish works speaking in their own voice stretched back some distance in the region and could be regularly found in dedications and editorial forewords, epigrams and prooemia, as well as more recently in various printed textual products keen to perform their own autonomous sense of self. When speaking, such print works were rarely humble: one 1479 Latin Bible printed in Basel by Johann Amerbach states, "*Est impressa nec in orbe mihi similis*" (Nothing in the world has been printed like me).[30] This is a trope to which Gersdorff's *Feldtbuch* would itself succumb in its 1526 second edition, which opens with the refrain, "*Das Feldbůch binn ich wol bekannt, wie mich Schylhans am ersten nannt*" (I am the well-known *Field Book*, as Schylhans first called me).[31]

Equally likely inspiration for the *Feldtbuch* Wound Man's voice can be found in contemporary medical objects. We find kindred vocalized poetry displayed three-dimensionally on surgical accoutrements of the period, in particular sixteenth-century amputation saws. These speaking tools were crafted from iron or steel into their typical bow-shaped forms, often with surprisingly intricate and animated decoration. Ornamental patterns gravitate toward the foliate, with petal-shaped gilding and vine-scroll inlay, while others sport animal features, hawk-headed handles or frilled elephantine trunks that spiral out from the main body of the design. Human faces abound too, morphing eloquently from handles and joints, with several reflecting the animalistic actions of the saw itself by utilizing the mouths of fantastical creatures to hold their blades in place: grinning wide to bear the jagged shapes of the blade beneath, the saw's teeth pose as their own. Such orally fixated animation is especially fitting given that contemporary surgical treatises often designated the act of surgery itself as a "biting" craft, with writers returning repeatedly to the action of chewing, munching, and gnawing in their texts to describe the actions of diseases, surgical operations, and surgery's own instruments.[32] One saw from Germany, now in Vienna, even pleads for the

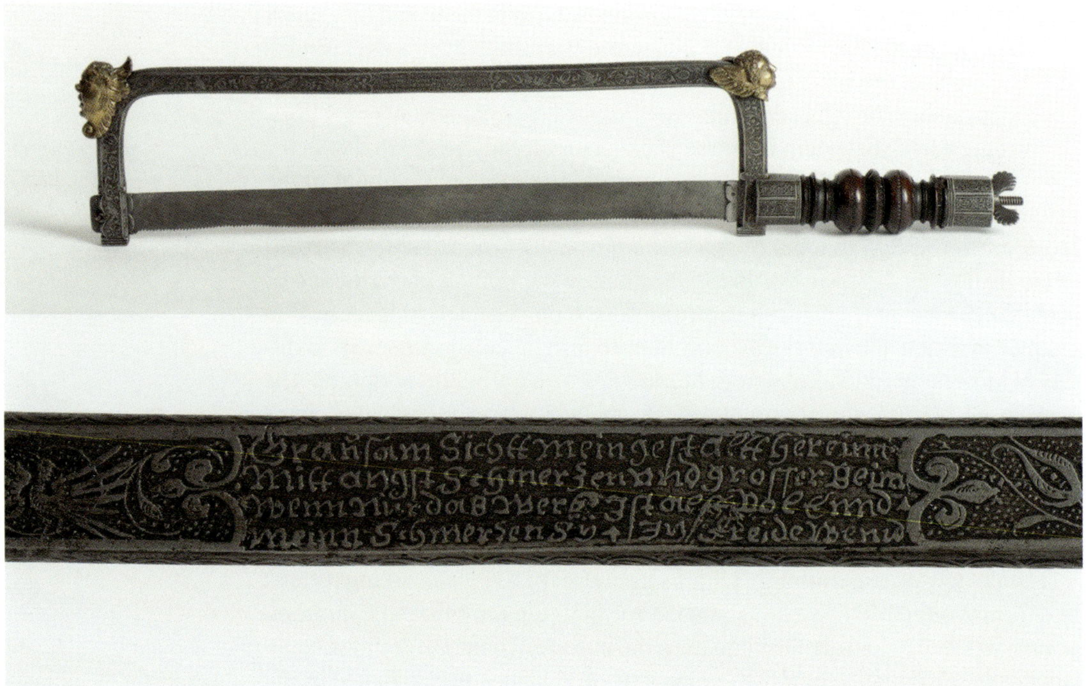

Fig. 5.7. Surgical saw with detail of poem, c. 1550, Germany. Iron, bronze, and wood, length 61 cm. Vienna, MAK – Museum of Applied Arts, Inventarnummer F 1033.

craft of its maker in a now-familiar first-person mode (fig. 5.7).[33] A pun on the double meaning of the German word *spruch*—translating as both the instrument of a "saw" and as a "motto"—frames a short poetic verse etched onto a similar saw's bow, which again talks of the simultaneous fear and hope that surgery could inspire:

Spruch: Grausam sieht mein Gestalt herein,
mit Angst, Schwäche, und großer Pein,
wann das Werk nun ist vollendt,
das trauern sich in Freude wendt.

Saw/Motto: My form looks horribly within,
with fear, trembling, and great pain,
but when the work is completed,
the sorrow is turned to joy.

Also intimately connected to the 1517 Wound Man in this regard was the chorus of first-person medical poetry issuing from elsewhere in Schott's own oeuvre. This appears most notably in a pair of large-format broadsheets that he printed in the same year as the *Feldtbuch*, designed both for independent circulation and for specific inclusion in Gersdorff's work and found bound into several surviving editions of the book (fig. 5.8).[34] They present two different specifically anatomical takes on the body, designed for Schott by the artist Hans Wächtlin.[35] One shows a skeleton, complete with Latin labels for many of its bones, entitled "*Ein contrafacter Todt*" (A Counterfeit of Death), and we learn from an accompanying caption that its form was

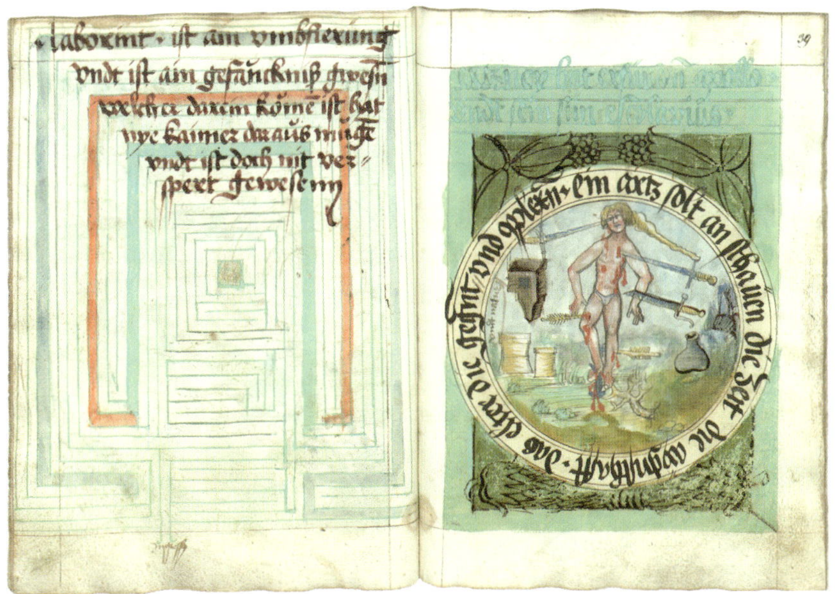

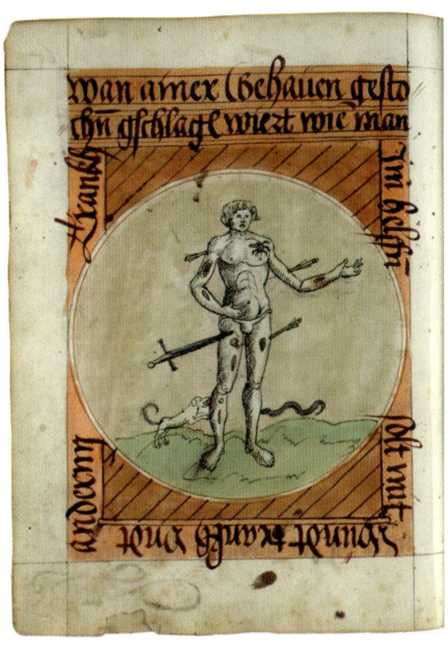

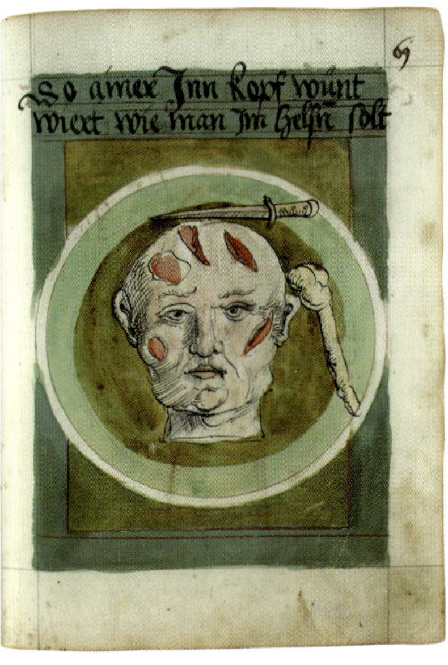

Fig. 5.9. Wound Men in two German *Bild-Enzyklopädien*. *Above:* Labyrinth and Wound Man, c. 1515–19, probably Bavaria. Ink and paint on paper, 30 x 23 cm (each folio). Kraków, Biblioteka Jagiellońska, BJ Rkp. Przyb. 35/64, fols. 38v–39r. *Below:* Wound Man and a Wound Man's head, 1524, probably Vienna. Ink and paint on paper, 29 x 21 cm. Erlangen, Friedrich-Alexander-Universität, Universitätsbibliothek, MS B 200, fols. 65v, 69r.

lengthy prose but through a colorful central picture around which sit short catchwords, statements, and poems that provide only brief elaborations on what the image has to say. Medicine features in several parts of these manuscripts' visual assortments, often with a theoretical dimension. On one folio of the Bavarian example, a floating head shows the different regions of the brain, while on other pages a skeleton displays its bones, a figure presents thirty-six points for bloodletting, urine flasks offer differently colored contents for diagnostic judgment, and—just as it does on Brunschwig's printed title page—the Wound Man heralds the manuscript's turn toward surgical information.[43] Several details of this figure in fact match very closely the 1497 woodblock from the front of the *Cirurgia*, including his long hair and the placement of his injurious instruments, suggesting that the image was once again copied directly from the original print. The Wound Man's literary staging here, however, is far more mythic than empirical: he sits across the page from an image of the Ancient Greek Labyrinth, whose turquoise palette is carried through to both the hazy landscape background of the Wound Man page and a short, faded inscription above him stating that "*Ertzney hat erfünden apollo undt sein sun escolapius*" (Medicine was invented by Apollo and his son Asclepius).[44] Presented with a heritage stretching back to the gods, this Wound Man is lent a distinctly epic quality conveying the sense that, like his mythical forebears, the figure's mere presence should be read as sufficiently symbolic of the surgical enterprise.

Other printed German Wound Men found their way into similar contemporary artistic projects. In a different early sixteenth-century *Bild-Enzyklopädie*—written a few years later, in 1524, most likely in Vienna in connection with a patron named Benedictus Rughalm—not one but two versions of the Wound Man have been hand-illustrated with significant skill: the first is a simplified, full-page Wound Man, and the second is just the figure's head.[45] Both are copied from the same printed source, namely one of the short booklets printed by Gengenbach, Aich, and Froschauer in the 1510s, which favored multiple detailed views of the figure and would have been busily circulating in the region. Meanwhile, sixteenth-century German medics and artists working on other kinds of books clearly also felt empowered to lift yet more Wound Men from the printed world and use them as a stand-alone medical trope for their own means whenever they liked. One user from the 1540s took this idea quite literally, cutting out the Wound Man from a copy of Gersdorff's *Feldtbuch* and pasting it into their own Latin translation of the work.[46] But such reworkings could be not only expedient but also artful, even beautiful. Only a few decades later, around 1580, another Viennese manuscript presents the reader with a rich compendium of techniques, treatments, and recipes. Recorded in the thick, confident penmanship of a barber-surgeon named Sebastien Jäger, the work's quality and contents suggest that it was created as a showpiece to ensure entry into his local guild.[47] It is telling, then, that in addition to the accumulated cures of his profession, Jäger chose to include a colorful Wound Man on this socially potent manuscript's very first page (fig. 5.10). Produced to such a high standard that we can safely assume it was commissioned from a local professional artist, this figure is yet another reimagining of the Wound Man from Gersdorff's *Feldtbuch*, complete with golden highlights and smudged artillery explosions.

The presence of this hand-illustrated copy of the *Feldtbuch* figure in Jäger's manuscript is all the more impressive given that the print run of Gersdorff's book had ended some thirty years prior, in 1551.[48] Clearly, in becoming allied to key surgical texts such as the *Feldtbuch* and the *Cirurgia*, the Wound Man had been granted real longevity. The figure recurred across the century and throughout the region in association with medical experience and authority, reproduced to evoke these authors' learned models of medical understanding. Yet at the same time, Jäger's book—just like the *Biechlin* and *Bild-Enzyklopädien*—reveals the Wound Man as an independent actor in his own right: an intellectualized but also specifically aesthetic collector's item, considered of the highest caliber by medics and artists alike.

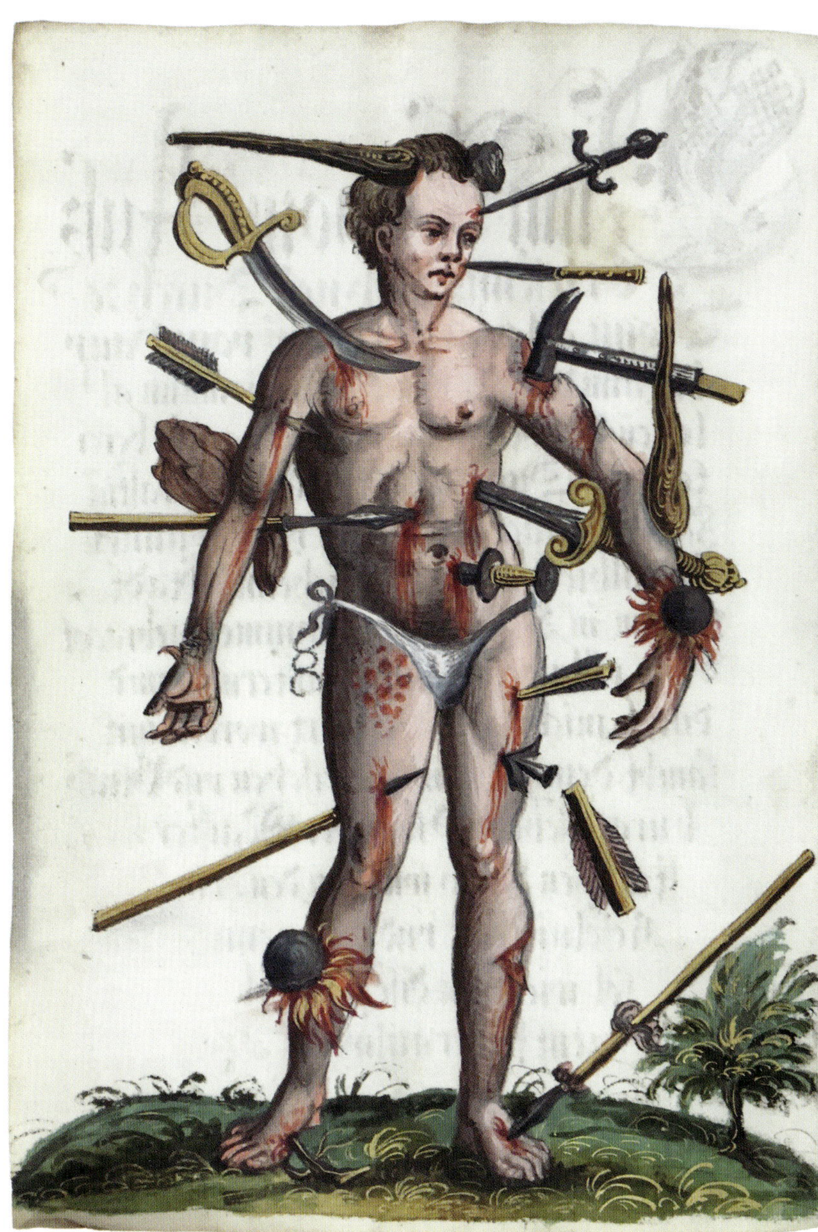

Fig. 5.10. Sebastian Jäger's Wound Man, c. 1580, Vienna. Ink and paint on parchment, 20 x 14 cm. Los Angeles, UCLA, Louise M. Darling Medical Library, MS Benjamin 8, fol. IVv.

Three Late Wound Men

To speak of a Wound Man drawn and painted in the year 1580 is clearly to have moved some significant distance from the very first images of the figure that emerged in Bohemian medical manuscript culture of the late 1300s. Yet even a sixteenth-century book like that of Sebastian Jäger was far from the last word on the Wound Man's early modern life.

Many of the traditions that we have already identified for the figure across both manuscript and print have timelines that extend further still.

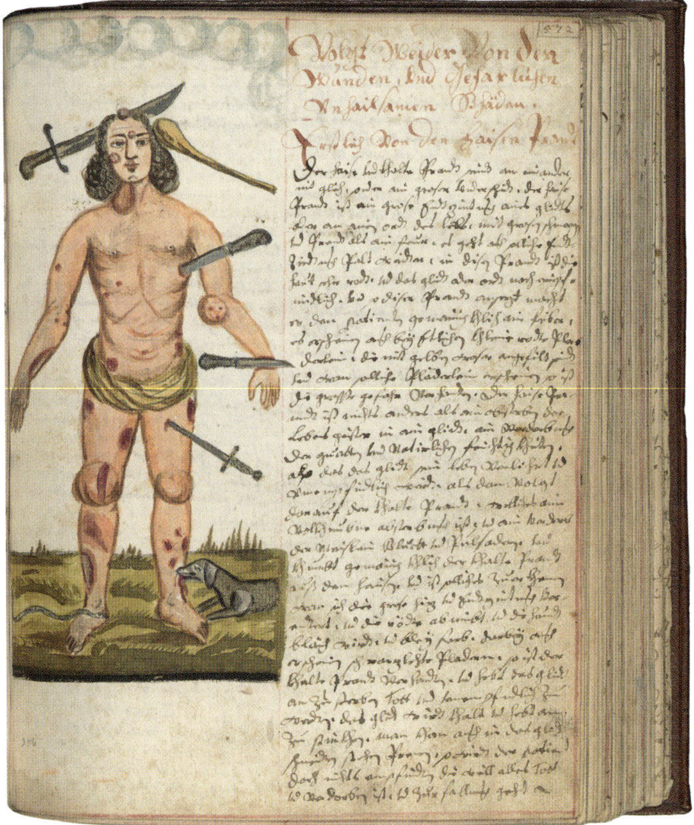

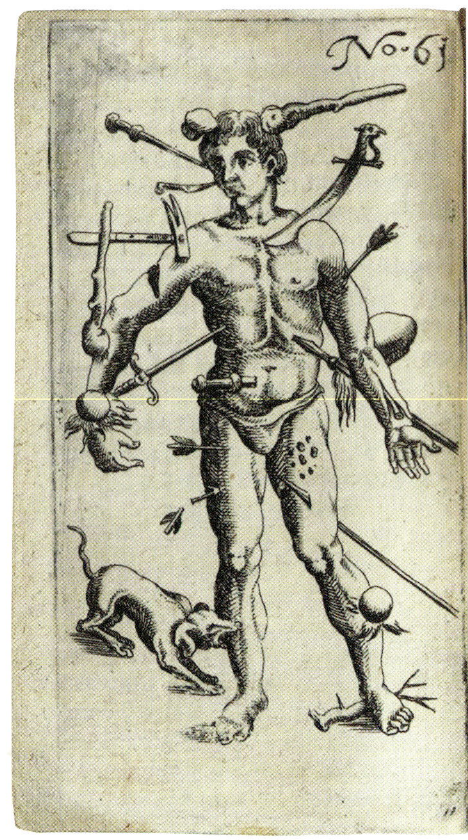

Fig. 5.11. Two quotidian Wound Men. *Left:* Wound Man, c. 1675, Germany. Ink and paint on paper, 20 x 15 cm. London, Wellcome Library, MS 990, 572. *Right:* Wound Man from Joseph Schmid's *Examen chirurgicum* (Augsburg: Johann Weh, 1649). Copperplate engraving, 13 x 8 cm. Augsburg, Staats- und Stadtbibliothek, Med 3998, plate inserted between pages 60 and 61.

Gersdorff's *Feldtbuch* continued to circulate in translation for decades, especially a Dutch edition known as *Scheel-Hans' Veldt Boeck*, which saw at least five printings in Amsterdam between 1591 and 1651, the last of which commissioned an entirely new, muscular Wound Man for the title page.[49] Likewise, the *Fasciculus medicinae*—as we have seen, a work already much reproduced across fifteenth-century Italy and Spain—reemerged once more onto the German market when, in 1530, the Strasbourg printer Christian Egenolff published the first of what would become many reissued translations of the text sporting a simple new title, the *Wundartznei* (Surgery).[50] Editions of the *Fasciculus* also continued to be produced in the Netherlands until 1567, and a full century later, in 1668, as if out of nowhere, another Venetian version of the text was reprised, complete with a now chunky-thighed Wound Man surrounded by cures.[51] The figure also flourished in other arenas (fig. 5.11). The late seventeenth century saw the Wound Man appear in contexts as diverse as an enormous handwritten German housebook of medical recipes produced for Franciscan nuns and a newly devised examination booklet printed to test young trainee surgeons, both a reminder that the figure's more quotidian users had continued to stick with the image through the centuries.[52] And as well as appearing in different contexts, the Wound Man's medico-diagrammatic structure was even being applied to entirely different kinds of bodies, including illustrating wounds and diseases in horses and cattle (fig. 5.12).[53]

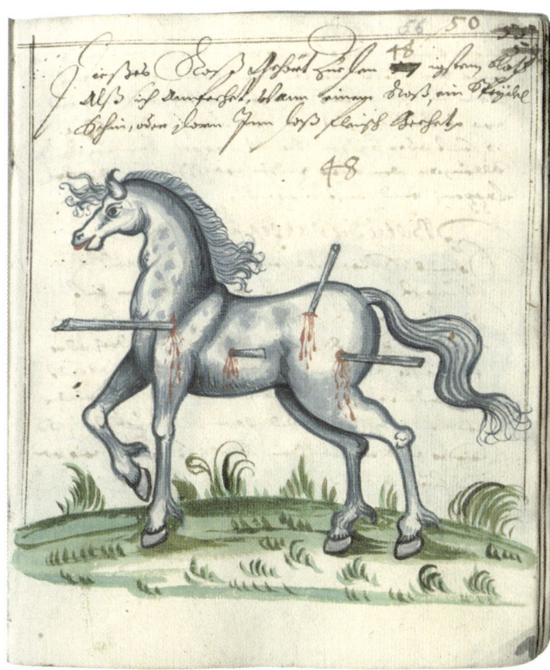

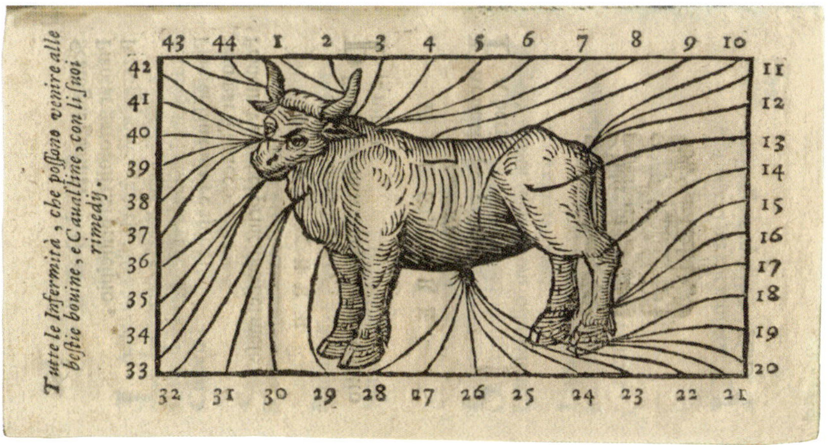

Fig. 5.12. Nonhuman bodies diagramming wounds. *Above:* Wound Horse, c. 1600–1650, southwestern Germany. Ink and paint on paper, 19 x 15 cm. Bethesda, National Library of Medicine, MS E 98, fol. 56r. *Below:* Injured and diseased cow from Giovanni Battista Ferraro's *Trattato utile e necessario ad ogni agricoltore* (Bologna: Giovanni Antonio Remondin, 1673). Woodcut, 15 x 9 cm. Bethesda, National Library of Medicine, WZ 250 F3764t 1673, 40.

The Wound Man's consistency across these decades is all the more surprising given that the practical and theoretical underpinnings of European medicine were of course themselves shifting.[54] To adapt a useful phrase from the historian of science Susan Lawrence, medicine's change throughout this period should not be understood as some grand, teleological corpus progressing inevitably toward the precepts of the modern day, a set of ideas standing separately from practitioners themselves. Rather, medicine should simply be defined as "that which medics do."[55] And medics of the sixteenth and seventeenth centuries were, at times, doing radically different things from the practices of their medieval forebears. Most frequently discussed is the rapidly changing structural understanding of the early modern body developing in the work of early anatomists such as Jacopo Berengario da Carpi and Johann Dryander, in which greater attention was called to observing the actual mechanics of the bodily interior, ideas that were later developed by practitioners such as Andreas Vesalius and William Harvey into full-fledged revisions of the body's internal systems.[56] At the same time, other medics were pulling the healing arts in less familiar directions, such as the controversial Swiss revisionist Theophrastus von Hohenheim, better known as Paracelsus, who argued against increasing investment in anatomical knowledge and advocated instead for the systematic dismantling of the university medical system.[57] In its place, Paracelsus and his followers offered a revised understanding of physiology viewed through more cosmological and alchemical lenses, and they also claimed a new approach to disease as exclusively ontologically distinct, the work of individual invasive agents thought to originate outside of the body. Although not dominating the center stage of this evolving medical debate, it is notable that the Wound Man was mobilized by both factions, making appearances in both a later edition of Paracelsus's *Große Wundarznei* (Great Surgery) and a *Chirurgia magna* (Great Surgery) published under Vesalius's name.[58]

As well as in writings by these much-promoted medical personalities, other forms of thinking being undertaken by less well-documented practitioners were also changing the frame of medical endeavor. A recognition was emerging of the hands-on medical learning being generated by a whole host of artisanal craftspeople, whose knowledge was gleaned through observation and experimentation that filtered upward, not down, to inform all sorts of developments in pharmacy, surgery, and other healing arenas.[59] The kinds of questions these practitioners were asking of the human body and the natural world were of a different texture from the parallel agendas of medical elites, as were the varying methods they used to answer them, with artisans and artists of many types implicated alongside physicians, surgeons, and other medics as the makers of healing knowledge.

This broadening of medicine's personnel in turn diversified the vehicles for communicating medical understanding, especially the written word. Produced in ever larger numbers and for ever broader audiences, early modern medical books were increasingly likely to contain the novel output of living authors rather than revised takes on canonical works, and the buzzing diversity of contemporary ideas was reflected in a host of newly emerging literary forms for medicine: case notes with expert commentary, extensive recipe collections, medical encyclopedias, shortened epitomes of more complex theoretical treatises, histories of the medical craft itself, and works covering diseases that were either new to the early modern world or had recently increased in spread, such as syphilis, smallpox, and tuberculosis. The latter genre in particular draws attention to the widening geographies of early modern medicine, forming a worldwide network connected more and more through developing trade routes and expansive settler-colonialism. As with their fifteenth-century precursors, illustrated medical works formed only a relatively small proportion of the overall printed and manuscript medicine circulating on this newly globalized scale. But even so, a snapshot of the period would reveal Spanish bloodletting figures being reproduced in Mexican Nahuatl codices, Indian manuscripts diagramming medical automata cribbed from Middle Eastern Arabic originals, and Vesalian-inspired skeletons standing proudly on the paper of both Persian anatomical treatises and Chinese decorated handscrolls.[60] Art historians have also carefully traced how the spread of such images was in turn enabled by rapidly developing contemporary vehicles for visual translation and transplantation. This evolving set of diverse technical practices kick-started an increasingly divergent sense of early modern visual culture, and encouraged images to shift and change ever more quickly in response to novel demands and novel purposes.[61]

To find a clear route for the Wound Man through this ever-broader set of contexts in early modernity is therefore a highly complicated task. To simply trace the iconographic lineage of the image through the general medical melee of the period, besides being an unsatisfying mix of references and counterreferences, would run the risk of diluting the various rich surgical and technological functions we have already found in the figure so far. Instead, in what follows, we turn to look in detail at three particular occasions for the Wound Man that speak more thematically to the image's later history. Each of these instances is at a further remove than the last in both time and space from the late medieval German-speaking lands where the figure first originated, beginning with sixteenth-century France, then seventeenth-century England, and finally eighteenth-century Japan. Moreover, the effect is speedy, a necessity to keep pace with an image that could itself move extremely quickly between circumstances, becoming ever stranger as it progressed. But as well as having the advantage of underlining the rapid diffusion and geographically extreme breadth of the Wound Man's international appeal, carefully exploring each of these discrete contexts also tells us something deeper about what these varied medico-visual cultures chose to do with the image. It reveals how they slotted the figure into their own immediate discourses and the different things the Wound Man became for each culture as a result.

France: The Wound Leg

As well extending the Wound Man's overall European legacy, the French history of the figure provides a rare opportunity to trace its impact on a more local level. France was a late adopter of the Wound Man. The figure's first print appearance in the country would not be until 1543, when it featured as part of the Parisian publisher Chrétien Wechel's printing of the *De chirurgica institutione libri quinque* (Five Books on Surgical Training), a major work by the eminent French surgeon Jean Tagault.[62] When it did appear, though, French surgeons and printers utilized the Wound Man not just as an important node in international medico-visual networks but also, more unusually, as a canvas on which highly specific regional interests could play out, a matter at once of image and language.

The character of Jean Tagault helps us first to take a step back and appreciate the unique nature of France's medical ecosystem at the time of the Wound Man's French debut in his *De chirurgica institutione,* a notably different framework for medicine when compared to parallel arenas in nearby Germany and Italy. In many ways, Tagault's book was typical of a mid-sixteenth-century surgical work produced by a member of what by the 1540s had become a firmly entrenched French medical establishment. The University of Paris, where Tagault was a doctor of medicine and later dean, held significant sway over both the central theoretical precepts of French medical training and the political appointments of its trainees. Its faculty had also long waged what historian Iain Lonie has characterized as an "unremitting war" against practitioners whom they felt had insufficient scholarly training or affiliation.[63] Seen within this institutional context, the elegant Latin of Tagault's *De chirurgica institutione* presents a highfaluting and somewhat confined vision of surgery. First, the book frames the field theoretically, charting humoral pathologies, rough anatomies of the body's parts, and ideas drawn from long-standing surgical authorities. Thereafter, it attends directly to the hands-on mechanics of surgery, including descriptions of various surgical instruments and six sections that in turn cover the treatment of tumors, wounds, ulcers, fractures, and dislocations, before finally offering an antidotary of *materia medica* written by a student of Tagault's, Jacques Houllier.[64] In short, the book is a formal text by a thoroughly institutionalized surgeon.

The book's visual language, by contrast, was more unusual, at least by French standards. This was largely down to its printer, Wechel, a Dutchman and humanist whose pan-European connections had helped him emerge as one of the foremost publishers of medical material in Paris.[65] Indicative of the early Parisian printing scene's particularly international flavor, Wechel's output often drew on German models. His workshop regularly produced editions of the same works as contemporary German printers, and he traded individual books and woodblocks with his German counterparts, including Herman Walter Ryff and Balthasar Beck.[66] In the *De chirurgica institutione*, this international influence was direct and unfiltered. Among the first few pages of Tagault's chapter on wounds, Wechel nestled woodcut replicas of images copied directly from Johann Schott's edition of Hans von Gersdorff's *Feldtbuch der Wundtartzney*, including reproductions of surgical instruments, scenes of battlefield bullet extraction, and the *Feldtbuch*'s much-reproduced Wound Man, generously allotted an entire page to itself (fig. 5.13).[67] The figure is labeled "*Corpus multifariam vulneratum*" (Body wounded in many parts), but besides this open-ended and ambiguous caption—and perhaps an echoing reference in the title of the subsection in which he appears, "*De sagittis, plumbeis, glandibus, & globis ferreis, ac quibuscunque aliis telis, e corpore extrahendis*" (On arrows, spears, bullets, and cannonballs, and any other missile weapons to be extracted from the body)—the image goes entirely unreferenced in the book. We get the sense that the Wound Man's appearance here was more about importing a novel and potentially marketable German artistic image into Wechel's output than teasing out the medical subtleties from Tagault's accompanying text.

Nonetheless, it was through appearances in the *De chirurgica institutione* that sixteenth-century audiences in France would have first become familiar with the figure, although not without deviation. Tagault's work was popular, and in a pattern to which we have now become accustomed, his text bounced back and forth between competing European printers and print centers to total more than thirty editions before the end of the century, its audience

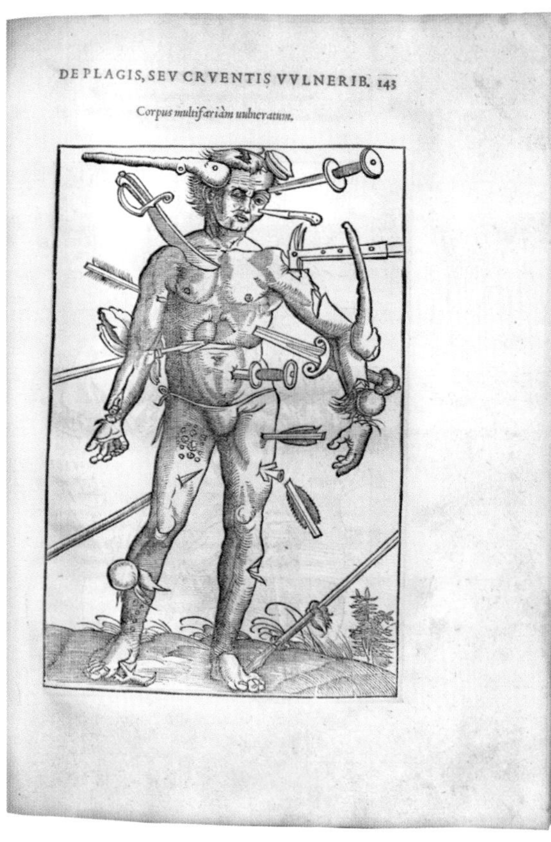

Fig. 5.13. Wound Man from Jean Tagault's *De chirurgica institutione libri quinque* (Paris: Chrétien Wechel, 1543). Woodcut, 29 x 21 cm. Paris, Bibliothèque nationale de France, RES FOL-TD73-44, 143.

growing all the while and its imagery likewise evolving. Just one year after Wechel's initial publication, the Venetian printer Vincenzo Valgrisi engaged a professor of medicine at Padua, Bassiano Landi, to re-edit the book and to better synthesize the scholarly references of Tagault's chapters. Lacking the same access to German woodblocks, or perhaps being reluctant to copy them quite as unashamedly as his Parisian counterpart had done, Valgrisi commissioned a new set of images for the volume that replicated Wechel's original choice of figures. Included among them was a new and particularly Italianate-looking Wound Man, a Triton-esque figure with aquiline features and a curly beard whose sculptural form is presented in far more elegant proportions than those of the Schott block (fig. 5.14).[68] Fittingly for the book's back-and-forth history, one year later, Valgrisi's image was in turn reimported back to France, where in 1545 the Lyonnaise merchant-publisher Guillaume Rouillé—himself a former Venetian apprentice whose shop was to be found in Lyon at "The Sign of Venice"—began the first of several further editions of the book produced in the country.[69] It was at this point that the image's relationship with Tagault's text became fully concrete. Whether in subsequent versions produced in France or Italy, or further European editions printed in Zürich in 1555, Antwerp in 1559, Frankfurt in 1610, Dordrecht in 1621, and Amsterdam in 1649, the reader would inevitably find a version of Valgrisi's windswept Wound Man gracing the pages of the *De chirurgia institutione*.[70] So far, so familiar. Firmly entangled with yet another hugely

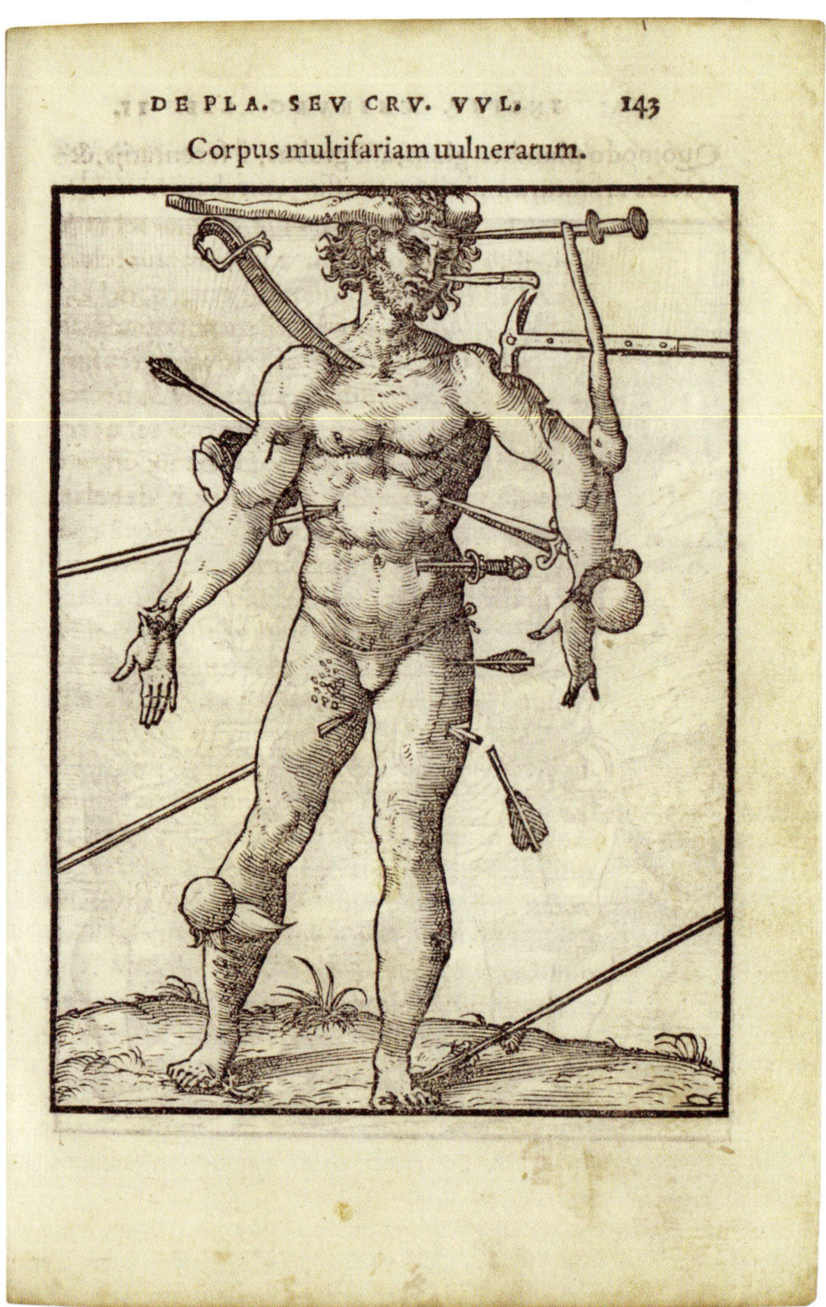

Fig. 5.14. Wound Man from Jean Tagault's *De chirurgica institutione libri quinque* (Venice: Vincenzo Valgrisi, 1544). Woodcut, 18 x 11 cm. London, Wellcome Library, EPB/A/6204, 143.

influential piece of surgical writing, the popularity of the Wound Man was ensured for yet another generation of European audiences.

Less typical, though, was the appearance of a peculiarly anatomized French offshoot of the figure: an isolated, floating appendage that we might call the Wound Leg. This image first appeared in 1549, when Rouillé's Lyon press published Tagault's book for the first time in a French-language edition, retitled *Les institutions chirurgiques* (Surgical Institutions) (fig. 5.15).[71] The decision to render Tagault's work in the vernacular was an important one. On the

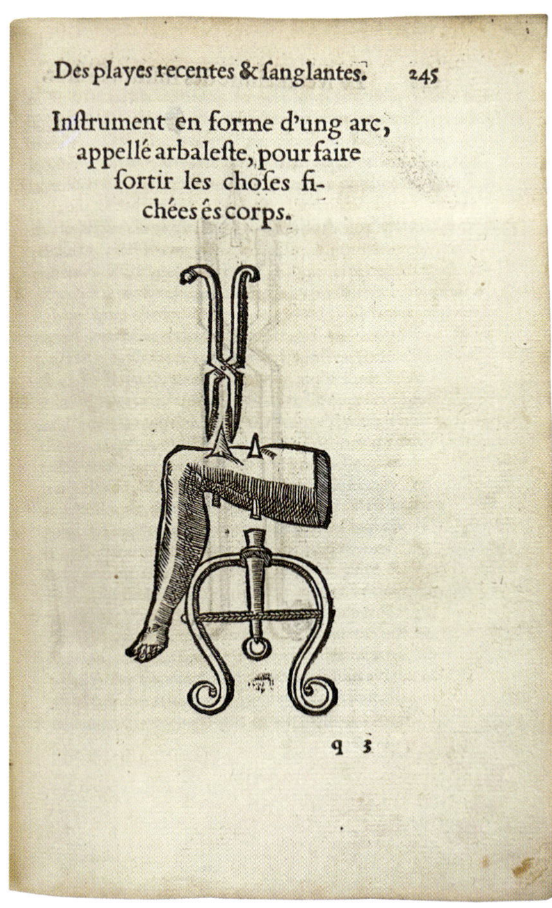
Des playes recentes & ſanglantes. 245

Inſtrument en forme d'ung arc, appellé arbaleſte, pour faire ſortir les choſes fichées ès corps.

q 3

Fig. 5.15. Wound Leg from Jean Tagault's *Les institutions chirurgiques* (Lyon: Guillaume Rouillé, 1549). Woodcut, 18 x 11 cm. London, British Library, C.97.bb.28, 245.

one hand, it was a move that slotted the surgeon—who had died three years earlier—into a long and esteemed tradition of vernacularized French surgical writers stretching back all the way to the later Middle Ages. Such a pedigree had clearly been important to Tagault himself, who, more than any other reference work, turned to the fourteenth-century *Chirurgia magna* (Great Surgery) of Gui de Chauliac, a fellow Frenchman and former incumbent of Tagault's own position at the University of Paris. On the other hand, the production of the vernacular *Institutions* fitted Rouillé's own agenda, expanding the work's potential readership beyond what must have been an entirely academic Latinate audience and making the work available to a far broader surgical community. This was part of a wider pattern of vernacular writing in France and a keen interest of Rouillé's specifically: in the coming years, he would steward to press French translations of Giovanni Boccaccio, Ludovico Ariosto, Herodian, and others, part of an overall project that he referred to in a preface to one of his books as "*la decoration et augmentation de la langue Françoise*" (the decoration and augmentation of the French language).[72]

Importantly, for Rouillé this concept of literary "augmentation" was as much visual as it was textual. On its first publication in 1543, Tagault had taken pains in the *De chirurgia institutione* to outline a list of eight key instruments that he considered critical to the surgical process, drawn in fact from Gui de

Chauliac's own advice on removing dangerous foreign bodies from wounds. Only some of these had found a match in Wechel's borrowed German woodcuts, and so, in his 1549 French edition, Rouillé refreshed the book's existing figures to match the newer, refined Venetian versions. He also offered a novel image of his own commission. This new figure, the eighth and final surgical instrument of Chauliac's to be highlighted by Tagault, is described as a tool "*in modum arcus illius, quem vulgo balistam vocant*" (in the shape of that bow that is popularly called a crossbow), used in a method of violently yet swiftly removing deep-set projectiles by firing them outward from the limb with a crossbow, or *arbaleste*, as Rouillé's French text names it.[73] Rather than simply leaving the reader to imagine such a dramatic instrument in use, Rouillé produces an image that clarifies this medical action. We see two arrows being prized out of the disembodied limb, the pair lodged in a similar position on the thigh to those shown in the book's earlier Wound Man, in a manner that implies that the leg could be a close-up detail of his injured body.

As we have seen in previous chapters, Rouillé was not the first to carve up the Wound Man in this way. Medieval Czech manuscripts had long before broken down the figure into discrete elements, as had early printed German books that drew inspiration from these same sources (figs. 2.6 and 5.5).[74] Works by more recent major surgical authors had also taken up an anatomized view of the Wound Man. In 1518, the famed surgeon-anatomist Jacopo Berengario da Carpi produced a short work on the subject of head trauma, the *Tractatus de fractura calve sive cranei* (Treatise on the Fracture of the Skull or Cranium), a text printed in Bologna that claimed to have its origins in Berengario's treatment of Lorenzo II de' Medici, who had suffered a fracture to the head from a gunshot fired in battle.[75] Berengario was himself no stranger to the direct consequences of wounding, responsible for a number of serious assaults on fellow doctors. We get a sense of his violent personality in the stinging "Farewell" with which he closes the *Tractatus*:

> *Proinde rabientem linguam idem caveat inserere, ne quando per artificii nostri scalpra relabens, caesim discindatur. Nos enim ad docti iudicis obeliscos opus reiicimus, facultatis nostrae studiosos ambimus, caeteros resecamus. Vale.*
>
> Therefore [the reader] should guard against inserting the raging tongue, lest at any time it is severed by the cuts made by the scapels of our trade. For we hand over the work to the critical reading of the learned judge, solicit the scholars of our faculty, and cut off the rest. Farewell.[76]

Perhaps it was for this reason that in the work's second edition of 1535, produced in Venice, the book's printer replaced the original title page with a new image, based closely on the Wound Man's head, that shows a twisting, bearded bust violently beset by the figure's familiar weapons (fig. 5.16).[77] It is possible that Rouillé, well connected in Venice, had seen this title page and chose to follow its lead in adopting a focused detail of the Wound Man to reflect the crossbow passage in the *Institutions*. Inspiration might likewise have come from the modular figures accompanying Johann Grüninger's editions of Brunschwig from the late 1490s onward, in which the printer either added

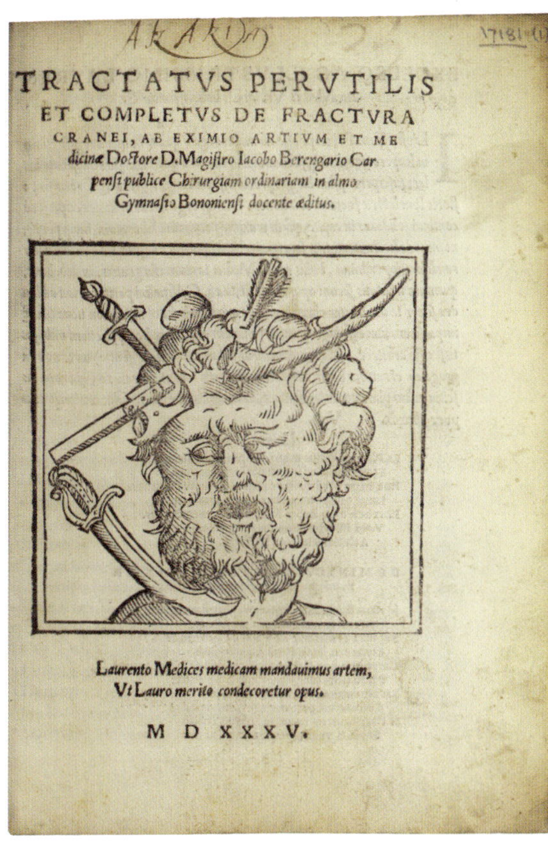

TRACTATVS PERVTILIS
ET COMPLETVS DE FRACTVRA
CRANEI, AB EXIMIO ARTIVM ET ME
dicinæ Doctore D. Magistro Iacobo Berengario Car
pensi publice Chirurgiam ordinariam in almo
Gymnasio Bononiensi docente æditus.

Laurento Medices medicam mandauimus artem,
Vt Lauro merito condecoretur opus.

M D XXXV.

Fig. 5.16. Title page of Jacopo Berengario da Carpi's *Tractatus perutilis et completus de fractura cranei* (Venice: Giovanni Antonio Nicolini, 1535). Woodcut, 19 x 13 cm. London, Wellcome Library, EPB/B/779/1.1, title page.

or removed whole limbs from the woodblock's figures to conceal or reveal new wounds. But even if not directly based on either source, the appearance of the Wound Leg nonetheless still correlates with a period of medical innovation in Rouillé's burgeoning publishing operation. In 1549 alone, he printed more than twenty medical works, ranging from contemporary writings by international authors such as Jacques Dubois and Sebastian Ostricher to a huge number of Galenic editions by Jean Vassés, Johann Winter, Marco Gattinara, Thomas Linacre, and others, covering works on muscles, bones, temperaments, bloodletting, uroscopy, and beyond. This boom suggests a growing base of medically inclined clientele eager for greater detail in their books, including new scenes of new instruments, the Wound Leg among them.

The unique aspect of the Wound Leg, however, is less the story of its initial appearance than the subsequent focus of its circulation. For despite being an image with typically international surgical origins—forged in the French translation of an Italian edition of a French work drawing on German imagery—this novel take on the Wound Man's isolated appendage remained distinct to France. Aligned specifically with a Francophone medical lineage, it never featured in later Venetian, Swiss, or German editions of Tagault's writing. Indeed, the "French-ness" of its usage only deepened as the image's history continued.

Consider the appearance of the Wound Leg in the work of the most influential French practitioner of the sixteenth century, Ambroise Paré, surgeon to four kings of France and best known for his innovations in the treatment of wounds, including major changes to the theorization of gunpowder injuries, the production of prosthetic limbs, and the design of surgical instruments.[78] It makes sense that Rouillé's vernacular translation of the *Institutions* would have appealed to Paré, a surgeon trained in artisanal, empirical contexts outside of Latinate academic confines, first in the field of barber-surgery and then supplemented by his short career as an army surgeon. Paré worked proudly and exclusively in French, a move that helped his texts find a particularly wide audience and stoked nationalist appeals to his royal patrons: one of his books, for instance, was dedicated to the "*seul profict de la posterité, & à l'ornement de l'Empire François*" (sole profit of posterity and to the ornament of the French Empire).[79] And as well as familiar language, in Rouillé's editions of Tagault, Paré would have found a kindred visuality.

We see this as early as Paré's second-ever publication, *La maniere de traicter les playes faictes tant par hacquebutes que par fleches* (The Manner of Treating Wounds Made by Gunshot and by Arrows), published in Paris by the widow of the printer Jean de Brie in 1552.[80] Here, writing in an introduction to his vernacular reader—whom he describes as an "*amateur de Chirurgie*" (surgical amateur)—Paré advocates for evaluating his efforts in surgical writing as much by his visual interventions as his technical ones:

> *Combien i'ay travaillé en la recognoissance & correction, tu en iugeras tant par les additions que par les figures & pourtraictz d'instrumentz de Chirurgie de nouveau adioustez & inserez. Lesquelz i'ay faict pourtraire au naturel comme verras.*
>
> How much I worked on recognition and correction [of his surgical text], you can judge from my additions and from the figures and portraits of surgical instruments, newly improved and inserted. These I had portrayed from life, as you will see.

Sure enough, Paré had the treatise packed with explanatory woodcuts organized by their practical use, including his own take on the Wound Leg (fig. 5.17). He seems to have conceived of the image in much the same manner as Tagault did: an accompanying phrase—"*comme tu peulx cognoistre par ceste figure*" (as you can understand from this figure)—clarifies that it is designed to elucidate instrumentation and procedure, once more enhancing the reader's understanding of the removal of arrow shafts and heads from a wound, a particularly pertinent specialism given Paré's army experience. Yet the visual treatment of Paré's newly commissioned woodblock of the Wound Leg is markedly different. Gone is the arc-shaped *arbaleste*, which has been replaced with even more elements drawn from the Wound Man's original body, including a whole range of broken arrows and arrowheads, a long spear, pincers, and forceps. Not only is the scene busier, but the unknown artist whom Paré commissioned to produce the image has offered a smart solution to the obvious problems of inelegance and oddness posed by Rouillé's original floating limb. Rather than flopping onto the page as if dropped out of nowhere, this upgraded leg emerges from a glorious frill of

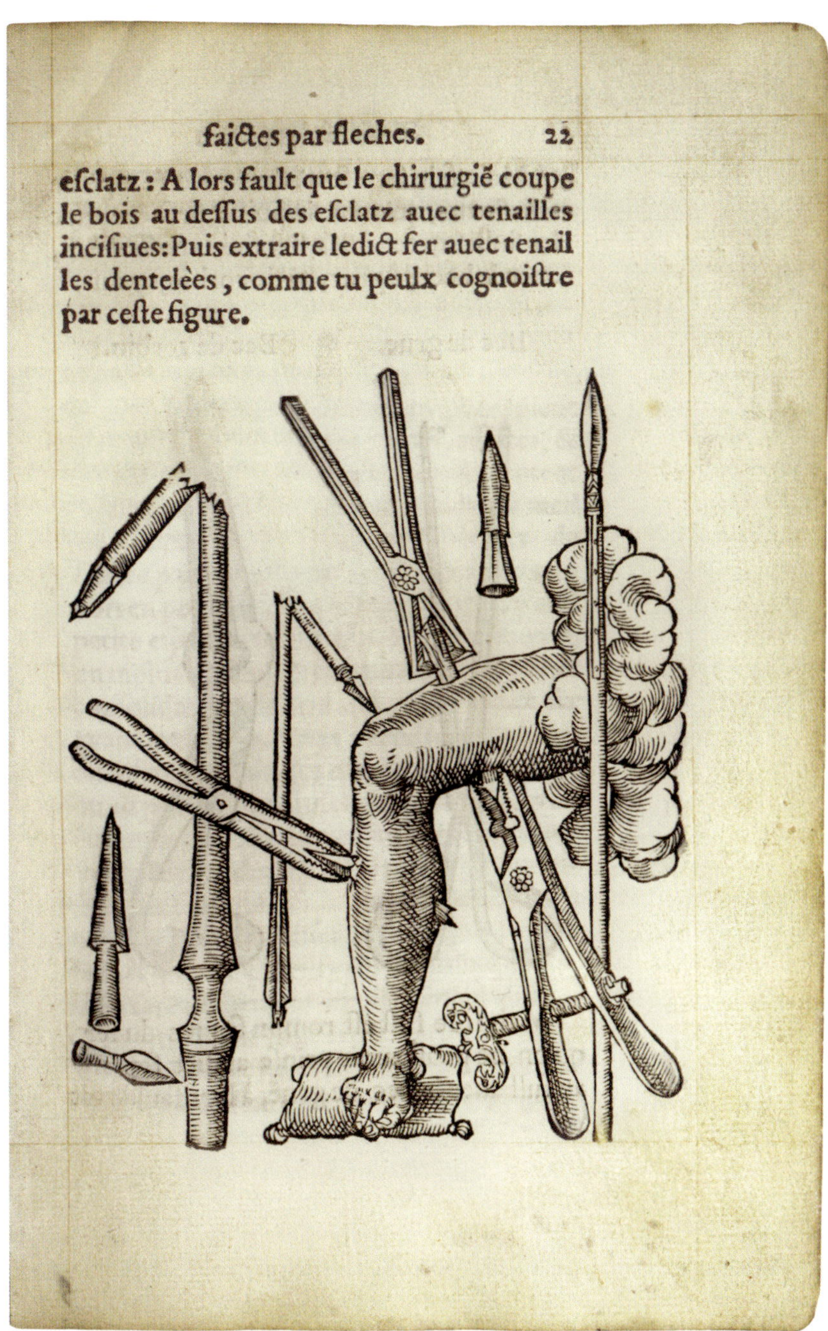
faictes par fleches. 22

eſclatz : A lors fault que le chirurgiē coupe le bois au deſſus des eſclatz auec tenailles inciſiues: Puis extraire ledict fer auec tenail les dentelèes, comme tu peulx cognoiſtre par ceſte figure.

Fig. 5.17. Wound Leg from Ambroise Paré's *La maniere de traicter les playes faictes tant par hacquebutes que par fleches* (Paris: Widow of Jean de Brie, 1552). Woodcut, 16 x 10 cm. Paris, Bibliothèque interuniversitaire de santé, Cote 35183-2, fol. 22r.

clouds and rests its foot on a tasseled pillow, a sophisticated appendage that emanates almost the same spiritual aura as a *manus Dei* from a contemporary Book of Hours.[81]

It was in this form that the image grew to become an integral part of French surgical vocabulary. Over the following decades, the Wound Leg passed through multiple Paré publications by multiple printers—including André Wechel, the son of Chrétien, Tagault's printer—all of whom remained faithful to the author's explicit goal of a highly visualized surgery. The importance of images clearly stayed with Paré too. Twenty-three years later, in 1575, we find the surgeon reiterating his long-standing commitment to the visual in the dedicatory opening of the first edition of his collected *Oeuvres*. Reflecting on what was by this point a career-long effort, Paré acknowledges that his achievements in improving the practice of surgery—his precise words are *augmentee* and *enrichie* (augment and enrich)—came both through technical development, born of his practical experience, and through his pictorial innovation.[82] To support his case, he references the more than three hundred plates included in the *Oeuvres*, which he proudly states that he "*faict tailler*" (had engraved) in order to aid the comprehension of the reader, a tradition that first began back in 1552 with his take on the Wound Leg.[83]

Once again, this situation stood in stark contrast to practice outside of France. In translations of Paré, the Wound Leg was still being removed. For instance, in a 1594 edition of *Les Oeuvres* produced in Frankfurt, the printers Johann Feyrabend and Peter Fischer chose to replace the image altogether, opting instead for a fully formed Wound Man. Printed in the very same spot in the book without even changing the caption, Feyrabend and Fischer clearly made the calculation that a German audience would appreciate the Wound Man in his entirety rather than one of his individualized parts. Yet back in France at around the same time, the image of the Wound Leg was popular enough to become a stand-alone showpiece. We find this difference eloquently affirmed in a book, now in London's Wellcome Collection, that on its opening folio bears a handwritten title in calligraphic letters naming it as a list of *Instrumenta chyrurgie et icones anathomice* (Instruments of surgery and anatomical images).[84] What follows are over two hundred pages of individual woodcut prints drawn both from Paré's *Oeuvres* and his other surgical works, each pressed entirely in isolation on the page with no accompanying text and lavished with careful, hand-applied color.[85] Among an opening tranche of surgical instruments we find the Wound Leg: presented as one of the book's most dramatically vibrant pictures, the limb is now emanating from a sapphire-colored cloud and resting on a plush red pillow whose tassels have been picked out in yellow (fig. 5.18).[86] The origins of this unique volume are not fully clear, although its early pages include a handwritten note naming one *N. Rassius Desneus chyrurgus regius*, the royal surgeon Nicolas Rasse des Neux, a well-connected Parisian contemporary of Paré's and most likely the book's commissioner.[87] The very fact that someone like Nicolas seems to have been interested in using his connections with the capital's printers and artists to have this bespoke suite of surgical images produced, devoid of their accompanying medicine and yet at significant expense, confirms just how firmly canonical the Wound Leg and its accompanying imagery had become within the French surgical establishment.

In France, therefore, we get a sense that the Wound Leg functioned as an image with its own specific microhistory. Cut off from the Wound Man's body, it sidestepped the figure's status when whole as a precise medical diagram and instead was enabled to function as both a surgically discrete and aesthetically interesting image. Buoyed by association over several generations with the country's most influential surgeons, it was in this form that

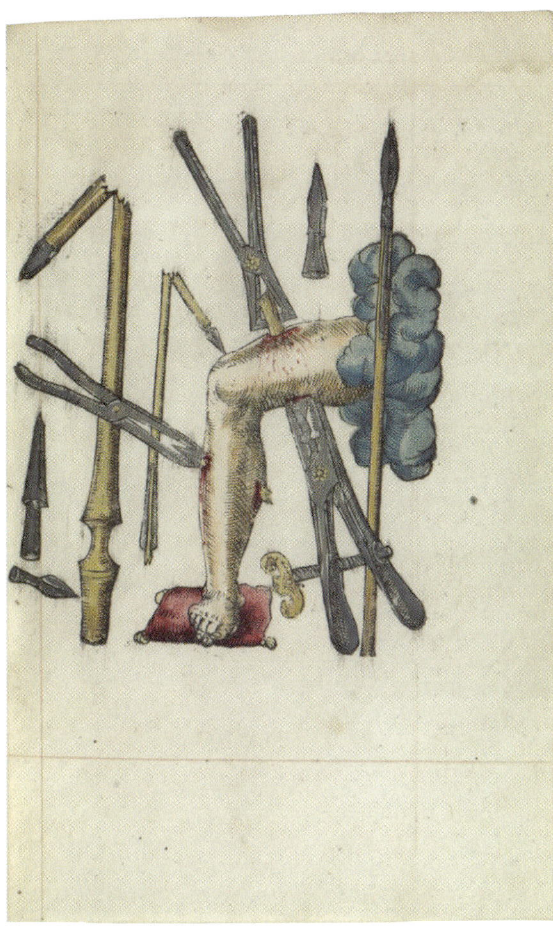

Fig. 5.18. Wound Leg from the album of Nicolas Rasse des Neux, after 1561, Paris. Hand-colored woodcut, 18 x 11 cm. London, Wellcome Library, EPB/B/4818, fol. b8r.

French medicine embraced the appendage. Indeed, by the fourth edition of Paré's *Oeuvres*, published in 1585, the Wound Leg was even being presented as if it had been a part of surgical practice for millennia.[88] Once again, in this edition the image appears deep in a section on surgical procedure, its familiar instruments sticking out from the shin and thigh in order to help clarify the treatment of arrow wounds. But this book's printer, Gabriel Buon, has also furnished the image with a new caption, a note to the reader claiming that a treatment for projectile injuries just like the one illustrated is mentioned by none other than Hippocrates in his *Epidemics*. Flanked by evidence from the Ancients, Buon presents the image as courting the approval not only of French experts but also of early modern medicine's most revered founding father, retrospectively folding the Wound Leg into a surgical tradition stretching back into time immemorial.

England: "Historicall Illustrations"

On the other side of the Channel, just as the French Wound Leg was first emerging, English engagements with the Wound Man were also afoot. As we saw at the start of this chapter, the figure must have been present in England

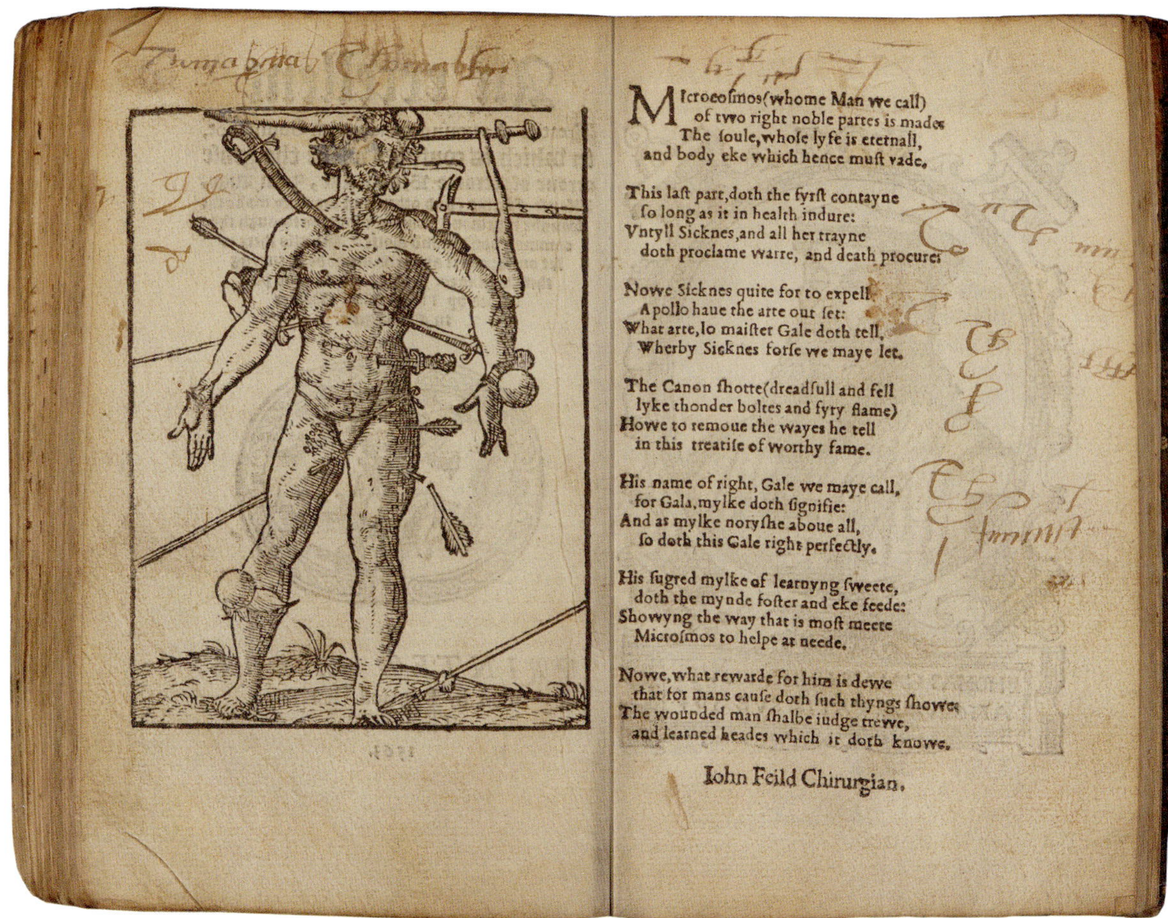

Microcoſmos(whome Man we call)
of two right noble partes is made:
The ſoule,whoſe lyfe is eternall,
and body eke which hence muſt vade.

This laſt part,doth the fyrſt contayne
ſo long as it in health indure:
Vntyll Sicknes,and all her trayne
doth proclame warre, and death procure:

Nowe Sicknes quite for to expell,
Apollo haue the arte out ſet:
What arte,lo maiſter Gale doth tell,
Wherby Sicknes forſe we maye let.

The Canon ſhotte(dreadfull and fell
lyke thonder boltes and fyry flame)
Howe to remoue the wayes he tell
in this treatiſe of worthy fame.

His name of right, Gale we maye call,
for Gala,mylke doth ſignifie:
And as mylke noryſhe aboue all,
ſo doth this Gale right perfectly.

His ſugred mylke of learnyng ſweete,
doth the mynde foſter and eke feede:
Showyng the way that is moſt meete
Microſmos to helpe at neede.

Nowe,what rewarde for him is dewe
that for mans cauſe doth ſuch thyngs ſhowe:
The wounded man ſhalbe iudge trewe,
and learned heades which it doth knowe.

Iohn Feild Chirurgian.

Fig. 5.19. Wound Man opposite a poem by John Field from Thomas Gale's *Certaine Workes of Chirurgerie* (London: Rowland Hall, 1563). Woodcut, 15 x 10 cm (each folio). London, Wellcome Library, EPB/2504/A/2, frontispiece to book III.

by around the end of the fifteenth century, when its hand-drawn likeness was being copied from circulating editions of the Italian *Fasciculus medicinae* into locally produced medical manuscripts (fig. 0.1). However, it was only sixty years later that an English press actually decided to reproduce the Wound Man in print.

Its first appearance was in a 1563 edition of the surgeon Thomas Gale's *Certaine Workes of Chirurgerie*, printed in London in the shop of Rowland Hall (fig. 5.19).[89] The image appears twice in the *Certaine Workes*, first on its title page and once again in the work's third section, on gunshot wounds, and in both instances Hall deploys a woodcut closely modeled on another work we have already explored, the title page of Tagault's *De chirurgica institutione*, which had been published by Valgrisi in Venice less than twenty years earlier (fig. 5.14). The London example is rougher in its finish, its lines a little less fine and crisp, but the debt to the Continental image is still clear in its casual pose and flowing locks. Nonetheless, this first English Wound Man is presented in rather different circumstances. Rather than parading alongside a specific set of surgical instructions, invoked to frame or represent trauma treatments, the Wound Man that opens the third section of Gale's work is instead accompanied by a page-long poem.

The verses in question are ascribed to Gale's friend, his fellow surgeon John Field, and across seven quatrains they paint a laudatory picture of the surgical profession, both the valiant efforts of surgical healers at large and Gale's work in particular. The poem reads:

Microcosmus (whome Man we call)
  of two right noble partes is made
The soule, whose lyfe is eternall,
  and body eke which hence must vade.

This last part, doth the fyrst contayne
  so long as it in health indure:
Vntyll Sicknes, and all her trayne
  doth proclame warre, and death procure.

Nowe Sicknes quite for to expell
  Apollo haue the arte out set:
What arte, lo maister Gale doth tell,
  Wherby Sicknes forse we maye let.

The Canon shotte (dreadfull and fell
  lyke thonder boltes and fyry flame)
Howe to remoue the wayes he tell
  in this treatise of worthy fame.

His name of right, Gale we maye call,
  for Gala, mylke doth signifie:
And as mylke noryshe aboue all,
  so doth this Gale right perfectly.

His sugred mylke of learnyng sweete,
  doth the mynde foster and eke feede:
Showyng the way that is most meete
  Microcosmos to helpe at neede.

Nowe, what rewarde for him is dewe
  that for mans cause doth such thyngs showe:
The wounded man shal be iudge trewe,
  and learned heades which it doth knowe.

IOHN FEILD CHIRURGIAN.[90]

This is not the first time in the Wound Man's history that we have come across poetry. Gersdorff's *Feldtbuch* saw the figure speak in its own rhyming verses, and the medieval Wound Man's accompanying *Wundarznei* contained short mnemonic ditties.[91] Yet this poetic intervention is by far the most extensive relationship forged between a piece of verse and the injured figure. Field certainly does not talk in subtle terms. Sickness, he professes, is a trouble of mythic proportions that Gale masterfully counters "right perfectly," pointing the "Microcosmos" of man back toward a healthy union of body and soul. The fact that the poem's final couplet makes direct mention of the figure standing across the page—"the wounded man," described as the "iudge trewe" of the surgical endeavor—clarifies that the image was not a decorative frivolity but something more integral and more intimate, the first of what would be a uniquely English set of engagements between the Wound Man, poetry, and the past.

It is relevant that this new direction for the figure relied on the imitation of an imported woodblock, for at this exact moment English medicine was engaged in a complicated relationship with Continental practice.[92] For some in early sixteenth-century England, especially the country's medical elite, a sense was growing that English medical knowledge lagged somewhat behind that of their European counterparts, with therapeutic production deemed peripheral and parochial in equal measure. Consider the much-cited founding charter of the Royal College of Physicians of London, established by Henry VIII in 1518, which framed the necessity of the institution very much in Continental terms. As well as acknowledging influential physicians of the time—such as John Chambers and the college's first president, Thomas Linacre—the document describes the college's mission as imitating the "*bene institutarum civitatum in Italia et aliis multis nationibus exemplum*" (the example of well-governed cities in Italy and many other nations), meaning universities in Padua, Bologna, Paris, and elsewhere in Europe.[93] The medical faculties at both Oxford and Cambridge were small, even when supplemented by study at college level, and most if not all of England's respected physicians completed their studies abroad.

This European influence was also felt particularly keenly in the production of English medical books, a fundamental publishing history that is crucial to stake out for our understanding of contemporary Wound Men. In the first decades of the sixteenth century, much of England's printed medical output consisted of translations of Continental writers such as Eucharius Rösslin, Gui de Chauliac, Ulrich von Hutten, Desiderius Erasmus, and Giovanni da Vigo, as well as collected bundles of works attributed to unnamed medics from major Continental centers such as Montpellier or Salerno.[94] The earliest of these Tudor translations to survive is in fact a 1525 rendering into English of a surgical work we have already considered, the *Buch der Cirurgia* of Hieronymus Brunschwig, whose original frontispiece bore the first printed Wound Man north of the Alps.[95] This translation typifies the international aspirations of English projects at the time. The circuitous route by which the original German text made its way to London is proudly proclaimed in a colophon by the book's printer, Peter Treveris, who, after singing the praises of the "noble experyence" and "vertuous handy warke" of the original author, indicates that Brunschwig's surgical treatments and antidotary were first "translated out of the speche of hye Almayne [the original German] and into lowe Duche [Low German]," before then moving "in to our moderstonge of Englysshe."[96] The illustrations that Treveris chose to place beside his translated text also make clear an even more diverse range of Continental prototypes: one, a squat skeleton posing with hand on hip, looks likely to have been copied from a 1513 edition of Brunschwig's German original; a pair of trepanation images that Treveris chose to grace the London edition's title page are copied from another German work, Gersdorff's *Feldtbuch*; and other diagrammatic sources include the German author Gregor Reisch's *Margarita philosophica*, Italian printed editions of Gui de Chauliac's *Cirurgia magna*, and multiple books produced by the Parisian printers Antoine Vérard and Jean du Pré.[97] Treveris's book thus goes above and beyond to showcase an awareness of the busy European marketplace for surgical ideas to the benefit of his new English readers, a truly Continental compendium in both text and image.

That said, for all that academic English medicine may have looked repeatedly to the Continent for inspiration, the image of England as exclusively a medical follower does not hold firm across all areas of healing expertise. The country was not without its own independent concentrations of significant practical specialisms, often arranged around increasingly powerful social collectives. Although London had always lacked a university, depriving it of a medical engine-house on the model of comparable Continental centers, its late fifteenth- and early sixteenth-century surgical scene was still vibrant, dominated by the influential Barbers' Company and a smaller group of master surgeons that had existed in various guises from the 1360s.[98] These were much larger and more influential collectives than those created by their physician counterparts: in 1514, seventy-two surgeons submitted themselves for examination by authorities in London, while in 1518, when the College of Physicians was founded, it contained only six members.[99]

Moreover, when in 1540 the barbers and surgeons combined their efforts to form the United Company of Barber-Surgeons, it became one of Tudor England's preeminent medical establishments, regulating practice and medical advertising, offering members sustained social support, and sponsoring teaching, often in collaboration with individuals from the College of Physicians. This educational effort in particular marked a departure from the late medieval image of surgery as predominantly—and proudly—a manual profession, a development clarified by the publishing efforts of individuals associated with the United Company, including learned works in English on uroscopy and anatomy.[100] Thomas Gale, author of the *Certaine Workes* and its first English Wound Man, was himself closely associated with the United Company, having been a member probably since its foundation and later its warden from 1555 and its master from 1561. It is fair to assume, therefore, that when John Field declares in the final lines of his grandiose poem that Gale's "wounded man" sits in conversation with "learned heades which it doth knowe," he had Englishmen in mind among the grandees of the surgical profession.

Key to this developing English medicine, as practiced by Gale and his contemporaries, was a slow return to the Classics, a movement that was to have significant sway over the English Wound Man. This idea relates closely to a broader rise in sixteenth-century English interests in Classical heritage and its influence, from the so-called Historical Revolution of writers rethinking

England's deep past to theologians struggling to adapt to changing religious relationships with Rome, to Antique influences on cultural works in performance, poetry, and visual culture.[101] Medical writers working in this tradition took ammunition from a humanistic project begun largely by members of the College of Physicians, especially Thomas Linacre, who eagerly advocated a return to the close, firsthand study of Classical texts on the healing arts.[102] English publishers struggled with Linacre's preferred source language, Greek, either through technical limitations of their type or because they simply did not see a significant market for such books among learned specialists, but a number of his Latin editions of Galen's writings did emerge immediately after the foundation of the College of Physicians in 1518, three of which were printed in London between 1521 and 1523.[103] And in the following decades, English printers were also increasingly willing to produce translations of Classical works into the vernacular, even if translators acknowledged that—to borrow a phrase from Linacre's contemporary, Humphrey Llwyd—certain Latin terms had to be left in the original as they "cannot be well Englyshed."[104]

The extent to which this Classical focus pioneered by learned physicians became a matter of concern more widely among practitioners in other parts of the healing profession is debatable, but it still had significant impact on medical books.[105] Survey, by way of example, some of the diverse markets at play over the course of a single influential decade, the 1540s, when multiple Classical influences jostled among the roughly sixty new English medical works printed, a key set of contexts for Gale and his Wound Man.[106] In 1543, the London printer Richard Grafton produced a translation of Plutarch's writings on health, retitled as *The Precepts of the Excellent Clerke Graue Philosopher Plutarche*.[107] The work had been translated from the original Greek into Latin by Erasmus in 1513 and was offered as a New Year's gift to the English diplomat John Young, a move that harnessed the learning of the Classics for the author's own social advancement. Thirty years later, the English edition sought to do much the same, matching both Erasmus's learning and his ambitious politicking in the dedication of the work to the Lord Chancellor Thomas Audley. In more academic developments, 1545 saw the physician Christopher Langton taking up the charge of his colleague Linacre. Drawing heavily on Classical originals, he published *An Introduction into Phisycke*.[108] Not only did this work claim to channel "the olde and aunciente phisitions among the Grekes whyche passed al other in phyisike," but in its introduction Langton brought to life an image of Phisycke herself, a powerful personification that over the course of several pages speaks of Greek mythological figures from Prometheus and Ixion to Paris and Pandora in order to set out the ethical expectations of physicians and the glories they might expect for good practice. As Phisycke concludes, "haue I not rewarded both Hypocrates & Gallene accordynglye?" Langton himself would turn again to Galenic writings two years later, when in 1547 he published his *Very Brefe Treatise Ordrely Declaring the Principal Partes of Physik*, a summary of the discipline's stance on physiology based almost entirely on Latin originals, a move probably encouraged by the appointment in 1546 of his fellow physician John Caius as lecturer to the United Company of Barber-Surgeons, where he proceeded to give lectures on the Classics to members in English.[109]

In a more shameless attempt to market the cachet this vernacularized learning of Ancient authorities could bring to a medical book, we might highlight publications throughout the decade by the London printer Robert Wyer, whose work regularly traded on exaggerated Classical pedigrees.[110] In 1542, he published *The Questyonary of Cyrurgyens with the Fourth Boke of the Terapentyke*, a work that claimed to contain the entirety of a book by Galen but in fact held only sparse pockets of translation.[111] In 1545, his *Prognosticacion, Drawen Out of the Bookes of Ipocras, Avicen, and Other Notable Auctours* held very little relation to the revered Classical authorities of its title.[112] And in both 1545 and 1549, Wyer produced books that claimed once more to translate full works by Plutarch, neither of which offered anything of the sort: one was only twelve pages long, and the English of both books is almost unreadably confusing in places.[113] Still, Wyer's Classicized marketing was polished and canny, harnessing the visual too. One of the volumes bore the Latin philosopher's name in enormous letters on its title page as part of a fanciful yet temptingly learned title, the *Practica Plutarche*, while the second reprised an old woodcut portrait of a generic ancient philosopher to give visual presence to the Classical authority and lend learned weight to its contents.

Returning specifically to Thomas Gale's *Certaine Workes*, we now get a better sense of why John Field's poem accompanying the Wound Man was so eagerly packed with Classical allusions. In fact, we should consider the entirety of Gale's book as very much part of this English Classical revival. As a learned surgeon and master of the United Company, Gale dedicated much of his publishing energy to the transmission of the Classics. His translation of Galen's *Methodus medendi* (Method of Healing)—what he jokingly called his "painefull booke"—was first published by Thomas East in 1566 and became a set text for the entrance examination of new surgeons.[114] And the *Certaine Workes* too reflects Gale's strong Classical commitments. From the very first sentence of his introductory dedication of the book to Robert Dudley, the Earl of Leicester, we find a cavalcade of references to the Ancients: Aristippus of Cyrene, the Trojan Wars, the centaur Chiron, Hercules and Telephus, Agamemnon, the Sophists, and so on. Gale decided to name the second treatise of the work using the Greek term invoked by contemporaries for a small-scale handbook, his *Enchiridion of Chirurgerie*, and as he notes in the treatise's conclusion, several of the medicinal ingredients are listed by their Latin name rather than being translated into English, so that the junior medic may "mervayll thereat."[115] It is writing like this that no doubt encouraged the Classical references in Field's poem beside the Wound Man. If mankind is a "Microcosmos," Field says, then Gale attacks our cosmic sickness in the guise of Apollo who "have the arte out set." Field's fifth quatrain even parses Gale's own name as stemming from the Greek word *Gala*, which "mylke doth signifie," nourishment for the wounded patient to whom Gale dispenses a "sugred mylke of learnyng sweete."

Thinking more broadly for a moment, we might even see the very inclusion of poetry in the *Certaine Workes* as itself a Classicizing move. Classical poetic references abound elsewhere in the book. Gale cites verses attributed to Homer and Horace, as well as twice offering a poetical Englishing of an aphorism by Galen, turning "*Assiduo illisu durum cauat undula saxum*" into

"The watry droppes, so moyst and Softe / Doth pearse harde Stones with falling ofte."[116] On one occasion we even find Gale engaged in live poetic translation. In the first book of the *Certaine Workes*—written in the form of a catechistic conversation between Gale, John Field, and a questioning student named John Yates—he parses for the aspiring surgeon an aphorism attributed to Propertius: "*Felix a tergo quem nulla Ciconia pinxit*" grows grandiloquently into a four-line piece of English verse, "O happie man that such happe hast / Thy path to treade so right / That no serpentyne tungue wyll carpe / Or longbild Storke eke Spite."[117] Thomas Elyot, a diplomat, scholar, and contemporary of Gale who also published an extremely popular medical work known as the *Castell of Helth*, opined that poetry itself had healing powers: speaking in defense of poets he paraphrases Horace to claim that, as well as entertain, "the nedy and sicke he [the poet] doth also his cure / To recomfort, if aught can amende."[118] By coupling his Wound Man with Field's verses, Gale was hoping to amplify the figure's curative reach.

Produced at a key moment of change in the framing of English medicine, one in which the intellectual ambition and social dynamics of surgery were evolving, Gale effectively fused the Wound Man with his interest in ancient poetics, forging an ongoing English association for the figure with the Classical past. His work had a substantial legacy. In an immediate sense, his books held significant material value: upon the surgeon's death in 1567, his will requested that 220 printed tomes be passed not to his wife or son but to a literate maidservant named Katherine in lieu of unpaid wages.[119] Another family employee, this time an unnamed man, was also similarly compensated when, according to the will, he inherited Gale's "written books of surgery in the English tonge and all the pamflitts and peces of written books or any written books of Surgery wherin any Englishe is written," a stress on popularizing the vernacular that seems to match Gale's intellectual aspirations. What became of these particular books and papers is not known, although their speedy distribution is surely testified in Gale's ongoing popularity. Nearly twenty years later, in 1586, the printer Thomas East decided to produce matching second editions of both the *Certaine Workes* and Gale's translation of Galen, while in 1588 Gale's contemporary William Clowes channeled several similar ideas into a new book of case studies aimed at apprentice practitioners, *A Prooved Practise for All Young Chirurgians*.[120] Clowes mentions "good Maister Gale" on occasion and favorably enough, even though he did not necessarily agree with his predecessor on matters of general theory or operative specifics. In fact, according to notebooks of the United Company, Clowes rarely agreed with any of his fellow members on much at all, the records showing regular transgressions of company rules and even open brawls with other surgeons.[121] Yet, in terms of rhetorical style, there are striking similarities between the *Prooved Practise* and the tone of the *Certaine Workes*. Classical references once more come thick and fast: Homer and Prometheus, Demosthenes and Chilon of Sparta, a poem on manly honor set in "Caesar's raigne," reference to an antediluvian Arcadia, an old woman at Newington beyond Saint George's Fields who has falsely set herself up as an oracle, and poetic fragments mentioning Cicero, Aesculapius, Apollo, and Mars. It is no surprise, then, that interspersed among Clowes's references—fronting a section on "instruments, good for young practizers of Chirurgerie"—we once more find the Wound Man.

Another copy of Tagault's figure, Clowes's image is put to more narrative didactic use, featuring alongside a number of firsthand case studies that resonate remarkably closely with the Wound Man's depicted injuries. In one case, Clowes cites a certain man who

> was thrust through his bodie with a sword, which did enter first under the cartilage or grisle ... the poynt of the sword passed thorowe his bodie, and so out at his backe, in such manner, that he which wounded the man did runne his way, and did leaue the sword sticking in his bodie: so the wounded man did with his owne hands pull out the sword.[122]

Another immediately follows concerning "a certaine traveiler into the East and West Indies," who was run through in a similar manner, the sword miraculously missing his vital organs. Clowes's cure for both is a concoction to be taken orally whose ingredients of plants and minerals he cites as having been recorded in "divers ancient copies" and invented by the "worthie Grecians." Even the Wound Man's medicine has been thoroughly Hellenized.

Infused with both the medical knowledge and rhetorical flare of the Classical past, the Wound Man's English allure continued into the seventeenth century. Evoking earlier German counterparts, contemporary surgeons saw the character as an appropriate title-page blazon for their newly Englished works, including translations of Ambroise Paré by Walter Hammond in 1617 and Thomas Johnson in 1634.[123] Physicians of the day appear to have been equally enchanted. Despite it being a rocky period for the professional standing of such healers, the Wound Man's status as a "Microcosmus," a term first coined by Gale and Field, was reaffirmed once again by the London physician Helkiah Crooke in his *ΜΙΚΡΟΚΟΣΜΟΓΡΑΦΙΑ: A Description of the Body of Man*, whose third edition of 1631 appended another translation of Paré with the figure on its opening page.[124]

We might even be tempted to read echoes of the figure surfacing with increasing regularity in contemporary English popular culture. In the 1602 play *A Larum for London*, the character of an amputee soldier who has "stumbled through a thousand shot" is throughout referred to simply as Stump, his tales of violent bodily defacement standing in for his actual name in much the same way as Field's poem speaks of the Wound Man.[125] In 1642, the author Daniel Lakin published *A Miraculous Cure of the Prusian Swallow-Knife*, a pseudo-medicalized account of an emergency operation undergone by one Andreas Grünheide, who had tried to use the butt of his knife to provoke vomiting but mistakenly swallowed it. The Dutchman is portrayed on the work's title page clutching the knife and gesturing to the counterpoint spot where it once sat poking at his belly (fig. 5.20).[126] Meanwhile, a ballad that was probably written at roughly the same time evokes a poetic combination of verse and wound familiar from the *Certaine Workes*. We read of a begging soldier who, couplet by couplet, claims to have accrued more and more fantastical wounds from different campaigns across Europe, their sum forming an impossibly mutilated body in precisely the mold of the Wound Man:

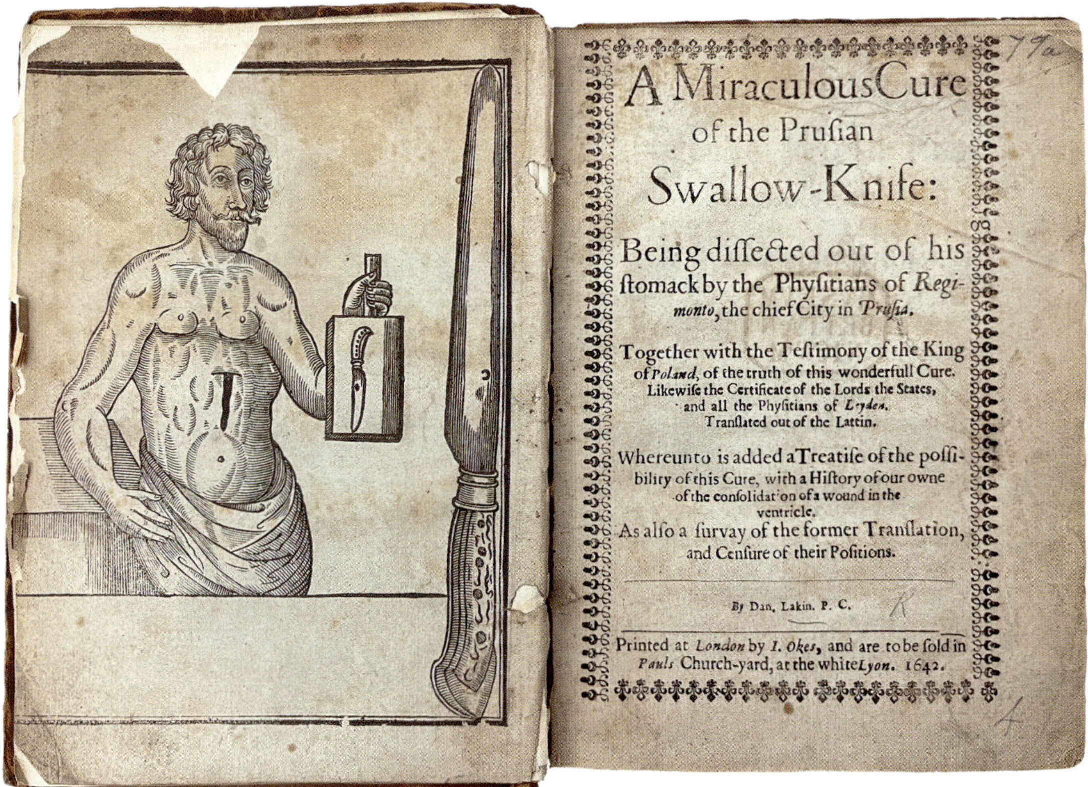

A Miraculous Cure
of the Pruſian
Swallow-Knife:
Being diſſected out of his
ſtomack by the Phyſitians of *Regimonto*, the chief City in *Pruſia*.

Together with the Teſtimony of the King
of *Poland*, of the truth of this wonderfull Cure.
Likewiſe the Certificate of the Lords the States,
and all the Phyſitians of *Leyden*.
Tranſlated out of the Lattin.

Whereunto is added a Treatiſe of the poſſibility of this Cure, with a Hiſtory of our owne of the conſolidation of a wound in the ventricle.
As alſo a ſurvay of the former Tranſlation, and Cenſure of their Poſitions.

By Dan. Lakin. P. C.

Printed at *London* by *I. Okes*, and are to be ſold in *Pauls* Church-yard, at the white *Lyon*. 1642.

Fig. 5.20. Frontispiece and title page of Daniel Lakin's *A Miraculous Cure of the Prusian Swallow-Knife* (London: John Oakes, 1642). Woodcut, 20 x 15 cm (each folio). London, British Library, General Reference Collection 1169.k.1, frontispiece and title page.

Twice through the Bulke I have been shot,
My braines have boyled like a Pot:
I have at lest these doozen times,
Been blowne up by those roguish Mines,
    under a Barracado
    in a Bravado,
throwing of a hand-Granado:
    Oh death was very neere,
    for it tooke away my eare ...

At push of Pike I lost mine eye,
At Bergen Siege I broke my thigh:
At Ostend, though I were a Lad,
I laid about me as I were mad ...

And since that made a Warlike Dance,
Both into Spaine, and into France,
    and there I lost a flood
    of Noble blood,
and did but very little good:
    and now I home am come,
    with ragges about my bumme,
God blesse you Sir, from this poore summe.[127]

As Alexander Wragge-Morley has convincingly shown, it was at this point in the later seventeenth century that images began to take on a particularly keen capacity for aesthetic thinking among the elite of England's scientific community, mobilized in debates around micrography, physiology, and even ancient history.[128] It is particularly interesting, then, that at precisely this moment the Wound Man appears to reach what we might consider its English apogee. Published in London in 1678, the *Compleat Discourse of Wounds* by John Browne, a Norwich anatomist and surgeon-in-ordinary to Charles II, contains one of the most unusual Wound Men to ever appear in print (fig. 5.21).[129] A full-page copperplate engraving, the figure is found in Browne's sixth chapter on removing extraneous bodies from wounds, placed opposite another full-page plate of surgical instruments. It is not, however, the extravagance of this Wound Man's injuries that catches the reader's attention, its wounds comparatively plain and somewhat sparse. Instead, it is his elaborate style that makes this figure leap off the page, his right arm thrown back dramatically and his left arm sweeping upward, hooking with it an incongruous piece of extravagant flowing cloth.

In his text, Browne is unusually clear about why he wanted the engraving included. Principally, he states, it was designed to act as a rhetorical aid in explanation of a key point in the treatment of wounds. As he notes:

> And since I have already declared to you how the Body of man may be variously assaulted by diversity of Instruments, I have here also expressed in this following Figure how his Parts may be contused, punged, incised and lacerated, by Clubs, Stones, Swords, Pikes, Faulchions, Arrows, Shot, and the like: against which, on the contrary side, I have also delineated such commodious Instruments, as are and have been allowed as most proper for the Extraction on and discharging of the same out of the wounded parts.[130]

Surgically speaking, Browne argues, a practitioner needs to decide which tools in their arsenal are most fitting to execute the cure of a particular injury, and this decision should be based on the correspondence of an instrument's "figure and shape" to that of the wound or lodged weapon they wish to cure, hence the pairing of Wound Man and instruments across the gutter. These were tools that Browne would have known well, having himself been appointed a naval surgeon in the Dutch War of 1665–1667, where he sustained a cannonball fracture to the arm, just as his Wound Man does.[131] But this particular Wound Man also offers a unique opportunity to consider another individual with clear stakes in the figure: its artist.

Up to this point we have looked at many images of the Wound Man both in manuscript and print, and while we might have been able to make certain assumptions about their artists' influences and training, their motivations and patrons, no traceable full names of any have survived. Here, though, Browne's Wound Man plate is signed "R. White sculpt.," indicating that the image was the work of the highly successful London artist Robert White, who was active from the late 1660s until around 1702.[132] Working as a draftsman and engraver and later in mezzotint, White is associated with several images

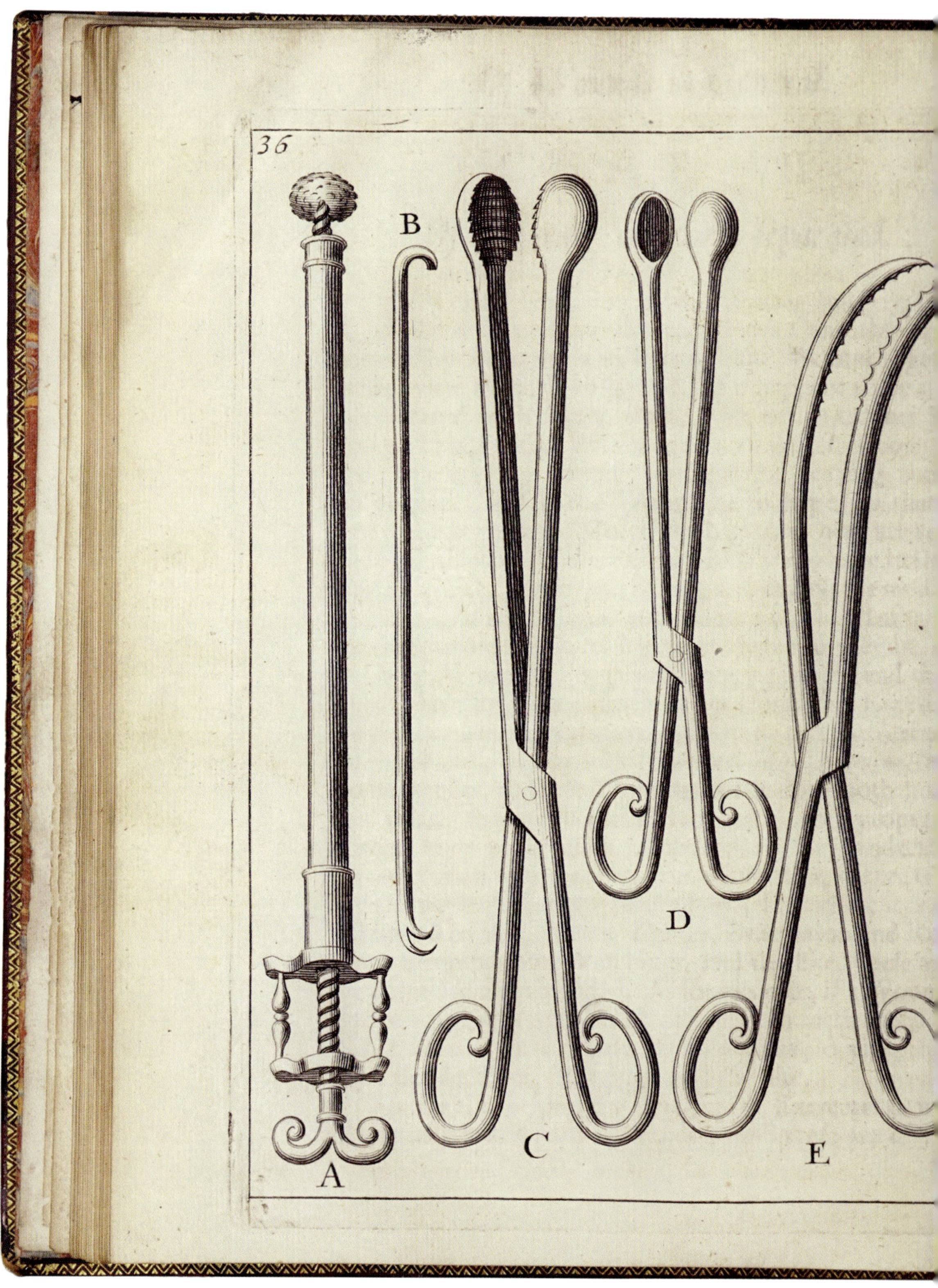

Fig. 5.21. Surgical instruments and Wound Man from John Browne's *A Compleat Discourse of Wounds* (London: E[lizabeth?] Flesher, 1678). Copperplate engraving, 21 x 15 cm (each folio). London, Wellcome Library, EPB/B/15691/1, 36–37.

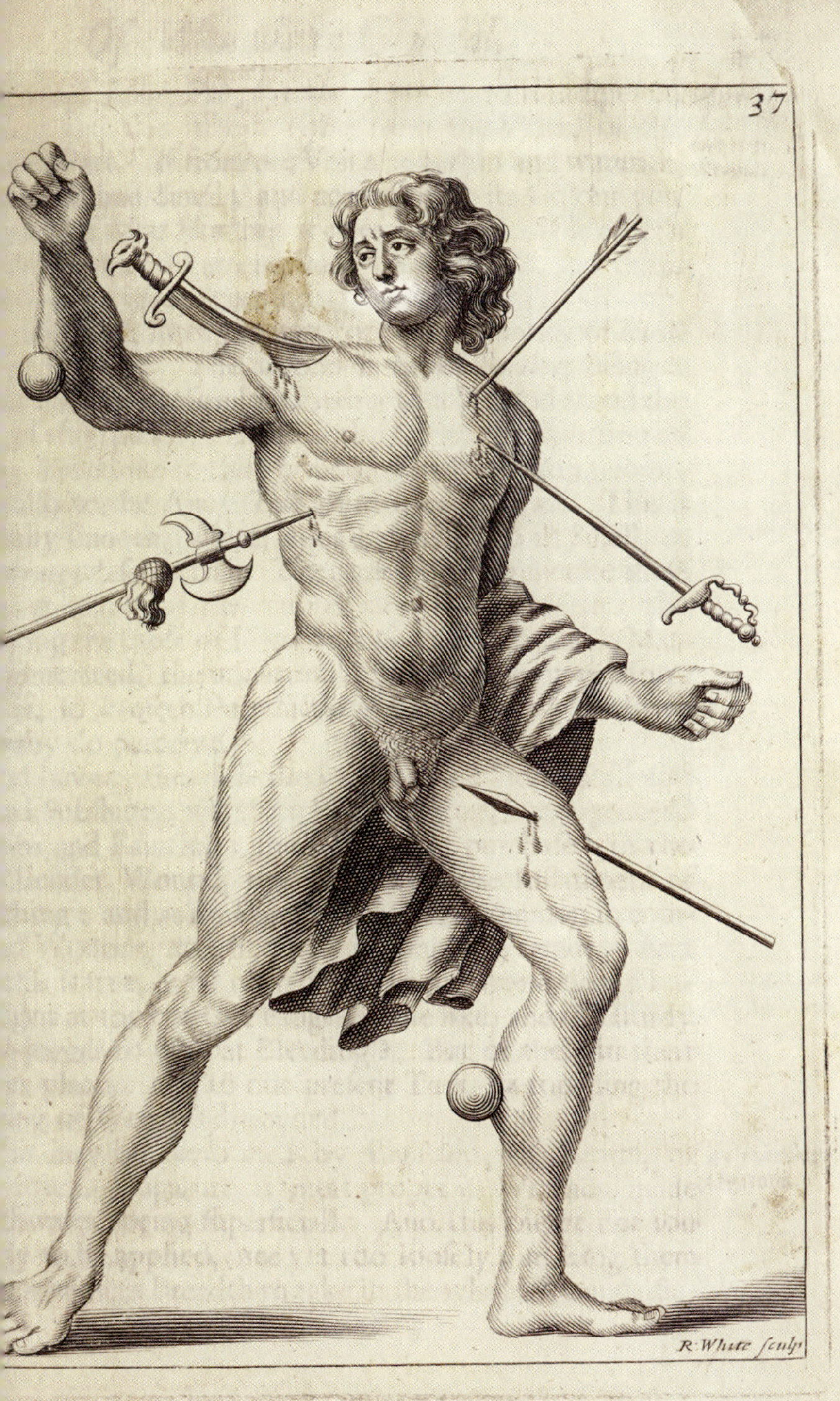
37
R: White sculp

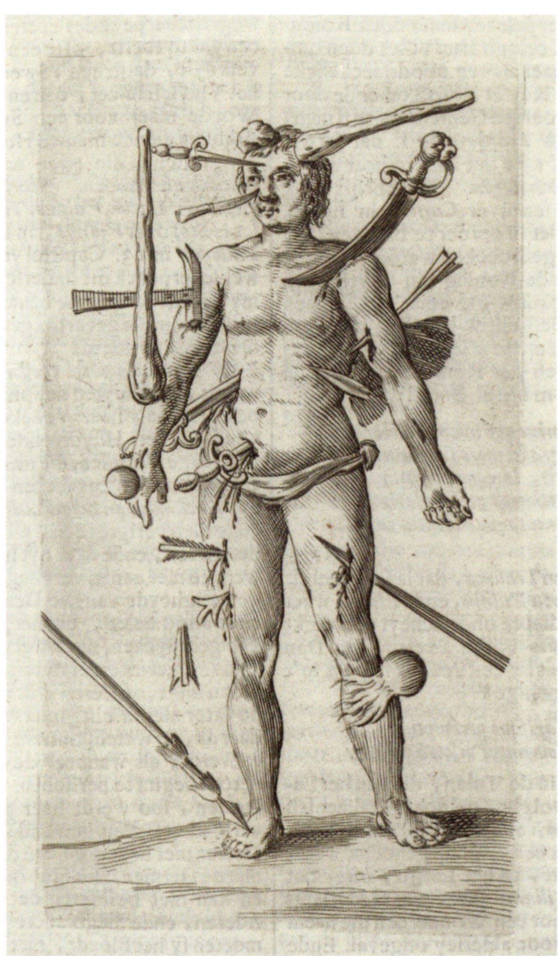

Fig. 5.22. Wound Man from Johan van Beverwijck's *Wercken der genees-konste* (Amsterdam: Widow of Jan Jacobsz. Schipper, 1672). Copperplate engraving, 25 x 18 cm. The Hague, Koninklijke Bibliotheek, KW 538 C 8, vol. 3, 127.

from works in the medical orbit, in particular an enormous 1677 print of the new buildings of Bethlem Hospital, which had recently been completed under the direction of Robert Hooke, as well as a detailed scene in another book by Browne showing Charles I curing scrofula by sacred touch.[133] However, he was far more famous among contemporaries as a keen-eyed producer of portrait miniatures depicting England's cultural and ruling elites, ranging from every post-Restoration monarch in his lifetime to writers, artists, and scientists such as John Milton, Henry Purcell, John Bunyan, and Robert Boyle.[134]

Many such portraits are noted in contemporary annotations as having been drawn "*ad vivum*," a term that both indicates their direct capture "from life" and connotes a contemporary interest in portraying the liveliness as well as a likeness of an individual, an idea White also brings to his Wound Man. Compare his figure with a Dutch Wound Man from just a few years earlier, printed in the 1672 edition of Johan van Beverwijck's *Wercken der genees-konste* (Works of Medicine) (fig. 5.22).[135] The Beverwijck image essentially reproduces with admirable clarity the very same figure that had been circulating in the Netherlands for nearly two centuries, reprising the same standard retinue of weapons, injuries, and skimpy briefs. White, by contrast, plays with the reader's focus. Despite having suffered some of the Wound Man's standard attacks by lance and cutlass, both of which still remain lodged in his skin and even pass entirely through his limbs, there is an obvious discordance between these weapons' long, poking forms and the minuscule entry and exit wounds they have generated. It is as if they are a set of flimsy tools pushed through a bloodless marble sculpture. Pulling the viewer's attention almost entirely away from the Wound Man's eponymous wounds, White instead trains our eye on the strange completeness of his underlying body, a twisting, muscular Adonis complete with fashionable contemporary haircut.

Specifically, this effect is achieved through White's mobilization of cutting-edge aesthetic currents from his own creative milieu, in particular a penchant for the Antique increasingly present in English artistic circles. This was a Classical correlative to contemporary ideas we have seen being embraced by England's medics, and at this point in the 1670s White would have had a number of potential routes to access objects and images from the distant past. His work as a portraitist included producing images for a number of English collectors of the Antique—including writer and antiquarian Sir John Marsham, book collector William Petyt, Classical translator Thomas Creech, and Joshua Barnes, the Regius Professor of Greek—and through David Loggan, White's influential teacher, the artist had become associated with publishing projects that recorded the antiquities of English universities.[136] White himself created a number of frontispieces for contemporary writers on the Antique, most notably a grandiose Classical facade with a central Homeric bust for the 1669 edition of John Ogilby's *Homer, His Odysses Translated, Adorn'd with Sculpture*, and a more explicitly English equivalent in Anthony Wood's 1674 *Historia et antiquitates universitatis Oxoniensis* (History and Antiquities of the University of Oxford), complete with a crowned King Charles shown beside a Classical column.[137]

It is unclear whether these connections would have granted White direct contact with the few pieces of Classical sculpture present in England at that time, but as a successful printmaker he would have had easy access to various prints and printed books that replicated Antique images, especially statuary that had for several centuries captivated European draftsmen and women. The 1670s, for instance, saw the publication of the German painter and antiquarian Joachim von Sandrart's *Teutsche Academie* (normally translated as the German Academy of the Noble Arts of Architecture, Sculpture, and Painting) and the Dutchman Jan de Bisschop's series *Signorum veterum icones* (Images of Ancient Figures), both collections of engravings showing famed Classical works.[138] One source, though, bears an unmistakable resemblance to White's Wound Man, an image from a slightly earlier collection of engravings made in 1638 by the Frenchman François Perrier and reprinted throughout the century as part of his *Segmenta nobilium signorum et statuarum* (Pieces of Noble Figures and Statues) (fig. 5.23).[139] Depicting a sculpture from Rome's Quirinal Hill, at the time thought to be an image of either Alexander the Great or one of the twin gods Castor and Pollux, the resonance with White's image is so close that the print was surely the figure's direct model, the very first Wound Man to take its source from outside of the surgical tradition. Trading the cuirass at the feet of Perrier's sculpture for the various weapons peppering the Wound

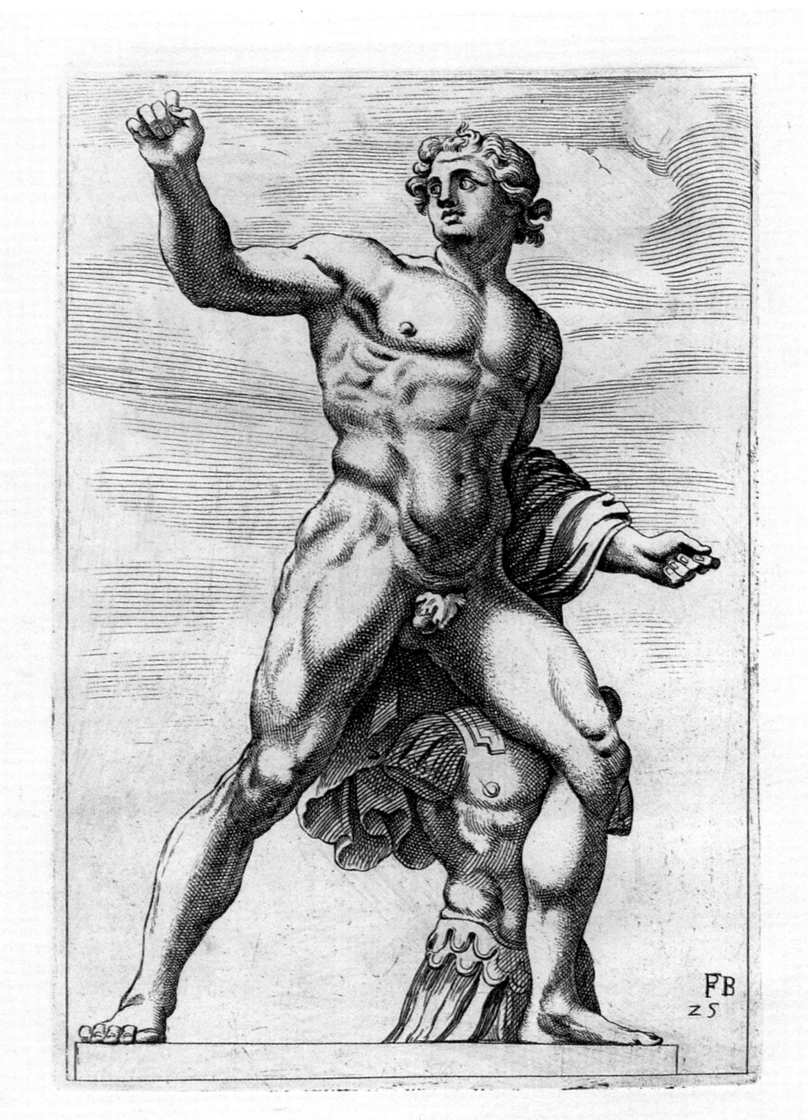

Fig. 5.23. Statue on the Quirinal Hill in Rome thought to be Alexander the Great, from François Perrier's *Segmenta nobilium signorum et statuarum* (Rome: printer unknown, 1638). Copperplate engraving, 24 x 16 cm. Heidelberg, Universitätsbibliothek, 80 B 392 RES, table 30.

Man's body, White shepherds the surgical image toward a uniquely Classical formula of perfection, drawing on ancient forms to lend a potentially pathetic figure a renewed and austere gravitas.

In a short letter included at the beginning of Browne's *Compleat Discourse*, a contemporary of the surgeon, the famed physician Thomas Browne, offered his praise for the volume, noting its breadth "across many subjects" and emphasizing both its use of various "approved Authours" and its impressive choice of "Effectuall Medicines, together with proper Historicall Illustrations." It is this "Historicall" purpose that White's artwork captures so perfectly: a long-standing English engagement with the Wound Man that, ever since the Classicizing poetic allusions of Gale's *Certaine Workes* a century earlier, once more slowly turned the figure away from the specifics of surgical cure and toward more local concerns, in this case building a glorious Antique past for England's aspirational surgeons.

Japan: Redhead-Style Surgery

The fate of the amputated French Wound Leg and Classicized English Wound Men demonstrates just two of the different ways in which the image of the Wound Man continued to evolve in discrete pockets of the European medical community throughout the early modern period. Rather than exclusively valued for its original diagrammatic clarity, we instead find the figure deployed across a multitude of changing local circumstances, just as likely to be evoked in the aid of social positioning or artistic experimentation as in medical communication. Nor was the Wound Man by this point an exclusively European phenomenon. As the story of one final later version of the image shows, at the turn of the eighteenth century the figure's early modern propensity for shifting chameleon-like across contexts had also helped it travel significant swaths of the globe.

The roots of this particular example are once more to be found in the work of a German surgeon, on this occasion a practitioner named Johannes Schultheiß, more commonly known by his Latin name, Scultetus. Born in Ulm in 1595, where he started life as a bricklayer's assistant, Scultetus turned to studying medicine in the second decade of the seventeenth century and learned under some of the most renowned specialists of his day, including the Dutchman Adriaan van den Spieghel in Vienna and the pioneering anatomist Hieronymus Fabricius in Padua.[140] Returning to Ulm in 1625, he quickly rose to become one of the most prominent surgeons in the entirety of the German-speaking lands, and shortly before his death in 1645 he completed the text of a book that was to form his most pervasive legacy. Published posthumously a decade later under the direction of his nephew Johannes Schultheiß the Younger, the work was entitled *ΧΕΙΡΟΠΛΟΘΗΚΗ, seu armamentarium chirurgicum XLIII tabulis* (Chiroplasty, or Surgical Arsenal in Forty-Three Tables).[141]

As the latter part of its title implies, this was a work geared entirely around images. Organizing the author's accumulated knowledge of the surgical field via a series of full-page plates—its eponymous "tables"—the book depicts a variety of procedures and instruments, each with a subsequent key of letters and Roman numerals to connect particular pictures with detailed written explanations on the following pages. This accompanying text normally included Scultetus's descriptions of specific operations, lists of relevant pharmaceuticals and recipes, and outlines of case histories drawn from the surgeon's own experience, many of which he elaborated on in an extensive *Observationes chirurgicae* (Surgical Observations) at the back of the book. As for the visual contents, the *Armamentarium*'s forty-three tables are rich and varied. The reader is presented with clusters of floating heads in various stages of the trepanning process, the dislocated limbs of patients shown being hauled back into place by groups of medics and assistants, and row

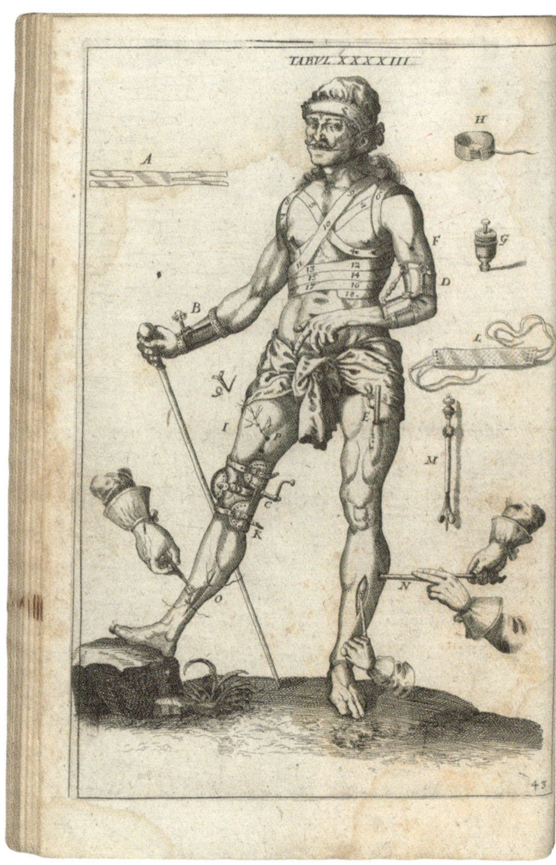

Fig. 5.24. Wound Man from Johannes Scultetus's *ΧΕΙΡΟΠΛΟΘΗΚΗ, seu armamentarium chirurgicum* (Ulm: Balthasar Kühne, 1655). Copperplate engraving, 35 x 22 cm. London, Wellcome Library, EPB/D/47562, table XXXXIII.

upon row of specialist tools for stitching, cutting, suturing, scraping, syringing, and more, most of which are depicted to realistic scale in the folio-sized book. One by one, the busy plates build to cumulative conclusion in the work's "*Tabula ultima*" (Final table), the only plate to contain just a single figure: a newly conceived Wound Man (fig. 5.24).

Standing in an unusual rocky landscape, supporting himself with a long cane, and sporting a tight silken nightcap, this novel version of the image feels less like a catalog of causes than a catalog of interventions. He wears complex bandaging and screw-tightened metallic splints, attended to from head to toe by the floating hands of multiple surgeons in midprocedure, each holding instruments that prod and pull at his wounds. The image might lack the graphic violence of earlier Wound Men, but this is only because the doctors have already begun their work. As we read in the table's subsequent description, this Wound Man is still suffering from a long list of woes:

> *TABULA ULTIMA*
> *De funda Galeni, cancro labiorum, arteriæ incisæ compressione, pedis contracti distensione, cubiti rigidi inflexione, sinus in femore magni apertione, locis & fasciis fonticulurum, glandium e vulneribus sclopetorum extractione, varicum sectione, labiorum vulneris per fibulas adductione, tibiæ cariosæ abrasione, & de ligatura pectoris, quam Galenus Cataphractam vocat.*

FINAL TABLE

On "Galen's Sling," cancer of the lips, compression of an incised artery, distension of a contracted foot, bending of a rigid elbow, opening of the great curve in the thigh, the places and bandaging of the fontanelle, extraction of bullets from gunshot wounds, bleeding of veins, bringing together the edges of the wound with clamps, abrasion of the decayed tibia, and on the binding of the breast, which Galen calls *Cataphracta*.

Substantial explanations of these instruments and procedures follow in effective combinations of image and text. The approach must have been prized by Scultetus's early readers, for by the time of the book's translation into German in 1666—under the title *Wund-Artzneyisches Zeug-Hauß* (Surgical Arsenal)—its roster of plates had grown in number to fifty-six.[142] With a firm eye on the aesthetic, these expanded designs were supplied by the Ulm painter Jonas Arnold the Younger, with the popular Wound Man himself also multiplied: he appears five times in one new plate, receiving treatment from the waist upward in different variations, while in another he is reimagined in a new and particularly grotesque guise in which he adopts the same pose to tabulate a variety of diseases and injuries, alongside an equally disturbing female equivalent (fig. 5.25).

Even before this German edition, Scultetus's book was extensively disseminated. His suite of images and their accompanying medicine was broadcast widely across Europe. In 1656, only one year after the initial printing in Ulm, a Latin edition was printed in The Hague, followed a year later in

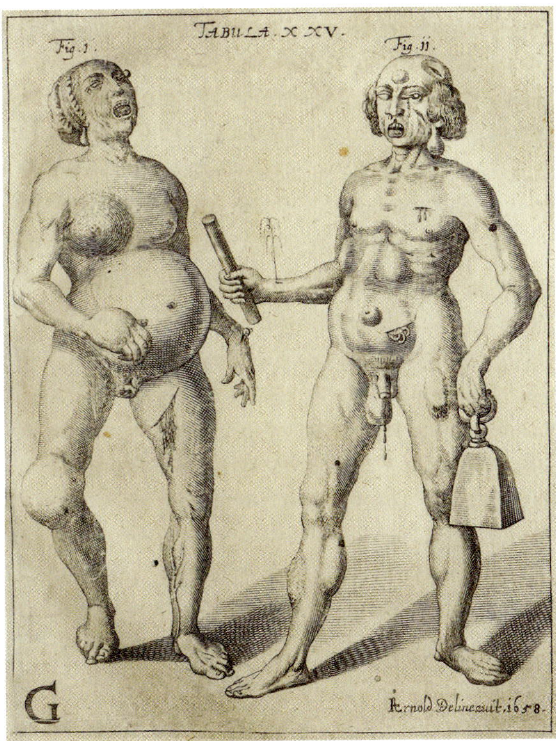

Fig. 5.25. Wounded and diseased male and female figure from Johannes Scultetus's *Wund-Artzneyisches Zeug-Hauß* (Frankfurt am Main: Johannes Gerlini, 1666). Copperplate engraving, 21 x 18 cm. Mannheim, Landesmuseum für Technik und Arbeit, no shelfmark, table XXV.

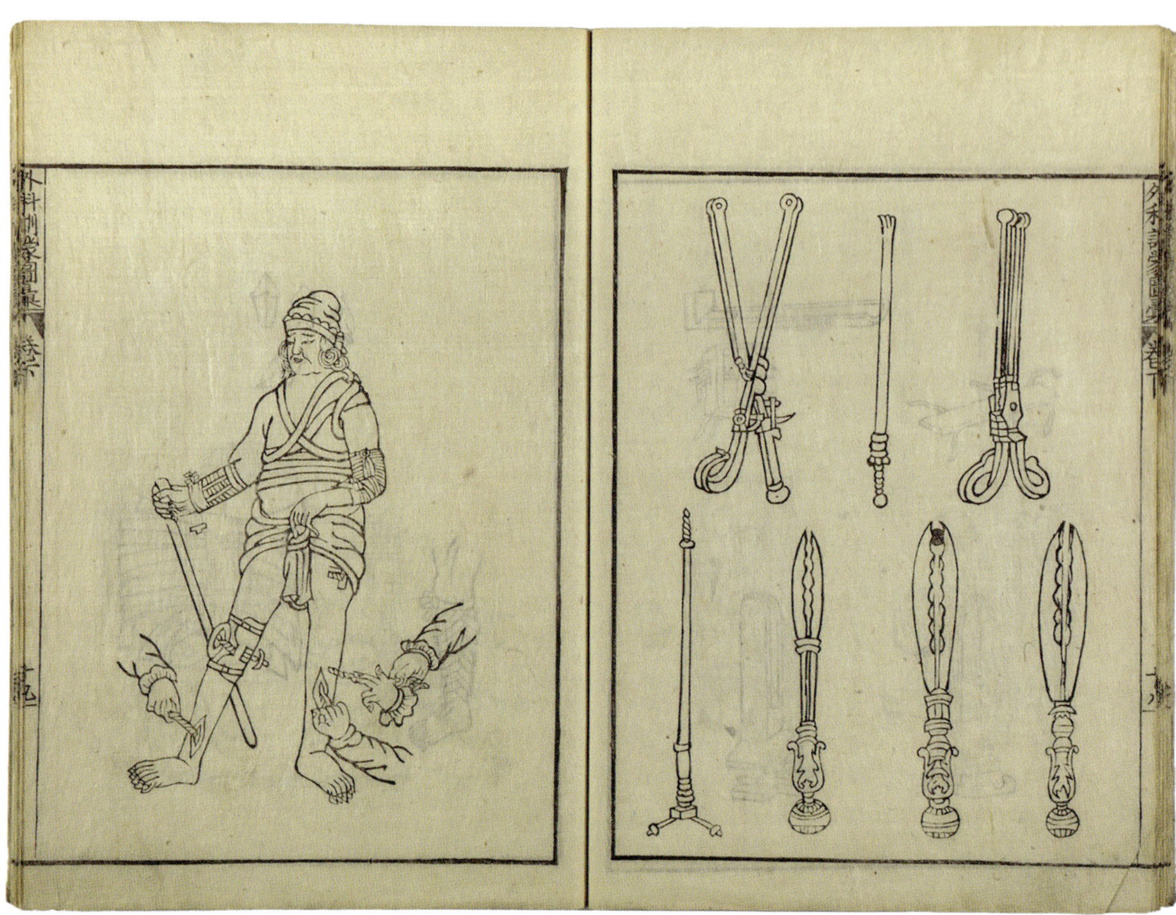

Fig. 5.26. Wound man from Irako Mitsuaki's *Geka kinmō zui* 外科訓蒙図彙 (Kyoto: unknown publisher, 1769). Woodcut, 26 x 17 cm (each folio). Kyoto, University Library, ケ/163, vol. 2, 36–37.

1657 by a Dutch translation, together marking the beginnings of a tradition of printing Scultetus in the Netherlands that would continue until at least 1748.[143] In 1672, a French translation was published in Lyon under the title *L'arcenal de chirurgie de Iean Scultet* (Johannes Scultetus's Surgical Arsenal), followed only two years later by the book's first English edition, *The Chyrurgeons Store-House Furnished with Forty-Three Tables Cut in Brass*.[144] And by the 1680s, further editions had been printed in Amsterdam, Dordrecht, Nuremberg, Venice, Frankfurt, Lyon, Leiden, and London, with the flexible nature of the book's combination of visual tables and explanatory text ensuring that across these different versions Scultetus's work could expand and contract with ease. While the 1666 German edition grew to accommodate fifty-six tables, editions in Amsterdam in 1669 and Leiden in 1692 instead shrank, crunching the original's forty-three tables down to a convenient ten. The result, a slim octavo book, could be carried by traveling specialists far more conveniently, allowing them to take the work and its imagery even further afield.

Such travel could be very far indeed, as evidenced by a figure in a book printed in 1769 not in Germany or England or France but in Japan (fig. 5.26).

The image appears in the second volume of a book printed in Kyoto entitled *Geka kinmō zui* (外科訓蒙図彙 Diagrams for Surgical Instruction), a work by the physician Irako Mitsuaki (伊良子光顕, also known as Irako Kōken) into which was channeled both Irako's own experience as a medic and a broader tradition of intercultural medical exchange between Japanese and European practitioners that had been building for roughly a century.[145] By the time Irako was writing in the 1760s, aggressive Portuguese, Spanish, British, and Dutch expansion had established numerous colonial holdings across Southeast Asia that operated largely through proxy companies, such as England's East India Company and the Dutch Verenigde Oostindische Compagnie (United East-India Company, or VOC), which in turn enforced extractive Western monopolies on textiles, spices, precious metals, slaves, and many other commodities.[146] One of Japan's responses to this violent colonial expansion was to bolster itself through increasingly strict isolationist foreign policies in relation to Europeans and restrict most forms of trade and exchange, especially with the Portuguese and Spanish, whose growing Catholic missionary activity in the country was viewed as a particular threat.[147] By the mid-seventeenth century, Westerners in Japan were almost entirely restricted to what became known by its inhabitants as Dejima (出島, sometimes translated as Exit Island), a man-made island in Nagasaki Harbor, occupied first by the Portuguese and subsequently by the Dutch from 1641.[148] Here, material trade took place alongside more cultural forms of exchange, including a slow but steady interchange of medical ideas and practices.

For Europeans, the presence on Dejima of Western doctors—mostly a single rotating Dutch or German medic in the employ of the VOC, with various levels of professional training—resulted in a growing importation of East Asian medical precepts and procedures, further encouraged by the inclusion of these doctors in annual diplomatic missions to meet with the shogun in Edo. The pharmacist Andreas Cleyer, for example, published multiple volumes of observations on Japanese plants between 1686 and 1695, while the Deventer physician Willem ten Rhijne spent enough significant time in direct communication with his Nagasaki counterparts to produce the first European treatise on the theory and practice of acupuncture in 1683.[149] On the other side of this exchange, Japanese medics were themselves able for the first time to engage in a sustained manner with Western medical texts and procedures, especially in areas less commonly the focus of local practice, such as pharmaceutical distillation, wound surgery, and in particular anatomical dissection, whose Japanese appropriation has its own particularly complex history, already much discussed in recent scholarship.[150] Although technically prohibited under the terms of the Dutch presence on Dejima, surgeons stationed there were occasionally authorized to give medical treatment in Nagasaki and beyond, and the successful cure of Japanese patients by figures such as Juriaen Henselingh or Caspar Schamberger generated substantial local interest in European techniques.[151] Equally significant were the relationships that Dutch and German surgeons were beginning to build with Japanese interpreters and translators, individuals who themselves had often been trained in medicine and who were increasingly being tasked by government officials with rendering selected elements of European surgical learning for a local audience.[152]

Practical imperatives did much to shape the parameters of this early medical translation movement. Several Japanese bureaucrats appear to have commissioned translations of European treatments in the hope of directly benefiting from them, for instance Inoue Masashige (井上政重), who in his time as *ōmetsuke* (大目付, sometimes translated as Grand Inquisitor) accumulated a large number of Dutch and Latin books on surgery in no small part because he suffered badly from bladder stones and hemorrhoids.[153] And beyond individual demands for novel techniques and cures, records associated with seventeenth-century Japanese physician-translators also suggest a broader interest in foreign medical structures. As early as the 1650s, local practitioners across Japan were angling to procure certificates of license to prove their qualifications in European surgery, a suite of techniques that were quickly becoming concretized under various specific Japanese terms: *Oranda geka* (阿蘭陀外科 Dutch surgery), *Kōmō-ryū geka* (紅毛流外科 Redhead-style surgery, a reference designed to distinguish the work of northern Europeans from that of the darker-haired Portuguese), and even *Kasuparu-ryū geka* (加斯巴流外科 Caspar-style surgery, in reference to the influential surgeon Caspar Schamberger).[154]

When we look too at the specifics of the earliest books produced on European surgery by these translators, both their physical format and linguistic tone suggest that they were being designed for the purpose of furthering foreign knowledge among a largely closed group of specialists. Such texts circulated in manuscript form rather than being produced in large-scale printed editions for mass consumption, and they were also written in kanbun (漢文), a Classicizing literary style using Chinese characters whose highly neologized vocabulary could often appear somewhat opaque, indicating a readership from more learned circles.[155] The fact that some of the earliest such texts bear titles emphasizing mysteriousness and confidentiality, such as *Kōmō-ryū geka hiyō* (紅毛流外科秘要 Secrets of Redhead-Style Surgery), *Oranda geka ihō hiden* (阿蘭陀外科醫方秘伝 Secret Transmission of Medical Formulas of Dutch Surgery), *Kōmō hiden geka ryōjishū* (紅毛秘傳外科療治集 Collection of Secretly Transmitted Redheaded Surgical Healing Methods), and *Nanban-ryū geka hidensho* (南蛮流外科秘伝書 Secret Transmission of the Southern Barbarian–Style Surgery), further contributes to the idea that for Japanese medics these manuscripts both showcased intellectual distinction and confirmed private allegiance to a novel—and potentially controversial—form of exciting intercultural medicine.[156]

Similar socio-medical concerns are present in the visual repertoire of these *Oranda geka* manuscripts. Paradigmatic here is the earliest and most influential of Japanese engagements with Western surgical imagery, the work of the Nagasaki interpreter Narabayashi Chinzan (楢林鎮山), whose writings Irako Mitsuaki would later draw on directly in producing the printed Wound Man of his *Geka kinmō zui*. Born in 1649, Chinzan is recorded as having studied Dutch from a young age, following the expectations of his interpreter family, with Nagasaki registers showing that by 1658 he had attained the rank of *kotsūji* (小通詞 junior interpreter) and by 1678 the rank of *ōtsūji* (大通詞 senior interpreter).[157] It was through this career that he came into close contact with a number of European medical specialists on Dejima, including the surgeon Daniel Busch, the botanist and physician Engelbert Kaempfer, and in particular Willem Hoffman, the island's senior surgeon from 1671 to 1676, under whom Chinzan claims to have studied for several months. Transcultural work of this sort always requires undertaking a social balancing act of subtle mediation, and as Wolfgang Michel notes, Chinzan clearly failed to maintain appropriate political equilibrium: in 1698, he was dismissed from his post following accusations of political scandal and conspiracy with the Dutch.[158] Nonetheless, his training and experience in European medical techniques were by this point substantial enough for Chinzan to pivot, setting up his own medical practice that channeled both European and Asian traditions alongside one another, effectively founding a school of intercultural translator-medics that was to be maintained well into the nineteenth century by his pupils, sons, and grandsons.

No autograph copies of Chinzan's writings are thought to survive, but a number of manuscripts reproduced by early copyists—most likely as objects to commemorate or certify training in Western methods—preserve a central corpus of texts attributed to him, his school, or close followers and today are spread widely across Japanese and American collections.[159] Together these writings are often grouped under the title *Geka sōden* (外科宗伝 Complete Manual of Surgery), a work consisting of four chapters that were probably written by Chinzan himself around 1706 and, in some manuscripts, further chapters probably added by early eighteenth-century followers.[160] Few *Geka sōden* manuscripts preserve the same precise order or contents, suggesting that these chapters were seen as a flexible bundle of texts to be differently employed depending on the needs and interests of particular users. Still, their collected chapter titles neatly illustrate the variety of European medical themes that were piquing the interest of contemporary Nagasaki practitioners: "*Shikake sho*" (仕掛書 On the Mechanics [of the Human Body]), "*Kinsō tetsuboku zu*" (金瘡趺撲図 Illustrated Treatment of Wounds), "*Oranda-koku yaku yu shūge*" (和蘭國薬油集解 Dutch Treatment by Medicinal Oils), "*Kōyaku sho*" (膏薬書 Treatment by the Application of Plasters), and "*Kinsō sho*" (金瘡書 Treatment of Wounds).

The level of direct similarity between Chinzan's *Geka sōden* and imported sources has been a matter of debate. Initially, early twentieth-century scholars framed Chinzan's work as simply passive translations of European texts present on Dejima. In part, this view has a surprisingly rich historiographical trail. Thanks to the deep roots of traditional Japanese family library collections, we can trace the existence of at least one European book formerly in the translator's direct personal possession, a Dutch edition of the French surgeon Ambroise Paré's collected works—a source for the French Wound Leg discussed earlier—that made its way, through the stewardship of the Narabayashi family, into a library in Tokyo in the late nineteenth century, only to be destroyed in the earthquake and fire of 1923.[161] Yet this long-standing assumption that Chinzan merely copied Paré into kanbun sits poorly with the actual evidence. In a plainly practical sense, the mere ownership of a European medical book did not mean that direct translation from it was necessarily at all easy: in 1724, the translator Namura Hachizaemon (名村八左衛門) was commissioned to produce a summary of certain sections of the same text by Paré, but the project was made tricky by the fact that only a fraction of the book's nine hundred pages remained legible due to heavy staining, presumably sustained during its transportation halfway around the world.[162] Moreover, a close reading of *Geka sōden* also clarifies that Chinzan was channeling influences well beyond Paré alone. As well as European writings, the work draws significantly on Asian traditions, especially the so-called *Waike zhengzong* (外科正宗 Orthodox Method of Surgery) of the sixteenth-century Chinese medic Chen Shigong (陳實功), from which Chinzan borrows various terminologies and descriptions of disease.[163] In addition, most manuscripts of *Geka sōden* open with a preface written by the botanist and scholar of neo-Confucianism Kaibara Ekiken (貝原益軒) in which he praises *Geka sōden* as an original work, evidence that learned contemporaries saw the text as simultaneously synthetic and original. Chinzan himself even openly acknowledges to the reader the selective nature of his translation. In the work's fourth chapter, he states that he is choosing to truncate his European sources because at this point they turn to consider internal medicine, an area he feels would hold little significance for Japanese audiences already well versed in more effective Asian traditions on the subject.

Crucially, we can also track this broad diversity of influence in Chinzan's work through its imagery. Many surviving *Geka sōden* manuscripts are packed throughout with detailed illustrations, ranging from simple forms in calligraphic line to figures that jump excitedly off the page. Paré's collected works appear once more to have been a significant influence. Among others, we find reproductions of the Frenchman's woodblocks showing surgical saws, amputation knives, arrow and bullet extractors, a dry suture to the cheek, and a skeleton posing as a gravedigger with a shovel, a detail that printers of Paré's book had themselves copied from the publications of Andreas Vesalius. Other European imagery appears too.[164] The work's very first picture depicts a figure with the skin of their head being peeled back in various stages to reveal the skull, an interpretation of an image from the combined work of Giulio Cesare Casseri and Adriaan van den Spieghel, whose *De humani corporis fabrica* (On the Fabric of the Human Body) would likely have been in the possession of the European surgeons on Dejima (fig. 5.27).[165]

The majority of images reproduced in *Geka sōden* in fact come from yet another European source: the *Armamentarium chirurgicum* of Scultetus. Nearly fifty details from Scultetus's various tables have been imported, a move that makes sense given that the work was after all designed around a flexible set of eminently transposable plates. Just like Chinzan's selective translation of his sources, so too the Japanese artists who illustrated his writings worked selectively, drawing from different parts of the *Armamentarium* as they saw fit. In some places they borrowed wholesale, replicating entire tables of instruments side by side in precisely the same order and orientation as Scultetus's printed plates. But elsewhere they focused their attention more creatively, selecting only choice single images from a given table:

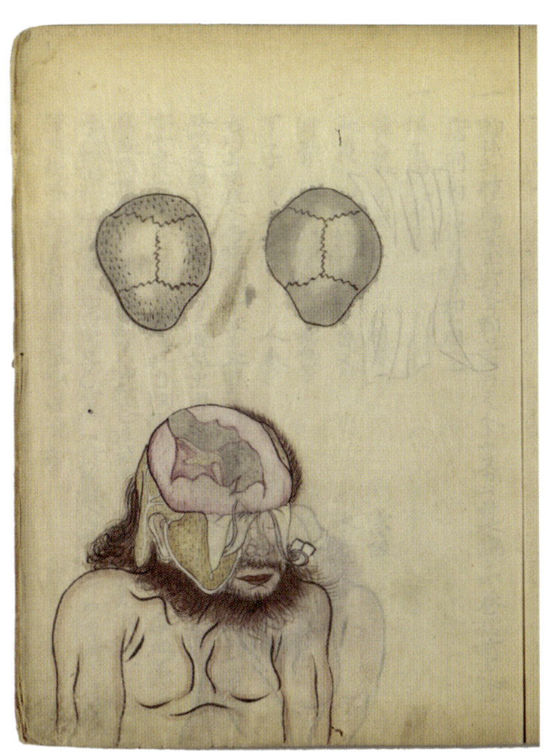

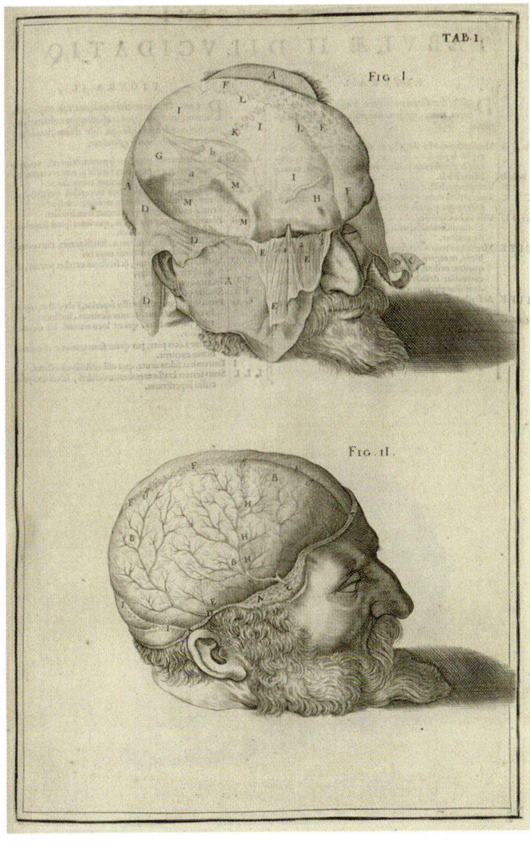

Fig. 5.27. Chinzan and one of his European sources. *Above:* The skull diagrammed and revealed from a manuscript of Narabayashi Chinzan's *Geka sōden* 外科宗伝, early 18th century, Nagasaki. Ink and paint on paper, 26 x 19 cm. Kyoto, University Library, ケ/165, 9. *Below:* Dissection of the skull from Adriaan van den Spiegel and Giulio Cesare Casseri's *Opera quae extant omnia* (Amsterdam: Johannes Blaeu, 1645). Copperplate engraving, 44 x 28 cm. Paris, Bibliothèque interuniversitaire de santé, Cote 260, "Tabulae anatomicae," book X, table I, 177.

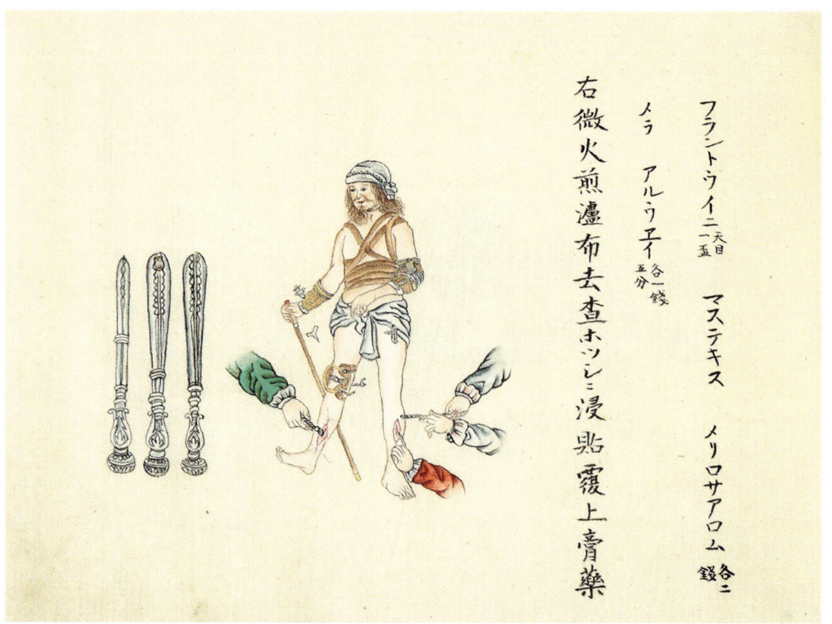

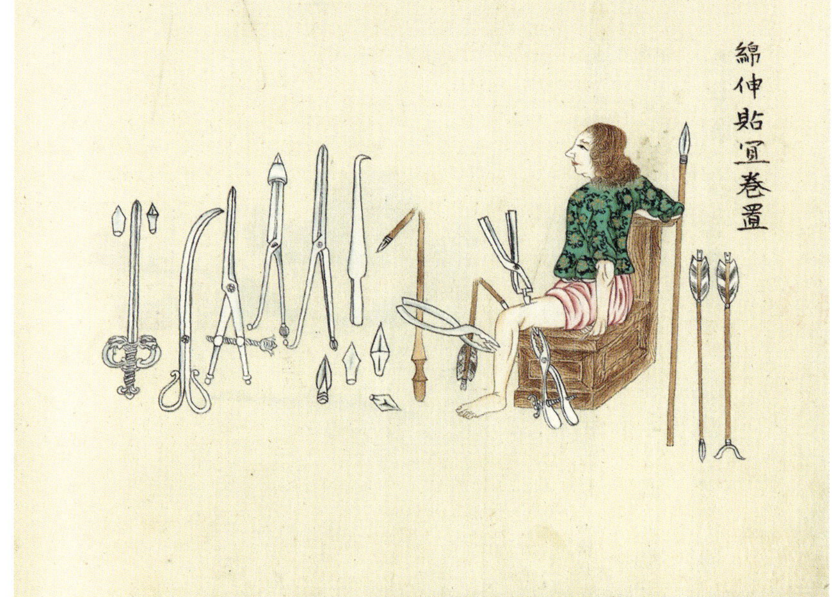

Fig. 5.28. Wound Man and elaborated Wound Leg from a manuscript of Narabayashi Chinzan's *Geka sōden* 外科宗伝, early 18th century, Nagasaki. Ink and paint on paper, 24 x 33 cm. Washington, DC, Library of Congress, R128.6 .N37 1706, n.p.

details of machinelike extenders for repairing broken limbs, figures with dislocated spines whose whole bodies are placed under torsion in long racks, and—present in every single illustrated copy of the Japanese text—Scultetus's cumulative Wound Man, complete with his heavy bandaging and metallic splints (fig. 5.28).

The consistent presence of the Wound Man across these Japanese manuscripts feels a pertinent parallel to the image's newfound status in Europe as an early modern artwork, gradually being brought into the service of aesthetic as well as medical currents. Initially, it seems that the quality of the woodcut illustrations that appeared in early modern Dutch scientific books proved a source of irritation to Japanese viewers. When the esteemed shogunal adviser Inaba Masanori (稲葉正則) was presented with a Western volume on botany, he declared that he found the images too small, requesting instead a volume with pictures in a larger format.[166] These highly illustrated *Geka sōden* manuscripts feel as if they are pulling in a similar direction, reproducing Western surgical woodcuts in sometimes physically larger and undoubtedly more colorful form than their original printers had ever attempted.

Indeed, as material objects, surviving manuscripts of Chinzan's text exhibit a deep commitment to artistry. No specific artists' names have survived on their pages, yet it is nonetheless clear that the individuals employed were highly skilled artisans, able to elegantly and accurately rework a Western printed source base in a variety of styles and regularly exercising their own discretion when it came to acts of visual translation. Some of their images are cumulative, formed by combining separate illustrative elements from different parts of a Dutch printed book into a single scene. Others have been more subtly edited, for instance by removing the intervening hands of the surgeon to allow details to stand alone with clarity. And yet more have been imaginatively extended from the original, taking small details of Scultetus or Paré and building outward. The image of the Wound Leg—which we know from our discussion of Paré earlier invariably appeared as an odd, pared-back element floating out from a cloud—was redesigned by its Japanese interpreters in precisely this manner. Extended to the right, they have reunited the rogue limb with a full body, adding the rest of an entirely realized person shown seated and gripping a wooden chair as they undergo the multiple simultaneous treatments.

It is through creative additions such as this that we also get a feel for these images' cross-cultural functioning within a Japanese context, increasingly co-opted into the contemporary colonial politics of the region as complicatedly racialized pictures. As with the originals on which they were based, the role of these images was at least in part to elucidate the medicine they accompanied. Pictures of surgical instruments or scenes of treatment would surely have helped showcase particular details to their Japanese owners, who quite reasonably may have been entirely unfamiliar with the European techniques on display. But the imagery of these *Geka sōden* manuscripts was also taking on a more delicate set of social obligations. If the medicine that these books contained was, as we have seen, the property of a tight-knit intellectual community, produced and shared not just for its basic healing functions but as a statement of intellectual alignment with potentially contraband Western concepts, then we can see these images too as harnessing a similar sense of cross-cultural performance. While some copies of *Geka sōden* take the form of typical codex books, wide-format works in which text and image chop and change across broad pages, at least ten manuscripts of the work survive in an entirely different configuration as horizontal *emaki* (絵巻 illustrated handscrolls), completely emptied of their medical text and

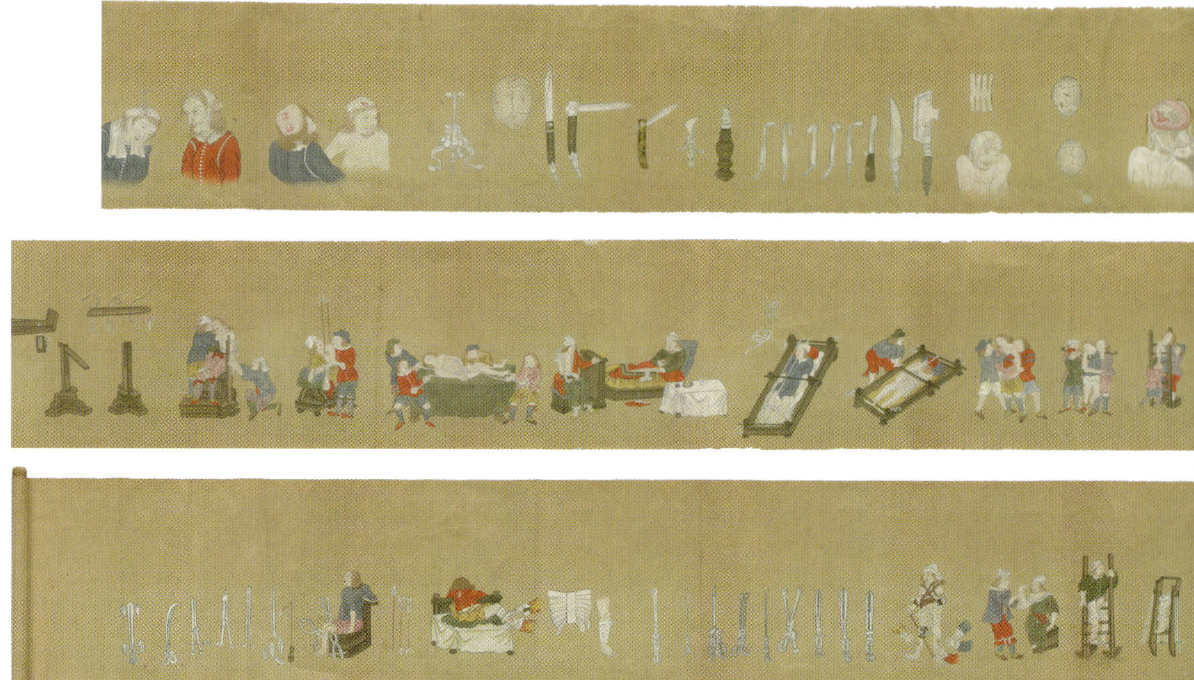

Fig. 5.29. Scroll of Narabayashi Chinzan's *Geka sōden* 外科宗伝, early 18th century, Nagasaki. Ink and paint on paper, 27 x 740 cm. Tokyo, National Diet Library, 本別 10–27.

reproducing only the illustrations that once accompanied Chinzan's writing (fig. 5.29).[167] Where they survive with firm provenance it is clear that these *emaki*, far from being inferior objects, hold exceptional pedigree, bearing either the names of Chinzan's direct descendants or those of his close followers. One even appears to have been produced for none other than Irako Mitsuaki, the author we met earlier who wrote *Geka kinmō zui* and through whom Chinzan's ideas would eventually make their way into print.[168] In elevating *Geka sōden* to the more aesthetic intellectual register in which *emaki* were commonly deployed within contemporary elite Japanese circles, these handscrolls opened up the work to more luxurious forms of musing. One can imagine Inaba Masanori, the councilor who had previously returned a Dutch book as pictorially insufficient, having his attention far more keenly held by elaborate objects such as these.

A picture-scroll of *Geka sōden* surviving today in Kobe City Museum offers the most direct evidence we have for these intriguing objects at work in this way.[169] As is typical, this scroll is comprised entirely of images inherited from the Narabayashi tradition, including bullet extractors, trepanation, facial surgery, and other details, all drawn from Scultetus and his fellow European authors. Only here these images are appended to a short text dated to the fourth lunar month of 1790, explaining that the scroll also acted as a license or diploma conferring what it calls "*tōryū hiji*" (當流秘事 our school's secrets) upon one Yoshio Kōgyū (吉雄耕牛, also named Kōsaku 耕作). Among the best-known translators of the late eighteenth century, Kōgyū was recognized among his Nagasaki peers for hosting fellow interpreters on the top floor of his house in a Dutch-style space spoken of colloquially as his *Kōmō zashiki* (紅毛座敷 Redhead parlor), a gathering place for Europhile contem-

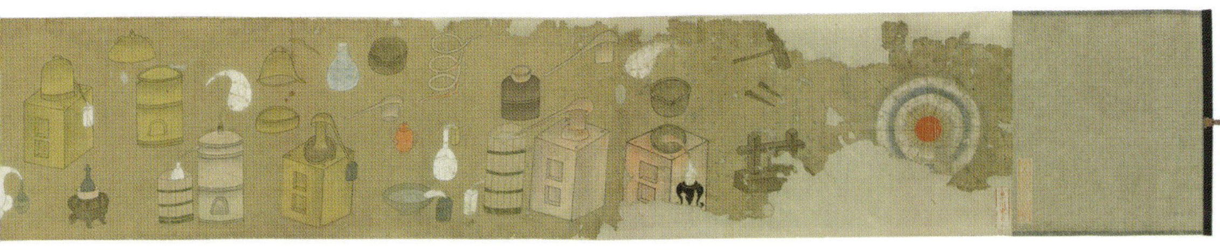

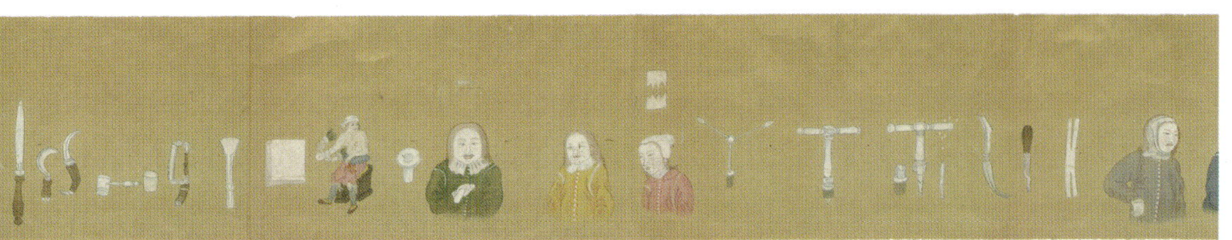

poraries to meet and discuss their work.[170] These were well-versed viewers who, as they watched the talking points of Kōgyū's scroll unfurl before their eyes—displayed at close quarters, perhaps accompanied by the narration of its owner—would have recognized all sorts of intercultural details. We might envisage them paying particularly careful attention to the ethnic calibration of figures in a *Geka sōden* scroll or codex, many of which have been visually coded by their artists to emphasize complexities of origin. Surviving examples from across the corpus present patients and doctors dressed in costumes ornamented with East Asian details, patterned with bold chrysanthemums or golden flowers, yet these clothes still bear the hallmarks of European designs, fitted with white ruffs and flowing cuffs. The Wound Man emerges as a particularly potent site for such medical hybridity (fig. 5.30). In one manuscript, the curly-ended handlebar mustache of the figure in Scultetus's final plate has been grown out into a long wispy goatee in an eighteenth-century Japanese style. In another, the figure has been entirely redressed and is presented wearing a rounded, white hat and black, flat-ended shoes, both markers of an overtly non-Japanese heritage. And in a third, particularly poignant case, the Wound Man's hair has been reworked from the dark shades of the original woodblock to a light orangey-blond set of curls: an artistic vision of "Redhead-style medicine" personified.

In their subtle coupling of a visual and literary intercultural medicine, these eighteenth-century Japanese images offer a fitting conclusion to this breakneck tour through the Wound Man's early modern legacy. On the one hand, the distinctiveness of the figure affords us an opportunity to track his printed presence across multiple geographical contexts, from Italy to Spain to Germany to France to England to the Netherlands to Japan. In fact, the remarkable consistency of his visual form across these different surgical environments enables the Wound Man to act as something of a benchmark for medical change. Through him we can chronicle the evolutions of surgical technique, procedure, and instrumentation over the course of some three hundred years, as transferred in the ebb and flow of intercultural medicine and its various evolutions. Yet, on the other hand, as historians of both art and medicine increasingly recognize, there are also crucial ethical questions

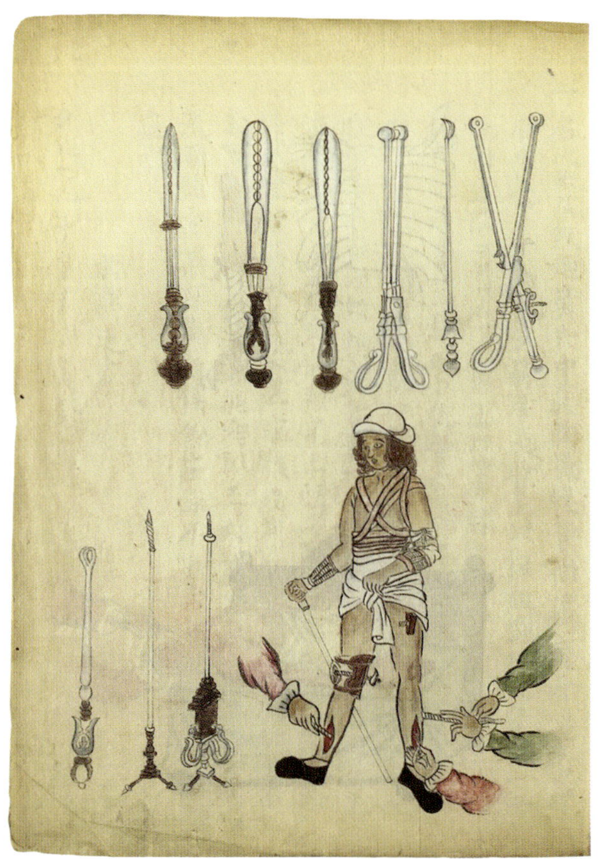

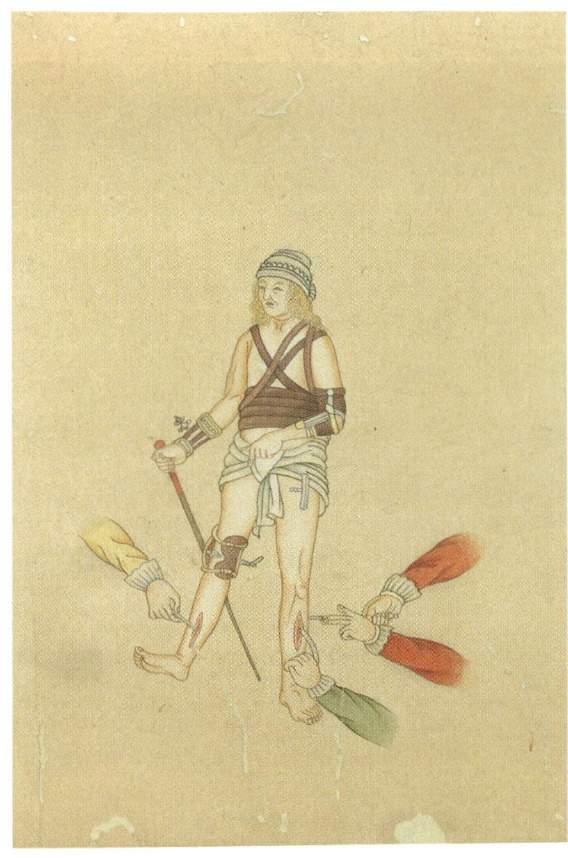

Fig. 5.30. Intercultural Wound Men. *Left:* Wound Man from a manuscript of Narabayashi Chinzan's *Geka sōden* 外科宗伝, early 18th century, Nagasaki. Ink and paint on paper, 26 x 19 cm. Kyoto, University Library, ケ/165, 46–47. *Right:* Wound Man from an illustrated scroll of Narabayashi Chinzan's *Geka sōden* 外科宗伝, 1790, Nagasaki. Ink and paint on paper, 22 x 552 cm. Tokyo, National Diet Library, 本別 10–26.

raised by texts and images that circulated so widely in this international early modern context, objects often morally freighted by their status as cultural exports amid a backdrop of aggressive politics at both the local and international levels. In a close study of smallpox imagery produced in China at roughly the same moment as Chinzan's handscrolls, Ari Larissa Heinrich has compellingly argued that early modern medical afterlives were not only lived in the abstract but had real-world consequences in the perception of others.[171] Whether it is the French receiving and amputating an image from Italy, the English reworking Continental pictures to promote their own new Classicizing values, or Japanese artists, medics, and translators creatively reimagining Dutch medicine for East Asian audiences, these moments of busy exchange demonstrate that the Wound Man's medical and artistic potential dwelled in its ability to speak for the surgical craft as a whole: a grisly yet lucid trademark of the profession through which users could express both their developing medical expertise and shifting cultural position.

EPILOGUE

Nuclear Wound Man

Epistemic diagram, medical tool, affective muse, technical spur, international artwork: the contention of this book has been that the image of the Wound Man occupies not just one of these positions but all of them. In tracing the figure's long history, the five previous chapters have made the case for this powerful surgical image as something regularly made and remade from the fourteenth century through to the eighteenth, to the benefit of numerous medical, social, and aesthetic ends. At once a tool for healing, for feeling, and for thinking—indeed, a tool that only begins to truly make sense when we consider all these positions at once—the Wound Man helped enable a multitude of concepts and contexts alive in the world surrounding it. But what if things worked the other way around too?

In his influential 1991 essay "The Manufacture of Bodies in Surgery," the sociologist Stefan Hirschauer argues that far from passive respondents to real-world concerns, modern anatomical illustrations are responsible for much more in medical practice than sociologists, historians, and even medics themselves give them credit for.[1] Acknowledging both the ritual aspects of scientific work and what he terms the "sculptural practices" of surgery, Hirschauer posits that the images through which today's surgeons first learn about the body play an outsized role in their fundamental conception of what a patient is and how they should look. His claim for modern surgical illustrations is radical: that these idealized pictures, encountered innocuously through the rigor of textbooks, are in fact so ingrained in the medical mindset that they come to govern the processes of practice itself. Tacitly, a surgeon's goal is transformed by such figures, which drive them to moderate the innate oddness and variation of the everyday patient by shaping them into the images of their training, artworks that end up demanding replication on real-life people. Instead of medical diagrams reflecting knowledge of the world, the world itself is remade in the form of a standardized medical diagram.

This twentieth-century take on the latent yet immense potential of medical imagery is an apposite coda to the Wound Man's own influential history, especially the figure's fleeting engagements in modernity. So, by way of both summary and conclusion, let us briefly consider one final life of the Wound

Man, its most abbreviated but perhaps its most unusual yet: its presence in an exhibition held in 1976 at the august United States Military Academy at West Point, New York, named by its organizers "The History of Military Medicine Together with a Graphic Display of the Wound Man through History."

Although its title is a mouthful, the show is intriguing as the only exhibition to ever present a comprehensive history of the Wound Man through a curatorial lens. It was the brainchild of Elizabeth Matthew Lewis, a sculptor who, when hired at West Point in 1968, was the first woman faculty member in the academy's 166-year history. Described patronizingly in an announcement of her appointment in *Time* magazine as "a soft-spoken art librarian," it was in fact Lewis's role to educate future military leaders far more widely in matters of aesthetics, art history, art appreciation, and related activities.[2] The role clearly also extended outside of the classroom into curating and display, hence Lewis mounting the 1976 "History of Military Medicine" exhibition in collaboration with the respected medical historian Gordon E. Mestler, whose son had graduated from the academy the previous year.[3]

A small catalog of the show, produced by Lewis with contributions from Mestler and others, preserves a statement of the exhibition's curatorial mission:

> Prevention . . . recognition . . . transport . . . treatment . . . repair . . . rehabilitation. All are the concern of the military surgeon, both at war and in peace. It is said that Albert Einstein, when asked what would be the weapon of World War III, replied, "I cannot tell you that, but I can tell you what will be the weapon of World War IV—stones!" And so, full circle. Thus, by means of artifacts, objects, pictures, books and the printed work, to exemplify the history and evolution of military medicine and surgery and the role of the military surgeon—that is the focus of the exhibit.[4]

This certainly chimes with the catalog's object list, which reveals that the exhibition treated West Point's cadets to a wild multimedia showcase, ranging from photographs of ancient skulls with arrow-point wounds to a copy of Brigadier General Edward Lyman Munson's 1917 page-turner *The Soldier's Foot and the Military Shoe*.

The inclusion of images of the Wound Man by Lewis and Mestler is likely to have been prompted by the figure's running presence in the midcentury American popular consciousness, where it was largely evoked in association with the military. Perhaps the most influential and certainly the most biting of these moments occurred in 1960, when the architect and industrial designer George Nelson took to the airwaves on the CBS anthology program *Camera Three*, fronting an episode he called "How to Kill People: A Problem of Design" (fig. 6.1).[5] Under the guise of a tour through historic weaponry, Nelson—already feted as one of the founders of American modernism—fired a provocative screed down the barrel of the camera, unveiling the design history of the military-industrial complex and highlighting the many hypocrisies therein. "The three areas of design," Nelson intones dryly in the piece's intro, "that receive the unquestioning support of society are design for fashion, design for homemaking, and design for killing." Printed large

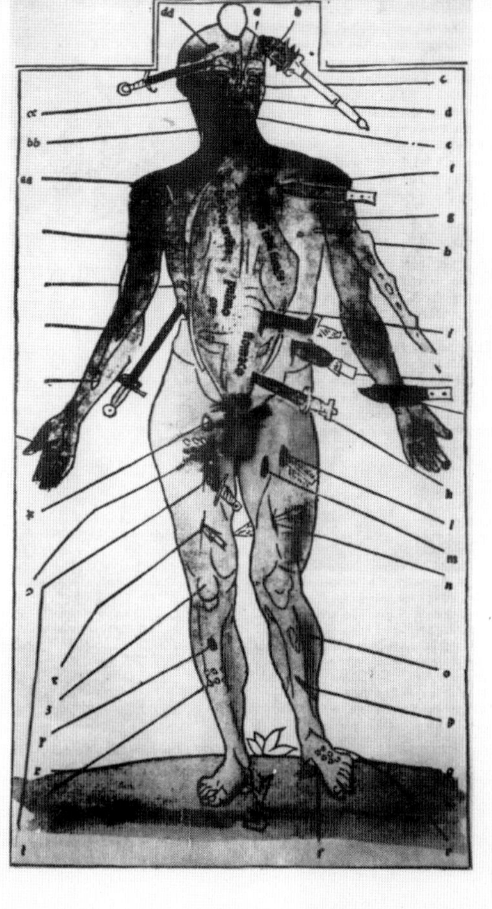

Fig. 6.1. Title page from a transcript of George Nelson's CBS *Camera Three* episode "How to Kill People: A Problem of Design," reproduced in *Industrial Design* 8, no. 1 (1961): 45.

so that the camera can slowly zoom in, an image of the Wound Man from a late fifteenth-century edition of the Venetian *Fasiculo di medicina* appears on screen. Conjured alongside a range of historic props, mostly weapons made by Indigenous makers from around the world, the figure is used by Nelson as a foil for the sleek abstraction of the monitors and missiles of the Cold War. Materials of push-button warfare, he claims, have become "too impersonal to be interesting and too complex to be comprehensible." The Wound Man, he implies by contrast, is a diagram designed to be individuated and, as a result, both empathetic and readable.

Sixty miles up the Hudson from Nelson's Manhattan design studio, Lewis and Mestler's West Point exhibition took to heart a similar synecdochal framing of the Wound Man and military character. The curators are pictured in Lewis's catalog in a grainy photograph that shows them engaged in cheerful conversation with Egon Weiss, the academy's military librarian, and Colonel

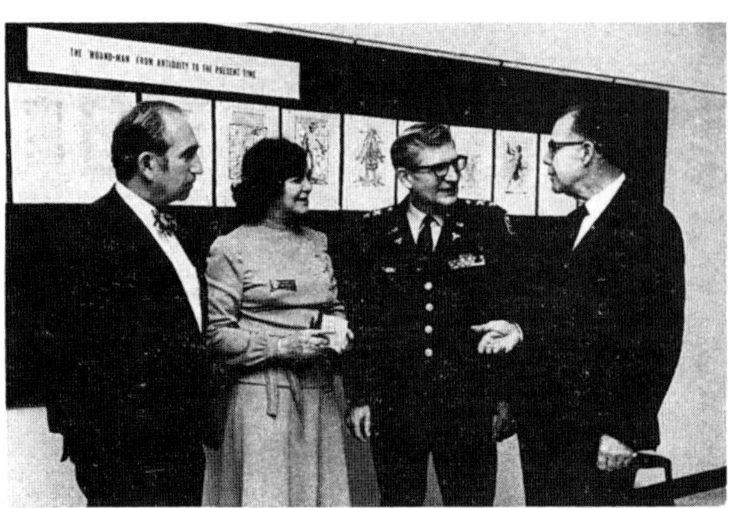

(Right to Left)

Mr. Gordon E. Mestler, Organizer of the Exhibit
COL Morton A. Pfotenhaur, Commander, Medical Activities, Surgeon, USMA
Dr. Elizabeth M. Lewis, Senior Lecturer and Fine Arts Librarian
Mr. Egon Weiss, United States Military Academy Librarian

Fig. 6.2. Elizabeth Matthew Lewis and her collaborators in front of the 1976 display "The Wound Man from Antiquity to the Present Time," from Elizabeth Matthew Lewis, *An Exhibition of Selected Landmark Books and Articles in the History of Military Medicine, Together with a Graphic Display of the Wound Man through History* (West Point, NY: United States Military Academy, 1976), iii.

Morton A. Pfotenhaur, a military surgeon and head of the academy's medical activities. And behind the group we see the only snippet that survives of their Wound Man display, a substantial chronological parade of figures in photographic reproduction (fig. 6.2).[6] Many of these Wound Men also appear in a section of Lewis's catalog specifically dedicated to a potted history of the figure, and although they often bear incorrect captions or out-of-date attributions, almost all are recognizable from the preceding five chapters of this book. The earliest Bohemian proto-Wound Men are present, as are a pair of figures from two fifteenth-century *Dreibilderserie* manuscripts, two Venetian Wound Men from editions of the printed *Fasciculus medicinae*, examples from the title pages of Hieronymus Brunschwig's *Cirurgia* and Hans von Gersdorff's *Feldtbuch*, and even John Browne's Classicizing English figure from 1678. Despite their presentation in rectangles of black-and-white, their sequence still oddly gels. In a snapshot, the argument is made that this was an image important to medical users for some time, but that the rationale behind this importance had itself shifted across the centuries. Together, the sweep of images shows the Wound Man's simultaneous consistency and variation, presenting the figure as somehow both momentous and malleable at the same time.

A note from Lewis in the catalog confirms that she and Mestler chose the examples for the display by thoroughly scouring assorted academic works on the history of surgery, principally the publications of Karl Sudhoff, the historian of medicine introduced at the beginning of this book whose work was foundational to the scholarly beginnings of the Wound Man. In fact, both the curators' selections and the unusual crops of the photographs displayed confirm that virtually every one of their images was drawn directly from the pages of Sudhoff's writings. These were figures from his articles in the *Archiv für Geschichte der Medizin,* blown up through the expediency of late 1960s reprographic technology to a fitting size for West Point's walls.[7] Yet for all this scrutinized historical effort, Lewis and Mestler's Wound Man display somehow seems more closely aligned with the approach of Sudhoff's intellectual counterpart and methodological opposite, the cultural historian Aby Warburg, whom we also met in the introduction to this book. The abstraction of their pin-up connections, surfing through the centuries on the back of a repeated visual trope, feels like the closest we might ever get to a realization of the Wound Man as part of a board in Warburg's thematic, interconnected *Bilderatlas*.

Also consistent with the transhistorical nature of a Warburgian approach is the West Point curators' insistence on looking forward in time as well as back. Indulging a perhaps inevitable sense of contemporary Cold War anxiety, Lewis and Mestler chose to bracket their historical display of Wound Men examples at both beginning and end with a pair of newly commissioned works: black ink drawings by a local artist named as one Ms. Adrienne K. Giebel. Neither of the new drawings is visible in the photograph of the exhibition, but both are reproduced in the catalog. Giebel's first image, titled "Wound Man of Primitive Times," depicts a lumbering neolithic caricature wielding a club and being bopped on the head with a large stone, evidence of the damage wrought by humanity's very earliest weapons. Her second image is more ominous, showing a semi-schematic figure midway through exploding at the stomach with a giant mushroom cloud emanating in the background behind him. Titled "The Ultimate Wound Man of Today," Lewis glosses the second drawing in the catalog as "the victim of thermonuclear warfare with its accompanying radioactive fallout." On the surface this might seem an extreme demand to make of the Wound Man, asking the framework of a medieval and early modern image some five hundred years old to stand simultaneously for the most violent tendencies of humankind's furthest past and, in the view of 1976 America, those of humankind's darkest future. Yet in a very real sense, speaking to contemporary concerns some distance beyond its surgical origins is precisely what the image of the Wound Man has always done, a strange body performing bridging maneuvers between opposing investments, temporalities, and audiences.

It is also in keeping with the Wound Man's spirit that in spite of the potential bleakness of this ending, Lewis's commentary in the exhibition's catalog remains insistently upbeat. Channeling what we have seen throughout the Wound Man's history to be a prevailing commitment to healing—and thus an image of hope amid medicine's travails—she concludes with a more positive parallel. Wound Men exhibit artistry in pen, paint, and print, and although "today the camera is preferred for making realistic duplications, the design of the human body, its vulnerable parts and the measures doctors must take, are based on the same principles, the dedication of talent and the same feeling for service."[8] The ending to this study of the Wound Man is likewise hopeful. It too has sought to show that when contemporary readers came across the figure's battered body, they did not only see aggression, pain, and loss. Rather, they could engage with the image through multifaceted creative modes. The Wound Man was an epistemic tool, encyclopedic as a visual repository of valuable surgical knowledge. It was a space for conflation, equating the surgeon's work with contemporary patterns of literary and religious discourse. It activated different forms of medical media, bouncing back and forth between manuscript medicine and the technologies of print. And perhaps above all, it was a cross-cultural artistic feat, a lavish emblem of practical medicine deployed to audiences across the world.

When we speak of historical objects as activating debate, inculcating power, or voyaging the oceans, our minds are far more likely to jump to the ricocheting histories of painting and sculpture, of diplomatic gifts, even of bulk goods, than they are to think of medical diagrams. Yet the Wound Man's history makes clear that healing images from before the modern era undertook all these roles and more: the varied stuff of this tangled figure's many, many lives.

Acknowledgments

I first started thinking and writing about the Wound Man nearly ten years ago, and as such I owe an enormous, heartfelt thanks to the input and guidance of many generous institutions, colleagues, mentors, and friends.

This project was first begun during my tenure as a Mellon Fellow at Columbia University in the Department of Art History and Archaeology. I offer my sincerest thanks to colleagues there who supported this work as my early ideas developed, and especially to Mellon Fellows Joseph Salvatore Ackley, Johanna Gosse, Daniel Greenberg, Mari Yoko Hara, Kevin Lotery, and Trevor Stark, for creating the warmest and most engaging research community one could hope for.

The bulk of this book was written during a year as Dibner Fellow in the History of Science and Technology in the inspiring surrounds of the Huntington Library, Art Museum, and Botanical Gardens in San Marino, California. I thank Steve Hindle and his team in the Research Department for nurturing such an open and stimulating intellectual environment, as well as the entire cohort of yearlong fellows. Even though the COVID-19 pandemic cut short our time together, it was an exceptional opportunity to learn from these colleagues' diverse disciplines and styles of thought, and I am hugely grateful for their generous feedback in steering this project toward publication.

A historian's job is simply not possible without the deep expertise of colleagues working in libraries, museums, and archives, especially their support in accessing and understanding materials from the collections they so graciously steward. I felt this debt especially keenly when I was compelled to write much of this book at a temporary remove from many primary sources during a string of pandemic lockdowns. For support with both their expertise and collections access during this period, as well as on many subsequent research visits, I wish to thank Nicole Baker (National Library of Medicine), Nicolas Bell and Anne McLaughlin (Trinity College, Cambridge), Mateja Demšar (Semeniška knjižnica, Ljubljana), Irene Friedl (UB LMU Munich), Julian Harrison (British Library), Ian David Holt (ZB Solothurn), Wolfgang-Valentin Ikas (Bayerische Staatsbibliothek), Russell A. Johnson (UCLA), Christoph Koschinski (DB Hildesheim), Martine Kreißler (Stadtarchiv Dessau-Roßlau),

James Lloyd (Royal College of Arms), Christoph Mackert (UB Leipzig), Claudia Minners-Knaup (HAB Wolfenbüttel), Karen Moran (Royal Observatory, Edinburgh), Jay Moschella (Boston Public Library), Ruth Ogden (St. John's College, Oxford), Jan Pařez (Royal Canonry of Premonstratensians at Strahov), Adam Poznański (UB Wrocław), Maria-Anna Schoderböck (Stift Klosterneuberg), Petr Slouka (Lobkowicz Collection), Katrien Smeyers (KU Leuven), David Speranzi (BNC Florence), Mark Statham (Gonville & Caius College, Cambridge), Rickey Tax (Huis van het Boek), Maximilian Alexander Trofaier (Schottenstifts Archiv), Jill Unkel (Chester Beatty Library, Dublin), Sandra Weidmann (ZB Zürich), and Liz Zanis (Metropolitan Museum of Art, New York). Two digital projects, the Handschriftencensus and the DMMapp, were also absolutely essential while researching manuscript materials from afar. I cannot thank the colleagues behind these inspirational projects enough. Their work represents the very best in academic collaboration and open-access scholarship, from which entire fields repeatedly benefit.

As this project progressed, it became clear that I would not be able to crisscross between the periods, geographies, and disciplines required for a full exploration of the Wound Man without the patient guidance of colleagues willing to share their own hard-won expertise in parallel fields. In particular, I want to thank the three colleagues whose language skills were absolutely integral to developing and honing this book's translations—Oren Margolis, Ben Pope, and Terumi Toyama—as well as many others who offered expert historical guidance as I moved further from my own area of expertise, especially Timon Screech, Sarah Monks, and Anita Guerrini.

I also thank colleagues who invited me to share excerpts of this research in seminars and at conferences. The communities in each of these institutions offered a huge amount of useful and engaging feedback that pointed the project in a host of previously unexpected directions. For such invitations, I thank the organizers of the Paul Mellon Centre–funded conference at the British Museum on "Invention and Imagination in British Art and Architecture," the Renaissance Skin Project conference on "The Porous Body" at King's College London, the "Ivory Mirror" symposium at Bowdoin College, and the "Body in History" conference at the Uniwersytet Gdański, as well as colleagues who invited me to share my work in the Department of History and Philosophy of Science at the University of Cambridge and the Department of History of Art at Yale University.

Right from our very first conversation, Michelle Komie at Princeton University Press was a tireless champion of this book. I thank her for generous advice and thoughtful guidance as this project crept from proposal to print. I also thank others at PUP who took such care with the manuscript and the book it became, including Annie Miller, Mark Bellis, Matt Avery, Jess Massabrook, Steve Sears, Sara Lerner, and Cynthia Buck. Innumerable errors in my text were caught by the surgical eye of the fantastic Jennifer Ottman, whose proofreading skills were absolutely invaluable. Financial support provided by a Publication Award from the Humanities Faculty of the University of East Anglia helped secure publication rights for some of this book's images. I also thank Nicholas Herman for sharing his extensive expertise and guidance in this area, especially for helping me find the right words to remind sometimes forgetful image-lenders of their ethical obligations when it comes to the free and open accessibility of historical materials and cultural heritage.

Once this book was in draft, it benefited enormously from the close reading and careful commentary of many colleagues who read either individual chapters or, in particularly generous cases, the entire manuscript. For this, I thank Jennifer Borland, Simon Dell, Sonja Drimmer, Lara Frentrop, Sivan Gottlieb, Monique Kornell, Aparna Kumar, Amanda Lanzillo, Taylor McCall, Lauren Rozenberg, and members of the "Objects, Images, and Spaces of Health" CHSTM Working Group, in particular my co-convenor Elaine Leong for her adventurous enthusiasm in producing such an engaging forum for sharing research. I also thank PUP's two anonymous peer reviewers for engaging so carefully and keenly with the book and providing such positive, supportive feedback.

For their constant support and encouragement, I thank my colleagues past and present in the Department of Art History & World Art Studies at the University of East Anglia: Jo Clarke, Simon Dell, Ed Krčma, Dan Rycroft, Sarah Wade, and Nick Warr. I am also indebted to the endlessly patient support and good advice of friends Lloyd de Beer, Alixe Bovey, Esther Chadwick, Nick Grant, Scott Nethersole, Tom Nickson, Stephanie O'Rourke, Sam Rose, and Allie Stielau.

Last, but by no means least, I want to thank my family for their support and patience, not only as I brought this project to a close but at all times and in all things. Writing this book would not have been possible without Anne Chmelewsky and Zoé, who appeared around the time of writing chapter 4. It is dedicated to the two of you.

Notes

ON TRANSLATION AND TRANSCRIPTION

This book contains many quotations transcribed and translated from non-English sources. All such transcriptions and translations are my own unless otherwise indicated in a note. Where non-English quotes appear in their original language they are rendered in italics, followed by an English translation. Because of the breadth of languages covered, my approach has been to adopt a more literal attitude to translation, emphasizing clarity of meaning and technical vocabularies. But I hope that by preserving the originals alongside the English, the reader can still appreciate their poetic and lyrical styles of expression.

INTRODUCTION. LONG, STRANGE HISTORIES

1. John Thurston, "How to Do It: How to Acquire a Coat of Arms," *British Medical Journal* 315, no. 7123 (1997): 1682–84.

2. Fergus Fleming, *The Man with the Golden Typewriter: Ian Fleming's James Bond Letters* (London: Bloomsbury, 2015), 177–78.

3. The band is the American hardcore four-piece Wound Man; the book of poems is Sheena Blackhall, *The Wound Man: Poems in Scots and English* (Aberdeen: Lochlands, 2015); *The Adventures of Wound Man and Shirley* was a 2009 work by theater-maker Chris Goode; the Wound Cat originated in Richard Malik et al., "Wound Cat," *Journal of Feline Medicine and Surgery* 8 (2006): 135–40.

4. Karl Sudhoff, *Tradition und Naturbeobachtung in den Illustrationen medizinischer Handschriften und Frühdrucke vornehmlich des 15. Jahrhunderts* (Leipzig: Barth, 1907), 82–85; Karl Sudhoff, "Der 'Wundenmann' in Frühdruck und Handschrift und sein erklärender Text: Ein Beitrag zur Quellengeschichte des 'Ketham,'" *Archiv für Geschichte der Medizin* 1, no. 5 (1908): 351–61.

5. On Sudhoff and the troubling politics that sit alongside his formidable scholarship, see Thomas Rütten, "Karl Sudhoff and 'The Fall' of German Medical History," in *Locating Medical History: The Stories and Their Meanings*, ed. Frank Huisman and John Harley Warner (Baltimore: Johns Hopkins University Press, 2004), 95–114.

6. Boyd H. Hill Jr., "A Medieval German Wound Man: Wellcome MS 49," *Journal of the History of Medicine and Allied Sciences* 20, no. 4 (1965): 334–57; Erltraud Auer and Bernhard Schnell, "'Der Wundenmann': Ein traumatologisches Schema in der Tradition der 'Wundarzenie' des Ortolf von Baierland: Untersuchung und Edition," in *"ein teutsch puech machen": Untersuchungen zur landessprachlichen Vermittlung medizinischen Wissens*, ed. Gundolf Keil (Wiesbaden: Reichert, 1993), 349–401; Klaus Neuhaus, "Der Wundenmann: Tradition und Struktur einer Abbildungsart in der medizinischen Literatur," PhD diss., Westfälische Wilhelms-Universität, 1982. In addition, I have previously published on a late fifteenth-century Wound Man discussed further in chapter 5: Jack Hartnell, "Wording the Wound Man," *British Art Studies* 6 (2017), https://doi.org/10.17658/issn.2058-5462/issue-06/jhartnell/000 (accessed August 1, 2024).

7. An important exception to this is Julie Orlemanski, *Symptomatic Subjects: Bodies, Medicine, and Causation in the Literature of Late Medieval England* (Philadelphia: University of Pennsylvania Press, 2019), which considers its Wound Man cover image in detail.

8. On Sudhoff and Warburg's relationship, see Xinyi Wen, "When Jupiter Meets Saturn: Aby Warburg, Karl Sudhoff, and Astrological Medicine in the Age of Disenchantment," *Journal of the History of Ideas* 84, no. 2 (2024): 321–55. I thank the author for sharing an advance copy of this article with me.

9. Referencing the wandering spirit of Jewish mythology, Georges Didi-Huberman captures something of this mystical quality when he calls Warburg a *dybbuk* in *L'image survivante: Histoire de l'art et temps des fantômes selon Aby Warburg* (Paris: Minuit, 2002), 28.

CHAPTER 1. DIAGRAM: AMBITIOUS FIGURES

1. Bert Hall similarly frames illustration's two poles as didactic on the one hand and elegant on the other: "The Didactic and the Elegant: Some Thoughts on Scientific

and Technological Illustrations in the Middle Ages and Renaissance," in *Picturing Knowledge: Historical and Philosophical Problems Concerning the Use of Art in Science*, ed. Brian Baigrie (Toronto: University of Toronto Press, 1996), 3–39. On Cicero's reception in the Middle Ages, see John O. Ward, "What the Middle Ages Missed of Cicero, and Why," in *Brill's Companion to the Reception of Cicero*, ed. William H. F. Altman (Leiden: Brill, 2015), 307–26; Jessica Ammer, *Der deutsche Cicero* (Göttingen: V&R Unipress, 2020). On medieval manuscripts of Cicero's work that appear to harness precisely the diagrammatic tensions discussed in this chapter, see Irene O'Daly, "Diagrams of Knowledge and Rhetoric in Manuscripts of Cicero's *De inventione*," in *Manuscripts of the Latin Classics 800–1200*, ed. Erik Kwakkel (Leiden: Leiden University Press, 2015), 77–106.

2. Vatican City, Biblioteca Apostolica Vaticana, MS Pal. Lat. 1225, fol. 423r. On Knab's life and work, see Steven J. Livesey, "Erhardus Knab, Medical Doctor and Secular Master of Arts, c. 1420–1480," in *International Encyclopaedia for the Middle Ages Online (IEMA): A Supplement to Lexikon des Mittelalters* (Turnhout: Brepols, 2005); Ludwig Schuba, "Knab, Erhard, von Zwiefalten," in *Die deutsche Literatur des Mittelalters: Verfasserlexikon*, ed. Wolfgang Stammler (Berlin: De Gruyter, 1983), 4:1264–71; Colette Jeudy and Ludwig Schuba, "Erhard Knab und die Heidelberger Universität im Spiegel von Handschriften und Akteneinträgen," *Quellen und Forschungen aus italienischen Archiven und Bibliotheken* 61 (1981): 60–108.

3. For an overview of Classical gynecology and its reception, see Helen King, *Hippocrates' Woman: Reading the Female Body in Ancient Greece* (London: Routledge, 1998). For overviews of medieval reproductive traditions and their social impact, see Monica H. Green, *Making Women's Medicine Masculine: The Rise of Male Authority in Pre-Modern Gynaecology* (Oxford: Oxford University Press, 2008); Joan Cadden, *The Meanings of Sex Difference in the Middle Ages: Medicine, Science, and Culture* (Cambridge: Cambridge University Press, 1993).

4. For recent work on breastfeeding in medieval Europe, see Maaike van der Lugt, "Nature as Norm in Medieval Medical Discussions of Maternal Breastfeeding and Wet-Nursing," *Journal of Medieval and Early Modern Studies* 49, no. 3 (2019): 563–88.

5. Faith Wallis, "What a Medieval Diagram Shows: A Case Study of *Computus*," *Studies in Iconography* 36 (2015): 1. A good historiographical overview of the diagram in visual studies is provided in Matthias Bauer and Christoph Ernst, *Diagrammatik: Einführung in ein kultur- und medienwissenschaftliches Forschungsfeld* (Bielefeld: Transcript, 2010). For a more didactic take from the perspective of data visualization, see Edward R. Tufte, *The Visual Display of Quantitative Information* (Cheshire, CT: Graphics Press, 1983).

6. On the final three Arabic terms, see Meekyung MacMurdie, "Proven Recipes: Geometry and the Art of Arabic Medicine," in *The Diagram as Paradigm: Cross-Cultural Approaches*, ed. Jeffrey F. Hamburger, David J. Roxburgh, and Linda Safran (Washington, DC: Dumbarton Oaks Publications, 2022), 334–35. For a discussion of diagrams in Hebraic traditions, especially Kabbalistic material of the early modern period, see Jeffrey H. Chajes, "We-ʿatah ʾatsayyer lekha ʿagulah u-mi-sham tavin mah she-tsarikh le-havin: ha-tarshim ha-qabbali ka-tsiyyur ʾepisṭemi ועתה אצייר לך עגולה ומשם תבין מה שצריך להבין: התרשים הקבלי כציור אפיסטמי," *Peʿamim* 150/152 (2018): 235–88.

7. Michael Evans, "The Geometry of the Mind: Scientific Diagrams and Medieval Thought," *Architectural Association Quarterly* 12, no. 4 (1980): 32–55.

8. However anachronistic, I use the word "diagram" in the analysis that follows, partly for clarity and partly in reflection of the long historiographical lineage of the medieval diagram. This formula is also utilized in two recent important edited volumes on the subject: Hamburger, Roxburgh, and Safran, *The Diagram as Paradigm*; Marcia Kupfer, Adam S. Cohen, and Jeffrey H. Chajes, eds., *The Visualization of Knowledge in Medieval and Early Modern Europe* (Turnhout: Brepols, 2020).

9. For a sample of recent work on argumentative diagrams in different medieval fields, see Jennifer M. Rampling, "Depicting the Medieval Alchemical Cosmos: George Ripley's *Wheel* of Inferior Astronomy," *Early Science and Medicine* 18, nos. 1/2 (2013): 45–86; Barbara Obrist, "Visual Representation and Science: Visual Figures of the Universe between Antiquity and the Early Thirteenth Century," *Spontaneous Generations* 6, no. 1 (2012): 15–23; Bruce Eastwood and Gerd Graßhoff, *Planetary Diagrams for Roman Astronomy in Medieval Europe, ca. 800–1500* (Philadelphia: American Philosophical Society, 2004). A very broad overview of these same issues is provided in Christoph Lüthy and Alexis Smets, "Words, Lines, Diagrams, Images: Towards a History of Scientific Imagery," *Early Science and Medicine* 14 (2009): 398–439. Although more than forty years old, invaluable case studies—many still insufficiently explored—are found in John Murdoch, *Album of Science: Antiquity and the Middle Ages* (New York: Scribner's & Sons, 1984).

10. Reviel Netz, *The Shaping of Deduction in Greek Mathematics: A Study in Cognitive History* (Cambridge: Cambridge University Press, 1999).

11. On stemmatic images, see Ayelet Even-Ezra, *Lines of Thought: Branching Diagrams and the Medieval Mind* (Chicago: University of Chicago Press, 2020). On related tree diagrams, see Andrea Worm and Pippa Salonis, eds., *The Tree: Symbol, Allegory, and Structural Device in Medieval Art and Thought* (Turnhout: Brepols, 2014), especially Annemieke R. Verboon, "The Medieval Tree of Porphyry: An Organic Structure of Logic," 83–101.

12. Paris, Bibliothèque de l'Arsenal, MS 1037 Rés., fol. 6v. On diagrammatic cherubim, see Mary Carruthers, "*Ars oblivionalis, ars inveniendi*: The Cherub Figure and the Arts of Memory," *Gesta* 48, no. 2 (2009): 99–119. This particular image comes from an extraordinary booklet exclusively populated with large-scale diagrams, part of a group of manuscripts known as the *Speculum theologie* (Mirror of Theology). On these books, see Lynn Ransom, "The '*Speculum theologie*' and Its Readership: Considering the Manuscript Evidence," *Papers of the Bibliographical Society of America* 93, no. 4 (1999): 461–83.

13. Aristotle states this in *De memoria et reminiscentia* (On Memory and Reminiscence), cited here from Joseph Dyer, "Didactic Images in a Thirteenth-Century French Music Theory Treatise: The *Scientia artis musice* of Hélie Salomon," *Plainsong and Medieval Music* 28, no. 1 (2019): 1–27. This sentiment is shared by various Classical and medieval theoreticians alike. For instance, Macrobius

states in his *Commentarii in somnium Scipionis* (Commentary on the Dream of Scipio) that "reason sinks into the mind more easily when expressed by drawing than by speech," as discussed in Isabelle Draelants, "*Depingo ut ostendam, depictum ita est expositio*: Diagrams as an Indispensable Complement to the Cosmological Teaching of the *Liber Nemroth de astronomia*," in *Inscribing Knowledge in the Medieval Book: The Power of Paratexts*, ed. Rosalind Brown-Grant et al. (Berlin: De Gruyter, 2019), 56–92.

14. Both Müller and Obrist focus on astronomical and cosmological works. See Kathrin Müller, *Visuelle Weltaneignung: Astronomische und kosmologische Diagramme in Handschriften des Mittelalters* (Göttingen: V&R Unipress, 2009); Barbara Obrist, "Démontrer, montrer, et l'évidence visuelle: Les figures cosmologiques, de la fin de l'Antiquité à Guillaume de Conches et au début du XIIIe siècle," in *Diagramm und Text: Diagrammatische Strukturen und die Dynamisierung von Wissen und Erfahrung*, ed. Eckart Conrad Lutz, Vera Jerjen, and Christine Putzo (Wiesbaden: Reichert, 2014), 45–78. Comparable astronomical diagrams are also discussed in John North, "Diagram and Thought in Medieval Science," in *Villard's Legacy: Studies in Medieval Technology, Science and Art*, ed. Marie-Thérèse Zenner (Burlington: Ashgate, 2004), 265–87.

15. Müller, *Visuelle Weltaneignung*, 18. For more on epistemic images, especially Lorraine Daston's coining of the term within the field of the history of science, see chapter 4.

16. Mary Carruthers, *The Book of Memory: A Study of Memory in Medieval Culture* (Cambridge: Cambridge University Press, 2008); Mary Carruthers, *The Craft of Thought: Meditation, Rhetoric, and the Making of Images, 400–1200* (Cambridge: Cambridge University Press, 1998). Other useful works are Flocel Sabaté, *Memory in the Middle Ages: Approaches from Southwestern Europe* (Leeds: Arc Humanities, 2020); Anna Maria Busse Berger, *Medieval Music and the Art of Memory* (Berkeley: University of California Press, 2005). For images and their role in medieval schooling, see Karl-August Wirth, "Von mittelalterlichen Bildern und Lehrfiguren im Dienste der Schule und des Unterrichts," in *Studien zum städtischen Bildungswesen des späten Mittelalters und der frühen Neuzeit*, ed. Bernd Moeller et al. (Göttingen: V&R Unipress, 1983), 256–370.

17. On these Bibles, see Susanne Rischpler, "*Biblia Sacra figuris expressa*": *Mnemotechnische Bilderbibeln des 15. Jahrhunderts* (Wiesbaden: Reichert, 2001).

18. Carruthers notes that Hugh even goes so far as to describe his pictures as full and complete "chapters" in their own right: *The Book of Memory*, 303ff.

19. Hugh claims that he wrote this text for a struggling friend who was finding it difficult to cope with his responsibilities as a newly installed head of a monastic community.

20. Melk, Stiftsbibliothek, Cod. 737 (23, A 26), fol. 100r.

21. For a reminder that color was never neutral in medieval understandings of memory, see Tanja-Isabel Habicht and Björn Reich, "Die Farbe der Erinnerung," in *Farbe im Mittelalter: Materialität—Medialität—Semantik*, ed. Ingrid Bennewitz and Andrea Schindler (Berlin: Akademie, 2011), 1:537–50.

22. Carruthers, *The Book of Memory*, 309.

23. Steffen Bogen, "Das Diagramm als Spiel: Semiotische Entdeckungen im Spielebuch von Alfons dem Weisen (1283 n. Chr.) mit einigen Beobachtungen zu Gudea als Architekt (2000 v. Chr.)," in Lutz, Jerjen, and Putzo, *Diagramm und Text*, 385–412.

24. On Alfonso's book, see Manuel González Jiménez et al., *Libro de los juegos de ajedrez, dados, y tablas de Alfonso X el Sabio*, 2 vols. (Valencia: Scriptorium, 2010).

25. Madrid, Real Biblioteca del Monasterio de El Escorial, MS T-I-6, fol. 96v.

26. John Bender and Michael Marrinan, *The Culture of Diagram* (Stanford, CA: Stanford University Press, 2010), 7.

27. For a more practical and active religious use of medieval diagrams, see Kathryn Vulić, "The Vernon Paternoster Diagram, Medieval Graphic Design, and the *Parson's Tale*," in *Chaucer: Visual Approaches*, ed. Susanna Fein and David Raybin (University Park, PA: Penn State University Press, 2016), 59–85.

28. Jeffrey F. Hamburger, *Haec figura demonstrat: Diagramme in einem Pariser Exemplar von Lothars von Segni "De missarum mysteriis" aus dem frühen 13. Jahrhundert* (Berlin: De Gruyter, 2013).

29. Hamburger, *Haec figura demonstrat*, 31. A complementary macrocosmic religious example can be found in Heymericus de Campo's *De sigillo eternitatis* (Seal of Eternity), discussed in Christel Meier-Staubach, "Die Quadratur des Kreises: Die Diagrammatik des 12. Jahrhunderts als symbolische Denk- und Darstellungsform," in *Die Bildwelt der Diagramme Joachims von Fiore: Zur Medialität religiös-politischer Programme im Mittelalter*, ed. Alexander Patschovsky (Berlin: De Gruyter, 2003), 23–53. Comparable visualizations also exist in Hebraic traditions, for instance Rashi's so-called Map-Diagram of the Holy Land, discussed in Kay Joe Petzold, "Die Kanaan-Karten des R. Salomo Ben Isaak (Raschi)—Bedeutung und Gebrauch mittelalterlicher hebräischer Karten-Diagramme," *Das Mittelalter* 22, no. 2 (2017): 332–50.

30. Davis Baird, *Thing Knowledge: A Philosophy of Scientific Instruments* (Berkeley: University of California Press, 2004).

31. For a recent English translation, see *Thomasin von Zirclaria: Der Welsche Gast (The Italian Guest)*, trans. Marion Gibbs and Winder McConnell (Kalamazoo, MI: Medieval Institute, 2009). See also the excellent "Welscher Gast Digital," Universität Heidelberg, https://digi.ub.uni-heidelberg.de/wgd/ (accessed August 1, 2024); Kathryn Starkey, *Courtier's Mirror: Cultivating Elite Identity in Thomasin von Zerclaere's "Welscher Gast"* (Notre Dame, IN: University of Notre Dame Press, 2013); Horst Wenzel and Christina Lechtermann, eds., *Beweglichkeit der Bilder: Text und Imagination in den illustrierten Handschriften des "Welschen Gastes" von Thomasin von Zerclaere* (Cologne: Böhlau, 2002). Despite various descriptions of Thomasin's writing as sporadic and unstructured, Vera Jerjen argues that the text of *Der Welsche Gast* itself can be considered a diagrammatically inclined "network" of structured exemplars: "Struktur und Erfahrung im 'Welschen Gast' Thomasins von Zerclaere," in Lutz, Jerjen, and Putzo, *Diagramm und Text*, 349–72.

32. Heinrich Rückert, ed., *Der wälsche Gast des Thomasin von Zirclaria* (Quedlinburg: Basse, 1852), line 8893.

33. As Jerjen and others have argued, the consistency of these images across all illustrated versions of *Der Welsche Gast* and their appearance among the very earliest copies

suggest that Thomasin himself probably guided their execution.

34. Munich, Bayerische Staatsbibliothek, Cgm 571, fol. 70v. In other examples of this image in manuscripts of *Der Welsche Gast*, figures to the right of each pairing can be identified as personifications of the relevant scientific areas, although given their variation in appearance, that seems not to be the case in this particular example. Jeffrey Hamburger neatly reframes these diagrams by elevating them from images containing theoretical information to the status of intellectual "attributes" of the disciplines depicted: *Diagramming Devotion: Berthold of Nuremberg's Transformation of Hrabanus Maurus's Poems in Praise of the Cross* (Chicago: University of Chicago Press, 2020), 253. We can track this trope of exchanging physicalized diagrams back at least as far as the twelfth century, for instance in a Parisian manuscript from around 1140—now Darmstadt, Universitäts- und Landesbibliothek, Hs. 2282, fol. 1v—where the outsized personification of *Dialectica* stands between discoursing philosophers holding a life-size version of the Tree of Porphyry.

35. Steffen Bogen and Felix Thürlemann, "Jenseits der Opposition von Text und Bild: Überlegungen zu einer Theorie des Diagramms und des Diagrammatischen," in Patschovsky, *Die Bildwelt der Diagramme Joachims von Fiore*, 1–22. On the role of practical diagrams in the training of medieval German surveyors, see Christina Lechtermann, "Die geometrischen Diagramme der *Geometria Culmensis*," *Das Mittelalter* 22, no. 2 (2017): 314–31.

36. Müller, *Visuelle Weltaneignung*, 9ff.

37. On *concordia*'s diagrammatic potential, see Jean-Claude Schmitt, "Qu'est-ce qu'un diagramme? A propos du *Liber floridus* de Lambert de Saint-Omer (ca. 1120)," in Lutz, Jerjen, and Putzo, *Diagramm und Text*, 81ff. For medieval concepts of balance, see Joel Kaye, *A History of Balance, 1250–1375: The Emergence of a New Model of Equilibrium and Its Impact on Thought* (Cambridge: Cambridge University Press, 2014).

38. For a broad popular history of this trope, see Manuel Lima, *The Book of Trees: Visualizing Branches of Knowledge* (New York: Princeton Architectural Press, 2014). For its more critical dimensions, see Franco Moretti, *Graphs, Maps, Trees: Abstract Models for a Literary Theory* (New York: Verso, 2004).

39. See, for instance, Cristina Noacco and Christophe Imbert, eds., *Le château allégorique: Image mentale et paysage d'autorité de l'Antiquité à nos jours* (Rennes: Presses Universitaires de Rennes, 2021); Christiania Whitehead, *Castles of the Mind: A Study of Medieval Architectural Allegory* (Cardiff: University of Wales Press, 2003); Jeffrey F. Hamburger, *Nuns as Artists: The Visual Culture of a Medieval Convent* (Berkeley: University of California Press, 1997), especially chap. 4, "The House of the Heart," 137–76; Elizabeth Sears, "Sensory Perception and Its Metaphors in the Time of Richard of Fournival," in *Medicine and the Five Senses*, ed. William F. Bynum and Roy Porter (Cambridge: Cambridge University Press, 1993), 17–39.

40. On the multiple medieval adaptations of these longer-standing strategies of personification, see Katharine Breen, *Machines of the Mind: Personification in Medieval Literature* (Chicago: University of Chicago Press, 2021).

41. Erich Auerbach, "*Figura*," *Archivum Romanicum* 22 (1938): 436–89. The most recent English translation appears in Erich Auerbach, *Time, History, and Literature: Selected Essays of Erich Auerbach*, ed. James I. Porter, trans. Jane O. Newman (Princeton, NJ: Princeton University Press, 2016), 65–113. For an extended critical reading of the essay and its place in Auerbach's work, see James I. Porter, "Disfigurations: Erich Auerbach's Theory of *Figura*," *Critical Inquiry* 44 (2017): 80–113.

42. For a detailed discussion of the personification of the seasons, see Barbara Obrist, "Le diagramme Isidorien des saisons, son contenu physique et les représentations figuratives," *Mélanges de l'École française de Rome* 108 (1996): 95–164.

43. Paris, Bibliothèque nationale de France, MS Latin 6734, fol. 1v. For comparable later examples, see the exhibition catalog by Claire Richter Sherman, *Writing on Hands: Memory and Knowledge in Early Modern Europe* (Washington, DC: Folger Shakespeare Library, 2000).

44. London, British Library, Harley MS 941, fol. 29v. Other examples of figural volvelles include a fourteenth-century figure on the inside cover of Oxford, Bodleian Library, MS Digby 46, and a fifteenth-century figure in London, British Library, Sloane MS 702, fol. 20v. For the interesting parallel case of the *navicula*, see Catherine Eagleton, *Monks, Manuscripts, and Sundials: The Navicula in Medieval England* (Leiden: Brill, 2010).

45. Michael Camille, "The Image and the Self: Unwriting Late Medieval Bodies," in *Framing Medieval Bodies*, ed. Sarah Kay and Miri Rubin (Manchester: Manchester University Press, 1994), 62–99.

46. Brussels, Koninklijke Bibliotheek van België, MS 19546, fol. 2r. For a modern Dutch translation, see Jacob van Maerlant, *Der naturen bloeme*, ed. Herman Thys (Antwerp: De Vries-Brouwers, 2011).

47. On Trees of Consanguinity, see Steffen Bogen, "Der Körper des Diagramms: Präsentationsfiguren, mnemonische Hände, vermessene Menschen," in *Bild und Körper im Mittelalter*, ed. Kristin Marek et al. (Munich: Fink, 2006), 63, where Bogen notes papal discussion of such trees. See also Christiane Klapisch-Zuber, *L'arbre des familles* (Paris: La Martinière, 2003); Christiane Klapisch-Zuber, *L'ombre des ancêtres: Essai sur l'imaginaire médiéval de la parenté* (Paris: Fayard, 2000). For their resonance in building genealogies, see Joan A. Holladay, *Genealogy and the Politics of Representation in the High and Late Middle Ages* (Cambridge: Cambridge University Press, 2019).

48. Vienna, Österreichische Nationalbibliothek, Cod. 2469, fol. 41r.

49. For more on the medieval use of micro- and macrocosmic figures, see Kellie Robertson, "Scaling Nature: Microcosm and Macrocosm in Later Medieval Thought," *Journal of Medieval and Early Modern Studies* 49, no. 3 (2019): 609–31; Ruth Finckh, *Minor mundus homo: Studien zur Mikrokosmos-Idee in der mittelalterlichen Literatur* (Göttingen: V&R Unipress, 1999).

50. Major survey studies of premodern medical imagery over the last fifty years include Taylor McCall, *The Art of Anatomy in Medieval Europe* (London: Reaktion, 2023); Peter Murray Jones, *Medieval Medicine in Illuminated Manuscripts* (London: British Library, 1998); Robert Herrlinger, *Geschichte der medizinischen Abbildung* (Munich: Heinz Moos, 1967); Loren C. MacKinney, *Medical Illustrations in Medieval Manuscripts* (London: Wellcome Historical Medical Library, 1965).

51. On stemmatic analyses in medicine, see Even-Ezra, *Lines of Thought*, 114ff. On the *Summaries* more generally, see Gerrit Bos and Y. Tzvi Langermann, *The Alexandrian Summaries of Galen's "On Critical Days"* (Leiden: Brill, 2015). For an unusual example of a medical book plotted in exclusively tabular form, see Vienna, Österreichische Nationalbibliothek, Cod. 2426.

52. On the Zodiac Man, see Sian Witherden, "Balancing Form, Function, and Aesthetic: A Study of Ruling Patterns for Zodiac Men in Astro-Medical Manuscripts of Late Medieval England," *Journal of the Early Book Society* 20 (2017): 79–110; John Wee, "Discovery of the Zodiac Man in Cuneiform," *Journal of Cuneiform Studies* 67 (2015): 217–33; Charles West Clark, "The Zodiac Man in Medieval Medical Astrology," PhD diss., University of Colorado, 1979; Harry Bober, "The Zodiacal Miniature of the *Très Riches Heures* of the Duke of Berry: Its Sources and Meaning," *Journal of the Warburg and Courtauld Institutes* 11 (1948): 1–34.

53. For the valency of color in another medieval diagrammatic context, see Jeffrey F. Hamburger, *Color in Cusanus* (Stuttgart: Hiersemann, 2021).

54. On the sphere, see Joanne Edge, *Onomantic Divination in Late Medieval Britain: Questioning Life, Predicting Death* (Woodbridge: Boydell & Brewer, 2024).

55. Charles Sanders Peirce, "Of Reasoning in General," number 2.282 of the collected papers reproduced in the Peirce Edition Project's *The Essential Peirce: Selected Philosophical Writings*, vol. 2, *1893–1913* (Bloomington: Indiana University Press, 1998), 13. For a close reading of Peirce in relation to medieval images, including several of Peirce's own diagrams, see Hamburger, *Diagramming Devotion*, 20ff.

56. Paris, Bibliothèque nationale de France, MS Hébreu 1181, fol. 265r.

57. For a general discussion of medieval eye anatomy and its internal logic, see Fernando Salmón, "The Body Inferred: Knowing the Body through the Dissection of Texts," in *A Cultural History of the Human Body in the Medieval Age*, ed. Linda Kalof (London: Bloomsbury, 2010), 77–98.

58. For a detailed overview of this history, see Debra L. Stoudt, "The Medical Manuscripts of the Bibliotheca Palatina," in *Manuscript Sources of Medieval Medicine: A Book of Essays*, ed. Margaret R. Schleissner (New York: Routledge, 1995), 159–81.

59. Peter Murray Jones, "Image, Word, and Medicine in the Middle Ages," in *Visualizing Medieval Medicine and Natural History, 1200–1550*, ed. Jean A. Givens, Karen M. Reeds, and Alain Touwaide (Aldershot: Ashgate, 2006), 8.

60. Vatican City, Biblioteca Apostolica Vaticana, MS Pal. Lat. 1264, fols. 49v–50r.

61. Vatican City, Biblioteca Apostolica Vaticana, MS Pal. Lat. 1105, fol. 9v.

62. Vatican City, Biblioteca Apostolica Vaticana, MS Pal. Lat. 1183, fols. 327v, 340v. On surgical imaging and al-Zahrāwī's text, see Jack Hartnell, "Tools of the Puncture: Skin, Knife, Bone, Hand," in *Flaying in the Pre-Modern World: Practice and Representation*, ed. Larissa Tracy (Woodbridge: Boydell & Brewer, 2017), 20–50; Monica H. Green, "Moving from Philology to Social History: The Circulation and Uses of Albucasis's Latin *Surgery* in the Middle Ages," in *Between Text and Patient: The Medical Enterprise in Medieval and Early Modern Europe*, ed. Florence Eliza Glaze and Brian K. Nance (Florence: SISMEL, 2011), 331–72.

63. Vatican City, Biblioteca Apostolica Vaticana, MS Pal. Lat. 1232, fol. 1r.

64. Vatican City, Biblioteca Apostolica Vaticana, MS Pal. Lat. 1232, fols. 3r, 178r.

65. Vatican City, Biblioteca Apostolica Vaticana, MS Pal. Lat. 1225, fol. 26r.

66. Vatican City, Biblioteca Apostolica Vaticana, MS Pal. Lat. 1264, fol. 244r–244v. As is typical of chiromancy treatises, the text here designates the first hand as a man's and the second hand as a woman's, although both outlines appear to be traced from Knab's own hands.

67. Vatican City, Biblioteca Apostolica Vaticana, MS Pal. Lat. 1181. For a description of this manuscript, see Ludwig Schuba, *Die medizinischen Handschriften der Codices Palatini Latini in der Vatikanischen Bibliothek* (Wiesbaden: Reichert, 1981), 151–52.

68. We cannot, of course, know the precise date of this insertion. The folding lines of the left-hand folio make clear it had separate origins from the booklet as a whole; these lines in fact match contemporary methods for folding letters and other correspondence, raising the intriguing possibility that the image was sent from one user to another. The German bloodletting text surrounding the man and its figural style suggest that it is an early example, perhaps as early as c. 1400.

69. Johann Christoph Friedrich, *Catalogus codicum scriptorum qui in Bibliotheca Regia ac Academica Wratislaviensi servantur* (1821–1823), 1:120, now Wrocław, Biblioteka Uniwersytecka, Akc. 1967/1.

70. Willi Göber, with Otto Günther, Joseph Klapper, and Karl Rother, *Katalog rękopisów dawnej Biblioteki Uniwersyteckiej we Wrocławiu* (c. 1920–1944), 2:71–77, now Wrocław, Biblioteka Uniwersytecka, Akc. 1967/2.

71. For bloodletting in the ancient world, see the classic work by Peter Brain, *Galen on Bloodletting* (Cambridge: Cambridge University Press, 1986).

72. On phlebotomical diagnostics and blood therapies, see Mariacarla Gadebusch Bondio, ed., *Blood in History and Blood Histories* (Florence: SISMEL, 2005), especially Ortrun Riha, "Die mittelalterliche Blutschau," 49–67, and Hartmut Bettin, "Der therapeutische Gebrauch von Blut im mittelalterlichen Abendland," 69–89; Johannes Mayer, "Die Blutschau in der spätmittelalterlichen deutschen Diagnostik: Nachträge zu Friedrich Lenhardt aus der handschriftlichen Überlieferung des 'Arzneibuchs' Ortolfs von Baierland," *Sudhoffs Archiv* 72, no. 2 (1988): 225–33; Friedrich Lenhardt, *Blutschau: Untersuchungen zur Entwicklung der Hämatoskopie* (Pattensen: Wellm, 1986).

73. Pedro Gil-Sotres, "Derivation and Revulsion: The Theory and Practice of Medieval Phlebotomy," in *Practical Medicine from Salerno to the Black Death*, ed. Luis García-Ballester et al. (Cambridge: Cambridge University Press, 2004), 110–55.

74. Linda Voigts and Michael McVaugh note that the *Epistula* contains a handful of corrupt Greek terms, suggesting at least some small connection to a Classical heritage: *A Latin Technical Phlebotomy and Its Middle English Translation* (Philadelphia: American Philosophical Society, 1984). Pearl Kibre has classified this text according to its five incipits, two of which begin with the characteristic question *Quid est flebotomia*: "Hippocrates

latinus: Repertorium of Hippocratic Writings in the Latin Middle Ages (V)," *Traditio* 35 (1979): 284–85.

75. See, for instance, Constantine the African's compilation of Galenic and Arabic translations, all of which touch on bloodletting. For more on his *Pantegni*, see Charles Burnett and Danielle Jacquart, eds., *Constantine the African and ʿAlī ibn al-ʿAbbās al-Maǧūsī: The "Pantegni" and Related Texts* (Leiden: Brill, 1994).

76. On processes of vernacularization in medicine, see Elizabeth W. Mellyn, "Passing on Secrets: Interactions between Latin and Vernacular Medicine in Medieval Europe," *I Tatti Studies* 16, nos. 1/2 (2013): 289–310; Michael R. McVaugh, "Academic Medicine and the Vernacularization of Medieval Surgery: The Case of Bernat de Berriac," in *El saber i les llengües vernacles a l'època de Llull i Eiximenis*, ed. Anna Alberini et al. (Barcelona: Publicacions de l'Abadia de Montserrat, 2012), 257–84; William Crossgrove, "The Vernacularization of Science, Medicine, and Technology in Late Medieval Europe," *Early Science and Medicine* 5 (2000): 47–63.

77. For relevant recent studies of the history of paper, see Daniel Bellingradt and Anna Reynolds, eds., *The Paper Trade in Early Modern Europe: Practices, Materials, Networks* (Leiden: Brill, 2021); Orietta Da Rold, *Paper in Medieval England: From Pulp to Fictions* (Cambridge: Cambridge University Press, 2020); Caroline Fowler, *The Art of Paper: From the Holy Land to the Americas* (New Haven, CT: Yale University Press, 2019).

78. Helen E. Valls, "Illustrations as Abstracts: The Illustrative Programme in a Montpellier Manuscript of Roger Frugardi's *Chirurgia*," *Medicina nei secoli* 8 (1996): 67–83. Such a tactic was used widely across different types of text and different medical cultures, as testified by bloodletting scenes in both the early fourteenth-century images that Valls examines and, for instance, a late fifteenth-century Hebrew medical manuscript that depicts a woman having blood let from her arm, now Cambridge, University Library, MS Dd.10.68, fol. 211r.

79. Paris, Bibliothèque nationale de France, MS Latin 15113, fol. 8v. Precise dating of the bloodletting material in this manuscript is difficult as it sits as a distinct quire at the beginning of a highly fragmented volume. On the book, see Danielle Jacquart, "Les sciences dans la bibliothèque de Saint-Victor," in *L'école de Saint-Victor de Paris: Influence et rayonnement du Moyen Âge à l'époque moderne*, ed. Dominique Poirel (Turnhout: Brepols, 2010), 197–225; Gilbert Ouy, *Les manuscrits de l'abbaye de Saint-Victor* (Turnhout: Brepols, 1999), 2:170–71.

80. This aesthetic is shared by one of the few bloodletting figures to survive in the Greek phlebotomical lineage, found in Paris, Bibliothèque nationale de France, MS Grec 2180, fol. 107v. Some have interpreted the title above this image as implying a Syrian prototype, although it seems more likely to be referring to a text of Middle Eastern origin that follows the figure rather than the figure itself. This likelihood and the figure's late fifteenth-century date make links to either a Classical Greek or Middle Eastern heritage difficult to trace with any confidence, as clarified in K. Marcelis, *De afbeelding van de aderlaat- en de zodiakman in astrologisch-medische handschriften van de 13de en 14de eeuw* (Brussels: Paleis der Academien, 1986), 57 (although Marcelis mistakenly cites the manuscript as Cod. Graecus 1180, not 2180).

81. Loren C. MacKinney, "The Beginnings of Western Scientific Anatomy: New Evidence and a Revision in Interpretation of Mondeville's Role," *Medical History* 6, no. 3 (1962): 233–39. On the *Chirurgie*, see Marie-Christine Pouchelle, *Corps et chirurgie à l'apogée du Moyen Âge* (Paris: Flammarion, 1983). On the impact of such illustrative drawing—or *Demonstrationszeichnung*, as it is termed in the German scholarship—in a particular series of surgical texts, see Gundolf Keil, "Ortolfs chirurgischer Traktat und das Aufkommen der medizinischen Demonstrationszeichnung," in *Text und Bild, Bild und Text*, ed. Wolfgang Harms (Stuttgart: Metzler, 1990), 137–49.

82. On the Nine-Figure Series, see Taylor McCall, "Functional Abstraction in Medieval Anatomical Diagrams," in *Abstraction in Medieval Art: Beyond the Ornament*, ed. Elina Gertsman (Amsterdam: Amsterdam University Press, 2021), 285–308.

83. Cambridge, Gonville and Caius College, MS 190/223, fol. 2v; Dessau-Roßlau, Anhaltische Landesbücherei, Georg Hs. 271, fol. 1r. On the Cambridge manuscript, see Taylor McCall, "Illuminating the Interior: The Illustrations of the Nine Systems of the Body and Anatomical Knowledge in Medieval Europe," PhD diss., Cambridge University, 2017, 44ff; Taylor McCall, "*Reliquam dicit pictura*: Text and Image in an Illustrated Anatomical Manual (Cambridge, Gonville and Caius College MS 190/223)," *Transactions of the Cambridge Bibliographical Society* 16 (2017): 1–22.

84. For a summary of the ways in which different bloodletting texts and bloodletting images could become coupled to and, crucially, uncoupled from each other, see Gundolf Keil, "Ein Schlesisches Aderlassbüchlein des 15. Jahrhunderts: Untersuchungen zum funktionsbedingten Gestaltwandel des Vierundzwanzig-Paragraphen-Textes," in *Fachtexte des Spätmittelalters und der Frühen Neuzeit: Tradition und Perspektiven der Fachprosa- und Fachsprachenforschung*, ed. Lenka Vaňková (Berlin: De Gruyter, 2017), 75–118.

85. Tracing textual transmission and identifying specific genealogical branches of both Latin and vernacular phlebotomical writing is a significant topic in German medical-historical circles, in spite of—or perhaps because of—the regular admission that the fractured nature of this corpus makes such a project extremely difficult. The Latin of this particular text appears related to various other named texts, including the so-called *24-Paragraph Text* and the *Venarum minutio Text*, although it has no specific precedent in the Hippocratic or Galenic corpus. For a good summary of these two texts in German and Latin, see Konrad Goehl and Johannes Gottfried Mayer, "Variationen über den Phlebotomie-Traktat 'Venarum minutio': Die Vorlage des sogenannten '24-Paragraphen-Textes,'" in *Editionen und Studien zur lateinischen und deutschen Fachprosa des Mittelalters*, ed. Konrad Goehl and Johannes Gottfried Mayer (Würzburg: Königshausen & Neumann, 2000), 45–66.

86. Paris, Bibliothèque nationale de France, MS Arsenal 2894, fol. 59r (the French manuscript); London, British Library, Additional MS 15582, fol. 61v (the Irish manuscript); Padua, Biblioteca storica di Medicina e botanica Vincenzo Pinali e Giovanni Marsili, MS Fanzago 2,I,5,28, fol. 1r (the Italian manuscript).

87. On folding almanacs, see Chelsea Silva, "Opening the Medieval Folding Almanac," *Exemplaria* 30 (2018): 49–65; Karen Eileen Overbey and Jennifer Borland,

"Diagnostic Performance and Diagrammatic Manipulation in the Physician's Folding Almanacs," in *The Agency of Things in Medieval and Early Modern Art: Materials, Power, and Manipulation*, ed. Grażyna Jurkowlaniec, Ika Matyjaszkiewicz, and Zuzanna Sarnecka (London: Routledge, 2017), 144–56; J. P. Gumbert, *Bat Books: A Catalogue of Folded Manuscripts Containing Almanacs or Other Texts* (Turnhout: Brepols, 2016); Hilary M. Carey, "What Is the Folded Almanac? The Form and Function of a Key Manuscript Source for Astro-Medical Practice in Later Medieval England," *Social History of Medicine* 16, no. 3 (2003): 481–509.

88. See, for instance, an unillustrated text from c. 1310, fancifully attributed to the Venerable Bede, which discusses strategies for letting blood; this text is contained within the so-called Insbrucker Arzneibuch—Munich, Bayerische Staatsbibliothek, Clm 14851—translated in Karl Sudhoff, *Beiträge zur Geschichte der Chirurgie im Mittelalter: Graphische und textliche Untersuchungen in mittelalterlichen Handschriften* (Leipzig: Barth, 1914–1918), 1:185–86. Similar texts have been the subject of focused study by Sudhoff's students, including Gerhard Eis, Wolfram Schmitt, Gerrit Bauer, and Hans Habernickel, working on the so-called *Bairisches*, *Genter*, *Haager*, and *Oxforder Aderlaßbüchlein*, among others. On Ortolf's bloodletting specifically, see Christine Boot, "*an aderlaszen ligt grosz gesunthait:* Zur Repräsentanz von Ortolfs Phlebotomie in deutschsprachigen Aderlaßtexten," in *"ein teutsch puech machen": Untersuchungen zur landessprachlichen Vermittlung medizinischen Wissens*, ed. Gundolf Keil (Wiesbaden: Reichert, 1993), 112–57.

89. Washington, DC, Library of Congress, Rosenwald Collection, MS 4.

90. Plague-bloodletting figures can be found in Munich, Bayerische Staatsbibliothek, Cgm 28, fol. 33v—a particularly arresting figure—and Munich, Universitätsbibliothek, 4° Cod. 885, fol. 8r, which is subject to a detailed treatment in Heinz Bergmann and Gundolf Keil, "Das Münchner Pest-Laßmännchen: Standardisierungstendenzen in der spätmittelalterlichen deutschen Pesttherapie," in *Fachprosa-Studien: Beiträge zur mittelalterlichen Wissenschafts- und Geistesgeschichte*, ed. Gundolf Keil et al. (Berlin: Schmidt, 1982), 318–30. One of the most graphic anatomical images is found in Venice, Biblioteca Nazionale Marciana, MS Lat. VII 32 (=3032), fol. 40r. Some examples receive this treatment in a startlingly realistic manner, the layers of their skin cut and pulled apart to expose the inner organs and diaphragm. A surviving figure in Wolfenbüttel, Herzog August Bibliothek, Cod. Guelf. 18.2 Aug 4°, fol. 110r, shows a more fanciful approach: perched on a three-legged stool, this man's entire torso has been opened up in a series of curving flaps and folds, treating the viewer to a fantasy of his innards, which, drained of any obstructing fluid, muscle, or tendon, float in the cavernous space of his body. For other, more sketchy examples, see Cologne, Historisches Archiv, MS Best. 7010, inside cover; Darmstadt, Universitäts- und Landesbibliothek, Hs. 266, fol. 69v.

91. These manuscripts are Vienna, Schottenstift, Cod. 160 (Hübl. 257), fol. 343r–343v; Trier, Stadtbibliothek, Hs. 1899/1472 8°, fols. 84v–85r. Uniquely among the corpus, one of the two figures contained in the Vienna manuscript depicts a woman. For more on the complex performance of gender in medical images, see chapter 2.

92. Heidelberg, Universitätsbibliothek, Cpg 5, fol. 13v. To date, nothing is known of Hans Grunawer besides this image, although in 1411 one "Hans Grunawer" is noted in the records of the Benedictine abbey in Einsiedeln. See P. Gallup Morel, *Die Regesten der Benediktiner-Abtei Einsiedeln* (Chur: Hitz, 1848), 51.

93. Karlsruhe, Badische Landesbibliothek, Cod. Lichtenthal 76, fol. 15v. The presence of unlabeled figures in several other surviving manuscripts suggests a similar scenario, including Philadelphia, University of Pennsylvania Special Collections, Schoenberg Institute, MS LJS 463, fol. 63r; Vienna, Österreichische Nationalbibliothek, Cod. 2826, fol. 179r; St. Louis, Concordia Seminary Library, no shelfmark ["Medizinisch-astrologisches Hausbuch"], fol. 76r; Munich, Bayerische Staatsbibliothek, Cgm 340, fol. 148r.

94. The figures are Oxford, Bodleian Library, MS Ashmole 789, fol. 365r; Oxford, Bodleian Library, MS Saville 39, fol. 10r. Also related is Oxford, Bodleian Library, MS Ashmole 391(5), fol. 8v. On specifically English traditions of phlebotomy, see Francisco Alonso Almeida, "A Middle English Text on Phlebotomy," *Revista canaria de estudios ingleses* 80 (2020): 29–49; Voigts and McVaugh, *A Latin Technical Phlebotomy*; Tony Hunt, "The Poetic Vein: Phlebotomy in Middle English and Anglo-Norman Verse," *English Studies* 77, no. 4 (1996): 311–22.

95. Cardiff, National Library of Wales, MS 3026C, fol. 11r. One of the Bodleian manuscripts noted here contains a sixteenth-century note of ownership that locates it in Hereford, suggesting a close relationship with this Welsh book.

96. For instance, Vatican City, Biblioteca Apostolica Vaticana, MS Pal. Lat. 1199, is a parchment book with a large paper sheet inserted at fol. 10, while Wrocław, Biblioteka Uniwersytecka, MS I F 334, is a paper book with a large parchment sheet inserted at fol. 262. Other books with large-scale tipped-in figures include Vatican City, Biblioteca Apostolica Vaticana, MS Pal. Lat. 1181 (discussed earlier); Vatican City, Biblioteca Apostolica Vaticana, MS Vat. Lat. 2411, with an insert at fol. 1.

97. Examples used as binding material include Klosterneuburg, Augustiner-Chorherrenstift, Cod. 278; Munich, Bayerische Staatsbibliothek, Cgm 5250(33 a); Leipzig, Universitätsbibliothek, Fragm. Lat. 368; Michelstadt, Nicolaus-Matz-Kirchenbibliothek, MS D 728, discussed in Konrad Goehl and Johannes Gottfried Mayer, "Der Aderlaßmann aus Michelstadt: Ein Plakat aus dem Mittelalter," in *Bewahren und Erforschen: Beiträge aus der Nicolaus-Matz-Bibliothek (Kirchenbibliothek) Michelstadt*, ed. Wolfgang Schmitz (Michelstadt: Stadt Michelstadt, 2003), 56–74. Another example from Beilngries is discussed later in this chapter, as well as in Max Künzel, "Beilngrieser Aderlaßmännlein," *Würzburger medizinhistorische Mitteilungen* 19 (2000): 153–75. In an interesting material twist, a fifteenth-century manuscript of Bohemian origin—now Los Angeles, UCLA, Louise M. Darling Biomedical Library, MS Benjamin 10—appears to contain two bloodletting figures pasted one atop the another: when lit from behind, both figures can be seen, the upper perhaps intended as a correction of the information in the lower.

98. Leipzig, Universitätsbibliothek, MS 1346, fol. 228v.

99. Třeboň, Státní Oblastní Archiv, MS A 17, fol. 417r.

On this manuscript, see Lucie Doležalová, "Personal Multiple-Text Manuscripts in Late Medieval Central Europe: The 'Library' of Crux of Telč (1434–1504)," in *The Emergence of Multiple-Text Manuscripts*, ed. Alessandro Bausi, Michael Friedrich, and Marilena Maniaci (Berlin: De Gruyter, 2020), 145–70.

100. Florence, Biblioteca Nazionale Centrale, MS Landau Finaly 221, fol. 3v. Marginal notes from both Francesco and Giovanni, the latter recording the birth of his children, confirm the passing of the prized book from father to son. On this manuscript, see Tiziana Pesenti, *Fasiculo de medicina in volgare: Venezia, Giovanni e Gregorio de Gregori, 1494* (Treviso: Antilia, 2001), 1:25.

101. Erfurt, Universitätsbibliothek, CA. 2° 257, fol. 56v.

102. One surviving English example—Oxford, Bodleian Library, MS Ashmole 789, fol. 365r—appears to be covered in three large drops of red liquid, which could be blood but are perhaps more likely to be wax stains or blooming mold. My thanks to Eleanor Baker for examining this manuscript in person on my behalf when pandemic travel restrictions did not allow me to do so, and to Daniel Wakelin for connecting us.

103. I have argued something similar for surgical tools: "Surgical Saws and Cutting-Edge Agency," in Jurkowlaniec, Matyjaszkiewicz, and Sarnecka, *The Agency of Things*, 157–69.

104. See, for example, Michael R. McVaugh, "Bedside Manners in the Middle Ages," *Bulletin of the History of Medicine* 71, no. 2 (1997): 201–23.

105. Ortrun Riha, "Der Aderlaß in der mittelalterlichen Medizin," *Medizin, Gesellschaft, und Geschichte* 8 (1989): 92–118.

106. These manuscripts are Vatican City, Biblioteca Apostolica Vaticana, MS Pal. Lat. 1376; Vienna, Schottenstift, Cod. 160 (Hübl. 257); Edinburgh, University Library, MS 126. For a case study of bloodletting in a monastic institution for women, see Gerhard Jaritz, "Aderlaß und Schröpfen im Chorfrauenstift Klosteneuburg (1445–1533)," *Jahrbuch des Stiftes Klosterneuburg* 9 (1975): 67–108.

107. Mary K. K. Yearl, "Bloodletting as Recreation in the Monasteries of Medieval Europe," in Glaze and Nance, *Between Text and Patient*, 217–44.

108. J.W.S. Johnsson, "Zur Geschichte des Rothaarigen Mannes im Manuskript Ny k. S. 846 in der Königlichen Bibliothek zu Kopenhagen," *Janus* 30 (1926): 304–17. For more on this manuscript, see chapter 2.

109. Munich, Bayerische Staatsbibliothek, Clm 206, fol. 24v. This enormous sheet has been folded down and bound within an extensive medical manuscript of over three hundred folios. The situation is complicated by writing on the back of the sheet outlining various astrological and phlebotomical matters; this suggests either that the writing was added in a later hand or that the sheet was on occasion taken down from the wall for further consultation. On this and similar astrological manuscripts in the same library, see Davide Juste, *Les manuscrits astrologiques latins conservés à la Bayerische Staatsbibliothek de Munich* (Paris: CNRS, 2011).

110. Künzel, "Beilngrieser Aderlaßmännlein," 153ff. Künzel notes that the same accounts also record the purchase of about 0.25 square meters of wood, perhaps a plank on which the calendar was mounted.

111. The tradition of Iatromathematical Housebooks is discussed further in chapter 4.

112. Riha, "Der Aderlaß," 110.

113. Zürich, Zentralbibliothek, MS Z VII 287, fol. 46r. The manuscript is discussed in Alfred Schmid, *Conrad Türsts Iatro-mathematisches Gesundheitsbüchlein für den Berner Schultheissen Rudolf von Erlach* (Bern: Haupt, 1947).

114. Paris, Bibliothèque nationale de France, MS Français 9141, fol. 55r. This visual strategy is found throughout the chapter headings of the manuscript, with scholars—perhaps representing the book's learned author—standing in different settings and pointing out natural philosophical features to wealthy elites. While this image might not necessarily represent the specifics of a scene from French daily life, it does suggest that the presence of such framed figures in physicians' studies and wealthy households was commonplace enough to stand in for anatomical or biological discussion as a whole. This figure is briefly discussed in more theoretical terms in Camille, "The Image and the Self," 66.

115. See, for instance, the relative chaos of a figure in Freiburg im Breisgau, Universitätsbibliothek, Hs. 57, fol. 135r.

116. See, for instance, Philadelphia, University of Pennsylvania Special Collections, Schoenberg Institute, MS LJS 449, fol. 26v. This figure and the three others in the book are almost certainly the product of the same workshop as a manuscript now in London, British Library, Additional MS 17987; the London book includes two figures on fol. 91r–91v with condensed red connecting lines of a style identical to the Philadelphia manuscript.

117. These two figures are Vatican City, Biblioteca Apostolica Vaticana, MS Pal. Lat. 1199, fols. 10v–11r; Vatican City, Biblioteca Apostolica Vaticana, MS Pal. Lat. 1376, fol. 299r.

118. Zürich, Zentralbibliothek, MS C 54, fol. 48v. For more on this manuscript, known as the Codex Schürstab, see Gundolf Keil's facsimile and commentary in Gundolf Keil, Friedrich Lenhardt, and Christoph Weisser, eds., *Vom Einfluss der Gestirne auf die Gesundheit und den Charakter des Menschen*, 2 vols. (Luzern: Faksimile, 1983).

119. These three figures are Vatican City, Biblioteca Apostolica Vaticana, MS Pal. Lat. 1452, fol. 127v; Berlin, Staatsbibliothek, Mgq 2021, fol. 181v ; Leipzig, Universitätsbibliothek, MS 1483, fol. 31v. All but one of the manuscripts with number keys come from German-speaking lands. Others include Heidelberg, Universitätsbibliothek, Cpg 644, fol. 63v; Berlin, Staatsbibliothek, Mgq 2021, fol. 181v; Cambridge, Trinity College, Wren Library, R.15.21, fol. 28v; Heiligenkreuz, Zisterzienserstift, Cod. 325, fol. 24v; Salzburg, Erzabtei St. Peter, Benediktinerstift, MS A VI 17, fol. 25v; Nuremberg, Germanisches Nationalmuseum, Hs. 18792, fol. 176r; Munich, Bayerische Staatsbibliothek, Clm 4394, fol. 115r; Munich, Bayerische Staatsbibliothek, Cgm 430, fol. 15v, which is the only survival currently known to use Roman numerals rather than Arabic figures.

120. Letter-keys had played a role in German didactic and legal texts for some time, for instance in early copies of the *Sachsenspiegel* (Saxon Mirror) from around 1300, such as Dresden, Sächsische Landesbibliothek, Staats- und Universitätsbibliothek, Mscr.Dresd.M.32. On the *Sachsenspiegel*, see the long-standing digital project based at the Herzog August Bibliothek Wolfenbüttel, Sachsenspiegel Online, https://www.sachsenspiegel-online.de/cms/ (accessed August 1, 2024).

121. These two figures are Kassel, Universitätsbibliothek, Landesbibliothek, und Murhardsche Bibliothek der Stadt Kassel, 2° MS Astron. 1, fol. 48r; Frankfurt am Main, Universitätsbibliothek, MS Barth. 160, fol. 9r. For a full analysis of the Kassel manuscript, see Markus Mueller, *Beherrschte Zeit: Lebensorientierung und Zukunftsgestaltung durch Kalenderprognostik zwischen Antike und Neuzeit: Mit einer Edition des Passauer Kalendars (UB/LMB 20 Ms. astron. 1)* (Kassel: Kassel University Press, 2009). Other figures with letter-keys include Karlsruhe, Badische Landesbibliothek, Cod. Lichtenthal 76, fol. 15v; Wrocław, Biblioteka Uniwersytecka, MS R 458, fol. 18v; Vienna, Österreichische Nationalbibliothek, Cod. 5511, fol. 3r; Prague, Národní knihovna České republiky, MS I E 39, fol. 145r; Berlin, Staatsbibliothek, Mgf 557, fol. 16r; Berlin, Staatsbibliothek, Mgo 710, fol. 25r; London, Wellcome Library, MS 508, fol. 57v; Vatican City, Biblioteca Apostolica Vaticana, MS Pal. Lat. 1451, fol. 80r; Vatican City, Biblioteca Apostolica Vaticana, MS Pal. Lat. 1376, inserted after fol. 298; Munich, Bayerische Staatsbibliothek, Clm 18294, fol. 282v; Munich, Bayerische Staatsbibliothek, Clm 14546, fol. 14r; Munich, Universitätsbibliothek, 8° Cod. 339, fol. 130v.

CHAPTER 2. MEDICINE: WOUND MECHANICS

1. Prague, Lobkowicz Collection, MS VI Fc 29, 97–99. Information on this manuscript is limited, as it has been largely restricted from view for researchers. On these three figures and the manuscript in general, see Miroslav Fendrych, "České rukopisné rostlináře," *Časopis Národního muzea: Oddíl přírodovědný* 131 (1962): 188; Sudhoff, *Beiträge zur Geschichte der Chirurgie im Mittelalter*, 1:72–74; Karl Sudhoff, "Abermals eine neue Handschrift der anatomischen Fünfbilderserie," *Archiv für Geschichte der Medizin* 3, no. 6 (1910): 353–68.

2. For a range of responses to this problematic term, see "Les miscellanées scientifiques au Moyen Âge," *Micrologus* 27 (special issue) (2019); Stephen G. Nichols and Siegfried Wenzel, eds., *The Whole Book: Cultural Perspectives on the Medieval Miscellany* (Ann Arbor: University of Michigan Press, 1996).

3. The note appears at the end of the text of Macer's *Herbal* on page 239 and reads "*anno domini Millesimo CCCXCViiij ipso Cinerum de xij mensis februarii Pontificatu Bonifacii noni.*"

4. On this group, see chapter 1.

5. This reasonable reconstruction is proposed in Sudhoff, *Beiträge zur Geschichte der Chirurgie im Mittelalter*, 1:73.

6. Paris, Bibliothèque nationale de France, MS Latin 6884, fols. 30v–34v. See also Arthur Morgenstern, "Das Aderlaßgedicht des Johannes von Aquila und seine Stellung in der Aderlaßlehre des Mittelalters," PhD diss., Universität Leipzig, 1917. Visually, another image—now Oxford, Bodleian Library, MS Canon. Misc. 559, fol. 2r—also links this trio back to phlebotomical practice: a particularly unusual figure from around 1400 whose body curls in a violent backbend at the center of a diagrammatic wheel, bloodlessly pierced with individuated arrows that link different bodily sites to the astronomical influence of different planets. The textual elements of this diagram, however, were never completed.

7. For recent overviews of the history of medieval surgery, see Lluís Cifuentes i Comamala, "Vernacular Surgery in the Medieval and Early Modern Latin West: Works, Individuals, and Research Methodologies," *Medicina nei secoli* 36, no.1 (2024): 103–32; Faith Wallis, "Pre-Modern Surgery: Wounds, Words, and the Paradox of 'Tradition,'" in *The Palgrave Macmillan Handbook of the History of Surgery*, ed. Thomas Schlich (London: Palgrave Macmillan, 2018), 49–70; Piers D. Mitchell, *Medicine in the Crusades: Warfare, Wounds, and the Medieval Surgeon* (Cambridge: Cambridge University Press, 2004); Michael R. McVaugh, "Therapeutic Strategies: Surgery," in *Western Medical Thought from Antiquity to the Middle Ages*, ed. Mirko D. Grmek (Cambridge, MA: Harvard University Press, 1998), 273–90. On Germany in particular, see Ortrun Riha, "Verwundungen aus der Sicht mittelalterlicher Chirurgen: Möglichkeiten und Grenzen der Behandlung," in *Verletzungen und Unversehrtheit in der deutschen Literatur des Mittelalters*, ed. Sarah Bowden, Nine Miedema, and Stephen Mossman (Tübingen: Narr Francke, 2020), 175–88.

8. For an extremely detailed account of this theoretical development, see Michael R. McVaugh, *The Rational Surgery of the Middle Ages* (Florence: SISMEL, 2006), 89–134.

9. Consider as well how much scholarship could be produced on bodily swelling in other contexts, for instance, the much-discussed issue of *apostemata* (apostemes). On this, see Michael R. McVaugh, "Surface Meanings: The Identification of Apostemes in Medieval Surgery," in *Medical Latin: From the Late Middle Ages to the Eighteenth Century*, ed. Wouter Bracke and Herwig Deumens (Brussels: Koninklijke Academie voor Geneeskunde, 2000), 13–29.

10. The medicine underpinning this concept is neatly explained in Karine van 't Land, "The Solution of Continuous Things: Wounds in Late Medieval Medicine and Surgery," in *Wounds in the Middle Ages*, ed. Anne Kirkham and Cordelia Warr (Aldershot: Ashgate, 2014), 89–109. Michael McVaugh discusses related dimensional ideas in "Spaces of Anatomy: Fistulas, the Knee, and the 'Three-Dimensional' Body," in *Medicine and Space: Body, Surroundings, and Borders in Antiquity and the Middle Ages*, ed. Patricia A. Baker, Han Nijdam, and Karine van 't Land (Leiden: Brill, 2012), 23–36.

11. Edouard Nicaise, *Chirurgie de maitre Henri de Mondeville* (Paris: Alcan, 1893), 227. The earliest known Latin manuscript of Mondeville is Paris, Bibliothèque nationale de France, MS NAL 1487.

12. Jon Clasper notes that vinegar is still used in hospital burns units even today: "The Management of Military Wounds in the Middle Ages," in Kirkham and Warr, *Wounds in the Middle Ages*, 22.

13. Michael Benskin, "For Wound in the Head: A Late Mediaeval View of the Brain," *Neuphilologische Mitteilungen* 86, no. 2 (1985): 199–215.

14. The repeated attempts by modern scientific trials to provide "proof" of medieval medicine's efficacy remain extremely problematic, not least because the teams carrying out this work often entirely lack historical consultation, leading to basic misreadings and an absence of key cultural contextualization.

15. On spiderwebs, see Hilde-Marie Gross and Gundolf Keil, "'*Wiltu die wunde wol bewarn*': Ein Leitfaden

feldärztlicher Notversorgung aus dem spätmittelalterlichen Schlesien," in *Medizin-, Pharmazie-, und Wissenschaftsgeschichte vom Mittelalter bis zur Gegenwart*, ed. Regine Pfrepper (Aachen: Shaker, 2007), 20.

16. On tree cuts, see Guido Majno, *The Healing Hand: Man and Wound in the Ancient World* (Cambridge, MA: Harvard University Press, 1975), 215–19. On myrrh and other aromatics in healing, see Paul Freedman, *Out of the East: Spices and the Medieval Imagination* (New Haven, CT: Yale University Press, 2008), 63.

17. This debate is neatly summarized in Clasper, "The Management of Military Wounds in the Middle Ages," 28ff.

18. Among the more useful translations of this work remains *The Surgery of Theodoric ca. A.D. 1267*, trans. Eldridge Campbell and James Colton (New York: Appleton-Century-Crofts, 1955–1960), with incarnatives noted at 1:47. For more on Borgognoni, see Francesca Roversi Monaco, ed., *Teoria e pratica medica nel basso Medioevo: Teodorico Borgognoni, vescovo, chirurgo, ippiatra* (Florence: SISMEL, 2019).

19. McVaugh, *The Rational Surgery of the Middle Ages*, 103.

20. The Latin here is from McVaugh, *The Rational Surgery of the Middle Ages*, 94n18, quoting Lanfranco's *Chirurgia magna*.

21. For dependable translations of al-Zahrāwī, see David Trotter, *Traitier de cyrurgie: Édition de la traduction en ancien français de la Chirurgie d'Abū-ʾl Qāsim Halaf Ibn ʿAbbās al-Zahrāwī du manuscrit BnF, Français 1318* (Berlin: De Gruyter, 2005); *Albucasis on Surgery and Instruments: A Definitive Edition of the Arabic Text with English Translation and Commentary*, ed. and trans. Martin S. Spink and Geoffrey L. Lewis (London: Wellcome Institute, 1973).

22. Spink and Lewis, *Albucasis*, 536ff.

23. Ian Naylor, "Medicines for Surgical Practice in Fourteenth-Century England: The Judgement against John Le Spicer," in Kirkham and Warr, *Wounds in the Middle Ages*, 175–96.

24. The fear of legal action is repeatedly enunciated by writers of medieval surgical texts, who urged fellow practitioners not to take responsibility for hopeless patients in case their death was attributed to failure on the practitioner's part. See the various accounts gathered in Wendy J. Turner and Sara M. Butler, eds., *Medicine and the Law in the Middle Ages* (Leiden: Brill, 2014).

25. Campbell and Colton, *The Surgery of Theodoric ca. A.D. 1267*, 2:212–13.

26. On opiates and other medieval pain relief, see Swen H. Brunsch, "Schmerzmittel im Mittelalter," *Der Schmerz* 21, no. 4 (2007): 331–38; Walton O. Schalick, "To Market, to Market: The Theory and Practice of Opiates in the Middle Ages," in *Opioids and Pain Relief: A Historical Perspective*, ed. Marcia L. Meldrum (Seattle: IASP, 2003), 5–20; Linda E. Voigts and Robert P. Hudson, "*A drynke þat men callen dwale to make a man to slepe whyle men kerven him*: A Surgical Anaesthetic from Late Medieval England," in *Health, Disease, and Healing in Medieval Culture*, ed. Sheila Campbell, Bert Hall, and David Klausner (New York: Palgrave, 1992), 34–56. For introductions to medieval conceptualizations of pain more generally, see Ashwak Hauter, "Madness, Pain, and *Ikhtilāṭ al-ʿaql*: Conceptualizing Ibn Abī Ṣādiq's Medico-Philosophical Psychology," *Early Science and Medicine* 25, no. 5 (2020): 453–79; Bianca Frohne and Jenni Kuuliala, "The Trauma of Pain in Later Medieval Miracle Accounts," in *Trauma in Medieval Society*, ed. Wendy J. Turner and Christina Lee (Leiden: Brill, 2018), 215–36; Esther Cohen, *The Modulated Scream: Pain in Late Medieval Culture* (Chicago: University of Chicago Press, 2010); Fernando Salmón, "Academic Discourse and Pain in Medieval Scholasticism," in *Medicine and Medical Ethics in Medieval and Early Modern Spain: An Intercultural Approach*, ed. Samuel S. Kottek and Luis García Ballester (Jerusalem: Magnes, 2009), 136–53.

27. McVaugh, "Bedside Manners in the Middle Ages," 219.

28. David Nicolle, "Wounds, Military Surgery, and the Reality of Crusading Warfare: The Evidence of Usāmah's Memoires," in Nicolle, *Warriors and Their Weapons around the Time of the Crusades* (Burlington: Ashgate, 2002), 39.

29. Currently, the only modern edition is Heinrich von Pfolsprundt, *Buch der Bündth-Ertznei*, ed. Heinrich von Haeser and Albrecht Middeldorpf (Berlin: Reimer, 1868).

30. Bologna, Biblioteca Universitaria, MS Greci 3632, fols. 384v–385r. This manuscript is explored in detail in Francesca Marchetti, "Le illustrazioni di uno Iatrosophion bizantino del XV secolo, cod. 3632 della Biblioteca Universitaria di Bologna," PhD diss., Università di Bologna, 2011.

31. In this, Mondeville is evoking a long-standing debate first staged by Galen between three medical camps: Methodists, Empiricists, and Dogmatists. For a summary, see McVaugh, "Therapeutic Strategies," 285–86; Nancy G. Siraisi, *Medieval and Early Renaissance Medicine: An Introduction to Knowledge and Practice* (Chicago: University of Chicago Press, 1990), 169–70.

32. This evidence is not without its methodological complications. Mitchell sensibly observes that hard science of this type offers a chance to combat various biases inherent to written sources—which are inevitably caught up in cultural acts of social and professional promotion—but he also notes that modern scientific failings might inject their own biases into proceedings: *Medicine in the Crusades*, 108. For the diversity of this kind of evidence, see Christopher Knüsel, "The Physical Evidence of Warfare: Subtle Stigmata?," in *Warfare, Violence and Slavery in Prehistory*, ed. Mike Parker Pearson and I.J.N. Thorpe (Oxford: BAR, 2005), 49–65.

33. Roberta Gilchrist, *Sacred Heritage: Monastic Archaeology, Identities, Beliefs* (Cambridge: Cambridge University Press, 2020), 71ff. The specific studies she cites include Dan-Axel Hallbäck, "A Medieval(?) Bone with a Copper Plate Support, Indicating an Open Surgical Treatment," *Ossa* 34 (1976): 63–82; Brian Connell et al., *A Bioarchaeological Study of Medieval Burials on the Site of St. Mary Spital: Excavations at Spitalfields Market, London E1, 1991–2007* (London: Museum of London Archaeology, 2012).

34. Mitchell, *Medicine in the Crusades*, 115–16, citing J. M. Lilley et al., *The Jewish Burial Ground at Jewbury* (York: Council for British Archaeology, 1994).

35. On battlefield contexts, see Mitchell, *Medicine in the Crusades*, 111.

36. Included in this category might be texts now known to scholars as the *Bamberg Surgery*, the *Chirurgia*

Salernitana, and the *Introductio sive Medicus*. For more on these early writings, see Gerhard Baader and Gundolf Keil, eds., *Medizin im mittelalterlichen Abendland* (Darmstadt: Wissenschaftliche Buchgesellschaft, 1982), especially Gerhard Baader, "Die Entwicklung der medizinischen Fachsprache in der Antike und im frühen Mittelalter (1970)," 417–42; Monica H. Green, "Rethinking the Manuscript Basis of Salvatore De Renzi's *Collectio Salernitana*: The Corpus of Medical Writings in the 'Long' Twelfth Century," in *La "Collectio Salernitana" di Salvatore De Renzi*, ed. Danielle Jacquart and Agostino Paravicini Bagliani (Florence: SISMEL, 2008), 15–60.

37. These social themes run throughout McVaugh, *The Rational Surgery of the Middle Ages*.

38. For general discussions of these wound charms and others in a German context, see chapter 3. See also Chiara Benati, "Charms and Blessings in the Middle Low German Medical Tradition," in *Medieval German Tristan and Trojan War Stories*, ed. Sibylle Jefferis (Göppingen: Kümmerle, 2017), 115–44; Christa M. Haeseli, *Magische Performativität: Althochdeutsche Zaubersprüche in ihrem Überlieferungskontext* (Würzburg: Königshausen & Neumann, 2011); Monika Schulz, "Wund- und Blutbeschwörungen," in *Verfasserlexikon* 11 (2004): 1683–90; Gundolf Keil, "Wundsegen," in *Lexikon des Mittelalters* (Munich: Artemis, 1998), 9:367–68.

39. Gundolf Keil, "Dreibilderserie," in *Lexikon des Mittelalters* (Munich: Artemis, 1986), 3:1373–74; Karl Sudhoff, "Neue Beiträge zur Vorgeschichte des 'Ketham,'" *Archiv für Geschichte der Medizin* 5, nos. 4/5 (1911): 280–301. The term *Dreibilderserie* has built into it a historiographical reference to the *Fünfbilderserie*, a term coined by Karl Sudhoff for a recurring series of medieval images addressing five core anatomical structures of the body, although recent studies have shown that this series in fact contained nine images, not five. On the *Fünfbilderserie* and its historiographical evolution, see McCall, "Illuminating the Interior"; Ynez Violé O'Neill, "The *Fünfbilderserie*: A Bridge to the Unknown," *Bulletin of the History of Medicine* 51, no. 4 (1977): 538–49; Sudhoff, *Tradition und Naturbeobachtung in den Illustrationen medizinischer Handschriften und Frühdrucke*, 49ff.

40. Seven known *Dreibilderserie* manuscripts survive that contain at least two of the series' three figures: Copenhagen, Kongelige Bibliothek, NKS 84 b 2°; Heidelberg, Universitätsbibliothek, Cpg 644; London, Wellcome Library, MS 49; Munich, Bayerische Staatsbibliothek, Cgm 597; Paris, Bibliothèque nationale de France, MS Latin 11229; Vatican City, Biblioteca Apostolica Vaticana, MS Pal. Lat. 1325; London, Sokol Books, no shelfmark ["Medicine"]. Eleven further manuscripts survive that contain one *Dreibilderserie* image in some form: Berlin, Staatsbibliothek, Mlq 275; Kassel, Universitätsbibliothek, Landesbibliothek, und Murhardsche Bibliothek der Stadt Kassel, 2° MS Med 7; Leipzig, Universitätsbibliothek, MS 1122; London, British Library, Arundel MS 251; Los Angeles, UCLA, Louise M. Darling Biomedical Library, MS Benjamin 10; Munich, Bayerische Staatsbibliothek, Clm 4394; Paris, Bibliothèque nationale de France, MS Latin 7138; Prague, Královská kanonie premonstrátů na Strahově, Strahovská knihovna, MS DC III 3; Prague, Národní knihovna České republiky, MS III C 2; Vatican City, Biblioteca Apostolica Vaticana, MS Pal. Lat. 1293; Würzburg, Universitätsbibliothek, M.ch.q.30. Four other manuscripts retain only traces of the series: Copenhagen, Kongelige Bibliothek, GKS 1658 4° (which contains two texts related to one of the *Dreibilderserie* images, but not the image itself); Berlin, Staatsbibliothek, Mlf 782 (which is a fragment of a large sheet, probably reused as binding material, with a slither of a single figure and its related text); Leipzig, Bibliothek des Instituts für Medizingeschichte, Cod. Txt. var. 41 (a book now lost, but recorded in Sudhoff, *Beiträge zur Geschichte der Chirurgie im Mittelalter*, 508–12); a lost text also mentioned briefly by Sudhoff (*Tradition und Naturbeobachtung in den Illustrationen medizinischer Handschriften und Frühdrucke*, illustrated at table XXI) as being in the private medical collection of Professor Gustav Klein in Munich.

41. For localization to Bohemia, see Auer and Schnell, "'Der Wundenmann,'" 355–56. The idea that these treatises might be related to medicine at the University of Prague has been repeated since the earliest scholarly work by Sudhoff and others, but not necessarily with much direct evidence. On the one hand, it certainly follows logically that the university might provide a locus for medical activity in the region, including the making of medical books and medical images. But on the other, little medical teaching appears to have taken place in Prague during the fourteenth and early fifteenth centuries in comparison with other major European centers. František Šmahel counts only ninety-nine professors and students between 1348 and 1420: *Alma mater Pragensis: Studie k počátkům Univerzity Karlovy* (Prague: Karolinum, 2016), 126ff. For more on academic medicine in the region, see Ota Pavlicek, ed., *Studying the Arts in Late Medieval Bohemia: Production, Reception, and Transmission of Knowledge* (Turnhout: Brepols, 2021); Vivian Nutton, "Medicine at the German Universities, 1348–1500: A Preliminary Sketch," in *Practical Medicine from the Black Death to the French Disease*, ed. Roger French et al. (Aldershot: Ashgate, 1998), 85–109.

42. Fifteenth-century Disease Men appear in the following manuscripts: Berlin, Staatsbibliothek, Mlq 275, fol. 16r; Heidelberg, Universitätsbibliothek, Cpg 644, fol. 1v; London, British Library, Arundel MS 251, fol. 37r; London, Wellcome Library, MS 49, fol. 39r–39v; Los Angeles, UCLA, Louise M. Darling Biomedical Library, MS Benjamin 10, fols. 90v–92r; Paris, Bibliothèque nationale de France, MS Latin 11229, fol. 37v; Prague, Královská kanonie premonstrátů na Strahově, Strahovská knihovna, MS DC III 3, 99; Prague, Národní knihovna České republiky, MS XIX C 49, fol. 176v; Vatican City, Biblioteca Apostolica Vaticana, MS Pal. Lat. 1293, fol. 1r; Vatican City, Biblioteca Apostolica Vaticana, MS Pal. Lat. 1325, fol. 346v; London, Sokol Books, no shelfmark ["Medicine"], fol. 264v.

43. Heidelberg, Universitätsbibliothek, Cpg 644, fol. 1v. A thorough catalog entry for this manuscript appears in Pamela Kalning, Matthias Miller, and Karin Zimmermann, *Die Codices Palatini germanici in der Universitätsbibliothek Heidelberg (Cod. Pal. germ. 496–670)* (Wiesbaden: Harrassowitz, 2014), 398–405.

44. In most manuscripts, this text is clearly identified by its opening discussion of alopecia, beginning "*Alopicia est casus capillorum cum ulceribus* . . . ." See Lynn Thorndike and Pearl Kibre, *A Catalogue of Incipits of Scientific Writings in Latin* (Cambridge: Cambridge

University Press, 1963), 85. In other manuscripts and several manuscript catalogs, it is given a variety of different titles: *Ad cognoscendam proprietatem morborum* (For the Knowledge of the Properties of Diseases), *Secuntur descriptiones diversarum infirmitatum* (Descriptions of Diverse Illnesses Follow), and *De aegritudinibus particularibus* (On Particular Illnesses).

45. For an excellent discussion of the etiologies and pathologies of these diseases as understood by medieval physicians, see Luke Demaitre, *Medieval Medicine: The Art of Healing from Head to Toe* (Santa Barbara, CA: Praeger, 2013). Also useful is Johani Norri, *Dictionary of Medical Vocabulary in English, 1375–1550* (New York: Routledge, 2016).

46. On premodern uterine thought across cultures, see Erica Couto-Ferreria and Lorenzo Verderame, eds., *Cultural Constructions of the Uterus in Pre-modern Societies, Past and Present* (Newcastle: Cambridge Scholars, 2018).

47. These manuscripts emphasize a quadripartite system, but other sources of the period speak of cognition as having three or even five individuated elements. On medieval brain function, see Annemieke R. Verboon, "Brain Ventricle Diagrams: A Century after Walther Sudhoff: New Manuscript Sources from the XVth Century," *Sudhoffs Archiv* 98, no. 2 (2014): 212–33; Ynez Violé O'Neill, "Diagrams of the Medieval Brain: A Study in Cerebral Localization," in *Iconography at the Crossroads*, ed. Brendan Cassidy (Princeton, NJ: Princeton Department of Art and Archaeology, 1993), 91–105; Edwin Clarke and Kenneth Dewhurst, *An Illustrated History of Brain Function* (Berkeley: University of California Press, 1972). On the relevance of memory in fifteenth-century Bohemia, see Lucie Doležalová, "*Fugere artem memorativam*? The Art of Memory in 15th c. Bohemia and Moravia (A Preliminary Survey)," *Studia Mediaevalia Bohemica* 2 (2010): 221–60.

48. Prague, Královská kanonie premonstrátů na Strahově, Strahovská knihovna, MS DC III 3, 99; Vatican City, Biblioteca Apostolica Vaticana, MS Pal. Lat. 1293, fol. 1r; Vatican City, Biblioteca Apostolica Vaticana, MS Pal. Lat. 1325, fol. 346v. On the Vatican manuscripts, see Schuba, *Die medizinischen Handschriften der Codices Palatini Latini*, 372–75, 431–34.

49. Paris, Bibliothèque nationale de France, MS Latin 11229, fol. 37v; Berlin, Staatsbibliothek, Mlq 275, fol. 16r; Prague, Národní knihovna České republiky, MS XIX C 49, fol. 176v; Los Angeles, UCLA, Louise M. Darling Biomedical Library, MS Benjamin 10, fols. 90v–92r. On the Paris manuscript, see Hilde-Marie Gross, "Illustrationen in medizinischen Sammelhandschriften: Eine Auswahl anhand von Kodizes der Überlieferungs- und Wirkungsgeschichte des 'Arzneibuchs' Ortolfs von Baierland," in Keil, *"ein teutsch puech machen,"* 273–75; Ernest Wickersheimer, *Maître Jean Gispaden: Chirurgien annécien et grenoblois de la fin du XVe siècle* (Genève: Kundig, 1926); Karl Sudhoff, "Eine Pariser 'Ketham'-Handschrift aus der Zeit König Karls VI. (1380–1422)," *Archiv für Geschichte der Medizin* 2, no. 2 (1908): 84–100. Written in a particularly neat hand and on thin, fine paper, this book is mostly in Latin but contains some texts in French, an indication that it was made in a Francophone locale; this would make it the only known *Dreibilderserie* manuscript with firm provenance outside of German-speaking lands. Judging by its mention of several specific historical individuals, Wickersheimer notes that it cannot have been made before 1417. On the UCLA manuscript, see Mirella Ferrari, *Medieval and Renaissance Manuscripts at the University of California, Los Angeles* (Berkeley: University of California Press, 1991), 15–17.

50. Bamberg, Staatsbibliothek, Msc.Med.6, fol. 142v. The book is a diverse compilation preserving the writings of the German encyclopedist and physician Northungus, alongside earlier texts drawn from the Italian translations of Constantine the African and a series of distinctly Germanic healing charms. For a preliminary description of the manuscript, see Burnett and Jacquart, *Constantine the African and ʿAlī ibn al-ʿAbbās al-Maǧūsī*, 197 and appendix II. For a recent evaluation of Northungus and his relation to the artistic traditions of Theophilus, see Ilya Dines, "The Theophilus Manuscript Tradition Reconsidered in the Light of New Manuscript Discoveries," in *Zwischen Kunsthandwerk und Kunst: Die "Schedula diversarum artium,"* ed. Andreas Speer (Berlin: De Gruyter, 2014), 3–10. In relation to earlier discussions of magical wound healing, this text also contains the so-called *Bamberger Blutsegen*, one of the earliest known groups of German wound charms.

51. For recent studies of Vindicianus's texts, see Fabio Stok, "Vindiciano e la teoria dei temperamenti," *Medicina nei secoli* 24, no. 1 (2012): 517–32; Louise Cilliers, "Vindicianus's *Gynaecia*: Text and Translation of the Codex Monacensis," *Journal of Medieval Latin* 15 (2005): 153–236.

52. The literature on women's medicine in the Middle Ages is extensive. Three particularly rich and useful recent volumes are Sara Ritchey, *Acts of Care: Recovering Women in Late Medieval Health* (Ithaca, NY: Cornell University Press, 2021); multiple essays in Sara Ritchey and Sharon Strocchia, eds., *Gender, Health, and Healing, 1250–1550* (Amsterdam: Amsterdam University Press, 2021); Monica H. Green, "Gender, Health, Disease: Recent Work on Medieval Women's Medicine," *Studies in Medieval and Renaissance History* 3, no. 1 (2005): 1–46.

53. Green, *Making Women's Medicine Masculine*.

54. On midwifery in a German context, see Theresa Hitthaler-Frank, *Hebammen, Ärzte und ihr "Rosengarten": Ein medizinisches Handbuch und die Umbrüche in der Obstetrik des 15. und 16. Jahrhunderts* (Berlin: Peter Lang, 2021); Elisheva Baumgarten, "Ask the Midwives: A Hebrew Manual on Midwifery from Medieval Germany," *Social History of Medicine* 32, no. 4 (2019): 712–33.

55. Images of pregnant women with female attendants appear in two manuscripts: Vienna, Österreichische Nationalbibliothek, Cod. Ser. n. 2641, fols. 40v–41v; Zürich, Zentralbibliothek, MS C 102b, fol. 108r. A cupping image appears in London, British Library, Sloane MS 6, fol. 177r. For more on these images, see Jennifer Borland, "Gendering Treatment: Cupping by Female Practitioners in Late Medieval Visual Culture," in *Gender and the "Natural" Environment in the Middle Ages: Bodies, Boundaries, and Belief*, ed. Patricia Skinner and Theresa L. Tyers (Cardiff: University of Wales Press, 2023), 36–62.

56. Venice, Biblioteca Nazionale Marciana, MS Lat. Zan. 320 (=1937), fol. 98r. It is worth noting that these images present no specifics of a woman's anatomy other than the womb, itself mostly abstracted either into simplistic circles or colorful flourishes. Compare this single tradition, surviving in only around twenty books, to the many hundreds of surviving figures from multiple

works that depict male bodies in diagrammatic explication or treatment. On the textual tradition of Muscio and its evolving images, see Francesca Marchetti, "Educating the Midwife: The Role of Illustrations in Late Antique and Medieval Obstetrical Texts," in *Pregnancy and Childbirth in the Premodern World: European and Middle Eastern Cultures from Late Antiquity to the Renaissance*, ed. Costanza Gislon Dopfel, Alessandra Foscati, and Charles Burnett (Turnhout: Brepols, 2019), 3–28; Green, "Moving from Philology to Social History," 351ff.

57. Fifteenth-century Disease Women appear in the following manuscripts: Copenhagen, Kongelige Bibliothek, NKS 84 b 2º, fol. 4r; Kassel, Universitätsbibliothek, Landesbibliothek, und Murhardsche Bibliothek der Stadt Kassel, 2° MS Med 7, inside front cover; Leipzig, Universitätsbibliothek, MS 1122, fol. 348v; London, Wellcome Library, MS 49, fol. 38r; Munich, Bayerische Staatsbibliothek, Cgm 597, fol. 259v; Munich, Bayerische Staatsbibliothek, Clm 4394, fol. 115v; Paris, Bibliothèque nationale de France, MS Latin 11229, fol. 31r; Paris, Bibliothèque nationale de France, MS Latin 7138, fol. 239v; Prague, Královská kanonie premonstrátů na Strahově, Strahovská knihovna, MS DC III 3, fol. 44v; Vatican City, Biblioteca Apostolica Vaticana, MS Pal. Lat. 1325, fol. 349v; Würzburg, Universitätsbibliothek, M.ch.q.30, fol. 259r; a partial figure surviving on a loose leaf, now Berlin, Staatsbibliothek, Mlf 782. A Disease Woman is recorded as being in the private medical collection of Professor Gustav Klein in Munich, but it appears to now be lost; it is illustrated in Sudhoff, *Tradition und Naturbeobachtung in den Illustrationen medizinischer Handschriften und Frühdrucke*, table XXI. Some of the images listed here are discussed further in Green, *Making Women's Medicine Masculine*, 153–58. Another is incorrectly stated as being present in Bruges, Bibliothèque de la Ville, MS 411, in Ginger Lee Guardiola, "Within and Without: The Social and Medical Worlds of the Medieval Midwife, 1000–1500," PhD diss., University of Colorado at Boulder, 2002, 62, but this is in fact the Würzburg image above. Sadly, the Universitätsbibliothek Würzburg was the only institution among the sixty-eight lenders of images to this book that was unwilling to follow best practice in the sharing of images for scholarly use; their practice of charging punitive fees for the reproduction of images from their collection—maintained despite being in direct contradiction of EU-wide legal frameworks governing the free sharing of historical documents—effectively censors manuscripts in their care from further scholarly work and greater public awareness. As a result, this image cannot be reproduced here.

58. When present, texts accompanying the Disease Woman in the *Dreibilderserie* typically include one of three potential elements. The first, sometimes titled *De mulieribus* (On Women), lists various cures, diseases, and recipes keyed to the illnesses inscribed on the figure. Sources for this material are highly varied: for instance, amid the medicine of Paris, Bibliothèque nationale de France, MS Latin 11229 and MS Latin 7138, is a paraphrasing of paragraph 123 of the *Trotula* ensemble discussing generation, while London, Wellcome Library, MS 49, opens with advice *Ad menstrua provocandum* (To provoke menstruation), material that appears in many contemporary texts on women's health. Christoph Ferckel has dug deeper into these cures and identifies elements of writings by Constantinus Africanus and the *De aegritudinum curatione* (On the Treatment of Diseases): "Zur Gynäkologie und Generationslehre im *Fasciculus medicinae* des Johannes de Ketham," *Archiv für Geschichte der Medizin* 6, no. 3 (1912): 205–22. The second potential element is a series of questions taken from the pseudo-Aristotelian *Problemata Aristotelis* or *Omnes homines*, renamed in these manuscripts the *Problemata Alberti* (Albert's Problems), which focus on various aspects of women's healthcare. This text appears in Copenhagen, Kongelige Bibliothek, NKS 84 b 2º, and Heidelberg, Universitätsbibliothek, Cpg 644; the latter manuscript is missing its Disease Woman, but a note—"*de ymagine mulierum*" (the image of women)—makes clear that it was once present, or was at least present in this manuscript's model. The third potential element is found in several *Dreibilderserie* manuscripts that include texts drawn from the pseudo-Albertine *Secreta mulierum* (Secrets of Women), in particular a section on conception that they title *Signa conceptionis*. This appears in at least three manuscripts: Heidelberg, Universitätsbibliothek, Cpg 644; Paris, Bibliothèque nationale de France, MS Latin 11229; Würzburg, Universitätsbibliothek, M.ch.q.30.

59. Copenhagen, Kongelige Bibliothek, NKS 84 b 2º, fol. 4r.

60. Vatican City, Biblioteca Apostolica Vaticana, MS Pal. Lat. 1325, fol. 349v; Munich, Bayerische Staatsbibliothek, Cgm 597, fol. 259v; London, Wellcome Library, MS 49, fol. 38r.

61. Katharine Park, *Secrets of Women: Gender, Generation, and the Origins of Human Dissection* (New York: Zone, 2006), 106–9.

62. On German sumptuary laws, see Ulinka Rublack, "The Right to Dress: Sartorial Politics in Germany, c. 1300–1750," in *The Right to Dress: Sumptuary Laws in a Global Perspective, c. 1200–1800*, ed. Giorgio Riello and Ulinka Rublack (Cambridge: Cambridge University Press, 2019), 44ff.

63. Berthold von Regensburg, *Predigten*, ed. Franz Pfeiffer and Joseph Strobl (Vienna: Braumüller, 1880), 60, lines 29–30.

64. Munich, Bayerische Staatsbibliothek, Clm 4394, fol. 115v. For reasons that remain unclear, the library allows this manuscript to be viewed in its reading room but not photographed, so it cannot be reproduced here. This folio contains both the unusual Disease Woman image and, on the recto, a bloodletting figure; the gazes of the figures appear to meet through the page. In keeping with several similar images, the folio is made of parchment, tipped into an otherwise paper book. For an overview of this manuscript, see Wolfgang Augustyn, "Zu einem astronomisch-medizinischen Handbuch aus dem Spätmittelalter (München, Bayerische Staatsbibliothek, cod. lat. mon. 4394): Ein Vorbericht," in *Rondo: Beiträge für Peter Diemer zum 65. Geburtstag*, ed. Wolfgang Augustyn and Iris Lauterbach (Munich: Zentralinstitut für Kunstgeschichte, 2010), 33–43.

65. Tübingen, Universitätsbibliothek, Md 2, fol. 42v. On this book, see Arthur Hénaff, "Le *Tübinger Hausbuch*: La miscellanée scientifique à l'épreuve de l'image," *Micrologus* 27 (special issue: "Les miscellanées scientifiques au Moyen Âge") (2019): 429–42; Gerd Brinkhus, David Juste, and Helga Lengenfelder, *Iatromathematisches Kalenderbuch / Die Kunst der Astronomie und Geomantie.*

Farbmikrofiche-Edition der Handschrift Tübingen, Universitätsbibliothek, Md 2 (Munich: Lengenfelder, 2005).

66. Prague, Národní knihovna České republiky, MS III C 2, fol. 44v. On this manuscript, see Lynn Thorndike, "Some Little Known Astronomical and Mathematical Manuscripts," *Osiris* 8 (1948): 54ff.

67. Kassel, Universitätsbibliothek, Landesbibliothek, und Murhardsche Bibliothek der Stadt Kassel, 2° MS Med 7, inside cover. On Geismar and his place in women's medicine, see Green, *Making Women's Medicine Masculine*, 206ff; Monica H. Green, "Gynäkologische und geburtshilfliche Illustrationen in mittelalterlichen Manuskripten: Sprechende Bilder halfen den Frauen," *Die Waage* 30, no. 4 (1991): 161–67.

68. Paris, Bibliothèque nationale de France, MS Latin 7138, fol. 239r. On this manuscript, see Wickersheimer, *Maître Jean Gispaden*.

69. Würzburg, Universitätsbibliothek, M.ch.q.30, fol. 259r. The lecture was a commentary on Albertus Magnus by a scholar named Laurentius Meissner de Dresden.

70. Camilla Luise Dahl and Isis Sturtewagen, "The Cap of St. Birgitta," in *Medieval Clothing and Textiles 4*, ed. Robin Netherton and Gale R. Owen-Crocker (Woodbridge: Boydell & Brewer, 2008), 125. It should be noted that the connection between veils and wedlock was not universal across the period, as discussed in Grzegorz Pac, "The Attire of the Virgin Mary and Female Rulers in Iconographical Sources of the Ninth to Eleventh Centuries: Analogues, Interpretations, Misinterpretations," in *Medieval Clothing and Textiles 12*, ed. Robin Netherton and Gale R. Owen-Crocker (Woodbridge: Boydell & Brewer, 2016), 5ff. For a book-length study of churching in a French context, see Paula M. Rieder, *On the Purification of Women: Churching in Northern France, 1100–1500* (New York: Palgrave MacMillan, 2006). On earlier European traditions of veiling, see Grace Stafford, "Veiling and Head-Covering in Late Antiquity: Between Ideology, Aesthetics, and Practicality," *Past & Present* 263, no. 1 (2024): 3–46.

71. This is discussed throughout Green, *Making Women's Medicine Masculine*, for example, in an Italian context at 249ff.

72. Fifteenth-century Wound Men appear in the following manuscripts: Copenhagen, Kongelige Bibliothek, NKS 84 b 2°, fol. 4v; Heidelberg, Universitätsbibliothek, Cpg 644, fol. 78v; London, Wellcome Library, MS 49, fol. 35r; Munich, Bayerische Staatsbibliothek, Cgm 597, fol. 244r; Paris, Bibliothèque nationale de France, MS Latin 11229, fol. 36v; Vatican City, Biblioteca Apostolica Vaticana, MS Pal. Lat. 1325, fol. 360v; Solothurn, Zentralbibliothek, Cod. S 474, fol. 238r; London, Sokol Books, no shelfmark ["Medicine"], fol. 291r. For a list of brief scholarly work on the Wound Man to date, see this book's introduction.

73. Munich, Bayerische Staatsbibliothek, Cgm 597, fol. 244r. An astronomical text on fol. 212r mentions its completion in the year 1485, a date we can tentatively extend to the manuscript as a whole. The manuscript is cataloged in Karin Schneider, *Die deutschen Handschriften der Bayerischen Staatsbibliothek München: Cgm 501–690* (Wiesbaden: Harrassowitz, 1978), 215–22; Gross, "Illustrationen in medizinischen Sammelhandschriften," 261–63; Pia Rudolph, "Medizin: Handschrift Nr. 87.6.4," in *Katalog der deutschsprachigen illustrierten Handschriften des Mittelalters (KdiH)*, vol. 9, ed. Kristina Freienhagen-Baumgardt, Pia Rudolph, and Nicola Zotz (Munich: Beck, 2022), http://kdih.badw.de/datenbank/handschrift/87/6/4 (accessed August 1, 2024).

74. The fact that the Wound Man's legs are busier than his torso could reflect the real-world frequencies of illness and accident: archaeological evidence from major battle sites in Sweden and Portugal has suggested that the majority of battle wounds were sustained on the lower legs rather than on the arms. Mitchell, *Medicine in the Crusades*, 110ff.

75. The *Wundarznei* in this Regensburg manuscript has unfortunately been cut short because of codicological meddling at some point in the book's history, stretching to only a single folio. The reverse is true for an unillustrated *Wundarznei* text we can now add to the corpus that appears in the final folios of Leipzig, Universitätsbibliothek, MS 1122, fols. 344r–347r. This manuscript includes no Wound Man, but the folio immediately preceding the text has been cut out. Perhaps this Wound Man is out there somewhere, circulating as a single page.

76. Given that the *Wundarznei* represents a living tradition, the precise length of the text fluctuates between manuscripts. Erltraud Auer and Bernhard Schnell's study of the text is the only work to produce a Latin and German edition from surviving manuscripts and later printed editions (although not Leipzig, Universitätsbibliothek, MS 1122, which they do not cite). In their edition, they create a text of forty-four paragraphs, although no single manuscript survives with all of these paragraphs intact in the order they present it. Instead, they range from over forty down to twenty-nine, with one unfinished example stopping short at only eight.

77. Auer and Schnell, "'Der Wundenmann,'" 351. Auer and Schnell also note that the text's plant names have strong Germanic and Bohemian roots, for instance, *zanikel*, *hintloufte*, *wontkraut*, *vinf finger krawt*, and *winter grun*. The Silesian witness, formerly Leipzig, Bibliothek des Instituts für Medizingeschichte, Cod. Txt. var. 41, is now lost. According to Sudhoff, it was written by the physician Pankratius Sommer in Hirschberg between 1451 and 1453: *Beiträge zur Geschichte der Chirurgie im Mittelalter*, 508–12.

78. We know little about Ortolf's life besides the internal evidence of his *Arzneibuch*, although two documents from February 1339 relating to a house in Würzburg note that it had once been the home of a well-established surgeon by the name of Ortolf. The house was owned by the Würzburg cathedral hospital, suggesting a possible close connection between Ortolf and the town's influential episcopal authorities. For a modern German translation of the *Arzneibuch*, see Ortrun Riha, *Mittelalterliche Heilkunst: Das Arzneibuch Ortolfs von Baierland (um 1300)* (Baden-Baden: Deutscher Wissenschaftsverlag, 2014). For a comprehensive Old German edition, see Ortolf von Baierland, *Das Arzneibuch Ortolfs von Baierland*, ed. Gundolf Keil and Ortrun Riha (Wiesbaden: Reichert, 2014). Also useful is the summary and bibliography in Ortrun Riha, "Arzneibuch des Ortolf von Baierland," Historisches Lexikon Bayerns Online, http://www.historisches-lexikon-bayerns.de/Lexikon/Arzneibuch_des_Ortolf_von_Baierland (accessed August 1, 2024). On the tricky terminological issues hiding behind the word *Arzneibuch*, see Ortrun Riha, *Wissensorganisation in medizinischen*

Sammelhandschriften: Klassifikationskriterien und Kombinationsprinzipien bei Texten ohne Werkcharakter (Wiesbaden: Reichert, 1992), 7–17.

79. From the authorities that Ortolf cites, as well as his lack of source material from contemporary Italian writers, it seems likely that he studied in France at some point in the mid-thirteenth century. On Ortolf's Latin sources, see Ortrun Riha, *Ortolf von Baierland und seine lateinischen Quellen: Hochschulmedizin in der Volkssprache* (Weisbaden: Reichert, 1992).

80. For a table of the correspondences between the two texts, see Auer and Schnell, "'Der Wundenmann,'" 355. They also note that "errors" have been introduced in the adaptation of Ortolf's text to the *Dreibilderserie*, for instance the mangling of certain plant names.

81. The Czech-Latin manuscript is Heidelberg, Universitätsbibliothek, Cpg 644; the Czech entry appears on fol. 82v, marked no. 17. The manuscript entirely in Old Czech is Prague, Národní knihovna České republiky, MS XVII H 22; it was written slightly later, around 1500, and has a proto-Wound Man on fol. 309r in the same style as the three early Lobkowicz figures, with points on the body marked and a note indicating that treatment either "can" or "cannot" be successfully given. The manuscript in Mittelhochdeutsch is London, Wellcome Library, MS 49, which has a Wound Man and *Wundarznei* on fols. 34r–35r.

82. This was first proposed by Gundolf Keil at the meeting of the Deutsche Gesellschaft für Geschichte, but only a brief abstract was subsequently published: "Zum Problem lateinisch-landessprachiger Verflechtung: Der 'Wunden-mann' des Kodex Wellcome 49," *Nachrichtenblatt der Deutschen Gesellschaft für Geschichte, Medizin, und Technik* 25, no. 2 (1975): 79–80.

83. The term "'How-To' Book" was first popularized in William Eamon, *Science and the Secrets of Nature: Books of Secrets in Medieval and Early Modern Culture* (Princeton, NJ: Princeton University Press, 1994). For a broader, cross-period take on this genre, see Angela N. H. Creager, Mathias Grote, and Elaine Leong, eds., "Learning by the Book: Manuals and Handbooks in the History of Science," *British Journal for the History of Science: Themes* 5 (special issue) (2020). The word holds some parallels with the German term *Fachprosa* (technical literature), the study of which in relation to medicine was pioneered by scholars such as Gerhard Eis, Gundolf Keil, Wolfram Schmitt, and others from the 1960s onward. For a recent cross-section of this material, see Lenka Vanková, ed., *Fachtexte des Spätmittelalters und der Frühen Neuzeit als Objekt der Fachsprachen- und Fachprosaforschung: Tradition und Perspektiven der Fachprosa- und Fachsprachenforschung* (Berlin: De Gruyter, 2014).

84. For instance, compare the tone of this text with that of the boastful fourteenth-century English surgeon John Arderne, whose works were being reproduced in England at the same time as the *Wundarznei* in Germany. On Arderne and surgical case histories more broadly, see Peter Murray Jones, "The Surgeon as Story-Teller," *Poetica* 72 (2009): 77–92.

85. Almuth Seebohm suggests that the size, contents, and expense of London, Wellcome Library, MS 49, point to its production for a monastic community, perhaps of Cistercians or Augustinian canons: *Apokalypse, Ars moriendi, medizinische Traktate, Tugend- und Lasterlehren: Die erbaulich-didaktische Sammelhandschrift London, Wellcome Institute for the History of Medicine, Ms. 49* (Munich: Helga Lengenfelder, 1995). Munich, Bayerische Staatsbibliothek, Cgm 597, seems to have close connections with a Dominican foundation in Regensburg. See Schneider, *Die deutschen Handschriften der Bayerischen Staatsbibliothek München*, 215–16.

86. Solothurn, Zentralbibliothek, Cod. S 474, fol. 238r. Elsewhere in this book, on fol. 320r, the owner records the birth of his son: "*Nota quod Johannes Hainczman filius meus natus est septimus in vigilia Johannis et Pauli anno Mcccc81*" (Note that my seventh son, Johannes Hainczman, was born on the eve of John and Paul in the year Mcccc81 [June 25, 1481]).

87. As with the *Wundarznei* itself, the sources of the *Antidotar* are surely broad. One recipe is explicitly attributed to Petrus Hispanus and another to Hippocrates. Auer and Schnell offer a full Latin edition in "'Der Wundenmann,'" 393–401.

88. On the medicinal role of gardens, see various essays in Peter Dendle and Alain Touwaide, eds., *Health and Healing from the Medieval Garden* (Woodbridge: Boydell & Brewer, 2008). On medieval gardens in a broader cultural context, see Michael Leslie, ed., *A Cultural History of Gardens in the Medieval Age* (London: Bloomsbury, 2013).

89. On a key contemporary Czech example, the Latin *herbarium* of Křišťan z Prachatic, see Dana Stehlíková, *Od anděliky po zimostráz: Latinský Herbář Křišťana z Prachatic a počátky staročeských herbářů* (Brno: Centrum pro studium demokracie a kultury, 2017).

90. The two classic studies addressing the ancient origins and subsequent spread of theriac are Thomas Holste, *Der Theriakkrämer: Ein Beitrag zur Frühgeschichte der Arzneimittelwerbung* (Hannover: Wellm, 1976); Gilbert Watson, *Theriac and Mithridatium: A Study in Therapeutics* (London: Wellcome Historical Medical Library, 1966). Jonathan Rubin uses one ingredient of the cure-all to track the Crusader importation of theriac from the Islamic Middle East to western Europe: "The Use of the 'Jericho Tyrus' in Theriac: A Case Study in the History of the Exchanges of Medical Knowledge between Western Europe and the Realm of Islam in the Middle Ages," *Medium Aevum* 83, no. 2 (2014): 234–53. For a reconstructive study of the drug, see Nils-Otto Ahnfelt, Hjalmar Fors, and Karin Wendin, "Making and Taking Theriac: An Experimental and Sensory Approach to the History of Medicine," *British Journal for the History of Science: Themes* 7 (2022): 39–62. On the visual qualities of theriac, see Winston Black, "Christ's Pharmacy: Theriac and Drug Jars in the Medieval Iconography of Disease Management," in *Materialities of Disease in the Global Medieval World: Images, Objects, and Remains*, ed. Lori Jones (York: Arc Humanities Press, forthcoming).

91. Three recent studies that shed useful light on sugar as a key material for medical and cultural exchange are Petros Bouras-Vallianatos, "Cross-Cultural Transfer of Medical Knowledge in the Medieval Mediterranean: The Introduction and Dissemination of Sugar-Based Potions from the Islamic World to Byzantium," *Speculum* 96, no. 4 (2021): 963–1008; Judith Bronstein, Edna J. Stern, and Elisabeth Yehuda, "Franks, Locals and Sugar Cane: A Case Study of Cultural Interaction in the Latin Kingdom of Jerusalem," *Journal of Medieval History* 45, no. 3 (2019): 316–30; Richard Jones, *Sweet Waste: Medieval Sugar Production in the Mediterranean Viewed from the*

2002 *Excavation at Tawahin es-Sukkar, Safi, Jordan* (Glasgow: Potingair, 2016).

92. It is no coincidence that these prized ingredients echo the Magi's gifts to Christ. For more on the relationship between spiritual and physical healing in this material, see chapter 3.

93. Freedman, *Out of the East*, 69.

94. Poems were not uncommon in contemporary Bohemian medical material. For the example of a poem attributed to a fourteenth-century Wrocław physician, see Donald Yates, "A Fourteenth-Century Latin Poem on the Art of the Physician," *Bulletin of the History of Medicine* 54, no. 3 (1980): 447–50.

95. This particular wording of the Latin and German comes from London, Wellcome Library, MS 49, fol. 34r.

96. For the most recent critical edition of the *Regimen sanitatis Salernitanum*, also known as the *Flos medicine*, see Virginia de Frutos Gonzalez, *Flos medicine (Regimen sanitatis Salernitanum): Estudio, edición crítica, y traducción* (Valladolid: Universidad de Valladolid, 2010). On the fate of the *Regimen* in Bohemian lands, see Milada Říhová, "*Regimen sanitatis* pro krále Václava," *Acta Universitatis Carolinae: Historia Universitatis Carolinae Pragensis* 35, nos. 1/2 (1995): 13–28. On non-naturals and holistic health specifically in a medieval German context, see Lucy C. Barnhouse, "From Helpful Gardens to Hateful Words: Moral and Physical Healthscaping in the Late Medieval Rhineland," in *Disease and the Environment in the Medieval and Early Modern Worlds*, ed. Lori Jones (New York: Routledge, 2022), 52–64.

97. On this idea, see Demaitre, *Medieval Medicine*, ixff.

98. On the diagrammatics of these figures, see chapter 1. For an introduction to this descriptive form of Arabic poetry, known as وصف (*wasf*), see Ali-Asghar Seyed-Gohrab, "Description (*Wasf*) and Ekphrasis in Anvari's Poetry," in *Studies on the Poetry of Anvari*, ed. Daniela Meneghini (Venice: Cafoscarina, 2006), 111–26. For the *Poetria nova*, see Edmond Faral, ed., *Les arts poétiques du XIIe et du XIIIe siècle* (Paris: Édouard Champion, 1924), 215, lines 598–99. For a broader sense of the cross-pollination between scientific and literary worlds in the Middle Ages, see Matthew Boyd Goldie, *Scribes of Space: Place in Middle English Literature and Late Medieval Science* (Ithaca, NY: Cornell University Press, 2019).

99. Clearly, the numbered diagrammatic bodies of contemporary bloodletting figures, a specifically Germanic phenomenon, have exerted an influence here. Two of these numerated Wound Men appear in close proximity to a bloodletting figure that uses the same technique.

100. Compare, for instance, Vatican City, Biblioteca Apostolica Vaticana, MS Pal. Lat. 1325, fol. 360v, with Heidelberg, Universitätsbibliothek, Cpg 644, fol. 78v. Ludwig Schuba catalogs the Vatican manuscript as being of a later date than Tiziana Pesenti: *Die medizinischen Handschriften der Codices Palatini Latini*, 431–34. Pesenti's more detailed study dates it on the basis of contents and watermarks to the last decade of the 1400s: *Fasiculo de medicina in volgare: Venezia, Giovanni e Gregorio de Gregori, 1494* (Treviso: Antilia, 2001), 1:8.

101. For a broad look at the concept of medical paratexts and a number of examples across periods, see Hannah C. Tweed and Diane G. Scott, eds., *Medical Paratexts from Medieval to Modern: Dissecting the Page* (London: Palgrave Macmillan Cham, 2018).

102. This is found alongside the left shin of the Wound Man in London, Wellcome Library, MS 49, fol. 35r.

103. London, Sokol Books, no shelfmark ["Medicine"], fol. 291r. This is an intriguing manuscript that only appeared on the market in 2023. Further close investigation is needed, but its contents and condition suggest that it was the personal notebook of a physician—or a number of physicians—who used it to record recipes, learned medical texts, and several *Dreibilderserie* texts and images. The presence of late fifteenth-century Bohemian authorities, Czech spellings of certain medicaments, and a mention of King Sigismund I makes clear its Central European origin, further linking the series with Bohemian lands. Other notes in the book suggest that its author, or at least an early annotator, brought the book to Padua and took notes while in lectures at the university there around 1500.

104. The sheet is now part of Copenhagen, Kongelige Bibliothek, NKS 84 b 2º, fol. 4v. This booklet is cataloged in Gross, "Illustrationen in medizinischen Sammelhandschriften," 233–35. For further discussion, see Sudhoff, "Neue Beiträge zur Vorgeschichte des 'Ketham,'" 288–98; J.W.S. Johnsson, "Zur Geschichte der Rothaarigen Mannes im Manuskript Ny k. S. 846 in der Königlichen Bibliothek zu Kopenhagen," *Janus* 30 (1926): 304–17.

CHAPTER 3. AFFECT: WOUNDS IN THE WORLD

1. Heidelberg, Universitätsbibliothek, Urk. Lehmann 185 (the charge) and 186 (the defense). For a brief summary of the case, see Johann Georg Lehmann, *Urkundliche Geschichte der Grafschaft Hanau-Lichtenberg* (Hanau-Lichtenberg: Schneider, 1863), 2:438–40.

2. Valentin Groebner, *Ungestalten: Die visuelle Kultur der Gewalt im Mittelalter* (Munich: Hanser, 2003), translated into English as *Defaced: The Visual Culture of Violence in the Late Middle Ages*, trans. Pamela Selwyn (New York: Zone, 2008).

3. Han Nijdam, "Compensating Body and Honor: The Old Frisian Compensation Tariffs," in *Medicine and the Law in the Middle Ages*, ed. Wendy J. Turner and Sara M. Butler (Leiden: Brill, 2014), 25–57. All Old Frisian terms used here are taken from Nijdam's table 2 listing different body parts. On similar medical references in the southern *Lex Baiuvariorum*, see Tamás Nótári, "Physicians, Patients, and Treatments in Early Medieval German (Especially Bavarian) Legislation," *Fundamina* 23, no. 1 (2017): 61–88.

4. On the legal frameworks in the various countries where these medieval and early modern medics were working, see Sara M. Butler, *Forensic Medicine and Death Investigation in Medieval England* (London: Routledge, 2014); Silvia De Renzi, "Medical Expertise, Bodies, and the Law in Early Modern Courts," *Isis* 98, no. 2 (2007): 315–22; Esther Fischer-Homberger, *Medizin vor Gericht: Gerichtsmedizin von der Renaissance bis zur Aufklärung* (Bern: Huber, 1983).

5. Han Nijdam, "Measuring Wounds in the *Lex Frisionum* and the Old Frisian Registers of Fines," in *Philologia Frisica Anno 1999*, ed. Piter Boersma et al. (Leeuwarden: Fryske Akademy, 2000), 181, 195.

6. On *Körperverletzung* more generally, see Groebner, *Ungestalten*, 94ff. For a useful summary of Scandinavian

and English wound legislation, see Jenny Benham, "Wounding in the High Middle Ages: Law and Practice," in *Wounds in the Middle Ages*, ed. Anne Kirkham and Cordelia Warr (London: Routledge, 2014), 151–74.

7. Gotha, Forschungsbibliothek, MS Chart. B 69, fol. 3r. Giles is here directly quoting from Book V of Aristotle's *Ethics*. For an overview of this philosophical tradition, see Katie L. Walter, "Peril, Flight, and the Sad Man: Medieval Theories of the Body in Battle," in *War and Literature*, ed. Laura Ashe and Ian Patterson (Woodbridge: Boydell & Brewer, 2014), 21–40.

8. For a broad theoretical take on the signifying capacities of medieval German literary classics, see Jan-Dirk Müller, "Writing—Speech—Image: The Competition of Signs," in *Visual Culture and the German Middle Ages*, ed. Kathryn Starkey and Horst Wenzel (New York: Palgrave Macmillan, 2005), 35–52. For a summary of the more aggressive side of courtliness across this literature, see Will Hasty, *Art of Arms: Studies of Aggression and Dominance in Medieval German Court Poetry* (Heidelberg: 2002).

9. These terms are discussed further in William C. McDonald, "Turnus in Veldeke's *Eneide*: The Effects of Violence," in *Violence in Medieval Courtly Literature: A Casebook*, ed. Albrecht Classen (New York: Routledge, 2004), 83–95.

10. Germanic wound symbolism has most recently been discussed in various essays in Sarah Bowden, Nine Miedema, and Stephen Mossman, eds., *Verletzungen und Unversehrtheit in der deutschen Literatur des Mittelalters* (Tübingen: Narr Francke, 2020), especially Wolfgang Haubrichs, "leid, harm und sêr: Zur Geschichte eines semantischen Komplexes der Verletzung," 17–34, and Simone Schultz-Balluff, "Das Wissen über Wunden: Zu Verwendungsweisen, Semantisierung und Konzeptualisierung von ahd. *wunti*/as. *wunda*/mhd. *wunde*," 35–80. Exploring the major literary role of wounding in medieval German writing has a long history, beginning with Margit M. Sinka, "Wound Imagery in the Medieval German Epic: Structural Significance of Wounds," PhD diss., University of North Carolina, 1974. The rest of this chapter focuses on German material, but several studies analyze similar ideas in related European languages and traditions from a variety of creatively abstract standpoints. See, for instance, Nicholas Ealy, *Narcissism and Selfhood in Medieval French Literature: Wounds of Desire* (New York: Palgrave Macmillan, 2019); Melissa Ridley Elmes, "Public Displays of Affliction: Women's Wounds in Sir Thomas Malory's *Morte Darthur*," *Modern Philology* 116, no. 3 (2019): 187–210; Peggy McCracken, *The Curse of Eve, the Wound of the Hero: Blood, Gender, and Medieval Literature* (Philadelphia: University of Pennsylvania Press, 2003).

11. For the most recent commentary and translation of *Willehalm* into modern German, see Wolfram von Eschenbach, *Willehalm*, trans. Werner Schröder (Berlin: De Gruyter, 2019). For further discussion of the work in various directions, see Martin H. Jones and Timothy McFarland, eds., *Wolfram's "Willehalm": Fifteen Essays* (Rochester, NY: Camden House, 2002). On the pictorial logic of early surviving illustrated copies of this epic, see Norbert H. Ott, "Nonverbale Kommentare: Zur Kommentarfunktion von Illustrationen in mittelalterlichen Handschriften," in *Schrift—Text—Edition*, ed. Christiane Henkes et al. (Berlin: De Gruyter, 2011), 116ff.

12. My transcription here is from a *Willehalm* manuscript written most likely in central Germany in 1334, now Kassel, Universitätsbibliothek, Landesbibliothek, und Murhardsche Bibliothek der Stadt Kassel, 2° MS Poet. et Roman. 1, fol. 75r.

13. Wolfenbüttel, Herzog August Bibliothek, Cod. Guelf. 30.12 Aug. 2°, fol. 80r.

14. Contemporary medicine is more often than not deployed by women in such epics. For more on this passage and other contemporary medical treatments that appear in German texts of the period, see Waltraut F. Dubé, "Medieval Medicine in Middle High German Epics," PhD diss., Indiana University, 1981.

15. On concepts of masculinity explored through German literary examples, see Jamie Page, "Masculinity and Prostitution in Late Medieval German Literature," *Speculum* 94, no. 3 (2019): 739–73; Ann Marie Rasmussen, "Masculinity and the *Minnerede*: Berlin, Staatsbibliothek Preussischer Kulturbesitz, Ms. germ. oct. 186 (Livonia, 1431)," in *Triviale Minne? Konventionalität und Trivialisierung in spätmittelalterlichen Minnereden*, ed. Ludger Lieb and Otto Neudeck (Berlin: De Gruyter, 2006), 119–38; Dorothea Klein, "Geschlecht und Gewalt: Zur Konstitution von Männlichkeit im 'Erec' Hartmanns von Aue," in *Literarische Leben: Rollenentwürfe in der Literatur des Hoch- und Spätmittelalters*, ed. Matthias Meyer and Hans-Jochen Schiewer (Tübingen: Max Niemeyer, 2002), 433–63; Mark Chinca, "Women and Hunting-Birds Are Easy to Tame: Aristocratic Masculinity and the Early German Love-Lyric," in *Masculinity in Medieval Europe*, ed. Dawn M. Hadley (London: Routledge, 1999), 199–213. For a recent general historiography of the subject, see Daniel F. Pigg, "Masculinity Studies," in *Handbook of Medieval Studies: Terms—Methods—Trends*, ed. Albrecht Classen (Berlin: De Gruyter, 2010) 1:829–35.

16. Eugene Vance, "Roland and the Poetics of Memory," in *Textual Strategies: Perspectives in Post-Structuralist Criticism*, ed. Josué V. Harari (Ithaca, NY: Cornell University Press, 1979), 374–403.

17. My transcription here is from the so-called Codex Manesse, now Heidelberg, Universitätsbibliothek, Cpg 848, fol. 230r, although given the significant damage to this page in the manuscript I have borrowed interpretation from Carl von Krause, ed., *Deutsche Liederdichter des 13. Jahrhunderts* (Tübingen: Niemeyer, 1952), 56, verse IV.

18. On wounds in siege literature, see Suzanne Conklin Akbari, "Erasing the Body: History and Memory in Medieval Siege Poetry," in *Remembering the Crusades: Myth, Image, and Identity*, ed. Nicholas Paul and Suzanne Yeager (Baltimore: Johns Hopkins University Press, 2012), 146–73. A reference to wounds as insignia appears as early as the tenth-century epic poem *Waltharius*, probably written by a monk at St. Gallen, as discussed in Scott E. Pincikowski, "Violence and Pain at the Court: Comparing Violence in German Heroic and Courtly Epics," in Classen, *Violence in Medieval Courtly Literature*, 95–96. For a case study in the breadth of wound imagery in a single text, see Margit M. Sinka, "Wound Imagery in Gottfried von Strassburg's 'Tristan,'" *South Atlantic Bulletin* 42, no. 2 (1977): 3–10. For two recent surveys of chivalric violence in different contexts, see Peter Sposato and Samuel Claussen, "Chivalric Violence," in *A Companion to Chivalry*, ed. Robert W. Jones and Peter Coss (Woodbridge: Boydell & Brewer, 2019), 99–118;

Richard W. Kaeuper, *Chivalry and Violence in Medieval Europe* (Oxford: Oxford University Press, 1999).

19. Siegfried R. Christoph, "Violence Stylized," in Classen, *Violence in Medieval Courtly Literature*, 115–25.

20. St. Gallen, Kantonsbibliothek, VadSlg MS 302, book II, fol. 35v. On this phenomenon, see Rachel E. Kellett, *Single Combat and Warfare in German Literature of the High Middle Ages: Stricker's* Karl der Grosse *and* Daniel von dem Blühenden Tal (London: Manley, 2008), 41; Scott E. Pincikowski, *Bodies of Pain: Suffering in the Works of Hartmann von Aue* (New York: Routledge, 2002), 23, 49.

21. St. Gallen, Kantonsbibliothek, VadSlg MS 302, book II, fol. 35r–35v. The passage appears in the recently published *Strickers "Karl der Große,"* ed. Johannes Singer (Berlin: De Gruyter, 2016), 141, lines 4934–40.

22. Literature on the *Nibelungenlied* is extremely extensive. For the best and most recent edition and commentary, see Hermann Reichert, ed., *Das Nibelungenlied: Text und Einführung*, 2nd ed. (Berlin: De Gruyter, 2017). For the most recent prose English translation, see Cyril Edwards, trans., *The Nibelungenlied: The Lay of the Nibelungs* (Oxford: Oxford University Press, 2010). On the specific significance of wounds in the *Nibelungenlied*, see H. B. Willson, "Blood and Wounds in the 'Nibelungenlied,'" *Modern Language Review* 55, no. 1 (1960): 40–50.

23. Riechert, *Das Nibelungenlied*, 158, verses 978–79.

24. As an early work, *Erec* survives poorly. It is preserved in full in only one sixteenth-century manuscript, the so-called Ambraser Heldenbuch, now Vienna, Österreichische Nationalbibliothek, Cod. Ser. n. 2663. Useful introductions are Joachim Bumke, *Der "Erec" Hartmanns von Aue: Eine Einführung* (Berlin: De Gruyter, 2006); Margreth Egidi, Markus Greulich, and Marie-Sophie Masse, eds., *Hartmann von Aue, 1230–1517: Kulturgeschichtliche Perspektiven der handschriftlichen Überlieferung* (Stuttgart: Hirzel, 2020). For the most recent edition, see *Ereck: Textgeschichtliche Ausgabe mit Abdruck sämtlicher Fragmente und der Bruchstücke des mitteldeutschen "Erek,"* ed. Andreas Hammer, Victor Millet, and Timo Reuvekamp-Felber (Berlin: De Gruyter, 2017).

25. My transcription is from Vienna, Österreichische Nationalbibliothek, Cod. Ser. n. 2663, XLIIIv.

26. Vienna, Österreichische Nationalbibliothek, Cod. 15478, fol. 291v.

27. New York, Morgan Library, MS M.763, fols. 257v–258r. On this scene more broadly, see Wolfgang Stechow, "Shooting at Father's Corpse," *Art Bulletin* 24, no. 3 (1942): 213–25.

28. Heidelberg, Universitätsbibliothek, Cpg 339, vol. II, fol. 425v. For more on medicine in *Parzival*, see Bernhard Dietrich Haage, *Studien zur Heilkunde im "Parzival" Wolframs von Eschenbach* (Göppingen: Kümmerle, 1992). On the Lauber workshop, see the extensive survey by Lieselotte Saurma-Jeltsch, *Spätformen mittelalterlicher Buchherstellung: Bilderhandschriften aus der Werkstatt Diebold Laubers in Hagenau*, 2 vols. (Wiesbaden: Reichert, 2002).

29. For an introduction to these and similar writers, see Tilman G. Moritz, *Autobiographik als ritterschaftliche Selbstverständigung: Ulrich von Hutten, Götz von Berlichingen, Sigmund von Herberstein* (Göttingen: V&R Unipress, 2019); Yuval Noah Harari, *Renaissance Military Memoirs: War, History and Identity, 1450–1600* (Woodbridge: Boydell & Brewer, 2004); Henry J. Cohn, "Götz von Berlichingen and the Art of Military Autobiography," in *War, Literature, and the Arts in Sixteenth-Century Europe*, ed. J. R. Mulryne and Margaret Shewring (New York: Palgrave Macmillan, 1989), 22–40. Also useful are various entries in the online resource by Gabriele Jancke et al., *Selbstzeugnisse im deutschsprachigen Raum: Autobiographien, Tagebücher und andere autobiographische Schriften 1400–1620*, https://www.geschkult.fu-berlin.de/e/jancke-quellenkunde/index.html accessed (August 1, 2024).

30. Jörg Rogge, "Kämpfer als Schreiber: Bemerkungen zur Erzählung von Kampferfahrung und Verwundung in deutschen Selbstzeugnissen des späten Mittelalters," in *Kriegserfahrungen erzählen: Geschichts- und literaturwissenschaftliche Perspektiven*, ed. Jörg Rogge (Bielefeld: Transcript, 2016), 86ff.

31. For an extensive bibliography of Ehingen's text, see its entry in the "Geschichtsquellen des deutschen Mittelalters," Bayerische Akademie der Wissenschaften, updated November 22, 2022, https://www.geschichtsquellen.de/werk/2438 (accessed August 1, 2024). The only English edition is nearly a century old and remains a useful guide but is an unreliable translation: *The Diary of Jörg von Ehingen*, trans. and ed. Malcolm Letts (London: Humphrey Milford, 1929).

32. This is transcribed from the earliest extant manuscript of the text in Stuttgart, Württembergische Landesbibliothek, Cod.hist.qt.141, 51–53.

33. An extensive bibliography on Diesbach's text can be found in the Bayerische Akademie der Wissenschaften's "Geschichtsquellen des deutschen Mittelalters." The most recent edition is Urs Martin Zahnd, ed., *Die autobiographischen Aufzeichnungen Ludwig von Diesbachs: Studien zur spätmittelalterlichen Selbstdarstellung im oberdeutschen und schweizerischen Raume* (Bern: Stämpfli, 1986); the lance injury is found at fol. 52ff.

34. The only illustrations associated with the text are found in Stuttgart, Württembergische Landesbibliothek, Cod.hist.qt.141; these are a series of accomplished portraits that supposedly depict the kings that Diesbach claimed to have met and served on his travels.

35. According to Rainer Leng in his survey for the *KdiH*, at least 48 manuscripts survive, with a total of more than 7,800 images: "Fecht- und Ringbücher (Nr. 38.)," in *Katalog der deutschsprachigen illustrierten Handschriften des Mittelalters (KdiH)*, ed. Ulrike Bodemann, Peter Schmidt, and Christine Stöllinger-Löser, vol. 4/2 (Munich: Beck, 2010), http://kdih.badw.de/datenbank/stoffgruppe/38 (accessed August 1, 2024). It is worth noting that Leng's categorization of these books has been questioned by subsequent scholars. Two good introductions to these works are Daniel Jaquet, Karin Verelst, and Timothy Dawson, eds., *Late Medieval and Early Modern Fight Books: Transmission and Tradition of Martial Arts in Europe (14th–17th Centuries)* (Leiden: Brill, 2016), especially Dierk Hagedorn, "German Fechtbücher from the Middle Ages to the Renaissance," 247–79; Sydney Anglo, *The Martial Arts of Renaissance Europe* (New Haven, CT: Yale University Press, 2000). On similar European materials from later periods, see Tobias Capwell, ed., *The Noble Art of the Sword: Fashion and Fencing in Renaissance Europe* (London: Wallace Collection, 2012). On German tournament culture in general, see Peter Jezler, Peter Niederhäuser, and Elke Jezler, eds., *Ritterturnier: Geschichte einer Festkultur* (Luzern: Quaternio, 2014).

A mass of material on German *Fechtbücher* has been accumulated by historical martial arts enthusiasts; this has rarely been written with a view to academic precision but can still be extremely useful. The best of these resources is the Wiktenauer project from the Historical European Martial Arts (HEMA) Alliance, https://wiktenauer.com (accessed August 1, 2024).

36. Eric Burkart, "Body Techniques of Combat: The Depiction of a Personal Fighting System in the Fight Books of Hans Talhofer (1443–1467 CE)," in *Killing and Being Killed: Bodies in Battle, Perspectives on Fighters in the Middle Ages*, ed. Jörg Rogge (Bielefeld: Transcript, 2017), 117.

37. The best introduction to the function of images in Talhofer's work is found in Burkart, "Body Techniques of Combat"; Eric Burkart, "Die Aufzeichnung des Nicht-Sagbaren: Annäherung an die kommunikative Funktion der Bilder in den Fechtbüchern des Hans Talhofer," *Das Mittelalter* 19, no. 2 (2014): 253–301.

38. Copenhagen, Kongelige Bibliothek, Thott 290, 2°, fol. 134v and 93v. Other important illustrated manuscripts of Talhoffer's work are Gotha, Forschungsbibliothek, MS Chart. A 558 (from 1448); Munich, Bayerische Staatsbibliothek, Cod. icon. 394a (from 1467); a manuscript now in a private collection known as MS XIX 17-3 (from 1446–1459).

39. On the secretive linguistics of these books in general, see Matthias Johannes Bauer, "Teaching How to Fight with Encrypted Words: Linguistic Aspects of German Fencing and Wrestling Treatises of the Middle Ages and Early Modern Times," in Jaquet, Verelst, and Dawson, *Late Medieval and Early Modern Fight Books*, 47–61.

40. Rachel E. Kellett, "Only a Flesh-Wound? The Literary Background to Medieval German Fight Books," in Jaquet, Verelst, and Dawson, *Late Medieval and Early Modern Fight Books*, 62–87.

41. Copenhagen, Kongelige Bibliothek, MS Thott 290, 2°, fol. 93v. Opposite, on fol. 94r, the narrative continues with a scene of the deceased being carried away in a coffin, headed by a couplet reading: "*Daz tragent in die fryheit hin weg inß grab / Daz got alle gelöbig selen hab amen*" (They carry away to freedom in the grave / may God have all devout souls. Amen).

42. Nicholas Pol's manuscript is now Nuremberg, Germanisches Nationalmuseum, Hs. 3227a. The *Fechtbuch* elements of this book, including writings by the famed fifteenth-century fencing master Johannes Liechtenauer, are explored in Eric Burkart, "The Autograph of an Erudite Martial Artist: A Close Reading of Nuremberg, Germanisches Nationalmuseum, Hs. 3227a," in Jaquet, Verelst, and Dawson, *Late Medieval and Early Modern Fight Books*, 451–80. Some of its medical elements are discussed in Trude Ehlert and Rainer Leng, "Frühe Koch- und Pulverrezepte aus der Nürnberger Handschrift GNM 3227a (um 1389)," in *Medizin in Geschichte, Philologie, und Ethnologie*, ed. Dominik Groß and Monika Reininger (Würzburg: Königshausen & Neumann, 2003), 289–320.

43. The Hebrew passages conclude the manuscript on fols. 149v–150v, although they appear incomplete. The manuscript also includes a portrait of a man labeled "*Jud Ebreesh*" (Hebrew Jew), whose relationship to the book is not yet clear.

44. On the specifics of this training, including its health-related elements, see Daniel Jaquet, "Six Weeks to Prepare for Combat: Instruction and Practices from the Fight Books at the End of the Middle Ages, a Note on Ritualised Single Combats," in Rogge, *Killing and Being Killed*, 131–64; Daniel Jaquet, "Fighting in the Fight-schools late XVth, early XVIth century," *Acta Periodica Duellatorum* 1, no. 1 (2013): 47–66.

45. My transcription is from Dresden, Sächsische Landesbibliothek, Staats- und Universitätsbibliothek, Mscr.Dresd.C.487, fol. 45v. The most recent critical edition of Ringeck's treatise is a work now sixty years old: Martin Wierschin, *Meister Johann Liechtenauers Kunst des Fechtens* (Munich: Beck, 1965). For more recent work on this text, see Rachel E. Kellett, "'... Vnnd schüß im vnder dem schwert den ort lang ein zů der brust': The Placement and Consequences of Sword-Blows in Sigmund Ringeck's Fifteenth-Century Fencing Manual," in *Wounds and Wound Repair in Medieval Culture*, ed. Larissa Tracy and Kelly DeVries (Leiden: Brill, 2015), 128–50.

46. London, Wellcome Library, MS 49, fol. 34v, item 23.

47. *Fachliteratur* (or *Sachliteratur*) is further discussed in chapter 2. On the specifically embodied nature of knowledge in the *Fechtbücher*, another element that links them closely with the "How-To" corpus, see Eric Burkart, "Mensch—Waffe—Körperwissen: Die bildliche und textliche Repräsentation von embodied knowledge in vormodernen Kampfbüchern," in *Objekte des Krieges: Präsenz und Repräsentation*, ed. Romana Kaske and Julia Saviello (Berlin: De Gruyter, 2019), 49–66.

48. On the terminological problems associated with this weaponry, see Iason-Eleftherios Tzouriadis, "'What Is the Riddle of Steel?': Problems of Classification and Terminology in the Study of Late Medieval Swords," in *The Sword: Form and Thought*, ed. Lisa Deutscher, Mirjam Kaiser, and Sixt Wetzler (Woodbridge: Boydell & Brewer, 2019), 3–11.

49. Elizabeth Coatsworth and Gale Owen-Crocker, *Clothing the Past: Surviving Garments from Early Medieval to Early Modern Western Europe* (Leiden: Brill, 2018), 277ff.

50. This and other clothing items were unearthed as part of a project run by the Universität Innsbruck's Institut für Archäologien. A summary of the work on the underpants is included in Beatrix Nutz and Harald Stadler, "Gebrauchsgegenstand und Symbol: Die Unterhose (Bruoch) aus der Gewölbezwickelfüllung von Schloss Lengberg, Osttirol," in *Neue Alte Sachlichkeit: Studienbuch Materialität des Mittelalters*, ed. Jan Keupp and Romedio Schmitz-Esser (Ostfildern: Jan Thorbecke, 2015), 221–50.

51. Just as with the Wound Man's underwear, the Lengberg briefs were secured around the waist with a knot at the side. While this pair are gray-white, the Wound Man's (where colored) are exclusively blue. This choice might simply have been a matter of economy: among the cheaper of dyed materials, blue linen was used most commonly for the lining of gowns or chasubles, as well as spun into thread for attaching decorative details.

52. Munich, Bayerische Staatsbibliothek, Cgm 1507, fol. 6r. Although a relatively central figure, little substantial scholarly work has been dedicated specifically to Paulus Kal. For more on his role in chronicling the personalities of the German *Fechtbücher* tradition, see

Hagedorn, "German Fechtbücher from the Middle Ages to the Renaissance," 253ff.

53. Contemporary figures found in a variety of settings follow sartorial suit. For instance, see an Alsatian manuscript telling the story of the Trojan Wars that shows a figure burning on a pyre, stripped down to his blue underwear, now Gießen, Universitätsbibliothek, Hs. 232, fol. 90r; a heraldic figure playfully punting through foliage and supporting an oversized coat of arms in the so-called Greiner Marktbuch, a gathering of laws and customs from the Austrian city of Grein, now Grein, Stadtarchiv, Urk. Nr. 1, fol. 1v; the figures of the Good and Bad Thieves in the Crucifixion scene of the Siebenhirter Hours, now Stockholm, Kungliga Biblioteket, MS A 225, fol. 158v; the twins of Gemini from a circular zodiacal diagram, folded and tipped into a prognosticatory manuscript from around 1514, now Vatican City, Biblioteca Apostolica Vaticana, MS Reg. Lat. 1309, fol. 33v.

54. The excavation and subsequent restoration of the sword and other grave goods was undertaken by researchers at the Universität Innsbruck's Institut für Archäologien, as described in Florian Messner and Ulrike Töchterle, "The Highest Art of Smithery: Research on a Tyrolean Sword," in Deutscher, Kaiser, and Wetzler, *The Sword*, 102–16.

55. The best broad introductions to the different material and religious aspects of this vast literature are Achim Timmermann, *Real Presence: Sacrament Houses and the Body of Christ, c. 1270–1600* (Turnhout: Brepols, 2009); Sarah Beckwith, *Christ's Body: Identity, Culture, and Society in Late Medieval Writings* (New York: Routledge, 1996); Miri Rubin, *Corpus Christi: The Eucharist in Late Medieval Culture* (Cambridge: Cambridge University Press, 1991).

56. On multicultural medieval medicine, see, for instance, the classic Spanish case study by Luis García Ballester, *Medicine in a Multicultural Society: Christian, Jewish, and Muslim Practitioners in the Spanish Kingdoms, 1222–1610* (Aldershot: Ashgate, 2001). For a more recent exploration of this phenomenon beyond Europe, see Ronit Yoeli-Tlalim, *ReOrienting Histories of Medicine: Encounters along the Silk Roads* (London: Bloomsbury, 2021).

57. The unpacking of this much-discussed Augustinian metaphor has a long history, stretching back to Rudolph Arbesmann, "The Concept of 'Christus Medicus' in St. Augustine," *Traditio* 10 (1954): 1–28. More recent studies include Jeremy J. Cîtrome, *The Surgeon in Medieval English Literature* (New York: Palgrave Macmillan, 2006), 23ff; Martin Honecker, "Christus medicus," in *Der kranke Mensch in Mittelalter und Renaissance*, ed. Peter Wunderli (Düsseldorf: Drosde, 1986), 27–43. On the specific history of *Christus medicus* in the Bohemian lands of the Wound Man, see Patrick Outhwaite, *Christ the Physician in Late-Medieval Religious Controversy: England and Central Europe, 1350–1434* (Woodbridge: Boydell & Brewer, 2024). Daniel McCann makes the important point that such spiritual healing was still no picnic, often invoking serious and increasing pain: *Soul-Health: Therapeutic Reading in Later Medieval England* (Cardiff: University of Wales Press, 2018), 310ff.

58. My transcription is from Cambridge, Corpus Christi College, MS 218, fol. 53r. On the *Livre* more broadly, translated with notes and introduction, see Henry of Grosmont, *Le livre de seyntz medicines: The Book of Holy Medicines*, trans. Catherine Batt (Tempe: Arizona Center for Medieval and Renaissance Studies Press, 2014).

59. For more on Galvano and his Christological discourse, see Joseph Ziegler, *Medicine and Religion c. 1300: The Case of Arnau de Vilanova* (Oxford: Clarendon, 1998), 143ff.

60. This is taken from the standard edition, which remains *Die Chirurgie des Heinrich von Mondeville*, ed. Julius Pagel (Berlin: Hirschwald, 1892), 79–80. For more on this idea in Mondeville, see Simone C. Macdougall, "The Surgeon and the Saints: Henri de Mondeville on Divine Healing," *Journal of Medieval History* 26, no. 3 (2000): 253–68. On Christ the Surgeon more generally, see Virginia Langum, "'The Wounded Surgeon': Devotion, Compassion, and Metaphor in Medieval England," in Tracy and DeVries, *Wounds and Wound Repair in Medieval Culture*, 269–90; Gerhard Fichtner, "Christus als Arzt: Ursprünge und Wirkungen eines Motivs," *Frühmittelalterliche Studien* 16, no. 1 (1982): 1–18.

61. London, British Library, Sloane MS 1977, fols. 2v–3r. For a detailed reading of this image, see Karl Whittington, "Picturing Christ as Surgeon and Patient in British Library MS Sloane 1977," *Mediaevalia* 35 (2014): 83–115.

62. On the specifics of such eucharistic healing, see Alessandra Foscati, "Healing with the Body of Christ: Religion, Medicine, and Magic," in *Il "Corpus Domini": Teologia, antropologia, e politica*, ed. Laura Andreani and Agostino Paravicini Bagliani (Florence: SISMEL, 2015), 209–27. On Christological bloodletting, see Mary K. K. Yearl, "Medieval Monastic Customaries on *Minuti* and *Infirmi*," in *The Medieval Hospital and Medical Practice*, ed. Barbara S. Bowers (Aldershot: Ashgate, 2007), 189. The precise text covering this issue in the Rule of Saint Benedict is found in chap. 36: "*Infirmorum cura ante omnia et super omnia adhibenda est, ut sicut revera Christo ita eis serviatur*" (The care of the sick must be taken first and above all, so that they will be served as if they were Christ in person).

63. This section of John Bromyard's *Summa predicantium* is summarized and cited in Ziegler, *Medicine and Religion c. 1300*, 238.

64. This language appears in Hildegard's *Scivias* twice: in Part 1, Vision 3, and in Part 3, Vision 13. On the *Scivias*, see Hildegard von Bingen, *Scivias*, ed. Barbara Newman, trans. Columba Hart and Jane Bishop (New York: Paulist, 1990); Adelgundis Führkötter and Angela Carlevaris, eds., *Hildegardis Bingensis: Scivias* (Turnhout: Brepols, 1978), 58, 627.

65. Baierland, *Das Arzneibuch Ortolfs von Baierland*, 41.

66. The classic work on *Wundsegen* remains Oskar Ebermann, *Blut- und Wundsegen in ihrer Entwicklung dargestellt* (Berlin: Mayer & Müller, 1903). A useful summary is Keil, "Wundsegen," 9:367–68. The clearest recent introduction to the medical use of medieval charms is Lea Olsan, "Charms and Prayers in Medieval Medical Theory and Practice," *Social History of Medicine* 16, no. 3 (2003): 343–66. Also relevant here is a parallel charm tradition claiming to offer magical protection against the weapons of enemies, discussed at length in Chiara Benati, "*À la guerre comme à la guerre* but with Caution: Protection Charms and Blessings in the Germanic Tradition," *Brathair* 17, no. 1 (2017): 155–91.

67. On the Three Good Brothers Charm specifically,

see Eleonora Cianci, *The German Tradition of the "Three Good Brothers" Charm* (Göppingen: Kümerle, 2013); Lea Olsan, "The Three Good Brothers Charm: Some Historical Points," *Incantatio* 1, no. 1 (2011): 48–78.

68. My transcription is taken from Bamberg, Staatsbibliothek, Msc.Med.6, fol. 139r. This text is known as the *Bamberger Blutsegen*, one of several *Blutsegen* (blood charms) that have been better explored in the literature than their parallel *Wundsegen*. The German tradition is neatly summarized in Gundolf Keil, "Blutsegen," in *Lexikon des Mittelalters* (Munich: Artemis, 1998), 2:291–92. On related texts in English and Dutch, see T. M. Smallwood, "A Charm-Motif to Cure Wounds Shared by Middle Dutch and Middle English," in *Cultuurhistorische Caleidoscoop*, ed. Christian De Backer (Ghent: Stichting Mens en Kultuur, 1992), 477–505.

69. For more on this figure, see chapter 2.

70. Bamberg, Staatsbibliothek, Msc.Med.6, fol. 142v.

71. We might recall from chapter 2 that several of these books were made or owned by religious individuals, for instance Brother Wilhelm de Rang in the Benedictine abbey of Saints Ulrich and Afra in Cologne, or Martin von Geismar, the head of the chapter of Saint Peter's in Fritzlar. In many cases, the *Dreibilderserie*'s medical texts also abut material of conspicuously Christian persuasion, their medicine colored by this religious affiliation. Of the sixty-five-folio *Dreibilderserie* manuscript now in the Wellcome Library, likely made in 1420s Bavaria, only eleven of its enormous pages actually focus on medical texts; the rest are given over to illustrated works on the Apocalypse, holy prophecy, virtues and vices, and *Ars moriendi* writings. Meanwhile, between the Wound Man and the Disease Woman of the fifteenth-century Munich *Dreibilderserie* book we find wedged a German translation of the *Somniale Danielis*, a book on dream divination dedicated to the Old Testament prophet Daniel.

72. Vatican City, Biblioteca Apostolica Vaticana, MS Pal. Lat. 1325, fol. 364r.

73. Heidelberg, Universitätsbibliothek, Cpg 644, fol. 62v (for hermaphrodites) and fol. 59r (for Exodus).

74. Vatican City, Biblioteca Apostolica Vaticana, MS Pal. Lat. 1325, fol. 364r (for the pleas to God and *Apostolicon*), fol. 364v (for *Gratia Dei*).

75. Paris, Bibliothèque nationale de France, MS Latin 11229, fol. 37v.

76. Vatican City, Biblioteca Apostolica Vaticana, MS Pal. Lat. 1325, fol. 346v.

77. The literature on this concept is vast, and so the focus here is on German contexts rather than summarizing the phenomenon at large. That said, the clearest outline of medieval European violent imagery as a whole remains Caroline Walker Bynum, "Violent Imagery in Late Medieval Piety," *Bulletin of the German Historical Institute* 30 (2002): 3–36, paired with a response in the same volume by Mitchell B. Merback, "Reverberations of Guilt and Violence, Resonances of Peace: A Comment on Caroline Walker Bynum's Lecture," 37–50.

78. Again, scholarship on medieval *compassio* is extensive, but a foundational summary remains Giles Constable's "The Ideal of the Imitation of Christ," the second part of his *Three Studies in Medieval Religious and Social Thought* (Cambridge: Cambridge University Press, 1995), 143–248. For an important revision of previously accepted thinking about *compassio*, see Sarah McNamer, *Affective Meditation and the Invention of Medieval Compassion* (Philadelphia: University of Pennsylvania Press, 2010), 59–85.

79. The encyclopedic authority on medieval Passion writing is Tobias A. Kemper, *Die Kreuzigung Christi: Motivgeschichtliche Studien zu lateinischen und deutschen Passionstraktaten des Spätmittelalters* (Berlin: Niemeyer, 2006), which addresses German-language materials from 144ff. Other important works that discuss similarly broad anthologies of texts are Sarah Bowden and Annette Volfing, eds., *Punishment and Penitential Practices in Medieval German Writing* (Woodbridge: Boydell & Brewer, 2018); Thomas H. Bestul, *Texts of the Passion: Latin Devotional Literature and Medieval Society* (Philadelphia: University of Pennsylvania Press, 1996); Walter Haug and Burghart Wachinger, eds., *Die Passion Christi in Literatur und Kunst des Spätmittelalters* (Berlin: Niemeyer, 1993); James H. Marrow, *Passion Iconography in Northern European Art of the Late Middle Ages and Early Renaissance* (Kortrijk: Van Ghemmert, 1979).

80. On activated wounds, see Sara Ritchey, "The Wound's Presence and Bodily Absence: Activating the Spiritual Senses in a Fourteenth-Century Manuscript," in *Sensory Reflections: Traces of Experience in Medieval Artifacts*, ed. Fiona Griffiths and Kathryn Starkey (Berlin: De Gruyter, 2019), 163–80. On antisemitic narratives, especially their visualized form, see Sara Lipton, *Dark Mirror: The Medieval Origins of Anti-Jewish Iconography* (New York: Metropolitan, 2014). Also relevant to this discussion are recent works on blood in German religious contexts: Bettina Bildhauer, *Medieval Blood* (Chicago: University of Chicago Press, 2009); Caroline Walker Bynum, *Wonderful Blood: Theology and Practice in Late Medieval Northern Germany and Beyond* (Philadelphia: University of Pennsylvania Press, 2007).

81. On the *Christi Leiden* and its highly complex textual stemma, see Kemper, *Die Kreuzigung Christi*, 147–49.

82. Quoted from the edited version of Harvard, Houghton Library, MS Ger. 69, published in Steven Rozenski and Claire Taylor Jones, "Christ's Passion Shown in a Vision: A Newly Identified Acephalous Fragment from Cambridge, Massachusetts, Houghton Library MS Ger. 69, fol. 101r–106v," *Journal of Medieval Religious Cultures* 45, no. 2 (2019): 113–38.

83. The *Künzelsauer Fronleichnamspiel* is preserved in Schwäbisch Hall, Stadtarchiv, HV HS 40; the quotation is from Peter K. Liebenow, ed., *Das Künzelsauer Fronleichnamspiel* (Berlin: De Gruyter, 1969), line 3705. The Innsbruck play is preserved in Innsbruck, Universitäts- und Landesbibliothek, Cod. 960. The Eger example is now Nuremberg, Germanisches Nationalmuseum, Hs. 7060. On similar texts, see Jutta Eming, "Gewalt im Geistlichen Spiel: Das *Donaueschinger* und das *Frankfurter Passionsspiel*," *German Quarterly* 78 (2005): 1–22. For a broader overview of violent performance in medieval Europe, in particular in France, see Jody Enders, *The Medieval Theater of Cruelty: Rhetoric, Memory, Violence* (Ithaca, NY: Cornell University Press, 1999).

84. "Im Oberreich" is now numbered Kl 111 in Wolkenstein's complete canon of poems. The German citation is taken from Oswald von Wolkenstein, *Das poetische Werk*, trans. Wernfried Hofmeister (Berlin: De Gruyter, 2011), 280, verse XI, lines 199–204; the English translation is taken from Albrecht Classen, *The Poems of Oswald von*

Wolkenstein: An English Translation of the Complete Works (New York: Palgrave Macmillan, 2009), 196. On the idea of violence elsewhere in Wolkenstein's *lieder*, see Eva Rothenberger, "Die Performanz des Schmerzes: Poetische Inszenierungsstrategien von *passio* und *compassio* bei Oswald von Wolkenstein," in *Geistliche Liederdichter zwischen Liturgie und Volkssprache: Übertragungen, Bearbeitungen, Neuschöpfungen in Mittelalter und Früher Neuzeit*, ed. Andreas Kraß and Matthias Standke (Berlin: De Gruyter, 2020), 107–24.

85. On the Man of Sorrows, see Bernhard Ridderbos, "The Man of Sorrows: Pictorial Images and Metaphorical Statements," in *The Broken Body: Passion Devotion in Late-Medieval Culture*, ed. Alasdair A. MacDonald, Bernhard Ridderbos, and Rita M. Schlusemann (Groningen: Egbert Forsten, 1998), 145–81; Catherine R. Puglisi and William L. Barcham, eds., *New Perspectives on the Man of Sorrows* (Kalamazoo: Medieval Institute, 2013).

86. On the *crux horribilis* and its context, see Paul Binski, "The Crucifixion and the Censorship of Art around 1300," in *The Medieval World*, ed. Peter Linehan and Janet L. Nelson (London: Routledge, 2001), 342–60.

87. On the details of the paint layers and subsequent restoration, as well as a brief summary of the sculptural type in the region, see Godehard Hoffman, *Das Gabelkreuz in Santa Maria im Kapitol zu Köln und das Phänomen der "Crucixifi dolorosi" in Europa* (Worms: Wernersche, 2006).

88. For a useful summary of this tradition, see Adrian Wilson and Joyce Lancaster Wilson, *A Medieval Mirror: "Speculum humanae salvationis" 1324–1500* (Berkeley: University of California Press, 1985).

89. Madrid, Biblioteca Nacional de España, VITR/25/7, fol. 35v. For a recent English translation of a Latin *Speculum* manuscript, see Melinda Nielsen, *An Illustrated Speculum humanae salvationis: Green Collection MS 000321* (Leiden: Brill, 2022), with the section comparing Christ and Antipater beginning at 293.

90. Foundational studies on the *Arma Christi* are Robert Suckale, "Arma Christi: Überlegungen zur Zeichenhaftigkeit mittelalterlicher Andachtsbilder," *Städel-Jahrbuch* 6 (1977): 177–208; Rudolf Berliner, "Arma Christi," *Münchner Jahrbuch der bildenden Kunst* 6 (1955): 35–152. The most useful recent explorations include Lisa H. Cooper and Andrea Denny-Brown, eds., *The Arma Christi in Medieval and Early Modern Material Culture* (Abingdon: Taylor & Francis, 2014); Marius Rimmele, "Geordnete Unordnung: Zur Bedeutungsstiftung in Zusammenstellungen der Arma Christi," in *Das Bild im Plural: Mehrteilige Bildformen zwischen Mittelalter und Gegenwart*, ed. David Ganz and Felix Thürlemann (Berlin: Reimer, 2010), 219–42. The *Arma* hold interesting medical parallels, especially in fifteenth-century German medical books, where visualized weapons float alone among texts on their cure; for instance, see the various images of arrows, clubs, and swords accompanying a fifteenth-century copy of Roger Frugardi's *Chirurgia*, now Hildesheim, Dombibliothek, Hs. 750.

91. The altarpiece illustrated here has been attributed to the so-called Master of the Holy Kinship (the Elder) and is the left exterior panel of the Triptych of the Holy Kinship, produced around 1420 in Cologne, now Wallraf-Richartz-Museum, WRM 59. The early Prague manuscript mentioned is the Passional of Abbess Kunigunde, now Prague, Národní knihovna České republiky, MS XIV A 17, where the *Arma* appear twice, on fols. 3r and 10r.

92. Bettina Bildhauer, *Medieval Things: Agency, Materiality, and Narratives of Objects in Medieval German Literature and Beyond* (Columbus: Ohio State University Press, 2020), 107.

93. This Latin is transcribed from Hugo de Sancto Victore, *De sacramentis* (Strassburg: Georg Husner, 1485), ISTC ih00535000, 2:16, part III; the English translation here is taken from *Hugh of Saint Victor on the Sacraments of the Christian Faith (De sacramentis)*, trans. Roy J. Deferrari (Cambridge, MA: Medieval Academy, 1951), 439. Hugh's ideas are discussed further in Esther Cohen, "The Animated Pain of the Body," *American Historical Review* 105, no. 1 (2000): 44ff.

94. For a good example of the textual side of this practice in the German tradition, see Marquard von Lindau's German treatise *De anima Christi*, as discussed in Stephen Mossman, *Marquard von Lindau and the Challenges of Religious Life in Late Medieval Germany: The Passion, the Eucharist, the Virgin Mary* (Oxford: Oxford University Press, 2010), 45ff.

95. This ivory was originally produced in southern Germany around 1360 to be used as a pax and is now New York, Metropolitan Museum of Art, accession no. 1970.324.9. On this Marian visual phenomenon more generally, see Carol M. Schuler, "The Seven Sorrows of the Virgin: Popular Culture and Cultic Imagery in Pre-Reformation Europe," *Simiolus* 21, nos. 1/2 (1992): 5–28.

96. The most extensive analysis and catalog of Sunday Christ images is Dominique Rigaux, *Le Christ du Dimanche: Histoire d'une image médiévale* (Paris: Harmattan, 2005). Other useful publications are Diana Hiller, "Some Italian Wall Paintings of the Sunday Christ: Monitory and Redemptory Iconographies and the Effect of Position," *Parergon* 37, no. 1 (2020): 79–112 (on Italian examples); Athene Reiss, *The Sunday Christ: Sabbatarianism in English Medieval Wall Painting* (Oxford: Archaeopress, 2000) (on English examples). On several Italian images of Mary employing a similar Sabbatarian trope, see Alberto Zaina, "Il precetto festivo tra ammonizione e devozione: Il 'Cristo della domenica' negli affreschi bresciani," *Brixia Sacra* 12, nos. 3/4 (2008): 33–63.

97. This example is notice no. 3 in Rigaux, *Le Christ du Dimanche*, 250–51. I thank Renzo Dionigi for generously sharing his excellent images of Sogn Gieri with me.

98. The visual heritage of such lines also finds precedent in late medieval painting, as discussed in Karl Whittington, *Trecento Pictoriality: Diagrammatic Painting in Late Medieval Italy* (London: Harvey Miller, 2023), 205–33. A similar pattern can be observed in images of Christ more generally. For instance, in a group of late fifteenth-century images of the Mass of Saint Gregory found in Brigittine Books of Hours from Sweden, the Five Wounds of Christ, linked to a chalice with thick red ink, are part streams of blood and part diagrammatic annotation. Examples include Berlin, Staatsbibliothek, Mtlo 71, fol. 123v; Uppsala, Universitetsbibliotek, C 420, fol. 11v. These Books of Hours have been surveyed in Eva Lindqvist Sandgren, "Birgittinska bönboksbilder," *Nordisk Tidskrift för Bildtolkning* 2 (2014): 19–48.

99. Achim Timmermann, "Vain Labor(?): Things, Strings, and the Human Condition in the Art of Giovanni Baleison," *RES: Anthropology and Aesthetics* 65/66

(2014–2015): 224–41. On a related topographical religious image, the visual allegory of Good and Bad Prayer, see Achim Timmermann, "Good and Bad Prayers, before Albertus Pictor: Prolegomena to the History of a Late Medieval Image," *Baltic Journal of Art History* 5 (2013): 131–77.

100. Karl Sudhoff, "Der 'Wundenmann' in Frühdruck und Handschrift und sein erklärender Text: Ein Beitrag zur Quellengeschichte des 'Ketham,'" *Archiv für Geschichte der Medizin* 1, no. 5 (1908): 351.

101. Assaf Pinkus, *Visual Aggression: Images of Martyrdom in Late Medieval Germany* (University Park, PA: Penn State University Press, 2021). For a summary of similar saintly ideas in contemporary painting, see Daria Dittmeyer, *Gewalt und Heil: Bildliche Inszenierungen von Passion und Martyrium im späten Mittelalter* (Cologne: Böhlau, 2014).

102. On this subject, including Bonaventure, see the classic work by Caroline Walker Bynum, *The Resurrection of the Body in Western Christianity, 200–1336* (New York: Columbia University Press, 1995), 247ff. By way of chivalric connection to earlier material in this chapter, we might observe that in Thomas Mallory's *Morte d'Arthur*, Lancelot is discovered so badly wounded that he is mistaken for a "man of worship." On this incident, see Richard W. Kaeuper, *Medieval Chivalry* (Cambridge: Cambridge University Press, 2016), 35. I thank John Renner for drawing this aspect of Bonaventure to my attention.

103. See, for example, the much-discussed woodcut of Sebastian dated c. 1420, now Munich, Staatliche Graphische Sammlung, Inv. Nr. 171 505. This image is described in Peter Parshall and Rainer Schoch, *Origins of European Printmaking: Fifteenth-Century Woodcuts and Their Public* (New Haven, CT: Yale University Press, 2005), 124–27. For more on early print medicine, including Sebastian, see chapter 4.

104. See the sweeping history outlined in Sheila Barker, "The Making of a Plague Saint: Saint Sebastian's Imagery and Cult before the Counter-Reformation," in *Piety and Plague from Byzantium to the Baroque*, ed. Franco Mormando and Thomas Worcester (Kirksville, MO: Truman State University Press, 2007), 90–131. For similar later material, see Louise Marshall, "Reading the Body of a Plague Saint: Narrative Altarpieces and Devotional Images of St. Sebastian in Renaissance Art," in *Reading Texts and Images: Essays on Medieval and Renaissance Art and Patronage*, ed. Bernard J. Muir (Exeter: University of Exeter Press, 2002), 237–72.

105. Extant Lauber manuscripts of the *Elsässische Legenda aurea* are Augsburg, Staats- und Stadtbibliothek, 2° Cod 158 and 159; Berlin, Staatsbibliothek, Mgf 495; Heidelberg, Universitätsbibliothek, Cpg 144. On the text, see the critical edition, *Die Elsässische "Legenda aurea,"* ed. Ulla Williams, Werner Williams-Krapp, and Konrad Kunze, 3 vols. (Tübingen: Niemeyer, 1980). On the work's images, see Werner Williams-Krapp, "Bild und Text: Zu den illustrierten Handschriften der *Legenda aurea* des französischen und deutschsprachigen Raums," *Archiv für Kulturgeschichte* 97 (2015): 89–107; Stephanie Rappl, *Text und Bild in der "Elsässischen Legenda aurea": Der Cgm 6 (Bayerische Staatsbibliothek München) und der Cpg 144 (Universitätsbibliothek Heidelberg)* (Hamburg: Kovač, 2015).

106. Augsburg, Staats- und Stadtbibliothek, 2° Cod 158, fol. 114v.

107. Frankfurt am Main, Universitätsbibliothek, MS Carm. 1, fol. 2v. On the *Buch der Natur*, see Claudia Märtl, Gisela Drossbach, and Martin Kintzinger, eds., *Konrad von Megenberg (1309–1374) und sein Werk: Das Wissen der Zeit* (Munich: Beck, 2006); Ulrike Spyra, *Das "Buch der Natur" Konrads von Megenberg: Die illustrierten Handschriften und Inkunabeln* (Cologne: Böhlau, 2005). Two further manuscript copies of the *Buch der Natur* survive from the Lauber workshop: Heidelberg, Universitätsbibliothek, Cpg 300 (which includes another bleeding figure, wearing the same white underpants as Albrecht von Berwangen); Stuttgart, Württembergische Landesbibliothek, Cod.med.et.phys.fol.14 (which is extensively illustrated but is missing the page immediately before the opening where any figure might have once stood).

108. Augsburg, Staats- und Stadtbibliothek, 2° Cod 158, fol. 47v (Stephen), fol. 118v (Agnes), fol. 295v (Felician), fol. 173v (Agatha), fol. 188v (Matthew), fol. 252r (Peter).

109. Strasbourg, Bibliothèque nationale et universitaire, MS 2929, fol. 57r. The codicology of this image within the manuscript, as well as the book's relation to other manuscripts of the same text, is complicated and uncertain; the situation is explained in Jeffrey F. Hamburger, "Heinrich Seuse, 'Das Exemplar' (Nr. 36.)," in *Katalog der deutschsprachigen illustrierten Handschriften des Mittelalters (KdiH)*, ed. Ulrike Bodemann, Kristina Freienhagen-Baumgardt, and Peter Schmidt, vol. 4/1 (Munich: Beck, 2012). This manuscript is KdiH Nr. 36.0.4.

110. Seuse's imagery has generated significant scholarship. In addition to Hamburger's extensive *KdiH* entries cited earlier and the bibliography therein, see, more recently, Ingrid Falque, "'*Daz man bild mit bilde us tribe*': Imagery and Knowledge of God in Henry Suso's *Exemplar*," *Speculum* 92, no. 2 (2017): 447–92; José van Aelst, "Visualizing the Spiritual: Images in the Life and Teachings of Henry Suso (c. 1295–1366)," in *Speaking to the Eye: Sight and Insight through Text and Image (1150–1650)*, ed. Thérèse de Hemptinne, Veerle Fraeters, and María Eugenia Góngora (Turnhout: Brepols, 2013), 129–51.

111. On contemporary German mystics more generally, see Bernard McGinn, *Mystik im Abendland*, vol. 4, *Fülle: Die Mystik im mittelalterlichen Deutschland (1300–1500)* (Freiburg: Herder, 2008).

112. Elaine Scarry, *The Body in Pain: The Making and Unmaking of the World* (Oxford: Oxford University Press, 1988), 16.

113. Orlemanski, *Symptomatic Subjects*, 9–12.

114. See, for instance, Peter Murray Jones, "The Surgeon as Story-Teller," *Poetica* 72 (2009): 77–92.

115. Eve Salisbury, *Narrating Medicine in Middle English Poetry: Poets, Practitioners, and the Plague* (London: Bloomsbury, 2022), especially her chap. 4, which considers household remedies in the manuscripts of the fifteenth-century landowner Robert Thornton.

116. Cohen's work remains the most wide-ranging discussion of medieval pain in the English scholarship: "'If You Prick Us, Do We Not Bleed?': Reflections on the Diminishing of the Other's Pain," in *Knowledge and Pain*, ed. Esther Cohen et al. (Amsterdam: Rodopi, 2012), 25–41; *The Modulated Scream*, especially her "Part I. Manipulating Pain." For more on medieval medical understandings of pain and pain relief, see chapter 2.

117. Rudolph Siegel, *Galen on the Affected Parts: Translation from the Greek Text with Explanatory Notes* (Basel: Karger, 1976), 50, 62. For more on this discussion, see Courtney Roby, "Galen on the Patient's Role in Pain Diagnosis: Sensation, Consensus, and Metaphor," in *Homo Patiens: Approaches to the Patient in the Ancient World*, ed. Georgia Petridou and Chiara Thumiger (Leiden: Brill, 2016), 304–22; Cohen, *The Modulated Scream*, 148ff. Late medieval medical theorists often played out rhetorical games of exhaustive reasoning, concluding that the diagnosis of different kinds of painful injury was impossible as it required infinite experience: only an individual who had suffered every possible type of pain—somehow in an emotionally objective manner—could offer actual comparison of its different levels and textures, and thus use it to form an accurate diagnosis. But who could come closer to this ideal medicalized position of infinite pain than the Wound Man, a figure covered in every conceivable injury from head to toe?

118. Anthony Bale, *Feeling Persecuted: Christians, Jews, and Images of Violence in the Middle Ages* (London: Reaktion, 2010), 10ff.

119. Mitchell B. Merback, *The Thief, the Cross, and the Wheel: Pain and the Spectacle of Punishment in Medieval and Renaissance Europe* (London: Reaktion, 1999), 126ff.

120. My transcription here is from Bamberg, Staatsbibliothek, Msc.Med.1, fol. 4v; the English translation is from Faith Wallis, *Medieval Medicine: A Reader* (Toronto: University of Toronto Press, 2010), 92.

121. The situation here is complex. Thirteenth- and fourteenth-century scholastic medics utilized the term *compassio* to differing degrees, even as the influences of earlier compassionate natural philosophers—for instance, Pietro d'Abano—remained strong in places. See Béatrice Delaurenti, *La Contagion des émotions:* Compassio, *une énigme médiévale* (Paris: Garnier, 2016). For similar ideas in Bonaventure's work, see Juanita Feros Ruys, "An Alternative History of Medieval Empathy: The Scholastics and *compassio*," *Emotions: History, Culture, Society* 2, no. 2 (2018): 192–213.

122. Freiburg im Breisgau, Universitätsbibliothek, Hs. 458. The dating of this manuscript is conflicted. Based on the colophon of one of its texts (fol. 346r), Frank Fürbeth dates the book to 1474 and attributes it to the Alsatian astrologer Johannes Liechtenberger; Winfried Hagenmaier instead cites studies of the book's watermarks that offer a more likely date of 1490–1493, a period that also coincides with several astrological tables in the manuscript. For the earlier dating, see Frank Fürbeth, *Johannes Hartlieb: Untersuchungen zu Leben und Werk* (Tübingen: Niemeyer, 1992), 19; for the later, see Winfried Hagenmaier, *Die deutschen mittelalterlichen Handschriften der Universitätsbibliothek und die mittelalterlichen Handschriften anderer öffentlicher Sammlungen (Kataloge der Universitätsbibliothek Freiburg im Breisgau 1,4)* (Wiesbaden: Harrassowitz, 1988), 89–98.

123. Fürbeth concedes that the attribution of the lunary to Hartlieb seems likely, but the evidence is conflicting. It survives in nine full or partial copies, each of which offers different information: some list Hartlieb as its author, others list him as its translator, and others simply mention him by name, stating that he was university orator; those naming him as the author variously date the text's original creation to 1433, 1434, and 1435; and texts likewise disagree on the work's patron, with some naming the knight Hans Kuchler and others a noblewoman named Katherina, possibly Kuchler's wife. For the situation in full, see Fürbeth, *Johannes Hartlieb*, 49ff.

124. On Hartlieb's text and for a close analysis of three surviving manuscripts, see Bodo Weidemann, "'Kunst der Gedächtnüß' und 'De mansionibus', zwei frühe Traktate des Johann Hartlieb," PhD diss., Freie Universität Berlin, 1964. On lunaries and lunar mansions in various contexts, see Aurelio Pérez Jiménez, "Las mansiones lunares: Adaptación árabe de una doctrina astrológica antigua," in *El Cielo del Islám*, ed. Fátima Roldán Castro (Seville: Universidad de Sevilla, 2014), 239–64; Charles Burnett, "Lunar Astrology: The Varieties of Texts Using Lunar Mansions, with Emphasis on Jafar Indus," *Micrologus* 12 (2004): 43–133; Irma Taavitsainen, *Middle English Lunaries: A Study of the Genre* (Helsinki: Société Néophilologique, 1988). For an enormous and virtually exhaustive survey of medieval prognostication in its many forms and across cultures, see Matthias Heiduk, Klaus Herbers, and Hans-Christian Lehner, eds., *Prognostication in the Medieval World: A Handbook* (Berlin: De Gruyter, 2020). On the same material but in a later period, see Robin B. Barnes, *Astrology and Reformation* (Oxford: Oxford University Press, 2016).

125. Freiburg im Breisgau, Universitätsbibliothek, Hs. 458, fol. 119r–119v.

126. In at least one instance, the *Mondwahrsagebuch* appears in a manuscript alongside surgical works including Ortolf von Baierland's *Arzneibuch*; this manuscript is now Vienna, Österreichische Nationalbibliothek, Cod. 5206.

127. Freiburg im Breisgau, Universitätsbibliothek, Hs. 458, fols. 120r–134r.

128. Paris, Bibliothèque nationale de France, MS Allemand 106, with Hartlieb's text beginning at fol. 178r. Much of the manuscript's contents are described thoroughly in two entries in the *Katalog der deutschsprachigen illustrierten Handschriften des Mittelalters*, but the *Mondwahrsagebuch* images are entirely overlooked in both: Pia Rudolph and Polina Gedova, "Medizin: Handschrift Nr. 87.2.14," in Freienhagen-Baumgardt et al., *Katalog der deutschsprachigen illustrierten Handschriften des Mittelalters (KdiH)*, vol. 9; Ulrike Bodemann, "Astrologie/Astronomie: Handschrift Nr. 11.4.16," in *Katalog der deutschsprachigen illustrierten Handschriften des Mittelalters (KdiH)*, ed. Norbert H. Ott, Ulrike Bodemann, and Gisela Fischer-Heetfeld, vol. 1 (Munich: Beck, 1991), https://kdih.badw.de/datenbank/handschrift/11/4/16 (accessed August 1, 2024).

129. Wolfenbüttel, Herzog August Bibliothek, Cod. Guelf. 29.14 Aug. 4°, fols. 1r–24v.

130. Vienna, Österreichische Nationalbibliothek, Cod. 4417*, fol. 19v.

CHAPTER 4. INTO PRINT: INTERNATIONAL INTERMEDIALITY

1. *Fasciculus medicinae* (Venice: Johannes and Gregorius de Gregoriis, 1491). This book is Incunabula Short Title Catalogue (hereafter ISTC) number ik00013000. All incunables in this chapter are cited with an ISTC number, their identifier in the key international online database of fifteenth-century European printing: Incunabula Short Title Catalogue, https://data.cerl

.org/istc/ (accessed August 1, 2024). ISTC entries also include links to further information on the same titles in the Gesamtkatalog der Wiegendrucke (hereafter GW), its German-language equivalent, which can be harder to search digitally but often includes more detailed information: Gesamtkatalog der Wiegendrucke, https://www.gesamtkatalogderwiegendrucke.de (accessed August 1, 2024). For consistency and to aid ISTC searching, I cite works using their title in the book's primary language specifically as given in their ISTC entry, as well as their printer's name using the ISTC's particular phrasing. However, while these details appear fixed and certain in such catalogs, they are in fact often a matter of debate within the scholarship. This process also results in some unusual historiographical quirks, for instance the frequent appearance of authors' or printers' names with atypical spellings or in their Latin derivation. These inconsistencies are often inherited from the changeable colophons or title pages of late medieval incunables themselves.

2. These ideas of early modern exchange are explored more fully in chapter 5. For recent art historical work on the virality and translation of early modern prints, especially across regional and national contexts, see Stephanie Porras, *The First Viral Images: Maerten de Vos, Antwerp Print, and the Early Modern Globe* (University Park, PA: Penn State University Press, 2023); Aaron M. Hyman, *Rubens in Repeat: The Logic of the Copy in Colonial Latin America* (Los Angeles: GRI, 2021); Suzanne Karr Schmidt and Edward H. Wouk, eds., *Prints in Translation, 1450–1750: Image, Materiality, Space* (London: Routledge, 2017).

3. Peter Parshall, "The Modem Historiography of Early Printmaking," in *The Woodcut in Fifteenth-Century Europe*, ed. Peter Parshall (New Haven, CT: Yale University Press, 2009), 9–15. The clearest English-language works introducing different aspects of Europe's early printed books and printed images are Falk Eisermann, "The Gutenberg Galaxy's Dark Matter: Lost Incunabula, and Ways to Retrieve Them," in *Lost Books: Reconstructing the Print World of Pre-Industrial Europe*, ed. Flavia Bruni and Andrew Pettegree (Leiden: Brill, 2016), 31–54; Parshall and Schoch, *Origins of European Printmaking*; Suzanne Karr Schmidt and Kimberly Nichols, *Altered and Adorned: Using Renaissance Prints in Daily Life* (New Haven, CT: Yale University Press, 2011); Kristian Jensen, ed., *Incunabula and Their Readers: Printing, Selling, and Using Books in the Fifteenth Century* (London: British Library, 2003); David Landau and Peter Parshall, *The Renaissance Print 1470–1550* (New Haven, CT: Yale University Press, 1994).

4. For instance, see the influential work by Elizabeth L. Eisenstein, *The Printing Press as an Agent of Change* (Cambridge: Cambridge University Press, 1979), whose arguments—and the critical responses to them—have been much discussed. Among the first and keenest to take issue with Eisenstein's picture of wholesale and speedy revolution were Paul Needham, "Review: The Printing Press as an Agent of Change," *Fine Print* 6 (1980): 23–35; Anthony T. Grafton, "The Importance of Being Printed," *Journal of Interdisciplinary History* 11, no. 2 (1980): 265–86. Eisenstein responded to Grafton and others in "An Unacknowledged Revolution Revisited," *American Historical Review* 107, no. 1 (2002): 87–105.

5. For a recent example of each of these respective approaches, see Oren Margolis, *Aldus Manutius: The Invention of the Publisher* (London: Reaktion, 2023); Lotte Hellinga, *Incunabula in Transit: People and Trade* (Leiden: Brill, 2018); Cristina Dondi, ed., *Printing R-Evolution and Society 1450–1500* (Venice: Ca' Foscari, 2020).

6. These useful numbers are taken from Cristina Dondi, "The European Printing Revolution," in *The Book: A Global History*, ed. Michael F. Suarez and Henry R. Woudhuysen (Oxford: Oxford University Press, 2013), 80–92.

7. Sabrina Minuzzi rightly bemoans that the lack of serious attention paid to fifteenth-century European medical material, especially in relation to the writing of early modern medical history at large, has left "Renaissance medicine" entirely synonymous with only the sixteenth century: "La stampa medico-scientifica nell'Europa del XV secolo: Con cenni sulla fruizione dei libri di materia medica e ricettari," in Dondi, *Printing R-Evolution and Society*, 199–251. As well as in Minuzzi's work, early printed medicine is surveyed in Jon Arrizabalaga, "Medical Genres in the Early Printing Press," in *Écritures médicales: Discours et genres, de la tradition antique à l'époque moderne*, ed. Laurence Moulinier-Brogi and Marilyn Nicoud (Lyon-Avignon: CIHAM, 2019), 311–34; Vivian Nutton, "Books, Printing, and Medicine in the Renaissance," *Medicina nei secoli* 17, no. 2 (2005): 421–42. Three classic surveys of the genre, now somewhat dated but that remain useful, are Thomas E. Keys, "The Earliest Medical Books Printed with Moveable Type," *Library Quarterly* 10, no. 2 (1940): 220–30; Arnold C. Klebs, *Incunabula scientifica et medica* (Bruges: Saint Catherine Press, 1938); William Osler, *Incunabula Medica: A Study of the Earliest Printed Medical Books 1467–1480* (New York: Garrison & Morton, 1923).

8. The earliest examples of printed works by these Classical medical authors currently known are Celsus, *De medicina* (Florence: Nicolaus Laurentii, 1478), ISTC ic00364000; Dioscorides, *De materia medica* (Colle di Val d'Elsa: Johannes de Medemblick, 1478), ISTC id00261000; Serapion, *Liber Serapionis aggregatus in medicinis simplicibus* (Milan: Antonius Zarotus, 1473), ISTC is00467000; Hippocrates, *De natura hominis* (Rome: Georgius Herolt, c. 1481), ISTC ih00277500.

9. The work's earliest known printing is *Articella* (Padua: Nicolaus Petri, c. 1476), ISTC ia01142500. On its printed emergence, see Jon Arrizabalaga, *The Articella in the Early Press, c. 1476–1534* (Cambridge: Wellcome Unit/CSIC, 1998); Tiziana Pesenti, "Editoria medica tra Quattro e Cinquecento: L'*Articella* e il *Fasciculus medicine*," in *Trattati scientifici nel Veneto fra il XV e XVI secolo*, ed. Ezio Riondato (Venice: Pozza, 1985), 1–29.

10. Mundinus, *Anatomia* (Padua: Petrus Maufer, c. 1475), ISTC im00871200; Gentilis Fulginas, *De balneis* (Padua: Johannes de Reno, 1473), ISTC ig00133000; Avicenna, *Canones medicinae* (probably Padua: printer unknown, 1472), ISTC ia01427400.

11. Mesue, *Opera* (Venice: Clemens Patavinus, after May 1471), ISTC im00508000; Nicolaus Salernitanus, *Antidotarium* (Venice: Nicolaus Jenson, 1471), ISTC in00160000. Evidence that healthy trade in medical books continued in Venice after this early date can be found in the so-called *Zornale* of the bookseller Francesco de Madiis, a key source for the history of

incunable printing in the city. There, Madiis lists sales, inventory, and barters relating to his Venetian bookshop over the course of three and a half years, including among them a line noting his acquisition in 1484 of a copy of the *Almansor Rasis*, an early medical work by al-Rāzī that had been circulating in print since the mid-1470s. For a summary of the *Zornale*, see Cristina Dondi and Neil Harris, "Oil and Green Ginger: The *Zornale* of the Venetian Bookseller Francesco de Madiis, 1484–1488," in *Documenting the Early Modern Book World: Inventories and Catalogues in Manuscript and Print*, ed. Malcolm Walsby and Natasha Constantinidou (Leiden: Brill, 2013), 341–406.

12. Rhasis, *Liber ad Almansorem* (Milan: Leonardus Pachel and Uldericus Scinzenzeler, 1481), ISTC ir00175000; Arnoldus de Villa Nova, *De arte cognoscendi venena* (Mantua: Johannes Vurster, 1473), ISTC ia01065900; Benevenutus Grassus, *De oculis eorumque aegritudinibus et curis* (Ferrara: Severinus Ferrariensis, c. 1474), ISTC ig00352000; Antonius Cermisonus, *Consiglio per preservar della peste* (Naples: Jodocus Hohenstein, 1475/1476), ISTC ic00401000; Moses Maimonides, *De regimine sanitatis ad Soldanum Babyloniae* (Florence: Apud Sanctum Jacobum de Ripoli, c. 1481), ISTC im00080000.

13. Ortolff von Bayerlandt, *Arzneibuch* (Augsburg: Günther Zainer, c. 1477), ISTC io00109000; *Die Ordnung der Gesundheit* (Nuremberg: Friedrich Creussner, c. 1472), ISTC ir00046000; Bartholomaeus Metlinger, *Ein Regiment der jungen Kinder* (Augsburg: Günther Zainer,1473), ISTC im00527000. The broadest survey of this German material remains Karl Sudhoff, *Deutsche medizinische Inkunabeln* (Leipzig: Barth, 1908). For an extensive discussion of the problems and opportunities afforded by the genre of single-sheet broadsides at large, see Falk Eisermann and Volker Honemann, "Die ersten typographischen Einblattdrucke," *Gutenberg-Jahrbuch* 75 (2000): 88–131; Volker Honemann et al., eds., *Einblattdrucke des 15. und frühen 16. Jahrhunderts: Probleme, Perspektiven, Fallstudien* (Tübingen: Niemeyer, 2000). On *Pestblätter* specifically, see Erik A. Heinrichs, *Plague, Print, and the Reformation: The German Reform of Healing 1473–1573* (Abingdon: Routledge, 2018).

14. Guilelmus de Saliceto, *De salute corporis* (The Netherlands: printer unknown, before 1472), ISTC is00029500.

15. Lanfrancus Mediolanensis, *Chirurgia* (Lyon: printer unknown, c. 1480), ISTC il00050900; Guido de Cauliaco, *Chirurgia* (Lyon: Nicolaus Philippi and Marcus Reinhart, 1478), ISTC ig00560700.

16. This percentage is cited in Dondi, "The European Printing Revolution," 85. Dondi's 15cBOOKTRADE Project cataloged some 940 works as "medical," from a total output of 30,243 fifteenth-century books: 15cBOOKTRADE, https://15cbooktrade.ox.ac.uk (accessed August 1, 2024).

17. The best summary of this genre is Richard L. Kremer, "Incunable Almanacs and *Practica* as Practical Knowledge Produced in Trading Zones," in *The Structures of Practical Knowledge*, ed. Matteo Valleriani (Cham: Springer, 2017), 333–69. Although outdated in some of its information, still useful for German materials is Karl Sudhoff, "Laßtafelkunst in Drucken des 15. Jahrhunderts," *Archiv für Geschichte der Medizin* 1, nos. 3/4 (1908): 219–88.

18. On this genre, see Jonathan Green, *Printing and Prophecy: Prognostication and Media Change 1450–1550* (Ann Arbor: University of Michigan Press, 2012).

19. On these ordinances, see Leonhard Hoffmann, "Almanache des 15. und 16. Jahrhunderts und ihre Käufer," *Beiträge zur Inkunabelkunde* 3, no. 8 (1983): 130–43.

20. *Aderlasskalender* (Mainz: Printer unknown, 1456), ISTC ia00051700.

21. The earliest editions of these texts currently known are Aristoteles, *De animalibus* (Venice: Johannes de Colonia and Johannes Manthen, 1476), ISTC ia00973000; Gaius Plinius Secundus, *Historia naturalis* (Rome: Conradus Sweynheym and Arnoldus Pannartz, 1473), ISTC ip00789000; Hrabanus Maurus, *Opus de universo* (Strassburg: The R-Printer, before July 1474), ISTC ir00001000.

22. See, for instance, Michael Puff von Schrick, *Von den ausgebrannten Wassern* (Augsburg: Johann Bämler, 1476), ISTC is00324500; Pseudo-Albertus Magnus, *Liber aggregationis* (Strassburg: Printer of the Breviarium Ratisponense, c. 1474–1479), ISTC ia00249500; Arnoldus de Villa Nova, *Von Bewahrung und Bereitung der Weine* (Esslingen: Conrad Fyner, after October 1478), ISTC ia01080000; Petrus de Crescentiis, *Ruralia commoda* (Augsburg: Johann Schüssler, c. 1471), ISTC ic00965000.

23. Albertus de Eyb, *Ehebüchlein* (Nuremberg: Friedrich Creussner, 1472), ISTC ie00180000; *Vocabularius* (Eltville: Nicolaus Bechtermüntze, 1469), ISTC iv00361800.

24. Minuzzi, "La stampa medico-scientifica nell'Europa del XV secolo," 200ff.

25. For a detailed general outline of images in early European printed books, see Andrea Franklin, "Woodcuts," in *Book Parts*, ed. Dennis Duncan and Adam Smyth (Oxford: Oxford University Press, 2019), 209–22; Paul Needham, "Prints in the Early Printing Shops," in Parshall, *The Woodcut in Fifteenth-Century Europe*, 38–91.

26. Why this particular genre has been the subject of so much interest is unclear. Perhaps it is the location of such herbals at an interdisciplinary nexus between art history, the history of medicine, and the history of technology. Or perhaps it is the role played by such technical pharmaceutical literature in broader debates about the "printing revolution," which feature prominently, for instance, in Eisenstein, *The Printing Press as an Agent of Change*, 453ff. Useful recent studies of the herbal tradition are Andrew Griebler, *Botanical Icons: Critical Practices of Illustration in the Premodern Mediterranean* (Chicago: University of Chicago Press, 2024); Brent Elliott, "The World of the Renaissance Herbal," *Renaissance Studies* 25, no. 1 (2011): 24–41; Minta Collins, *Medieval Herbals: The Illustrative Traditions* (London: British Library, 2000); Jerry Stannard, *Herbs and Herbalism in the Middle Ages and Renaissance* (London: Routledge, 1999).

27. Konrad von Megenberg, *Buch der Natur* (Augsburg: Johann Bämler, 1475), ISTC ic00842000. For more on the *Buch der Natur*, see chapter 3.

28. *Herbarium Apulei* (Rome: Johannes Philippus de Lignamine, c. 1481–1482), ISTC ih00058000. For an overview of this herbal and its unusual place in the history of early printing, see Dominic Olariu, "The Misfortune of Philippus de Lignamine's Herbal, or New Research Perspectives in Herbal Illustrations from an Iconological Point of View," in *Early Modern Print Culture in Central Europe*, ed. Stefan Kiedroń, Anna-Maria Rimm,

and Patrycja Poniatowska (Wrocław: Wydawnictwo Uniwersytetu Wrocławskiego, 2014), 39–62.

29. *Herbarius latinus* (Mainz: Peter Schoeffer, 1484), ISTC ih00062000.

30. *Herbarius latinus* (Speyer: Johann and Conrad Hist, 1484), ISTC ih00063000; *Herbarius latinus* (Leuven: Johann Veldener, after February 1486), ISTC ih00059000; *Herbarius latinus* (Paris: Jean Bonhomme, c. 1486), ISTC ih00061000; *Gart der Gesundheit* (Mainz: Peter Schöffer, 1485), ISTC ig00097000; *Hortus sanitatis* (Mainz: Jacob Meydenbach, 1491), ISTC ih00486000. On these works, see Andrea van Leerdam, "Popularising and Personalising an Illustrated Herbal in Dutch," *Nuncius* 36, no. 2 (2021): 356–93; Pia Rudolph, *Im Garten der Gesundheit: Pflanzenbilder zwischen Natur, Kunst und Wissen in gedruckten Kräuterbüchern des 15. Jahrhunderts* (Cologne: Böhlau 2020); Brigitte Baumann and Helmut Baumann, *Die Mainzer Kräuterbuch-Inkunabeln* (Stuttgart: Hiersemann, 2010).

31. Gutenberg himself was bankrupted by his printing, and medical works were significant culprits in the downfall of printers even at the end of the century. In 1500, the Venetian printers Zacharias Callierges and Nicolaos Vlastos produced a luxury Greek-language edition of Galen's *Method of Healing* that effectively ended their enterprise. On this affair, see Nutton, "Books, Printing, and Medicine in the Renaissance," 423. For the financial complexities of early printing more generally, see John L. Flood, "'*Volentes sibi comparare infrascriptos libros impressos* . . .': Printed Books as a Commercial Commodity in the Fifteenth Century," in Jensen, *Incunabula and Their Readers*, 139–51; Neil Harris, "Costs We Don't Think About: Rubrication and Illumination. An Unusual Copy of Franciscus de Platea, *Opus restitutionum* (1474), and a Few Other Items," in Dondi, *Printing R-Evolution and Society*, 511–40, although the very fact that Harris labels visual elements as a set of "costs we don't think about" only serves to emphasize the textual bias of most current incunable studies.

32. On the circulation of herbal woodblocks, especially in a sixteenth- and seventeenth-century context, see Bruce T. Moran, "Preserving the Cutting Edge: Traveling Woodblocks, Material Networks, and Visualizing Plants in Early Modern Europe," in Valleriani, *The Structures of Practical Knowledge*, 393–419. For a case study in reused French blocks, see Diane E. Booton, *Publishing Networks in France in the Early Era of Print* (London: Routledge, 2018), 53–80.

33. The manuscript is now Montecassino, Archivio della Badia, Cod. 97.

34. On the problem of reading the development of herbals as an inevitable part of the development of print technology, see Sabrina Minuzzi, "15th-Century Practical Medicine in Print: Beyond the Profession, Towards the *miscere utile dulci*," *Nuncius* 36, no. 2 (2021): 199–263.

35. Sachiko Kusukawa, *Picturing the Book of Nature: Image, Text, and Argument in Sixteenth-Century Human Anatomy and Medical Botany* (Chicago: University of Chicago Press, 2012). See also Florike Egmond, *Eye for Detail: Images of Plants and Animals in Art and Science 1500–1630* (London: Reaktion, 2016); Claudia Swan, "The Uses of Realism in Early Modern Illustrated Botany," in *Visualizing Medieval Medicine and Natural History, 1200–1550*, ed. Jean A. Givens, Karen M. Reeds, and Alan Touwaide (Burlington: Ashgate, 2006), 239–49; Brian W. Ogilvie, *The Science of Describing: Natural History in Renaissance Europe* (Chicago: University of Chicago Press, 2006).

36. Folz claimed his self-publishing as an act of proto-copyrighting, guarding against the false replication of his work. On Folz generally, see Caroline Huey, *Hans Folz and Print Culture in Late Medieval Germany* (New York: Routledge, 2017); Ursula Rautenberg, "Das Werk als Ware: Der Nürnberger Kleindrucker Hans Folz," *Internationales Archiv fur Sozialgeschichte der deutschen Literatur* 24 (1999): 1–40; Aaron E. Wright, "'*Die gotlich sterk gab daz der teutschen zungen*': Folz, Schedel, and the Printing Press in Fifteenth-Century Nuremberg," *Fifteenth Century Studies* 19 (1992): 319–49; Hans Folz, *Die Reimpaarsprüche*, ed. Hanns Fischer (Munich: Beck, 1961).

37. Hans Folz, *Kalenderparodie* (Nuremberg: Hans Folz, c. 1479), ISTC if00239150. On parody almanacs, see Silvia Pfister, *Parodien astrologisch-prophetischen Schrifttums 1470–1590: Textform—Entstehung—Vermittlung—Funktion* (Baden-Baden: Koerner, 1990).

38. Hans Folz, *Von einem griechischen Arzt* (Nuremberg: Hans Folz, 1479), ISTC if00239220.

39. Hans Folz, *Von der Pestilenz* (Nuremberg: Hans Folz, 1482), ISTC if00239550.

40. Hippocrates and Galen appear in *Von der Pestilenz*. Saint Sebastian appears in Folz's prose version of the same text, *Von der Pestilenz* (Nuremberg: Hans Folz, 1482), ISTC if00239200. Other images are known through reprinting of Folz's work by other nearby presses, including Hans Folz, *Vom Branntwein* (Bamberg: Marx Ayrer und Hans Bernecker, 1493), ISTC if00239290; Hans Folz, *Von den Bädern* (Nuremberg: Hans Mair, before 1495), ISTC if00239230; a version plagiarized by Clement von Graz, *Von den Bädern* (Brünn: Conrad Stahel and Mathias Preunlein, 1495), ISTC ic00740200.

41. Bartholomaeus Anglicus, *Van den proprieteyten der dinghen* (Haarlem: Jacob Bellaert, 1485), ISTC ib00142000.

42. On Blaubirer's example specifically, see Francis B. Brévart, "Johann Blaubirers Kalender von 1481 und 1483: Traditionsgebundenheit und experimentelle Innovation," *Gutenberg-Jahrbuch* 63 (1988): 74–83.

43. Francis B. Brévart, "The German 'Volkskalender' of the Fifteenth Century," *Speculum* 63, no. 2 (1988): 312–42. A summary of the Iatromathematical Housebook tradition, as well as discussion of the difficulties produced by this term, can be found in Bernhard Schnell, *Arzneibücher—Kräuterbücher—Wörterbücher: Kleine Schriften zur Text- und Überlieferungsgeschichte mittelalterlicher Gebrauchsliteratur* (Würzburg: Königshauses & Neuman, 2019), especially 223–54; Pia Rudolph, "Hausbücher (Nr. 49a)," in *Katalog der deutschsprachigen illustrierten Handschriften des Mittelalters (KdiH)*, ed. Ulrike Bodemann et al., vol. 6 (Munich: Beck, 2015), https://kdih.badw.de/datenbank/stoffgruppe/49a (accessed August 1, 2024); Carmela Giordano, "Ruolo e funzione delle immagini nei testi scientifici del medioevo tedesco: Considerazioni su due Hausbücher," in *Testo e immagine nel medioevo germanico*, ed. Maria Grazia Saibene and Marina Buzzoni (Milan: Parole, 2001), 268–76; Keil, Lenhardt, and Weisser, *Vom Einfluss der Gestirne auf die Gesundheit und den Charakter des Menschen*. Xylographic printed precedents of this tradition remain poorly understood,

but they include Heidelberg, Universitätsbibliothek, Cpg 438; Wolfenbüttel, Herzog August Bibliothek, Cod. Guelf. 1189 Helmst.; Washington, DC, Library of Congress, Rosenwald Collection, Incun. 1474 .M82.

44. *Kalender* (Augsburg: Johann Blaubirer, 1483), ISTC ik00001500.

45. These figures are calculated from works in the Gesamtkatalog der Wiegendrucke listed under "Kalender, Deutscher."

46. *Calendrier des Bergers* (Paris: Guy Marchant, 1491), ISTC ic00053800. For a summary of the *Calendrier* tradition and a facsimile of an edition of 1493, see Max Engammare, ed., *Calendrier des Bergers* (Paris: Fondation Martin Bodmer, 2008).

47. Heinrich von Laufenberg, *Versehung des Leibes* (Augsburg: Erhard Ratdolt, 1491), ISTC ih00013000. This figure is a decorative herald of bloodletting rather than a specifically functional figure, similar to several manuscript images discussed in chapter 3. For more on Laufenberg, see the historical materials accompanying an edition of his *Regimen de Gesundheit* in Bernhard Schnell and Marlis Stähli, eds., *Heinrich Laufenberg: Regimen der Gesundheit* (Munich: Lengenfelder, 1998), 7–28.

48. Johannes Stöffler, *Calendarium Romanum magnum* (Oppenheim: Jakob Köbel, 1518). As a work produced after 1501, Stöffler's book falls outside the remit of the ISTC but is included in the Universal Short Title Catalogue (hereafter USTC) as number 617753. Works after this date will be cited here with their USTC numbers. If not present in the USTC, they will instead be listed alongside the shelfmark of a copy held in a major library collection, for ease of location. On calendrical debates in this and earlier periods, see C. Philipp E. Nothaft, *Scandalous Error: Calendar Reform and Calendrical Astronomy in Medieval Europe* (Oxford: Oxford University Press, 2018).

49. That said, as Falk Eisermann has shown, the incunable market also often courted the same elite clientele as its manuscript forebears: "Mixing Pop and Politics: Origins, Transmission, and Readers of Illustrated Broadsides in Fifteenth-Century Germany," in Jensen, *Incunabula and Their Readers*, 159–77.

50. On Prüss, see Catarina Zimmermann-Homeyer, "Spuren eines drucktechnischen Experiments in den Holzschnitten der Terenz-Ausgaben des Straßburger Frühdruckers Johann Prüß," *Gutenberg-Jahrbuch* 94 (2019): 129–50; Miriam Usher Chrisman, *Lay Culture, Learned Culture: Books and Social Change in Strasbourg, 1480–1599* (New Haven, CT: Yale University Press, 1982), 16ff; François Ritter, "Les successeurs de l'imprimeur Jean Prüss (Père)," *Gutenberg-Jahrbuch* 26 (1951): 101–9.

51. *Kalender* (Strassburg: Johann Prüss, c. 1483), ISTC ik00002500. Other medical works produced by Prüss include the *Antidotarium* of Nicholas of Salerno—which in c. 1483 he combined with works by Ibn Māsawaiyh and al-Zahrāwī (ISTC in00163000)—and a *Hortus sanitatis* from c. 1497 (ISTC ih00488000).

52. *Martyrologium der Heiligen nach dem Kalender* (Strassburg: Johann Prüss, 1484), ISTC im00340000. According to the text's prologue, the work was translated into German by Alsatian Franciscans during Advent 1483.

53. Given their popularity, it is possible that Prüss's combination of religious and calendrical material here may have influenced other printers, such as the Parisians Antoine Vérard and Jean Du Pré, who from the late 1480s began to experiment with highly illustrated printed Books of Hours. These texts often opened their dense pages with a religious calendar fronted by a semi-anatomized Zodiac Man highly similar to Prüss's figure—sometimes known now as the Planetary Man—with a characteristic distended belly opened and connected by lines to miniature representations of the seven planets and personifications of the four temperaments. See, for instance, the figure in *Horae* (Paris: Antoine Caillaut for Antoine Vérard, 1488), ISTC ih00359642. In 1490, the Kirchheim printer Markus Reinhard produced a very similar Book of Hours whose imagery connects even more directly with German traditions. Fittingly for the town's location close to Prüss's Strasbourg, his Zodiac Man wears the same blue underpants as those sported by the *Dreibilderserie* figures: *Horae* (Kirchheim in Elsass: Marcus Reinhart, 1490), ISTC ih00366000. For a summary of early printed Books of Hours across Europe, see Cristina Dondi, "Books of Hours: The Development of the Texts in Printed Form," in Jensen, *Incunabula and Their Readers*, 53–70. The genre is exhaustively surveyed in the Gesamtkatalog der Wiegendrucke, listed under "Horae."

54. By this point in the century, almanacs contained a wide range of imagery. At the following ISTC numbers, images can be found depicting the Nativity (ISTC ih00484000), the moon (ISTC ia00503300), various saints (ISTC ih00484230), astrological diagrams (ISTC ia00508100), zodiacal imagery (ISTC if00000700, ISTC if00000750, ISTC ia00516830), planetary personifications (ISTC ia00517500), medical parodies (ISTC ia00157150), and gilded initials (ISTC ia00507900). Zodiac figures continued to be reproduced in almanacs well into the eighteenth century, especially in German-speaking lands. For a summary of images in early almanacs by iconography, see Catarina Zimmermann-Homeyer, "Illustrated Almanacs: Imaging Strategies in Bloodletting Calendars of the Incunabula Period," *Gutenberg Jahrbuch* 97 (2022): 118–45. On the pictorial puzzles posed by a single almanac, see Peter Amelung, "Zum Bilderschmuck der frühen Einblattkalender: Probleme um einen Augsburger Almanach auf das Jahr 1496 (GW 1513)," *Gutenberg-Jahrbuch* 55 (1980): 235–45. On the forms and prices of almanacs into the sixteenth century, see Sachiko Kusukawa, "Andreas Nolthius' *Almanach* for 1575," *Journal of the History of Astronomy* 42, no. 1 (2011): 91–110.

55. *Almanac* (Strassburg: Johann Prüss, c. 1484), ISTC ia00505200.

56. *Almanac* (Strassburg: Johann Prüss, c. 1494), ISTC ia00518150. Other printers were also taking note. Before the end of the century, bloodletting figures appeared in calendars printed by Johann Grüninger (ISTC ia00517930), Leinhart Ysenhut (ISTC iw00070040), Peter Wagner (ISTC ia00520450), Caspar Hochfeder (ISTC ia00520000), Peter Schöffer (ISTC ia00052000), Johann Schäffler (ISTC ia00051800), Martin Landsberg (ISTC if00004700), and Ambrosius Huber (ia00052850).

57. *Almanac* (Basel: Printer of the Form der Copyen, c. 1489–1490), ISTC ia00516050.

58. Konrad von Megenberg, *Buch der Natur* (Augsburg: Johann Bämler, 1475), ISTC ic00842000.

59. The Gregori brothers typically latinized their names in their books, printing as "Johannes et Gregorius de Gregoriis." For a useful short summary of the Gregoris'

career, see Natalie Lussey Seale, "The Gregori Brothers," in New York Academy of Medicine, "Facendo Il Libro: The Making of *Fasciculus medicinae*, an Early Printed Anatomy" (online exhibition), https://digitalcollections.nyam.org/digital/gregori (accessed August 1, 2024). A more detailed biography can be found in Tiziana Pesenti, "Di Gregori, Giovanni e Gregorio," *Dizionario Biografico degli Italiani* 36 (1988), https://www.treccani.it/enciclopedia/de-gregori-giovanni-e-gregorio_%28Dizionario-Biografico%29/ (accessed August 1, 2024). On early print in Venice more generally, see Rosa Salzberg, *Ephemeral City: Cheap Print and Urban Culture in Renaissance Venice* (Manchester: Manchester University Press, 2014); Angela Nuovo, *The Book Trade in the Italian Renaissance* (Leiden: Brill, 2013); Mario Infelise, "Book Publishing and the Circulation of Information," in *A Companion to Venetian History, 1400–1797*, ed. Eric R. Dursteler (Leiden: Brill, 2013), 651–74; Tiziana Plebani, *Venezia 1469: La legge e la stampa* (Venice: Marsilio, 2004); Dennis E. Rhodes, *Silent Printers: Anonymous Printing at Venice in the Sixteenth Century* (London: British Library, 1995); and the classic by Horatio F. Brown, *The Venetian Printing Press* (London: Nimmo, 1891).

60. For example, Cicero's *Tusculanae disputationes* (ISTC ic00637000), *De inventione* (ISTC ic00648000), and *Orationes* (ISTC ic00545500); Valerius Maximus's *Facta et dicta memorabilia* (ISTC iv00033000); Horace's collected *Opera* (ISTC ih00448000); and Terence's *Comoediae* (ISTC it00081230).

61. *Frottola di un Caligaro* (ISTC if00325500); *Storia della battaglia di Campo Morto* (ISTC is00791200).

62. The legal phase appears to have begun in 1484 with the printing of three large Justinianic legal texts and commentaries: *Digestum vetus* (ISTC ij00549500); *Codex Justinianus* (ISTC ij00580000); *Digestum inforiatum* (ISTC ij00557300).

63. The ISTC and the GW part ways on the attribution to the Gregori brothers of some of these early texts, but candidates for their early printed medical works include Franciscus Guasconus, *Prognosticon* (1482–1483), ISTC ig00539070; *Kalendarium* (c. 1486), ISTC ik00000543; Paulus de Middelburgo, *Prognosticon* (c. 1485–1486), ISTC ip00185400; Bernardus de Granollachs, *Lunarium* (1488–1489), ISTC ig00338000; Johannes Antonius Mahomerius, *Prognosticon* (1491–1492), ISTC im00056600; Guillelmus de Saliceto, *Summa conservationis et curationis* (1489), ISTC is00033000; Guillelmus de Saliceto, *Summa conservationis et curationis* (1490), ISTC is00034000; Michael Scotus, *Liber physiognomiae* (1490), ISTC im00561000; Albertus Magnus, *Physica* (1488–1489), ISTC ia00299000; Albertus Magnus, *De coelo et mundo* (1490), ISTC ia00227000; Antonius Gazius, *Corona florida medicinae* (1491), ISTC ig00111000.

64. Avenzohar, *Liber Teisir* (1490–1491), ISTC ia01408000; Aristoteles, *De animalibus* (1492), ISTC ia00974000; Bernardus de Gordonio, *Lilium medicinae* (1496–1497), ISTC ib00450000; Johannes Mesue, *Opera medicinalia* (1497), ISTC im00517000; Avicenna, *De animalibus* (c. 1500), ISTC ia01416000; *Articella* (c. 1500), ISTC ia01147000; *Articella* (1502), ISTC ia01147500; Alexander Benedictus, *De observatione in pestilentia* (1493), ISTC ib00320420; Alexander Benedictus, *Collectiones medicinae* (c. 1493), ISTC ib00320380.

65. On the *Fasciculus medicinae* generally, see Pia Eckhart, "Medial Translations and Material Manifestations: The *Fasciculus medicinae* in Physician-Patient Interaction," in *Between Manuscript and Print: Transcultural Perspectives, ca. 1400–1800*, ed. Sylvia Brockstieger and Paul Schweitzer-Martin (Berlin: De Gruyter, 2023), 43–88; Taylor McCall, "The *Fasciculus Medicinae*: An Introduction to the Images and Texts," Facendo Il Libro, https://digitalcollections.nyam.org/digital/fasciculusmedicinae (accessed August 1, 2024); Christian Coppens, *De vele levens van een boek: De Fasciculus medicinae opnieuw bekeken* (Brussels: Koninklijke Academie voor Geneeskunde van België, 2009); Pesenti, *Fasiculo de medicina in volgare; The Fasciculus medicinae of Johannes de Ketham, Alemanus: Facsimile of the First (Venetian) Edition of 1491*, trans. Charles Singer and Luke Demaitre (Birmingham: Classics of Medicine Library, 1988); *Der Fasciculus medicinae des Johannes de Ketham, Alemannus: Facsimile des Venetianer Erstdruckes von 1491*, with commentary by Karl Sudhoff (Milan: Lier, 1924).

66. On medieval uroscopic images, see Carly B. Boxer, "Uroscopy Diagrams, Judgment, and the Perception of Color in Late Medieval England," *Word & Image* 38, no. 4 (2022): 327–47. On the use of color in the *Fasciculus* uroscopic images specifically, see Stefanie Zaun and Hans Geisler, "Die Harnfarbbezeichnungen im *Fasciculus medicine* und ihre italienischen und spanischen Übersetzungen," in *Farbe im Mittelalter: Materialität—Medialität—Semantik*, ed. Ingrid Bennewitz and Andrea Schindler (Berlin: Akademie, 2011), 969–85.

67. This text, beginning *Vena in medio frontis* (Vein in the middle of the forehead), and a second phlebotomy treatise that follows, known to modern scholars as the *Venarum minutio* text, are both very close to texts that appear in phlebotomical manuscripts from earlier centuries, as discussed in chapter 1.

68. On the Disease Woman's accompanying texts, see Britta-Juliane Kruse, *Verborgene Heilkünste: Geschichte der Frauenmedizin im Spätmittelalter* (Berlin: De Gruyter, 2012), 23–30; Ferckel, "Zur Gynäkologie und Generationslehre im *Fasciculus medicinae* des Johannes de Ketham." See also discussion of the manuscript versions of the figure in chapter 2.

69. The *Fasciculus*'s final few pages are taken up by an unillustrated treatise on plague originally written by the late fourteenth-century physician Pietro da Tossignano, a professor of medicine and later private physician to the Visconti. Tossignano wrote his *Consilium pro peste evitanda* (Strategy for Evading the Plague) in the late fourteenth century, and it was first printed in Venice several decades before the *Fasciculus*: Petrus de Tussignano, *De peste* (Venice: printer unknown, c. 1472), ISTC ip00536000.

70. The colophons appear at the end of the Disease Man's associated texts but before the *Fasciculus*'s closing plague tract, emphasizing the booklet's conception of its *Dreibilderserie* material as a discrete and coherent unit.

71. On Monferrato, see Pesenti, *Fasiculo de medicina in volgare*, 1:54–67.

72. Sudhoff comments on Ketham in a number of locations, especially articles in the first two decades of the twentieth century published in the *Archiv für Geschichte der Medizin*, all of which found fruition in his commentary on a facsimile of the booklet: *Der Fasciculus medicinae*, 41–43.

73. The arguments are summarized in Coppens, *De vele levens van een boek*, 9ff; Pesenti, *Fasiculo de medicina in volgare*, 1:47ff.

74. Pesenti, *Fasiculo de medicina in volgare*, 1:43ff. The text reads: "*Ista residua deficiunt in aliquibus marginibus figure precedentis vbi consimiles littere alphabeti comprehenduntur*" (The remaining are missing in some of the margins of the previous figure, where similar alphabetical keys can be found).

75. Such a situation is not unusual, although, intriguingly, the Gregori brothers are associated with a rare case in which the original manuscript used to derive one of their printed works still survives. For a description of this case and further bibliography, see Pesenti, *Fasiculo de medicina in volgare*, 1:43n30.

76. Pesenti, *Fasiculo de medicina in volgare*, 1:46.

77. On Venetian-German publishing links, see Bettina Pfotenhauer, *Nürnberg und Venedig im Austausch: Menschen, Güter, und Wissen an der Wende vom Mittelalter zur Neuzeit* (Regensburg: Schnell & Steiner, 2016); Nuovo, *The Book Trade in the Italian Renaissance*; Marino Zorzi, "Stampatori tedeschi a Venezia," in *Venezia e la Germania: Arte, politica, commercio*, ed. Susanna Biadene (Milan: Electa, 1986), 115–40. On commercial connections between Venice and Germany, see Uwe Israel, "Brokers as German-Italian Cultural Mediators in Renaissance Venice," in *Migrating Words, Migrating Merchants, Migrating Law: Trading Routes and the Development of Commercial Law*, ed. Stefania Gialdroni et al. (Leiden: Brill, 2020), 95–117; Philippe Braunstein, *Les Allemands à Venise (1380–1520)* (Rome: École française, 2016).

78. The fragment appears in a copy of the Gregoris' edition of Horace's *Opera* (1483), ISTC ih00448000, now Princeton, Princeton University Library, 2865.1483q. On the survival of the Mainz *Donatus* more broadly, see Eric Marshall White, "Binding Waste as Book History: Patterns of Survival among the Early Mainz Donatus Editions," in Dondi, *Printing R-Evolution and Society*, 253–77.

79. Armstrong's useful summary of Venetian incunable imagery and its chronology is found in "The Decoration and Illustration of Venetian Incunabula: From Hand Illumination to the Design of Woodcuts," in Dondi, *Printing R-Evolution and Society*, 775–818.

80. Munich, Bayerische Staatsbibliothek, 2 Inc.c.a. 1453 and 2 Inc.c.a. 1588 d. These are copies, respectively, of the *Digestum vetus* (ISTC ij00549500) and *Infortiatium* (ISTC ij00557400). These two books were in the Benedictine Abbey of Tegernsee, south of Munich, by at least 1488, as were a number of the Gregoris' other printed works, although only a few have significant decoration.

81. Cambridge, University Library, Inc.2.B.3.45[1506]. On this book, see Laura Nuvoloni, "Un'aggiunta al catalogo di Antonio Maria da Villafora: Il *Corona florida medicinae* di Antonio Gazio (1491) della University Library di Cambridge," in *Miniatura: Lo sguardo e la parola*, ed. Federica Toniolo and Gennaro Toscano (Milan: Cinisello Balsamo, 2012), 330–35.

82. Early examples of Venetian incunables with images and diagrams include Johannes de Sacro Bosco, *Sphaera mundi* (Venice: Franciscus Renner, 1478), ISTC ij00402000; Werner Rolewinck, *Fasciculus temporum* (Venice: Georgius Walch, 1479), ISTC ir00260000; Euclides, *Elementa geometriae* (Venice: Erhard Ratdolt, 1482), ISTC ie00113000; Jacobus Publicius, *Artes orandi, epistolandi, memorandi* (Venice: Erhard Ratdolt, 1482), ISTC ip01096000. On Ratdolt's mathematical diagrams and their typographic innovation, see Emily R. Anderson, "Printing the Bespoke Book: Euclid's *Elements* in Early Modern Visual Culture," *Nuncius* 35, no. 3 (2020): 536–60; Renzo Baldasso, "Printing for the Doge: On the First Quire of the First Edition of the *Liber elementorum Euclidis*," *La Bibliofilía* 115, no. 3 (2013): 525–52; Gregg De Young, "Mathematical Diagrams from Manuscript to Print: Examples from the Arabic Euclidean Transmission," *Synthese* 186 (2012): 21–54; Victor Carter, Lotte Hellinga, and Tony Parker, "Printing with Gold in the Fifteenth Century," *British Library Journal* 9, no. 1 (1983): 1–13.

83. These texts and their respective problems include a small woodblock street scene at the front of their edition of *Frottola di un Caligaro* (ISTC if00325500), although the dating of the one surviving version of this text to around 1485 is questionable, being possibly closer to 1500; a *Lunarium* (ISTC ig00338000) from around 1488 whose frontispiece depicts a pair of astrologers but whose attribution to the Gregoris is contested; a *Breviarium Romanum* (ISTC ib01122500) from 1490 containing an image of Saint Jerome attributed to Gregorio alone rather than a brotherly collaboration, and in some cases to an entirely different printer altogether. Pesenti claims that the brothers did not use woodblock initials for the first time until 1492 and first used woodblock frames in 1495: *Fasiculo de medicina in volgare*, 1:79.

84. The debates over attribution of these early printed frontispieces are complex, and artists have been assigned to them often only on stylistic grounds. See, for instance, the various case studies collected in Lilian Armstrong, *Studies of Renaissance Miniaturists in Venice*, 2 vols. (London: Pindar, 2003).

85. Alchabitius, *Libellus isagogicus* (Venice: Johannes and Gregorius de Gregoriis, 1491), ISTC ia00364000. Many of the woodcuts in this edition were copied from Ratdolt's earlier Venetian edition: Alchabitius, *Libellus isagogicus* (Venice: Erhard Ratdolt, 1485), ISTC ia00363000.

86. Aristoteles, *De animalibus* (1492), ISTC ia00974000; Giovanni Boccaccio, *Decamerone* (1492), ISTC ib00728000.

87. Boethius, *Opera* (vol. 1: March 26, 1491; vol. 2: August 18, 1492), ISTC ib00767000. This effect is in part exaggerated by the fact that the first volume contains Boethius's works on geometry and mathematics, which, among all his writings, require the most extensive diagrammatic explanation. But it is still relevant that this highly illustrated first volume was printed second, out of order, and was only attempted over a year after the diagrammatic experimentation of the *Fasciculus*.

88. For a useful summary of this two-tone technique, pioneered in the city by the Ratdolt press, see Ad Stijnman and Elizabeth Savage, "Materials and Techniques for Early Colour Printing," in *Printing Colour 1400–1700: History, Techniques, Functions, and Receptions*, ed. Ad Stijnman and Elizabeth Savage (Boston: Brill, 2015), 11–22; Joseph Dane, *Blind Impressions: Methods and Mythologies in Book History* (Philadelphia: University of Pennsylvania Press, 2013), 149–55.

89. *Ars moriendi* (Venice: Johannes Clein and Piero Himel, 1490), ISTC ia01109000; Johannes de Sacro

Bosco, *Sphaera mundi* (Venice: Bonetus Locatellus for Octavianus Scotus, 1490), ISTC ij00409000.

90. There is at least a small possibility that the long linking lines of the *Fasciculus*'s woodblocks were not carved into the wood but instead formed by inset strips of copper wire, as is evidenced elsewhere in early printed materials. However, while the surviving evidence is not certain, the consistency of the printed lines across multiple editions of the booklet suggests that they were more likely xylographic features. I thank Elizabeth Savage for this observation and her support in getting to grips with the detail of these early printing techniques. On this technique in Ratdolt's press, see Anderson's citation of earlier observations by Renzo Baldasso and A. Hyatt Mayor: "Printing the Bespoke Book," 543. On a contemporary German book produced by Johann Prüss, whose images had xylographic diagrammatic lines added at a later date, see Zimmermann-Homeyer, "Spuren eines drucktechnischen Experiments."

91. Pesenti, *Fasiculo de medicina in volgare*, 1:40. Her precise words are: "*Ogni intento diagrammatico sembra inoltre abbandonato.... Questa figura non ha più nulla in comune con lo schematico, flaccido giovane uomo calvo e in mutande azzurre ... ha la prestanza, la postura, la fisionomia di un nudo disegnato dal Mantegna*."

92. Many of these suggestions originate with Charles Singer's translation of Sudhoff's readings and have spiraled into full-blown fact in later texts: Singer and Demaitre, *The Fasciculus medicinae*, 117ff.

93. Daston has explored the idea of epistemic images extensively, with the clearest summary of the concept appearing in "Epistemic Images," in *Vision and Its Instruments: Art, Science, and Technology in Early Modern Europe*, ed. Alina Payne (University Park, PA: Penn State University Press, 2015), 13–35.

94. *Fasiculo de medicina* (1494), ISTC ik00017000. The year of this edition can sometimes be confused, as the date is recorded using the *more Veneto*, the Venetian convention of beginning the year on March 1: the book's colophon reads "*Nel M.ccccIxxxxiii adi v Februario*" (February 5, 1493), but this would be February 1494 in today's calendar.

95. Francesco Petrarca, *Epistolae familiares* (1492), ISTC ip00399000; Aristoteles, *De animalibus* (1492), ISTC ia00974000.

96. On the role of translation in the life of early modern printed books, surveyed in various geographical contexts, see Andrea Rizzi, ed., *Trust and Proof: Translators in Renaissance Print Culture* (Leiden: Brill, 2017).

97. By this date, the *Anathomia* already had an extensive life in the vernacular. On its vulgarized manuscript tradition, see the edition and commentary by Maria Rosaria D'Anzi, ed., *Hanothomya del corpo humano: Volgarizzamento da Mondino de Liuzzi* (Rome: ARACNE, 2012).

98. Sabrina Minuzzi is certain that Montagnana is in fact one Pietro del Min, a lecturer in anatomy at both Padua and Ferrara: "La stampa medico-scientifica nell'Europa del XV secolo," 214–15. She cites Eleonora Gamba, "Pietro da Montagnana: La vita, gli studi, la biblioteca di un *homo trilinguis*," PhD diss., Università degli Studi di Padova, 2016, 83–84. The *Fasiculo* image of Montagnana clearly borrows from an established Venetian trope of a seated academic, seen, for example, in the frontispiece to Aesopus, *Aesopus moralisatus* (Venice: Manfredus de Bonellis, 1491), ISTC ia00151000.

99. This anatomy scene is much discussed in the literature, including Taylor McCall, "Anatomical Icon: The Dissection Scene across Manuscript and Print," *KNOW: A Journal on the Formation of Knowledge* 6, no.1 (special issue: "Anatomical Things") (2022): 7–46; Pesenti, *Fasiculo de medicina in volgare*, 1:114ff; Andrea Carlino, *La fabbrica del corpo: Libri e dissezione nel Rinascimento* (Turin: Einaudi, 1994), 15–25; Jerome J. Bylebyl, "Interpreting the *Fasciculo* Anatomy Scene," *Journal of the History of Medicine and Allied Sciences* 45, no. 3 (1990): 285–316. On early dissection culture in Venice specifically, see Cynthia Klestinec, *Theaters of Anatomy: Students, Teachers, and Traditions of Dissection in Renaissance Venice* (Baltimore: Johns Hopkins University Press, 2011).

100. On the reuse of images elsewhere in a Venetian context, see Cristina Dondi et al., "The Use and Reuse of Printed Illustrations in 15th-Century Venetian Editions," in Dondi, *Printing R-Evolution*, 839–870.

101. *Fasciculus medicinae* (Venice: Johannes and Gregorius de Gregoriis, 1495), ISTC ik00014000. This edition's text largely follows the Gregoris' 1491 Latin edition, although here Mondino's *Anathomia* includes a colophon naming the Imolese doctor Petrus Andreas Morsianus as its editor.

102. This copy is Washington, DC, Smithsonian Library, Dibner Library Special Collections, R128.6 .K43 1495 quarto.

103. It is certainly possible that as these blocks wore down over time they were repaired, although changes to details in the anatomy scene make clear that at least this image was significantly remodeled as early as 1495 to include an older lector, now more clearly reading aloud from an opened book, and an open window showing a landscape beyond. The Gregori editions post-1500 are *Fasciculus medicinae* (1500), ISTC ik00015000; *Fasciculus medicinae* (1501), ISTC ik00016000 (again, confusion over the Venetian calendar sometimes mistakenly places the latter book in 1500). From this point onward, the Venetian editions move beyond the chronological scope of the ISTC, and some, but not all, appear in the USTC. The Gregoris' two further editions are *Fasciculo di medecina vulgare* (Venice: Johannes and Gregorius de Gregoriis, 1508), USTC 813143; *Fasciculus medicine* (Venice: Johannes and Gregorius de Gregoriis, 1514), USTC 837017 (once again, the latter is sometimes confused through misreading of the Venetian calendar as 1513, including in the USTC).

104. Minuzzi, "La stampa medico-scientifica nell'Europa del XV secolo," 214.

105. Schedel's book is now Munich, Bayerische Staatsbibliothek, 2 Inc.c.a. 3894.

106. Zwingli's book is now Zürich, Zentralbibliothek, Ink K 120,2.

107. The contents of the Bishop of Odense's library are recorded in Wolfgang Undorf, "Lost Books, Lost Libraries, Lost Everything? A Scandinavian Early Modern Perspective," in Bruni and Pettegree, *Lost Books*, 101–19.

108. Gessner's book is now Zürich, Zentralbibliothek, 3.11,2.

109. Knyvett's book is now Cambridge, University Library, Inc.3.B.3.45[1519].

110. Richard J. Durling, "An Early Manual for the Medical Student and the Newly-Fledged Practitioner: Martin Stainpeis' *Liber de modo studendi seu legendi in medicina* ([Vienna] 1520)," *Clio Medica* 5 (1970): 7–33.

111. *Compendio de la salud humana* (Zaragoza: Paul Hurus, 1494), ISTC ik00017600. An edition of the Spanish text, with commentary, appears in María Teresa Herrera, *Compendio de la humana salud* (Madrid: ARCOS/LIBROS, 1990), and a transcription also appears online in the Hispanic Seminary of Medieval Studies' "Spanish Medical Texts," http://www.hispanicseminary.org/t&c/med/index-en.htm (accessed August 1, 2024). Two other texts preserved in Spanish editions of the book include a Castilian *Liber physiognomiae* (Book of Physiognomy) and the *Tratado de la formación o generación* (Treatise on Formation or Generation), both discussed in María Nieves Sánchez González de Herrero and María Concepción Vázquez de Benito, *Tratado de fisonomía: Tratado de la forma de la generación de la criatura* (Salamanca: DLE, 2009). On early medical printing on the Iberian Peninsula more generally, see Jon Arrizabalaga, "El libro científico en la primera imprenta castellana (1485–1520)," in *Historia de la ciencia y de la técnica en la Corona de Castilla*, ed. Luis García Ballester (Valladolid: Junta de Castilla y León, 2002), 2:619–50. A useful list of early medical works in Spanish vernaculars can be found in Michael R. Solomon, *Fictions of Well-Being: Sickly Readers and Vernacular Medical Writing in Late Medieval and Early Modern Spain* (Philadelphia: University of Pennsylvania Press, 2010), 131–65.

112. Hurus and printing in Zaragoza are discussed as part of the extremely useful survey by Julián Martín Abad, *Los primeros tiempos de la imprenta en España* (Madrid: Laberinto, 2003), 102–5. On early printing in various other Spanish locations, see Julián Martín Abad, *Cum figuris: Texto e imagen en los incunables españoles. Catálogo bibliográfico y descriptivo* (Madrid: Arco Libros, 2018); Benito Rial Costas, ed., *Print Culture and Peripheries in Early Modern Europe: A Contribution to the History of Printing and the Book Trade in Small European and Spanish Cities* (Leiden: Brill, 2013).

113. Hurus's work and movements in this period are reconstructed alongside those of other incunable printers of Zaragoza in the extremely detailed archival work of Miguel Ángel Pallarés Jiménez, *La imprenta de los incunables de Zaragoza y el comercio internacional del libro a finales del siglo XV* (Zaragoza: IFC, 2008), 61ff. He notes, for instance, that in 1495 the merchant Climent Angorrita oversaw the importation of over thirty German woodblocks, several of which ended up in the Hurus press. For more on the exchange of such images in early Spanish printing, see Manuel-José Pedraza-Gracia, "Illustrating and Publishing on the Hand-Press in Spain from the Fifteenth to the Eighteenth Century: The Ownership of Icono-Typographic Resources," in *Illustration and Ornamentation in the Iberian Book World, 1450–1800*, ed. Alexander Samuel Wilkinson (Leiden: Brill, 2022), 61–86.

114. Zaun and Geisler argue, for instance, that small changes made in the translations of the *Fasciculus*'s urine text reveal a more subtle understanding of the mechanics of medieval urology than the Latin original: "Die Harnfarbbezeichnungen im *Fasciculus medicine*," 979–81. Hurus or his editor instigated further small changes to make the work their own. The plague treatise of Pietro da Tossignano that was originally included by the Gregoris is replaced by an older tract on the same topic, Vasco de Taranta's *Tratado de la peste*, as well as the first Castilian translation of Michael Scotus's *Liber physiognomiae*. Visually, some small but new elements are also added: a half-page image of two doctors in discussion, marginalia of urine flasks, small details of the twelve signs of the zodiac, and an image of the pierced Saint Sebastian, a detail that evoked both plague treatises and Hurus's own printer's mark, which appears at the end of the book. The figure of the Disease Woman does not appear in any of the three surviving copies of the work; this could be a conscious decision reflecting the medico-visual tastes of the printers and their audiences, although all surviving copies of these works are somewhat defective, and a letter-key referring to the figure remains in all cases.

115. On this mystery woodcutter, Jimenez cautiously cites a brief note in Agustín Millares Carlo, *Introducción a la historia del libro y de las bibliotecas* (Mexico City: Fondo de Cultura Económica, 1993), 127.

116. Johannes de Capua, *Exemplario contra los engaños y peligros del mundo* (Zaragoza: Paulus Hurus, 1493), ISTC ij00271500. Earlier editions are Johannes de Capua, *Buch der Weisheit der alten Weisen* (Urach: Conrad Fyner, c. 1482), ISTC ij00269000; Johannes de Capua, *Buch der Weisheit der alten Weisen* (Augsburg: Johann Schönsperger, 1484), ISTC ij00270200; Johannes de Capua, *Directorium humanae vitae* (Strassburg: Johann Prüss, c. 1489), ISTC ij00268000.

117. *Epilogo en medicina* (Burgos: Juan de Burgos, 1495), ISTC ik00018000. On Juan de Burgos, see Abad, *Los primeros tiempos de la imprenta en España*, 74ff. The Burgos edition also adds a short treatise on generation to the end of the book, illustrated by a small image of the Annunciation. Coppens suggests that this text might be a translation of Arnau de Villanova's *De conceptione: De vele levens*, appendix 1.1.

118. *Epilogo en medicina y en cirurgia conveniente ala salud* (Pamplona: Arnaldo Guillen de Brocar, 1495), ISTC ik00018300. On Brocar, see Abad, *Los primeros tiempos de la imprenta en España*, 81ff.

119. Folke Gernert, *Fictionalizing Heterodoxy: Various Uses of Knowledge in the Spanish World from the Archpriest of Hita to Mateo Alemán* (Berlin: De Gruyter, 2019), 25–28.

120. Guido de Cauliaco, *Die Cyrurgie van meester Guido de Cauliaco* (Antwerp: Henrick Eckert van Homberch, 1508), USTC 400275. Coppens notes that although the colophon reads 1507, the printing must in fact have been in 1508. On this text and its relation to the *Fasciculus*, see Christian Coppens, "'For the Benefit of Ordinary People': The Dutch Translation of the *Fasciculus medicinae*, Antwerp 1512," *Quaerendo* 39, no. 2 (2009), 168–205. On the role of images in the Dutch *Fasciculus* and related early sixteenth-century Dutch books, see Andrea van Leerdam, *Woodcuts as Reading Guides: How Images Shaped Knowledge Transmission in Medical-Astrological Books in Dutch (1500–1550)* (Amsterdam: Amsterdam University Press, 2024).

121. *Fasciculus medicine* (Antwerp: Claes de Grave, 1512), USTC 400312.

122. Coppens convincingly suggests that the model for this figure is a Zodiac Man found on a Nuremberg almanac from c. 1495–1496, printed by Caspar Hochfeder (ISTC ia00520000): "'For the Benefit of Ordinary People,'" 181. Both share the same distribution of figures and framed arches, as well as a pair of faces—one old and one young—on either side of the Zodiac Man's own face, symbolizing the different ages of a human life.

123. *Fasciculo di medicina vulgare* (Milan: Giovanni de Castellione, 1509), USTC 762556. Interestingly, this edition's Zodiac Man has an unusual style, with heavy linear shading that feels more reminiscent of the Spanish *Compendio* images than its Italian predecessors, perhaps indicating an even more complicated cross-pollination.

124. These texts are listed in the *Verzeichnis der im deutschen Sprachbereich erschienenen Drucke des 16. Jahrhunderts* (hereafter VD16) as numbers J619–J621. Their grouping and relation to the *Fasciculus* is discussed in Eckhart, "Medial Translations and Material Manifestations," 55ff.

125. *Fasciculo di medicine vulgare* (Milan: Giovann'Angelo Scinzenzeler, 1516), USTC 837018.

126. *Conpendio [sic] de la salud humana* (Seville: Jacob Cromberger, 1517), USTC 339382. On reuse in the Cromberger press, see Nuria Aranda García, "Book Illustration in the Late Fifteenth and Early Sixteenth Centuries: The First Editions of the Siete Sabios de Roma," in Wilkinson, *Illustration and Ornamentation in the Iberian Book World*, 249ff.

127. *Fasciculo de medicina* (Venice: Cesare Arrivabene, 1522), USTC 837019; *Fasciculus medicie [sic]* (Venice: Cesare Arrivabene, 1522), USTC 837020. Occasional mention is made of a further edition in 1515, but this is only known secondhand; Coppens dubs it a *spookedite* (ghost edition). From early on in Venice's print history, it was common practice for publishers to sell or share woodblocks; in many cases these were not owned by publishers or the engravers who made them but by the local guild, the Fraglia di Pittori, who leased them for a fee. For more on the Arrivabene specifically, see Natalie Lussey Seale, "The Arrivabene Family," in New York Academy of Medicine, "Facendo Il Libro: The Making of Fasciculus medicinae, an Early Printed Anatomy" (online exhibition), https://digitalcollections.nyam.org/digital/arrivabene (accessed August 1, 2024); Erika Saccocci, "Arrivabene, Andrea," in *Dizionario dei tipografi e degli editori italiani*, ed. Marco Menato, Ennio Sandal, and Giuseppina Zappella (Milan: Editrice Bibliografica, 1997), 1:45–46.

128. *Fasciculus medicine* (Antwerp: Claes de Grave, 1529), USTC 437444. Coppens notes that the *Fasciculus* text remained popular in Antwerp well into the second half of the century, as testified by its reprinting as late as 1567: *Het licht der medecijnen ende cyrurgien* ... (Antwerp: Jan II van Ghelen, 1567), USTC 401306.

129. Intermediality as a concept has received extensive treatment, but for terminological discussions in relation to European print, see various essays in Alfred Messerli and Michael Schilling, eds., *Die Intermedialität des Flugblatts in der Frühen Neuzeit* (Stuttgart: Hirzel, 2015).

130. Sonja Drimmer, "The Manuscript Copy and the Printed Original in the Digital Present," *Digital Philology* 9, no. 2 (2020): 93–119.

131. In addition to the extensive bibliography gathered by Drimmer in "The Manuscript Copy and the Printed Original in the Digital Present" and work by other authors already mentioned, for German-language scholarship see Arno Mentzel-Reuters, "Das Nebeneinander von Handschrift und Buchdruck im 15. und 16. Jahrhundert," in *Buchwissenschaft in Deutschland: Ein Handbuch*, ed. Ursula Rautenberg (Berlin: De Gruyter, 2010), 411–42; for English-language scholarship, see Zeynep Tenger and Paul Trolander, "From Print versus Manuscript to Sociable Authorship and Mixed Media: A Review of Trends in the Scholarship of Early Modern Publication," *Literature Compass* 7, no. 11 (2010): 1035–48. For the place of images specifically in this landscape of media change, see Jeffrey F. Hamburger and Maria Theisen, eds., *Unter Druck: Mitteleuropäische Buchmalerei im 15. Jahrhundert* (Peterberg: Imhof, 2018); Jeffrey F. Hamburger, Robert Suckale, and Gude Suckale-Redlefsen, eds., *Painting the Page in the Age of Print: Central European Manuscript Illumination of the Fifteenth Century* (Toronto: PIMS, 2018); David S. Areford, *The Viewer and the Printed Image in Late Medieval Europe* (Aldershot: Ashgate, 2010); Peter Schmidt, *Gedruckte Bilder in handgeschriebenen Büchern: Zum Gebrauch von Druckgraphik im 15. Jahrhundert* (Cologne: Böhlau, 2003). For a specific case study in the potential importance of interdependent media for one fifteenth-century printer, see Jeffrey F. Hamburger, "Between Basel and Lyon: Bernhard Richel, Martin Huss, and a Possible Printer's Vade Mecum (The Morgan Library & Museum, MS M.158)," *Gutenberg-Jahrbuch* 97 (2022): 16–37.

132. These blank spaces seem to have specifically been left in printed editions of Hyginus, *Poetica astronomica* (Ferrara: Augustinus Carnerius, 1475), ISTC ih00559000. See David McKitterick, "What Is the Use of Books without Pictures? Empty Space in Some Early Printed Books," *La Bibliofilía* 116, nos. 1–3 (2014): 67–82.

133. Kathryn Rudy presents a detailed investigation of these compilations in various works: *Image, Knife, and Gluepot: Early Assemblage in Manuscript and Print* (Cambridge: Open Book Publishers, 2019); Kathryn Rudy, *Piety in Pieces: How Medieval Readers Customized their Manuscripts* (Cambridge: Open Book Publishers, 2016). Particularly interesting examples in a German medical context can be found in Munich, Bayerische Staatsbibliothek, Cgm 328, and Vienna, Österreichische Nationalbibliothek, Cod. 13106, to mention only two.

134. Prague, Národní knihovna České republiky, MS XVII D 10.

135. On the *Františkánova kompilace* and its place in Old Czech medical literature, see Stehlíková, *Od andělíky po zimostráz*; David Tomíček, *Víra, rozum a zkušenost v lékařství pozdně středověkých Čech* (Ústí nad Labem: UJEP, 2009); Alena Černá, *Staročeské knihy lékařské* (Brno: Host, 2006).

136. The only almanacs currently known to have survived from this shop are dated 1507, although this is not necessarily a reason to assume that Höltzel or other Nuremberg printers were not using this block earlier. The surviving broadsheet contains the almanac of Konrad Tockler and is now Prague, Národní knihovna České republiky, Teplá fragm. 502.

137. Karl Sudhoff, "Zwei deutsche Reklamezettel zur Empfehlung von Arzneimitteln—Petroleum und Eichenmistel—gedruckt um 1500," *Archiv für Geschichte der Medizin* 3, no. 6 (1910): 397–402, describing *Die Tugend des edlen Öls Petroleum* (Nuremberg: Ambrosius Huber, c. 1500), ISTC ip00421500.

138. The pasted zodiac images match the woodblocks used for a single-sheet almanac of 1518 by the Vienna printer Johannes Singriener, now Vienna, Österreichische Nationalbibliothek, F 000008-B ALT FLUG.

139. Basel, Universitätsbibliothek, O IV 38. For more on this manuscript, see Rudolph, "Medizin: Handschrift Nr. 87.2.1."

140. Budapest, Országos Széchényi Könyvtár (Széchényi-Nationalbibliothek), Cod. Germ. 56. This book's owner was clearly interested in media diversity, for they inserted a single-page, printed bloodletting figure a few pages later. For more on this manuscript, see Pia Rudolph, "Medizin: Handschrift Nr. 87.2.4," in Freienhagen-Baumgardt et al., *Katalog der deutschsprachigen illustrierten Handschriften des Mittelalters (KdiH)*, vol. 9. That the book's calendar is from Salzburg and its dialect is Bavarian-Austrian helps with its localization, although its coat of arms has not yet been identified.

141. Cambridge, Trinity College, Wren Library, O.9.31.

142. The incunable is Guilelmus de Saliceto, *De salute corporis* (The Netherlands: printer unknown, before 1472), ISTC is00029500.

143. The urine treatise starts on fol. 28 and includes elements of the *Fasciculus*'s urine wheel, here reduced to text alone. The phlebotomy treatises start on fol. 30r. Immediately after the phlebotomical material on fol. 33r is a short fragmentary passage from the end of another treatise, indicating that the book once contained more texts than currently survive.

144. The hairline is a detail found only in the 1491 edition of the *Fasciculus*, suggesting that this edition was the source of the Cambridge manuscript.

145. The *Fasciculus*'s phlebotomy text concludes with item dd, whereas the Trinity manuscript adds items ee to kk.

146. Ann M. Blair, "Reflections on Technological Continuities: Manuscripts Copied from Printed Books," *Bulletin of the John Rylands Library* 91, no. 1 (2015): 7–33. On the relevance of copying for early modern knowledge practices, see Sietske Fransen and Katherine M. Reinhart, eds., "The Practice of Copying in Making Knowledge in Early Modern Europe," *Word & Image* 35, no. 3 (special issue) (2019).

147. Marcatellis's case is discussed most extensively in Albert Derolez, *The Library of Raphael de Marcatellis, Abbot of St. Bavon's, Ghent, 1437–1508* (Ghent: Story-Scientia, 1979).

148. London, British Library, Sloane MS 345; the texts reproduced relate to wound surgery (fols. 118r–127v), women's medicine (fols. 128r–130r), and disease (fols. 131r–136v). Despite not reproducing the original work's images, the author has chosen to keep the printed version's alphabetized key, reformulated from a device originally for cross-referencing text and image into a way of generating order among the assembled texts. Eckhart notes two other text-only translations of the *Fasciculus:* Leiden, Universiteitsbibliotheek, MS VCO 6; Madrid, Biblioteca Nacional de España, 2.328. See "Medial Translations," 68–69.

149. Vienna, Österreichische Nationalbibliothek, Cod. 14034.

150. The design of the copied figures makes clear that the creator of this book was working from one of the Gregoris' later Latin editions from 1495, 1500, or 1501. As evidence of the tracing, compare the combinatory figure's face with that of the Zodiac Man copied on fol. 10v and the body with the bloodletting figure on fol. 8v.

151. Leiden, Universiteitsbibliotheek, MS BPL 1905.

152. The one exception here is the image of the Disease Woman and a large portion of her gynecological treatise, which is missing from this book. Whether this is a deliberate omission or the result of the book's somewhat dilapidated condition is unclear, although it remains a feature of several later works inspired by the *Fasciculus*, perhaps suggesting the shifting tastes and audiences for gynecological materials.

153. Ljubljana, Semeniška knjižnica, SKLJ Rkp. 2.

154. The signed and dated image is that of Petrus de Montagnana at his desk, the *Fasciculus*'s former frontispiece, relocated to the end of the book in the Arrivabene Latin edition and found in this German manuscript on fol. 201r. The narrative scene of a doctor being brought urine to examine beneath a portico at fol. 159v, the penultimate image in this book, also contains the artist's initials, N.P., which appear in a tiny central spandrel of the arches. The manuscript's translation follows the Arrivabene text closely, including its colophon mentioning the years 1522 (the date of the Arrivabene edition) and 1500 (the date of an earlier edition of the *Fasciculus* on which the 1522 version draws). These dates are not to be confused with the dating of this German translation, which we would do better to instead intuit from the dated illustrations. Again, no Disease Woman is present in the manuscript, only the notes surrounding her in the 1522 edition, although the treatises accompanying this figure in the Arrivabene edition have been translated in detail. This once more suggests that the manuscript was made in a context where a theoretical text on gynecology was more welcome than an image of a naked woman.

155. These colored figures bear some resemblance to a set of three images included in a book from c. 1560 belonging to the Regensburg physician Ambrosius Prechtl, now Vatican City, Biblioteca Apostolica Vaticana, MS Pal. Lat. 1241, fol. 315r ff.

CHAPTER 5. IMAGE: WOUND MAN AESTHETICS

1. London, Wellcome Library, MS 290, fol. 53v.

2. On these uses, see the introduction.

3. On this manuscript, see Jesús Romero-Barranco, *The Late Middle English Version of Constantinus Africanus' "Venerabilis anatomia" in London, Wellcome Library, MS 290 (ff. 1r–41v)* (Newcastle: Cambridge Scholars, 2015), whose linguistic analysis suggests that the treatises were written north of the Thames, in Essex near Chelmsford; Kathleen L. Scott, *Later Gothic Manuscripts 1390–1490* (London: Harvey Miller, 1998), 2:275–77.

4. On the *Anatomia porci*, see Ynez Violé O'Neill, "Another Look at the 'Anatomia porci,'" *Viator* 1 (1970): 115–24.

5. London, Wellcome Library, MS 290, fols. 49v–52v.

6. Samuel A. J. Moorat, *Catalogue of Western Manuscripts on Medicine and Science in the Wellcome Historical Medical Library* (London: Wellcome Library, 1962), 185–86. For more on the argument that these images are drawn from the *Fasciculus* rather than being its model, see Hartnell, "Wording the Wound Man."

7. Sonja Drimmer, "Discomforting Book History: An English Manuscript, an Italian Printed Book" (forthcoming). I thank the author for generously sharing their work in advance of publication. The manuscript is London, British Library, Arundel MS 66, and is precisely dated

in its colophon; the incunable from which it draws is Hyginus, *Poetica astronomica* (Venice: Erhard Ratdolt, 1482), ISTC ih00560000.

8. Nutton, "Books, Printing, and Medicine in the Renaissance"; Elisabeth Leedham-Green, Dennis E. Rhodes, and Frank H. Stubbings, *Garrett Godfrey's Accounts, c. 1527–1533* (Cambridge: Cambridge Bibliographical Society, 1992).

9. Hieronymus Brunschwig, *Buch der Cirurgia* (Strassburg: Johann Grüninger, 1497), ISTC ib01225000, title page.

10. On German university medicine and physicianship, see Michael Stolberg, *Gelehrte Medizin und ärztlicher Alltag in der Renaissance* (Berlin: De Gruyter, 2020); Hannah Murphy, *A New Order of Medicine: The Rise of Physicians in Reformation Nuremberg* (Pittsburgh: University of Pittsburgh Press, 2019); Nutton, "Medicine at the German Universities, 1348–1500." On German surgical guilds, especially in later periods, see Annamarie Kinzelbach, *Chirurgen und Chirugie-Praktiken: Wundärzte als Reichsstadtbürger 16. bis 18. Jahrhundert* (Mainz: Donata Kinzelbach, 2015).

11. On Brunschwig's biography and various aspects of his work, see Tillmann Taape, "Distilling Reliable Remedies: Hieronymus Brunschwig's *Liber de arte distillandi* (1500) between Alchemical Learning and Craft Practice," *Ambix* 61, no. 3 (2014): 236–56; Gundolf Keil, "Brunschwig, Hieronymus, Wundarzt (um 1450–1512/13)," *Enzyklopädie Medizingeschichte* 1 (2007): 217; Pierre Bachoffner, "Jérôme Brunschwig, chirurgien et apothicaire strasbourgeois, portraituré en 1512," *Revue d'histoire de la pharmacie* 298 (1993): 269–78; Henry E. Sigerist, *Hieronymus Brunschwig and His Work: A Fifteenth-Century Surgeon* (New York: Abrahamson, 1946). For the emphasis on craft alongside theory found in Brunschwig's work, as well as that of other related German medics, see Alisha Rankin, *Panaceia's Daughters: Noblewomen as Healers in Early Modern Germany* (Chicago: University of Chicago Press, 2013), 48ff.

12. Brunschwig's approach fits neatly into Miriam Usher-Chrisman's seminal model for the emergence of lay knowledge in the city, as presented in *Lay Culture, Learned Culture*.

13. Examples of these Grüninger works include Sebastian Brant, *Das Narrenschiff* (1494), ISTC ib01081000; *Biblia Sacra* (1485), ISTC ib00633000; Hieronymus Baldung, *Aphorismi compunctionis theologicales* (1497), ISTC ib00036000; *Navicula Sanctae Ursulae* (1497), ISTC iu00076000; for a broadside, Jacob Locher, *Carmen in faciem Aquile et laudem Maximiliani* (1497), ISTC il00260000. For recent work on Brant, including discussion of Grüninger's role in his works, see Peter Andersen and Nikolaus Henkel, eds., *Sebastian Brant (1457–1521): Europäisches Wissen in der Hand eines Intellektuellen der Frühen Neuzeit* (Berlin: De Gruyter, 2023).

14. *Gart der Gesundheit* (1485–1486), ISTC ig00099000; *Gart der Gesundheit* (1489), ISTC ig00108000; *Horae* (1494), ISTC ih00377500.

15. Tillmann Taape, "Common Medicine for the Common Man: Picturing the 'Striped Layman' in Early Vernacular Print," *Renaissance Quarterly* 74, no. 1 (2021): 1–58. Melanie Panse also suggests that the placement of Brunschwig's images reflected his intentions for the text and its broad audience: "Den Leser in Text und Bild begleiten: Formen der Wissensvermittlung in medizinischen Schriften des ausgehenden Mittelalters," in *Lehre und Schule im Mittelalter—Mittelalter in Schule und Lehre*, ed. Ursula Kundert (Berlin: De Gruyter, 2012), 126–38.

16. Terentius, *Comoediae* (Strassburg: Johann Grüninger, 1496), ISTC it00094000. The same blocks were reused for Jacobus Locher, *Panegyricus ad Maximilianum* (Strassburg: Johann Grüninger, 1497), ISTC il00264000. For a very early and somewhat less sophisticated example of this modular technique, see Albrecht Pfister's 1461 printing of Ulrich Boner, *Der Edelstein* (Bamberg: Albrecht Pfister, 1461), ISTC ib00974500. Zimmermann-Homeyer also notes in two studies that Grüninger's edition of the *Comedies* pioneers several other visual techniques: "Spuren eines drucktechnischen Experiments"; *Illustrierte Frühdrucke lateinischer Klassiker um 1500: Innovative Illustrationskonzepte aus der Strassburger Offizin Johannes Grüningers und ihre Wirkung* (Wiesbaden: Harrassowitz, 2018).

17. Taape notes that the makers of these half-blocks also used a system of interchangeable plugs to amend small details in repeated figures, for instance removing or replacing a patient's shoes to reveal or hide a wound on the foot beneath: "Common Medicine for the Common Man," 27ff.

18. Ursula Rautenberg, *Das Titelblatt: Die Entstehung eines typographischen Dispositivs im frühen Buchdruck* (Erlangen: FAU, 2004); Margaret M. Smith, *The Title-Page: Its Early Development, 1460–1510* (London: British Library, 2000). For a more statistical take on this material, see Ursula Rautenberg, "Die Entstehung und Entwicklung des Buchtitelblatts in der Inkunabelzeit in Deutschland, den Niederlanden und Venedig: Quantitative und qualitative Studien," *Archiv für Geschichte des Buchwesens* 62 (2008): 1–105. On French parallels, see Malcolm Walsby, "The Creation of the Title Page in French Incunabula," *Gutenberg-Jahrbuch* 97 (2022): 38–46. For a recent discussion of the phenomenon across a variety of early modern works, see Gitta Bertram, Nils Büttner, and Claus Zittel, eds., *Gateways to the Book: Frontispieces and Title Pages in Early Modern Europe* (Leiden: Brill, 2021).

19. Sebastian Brant, *De monstruoso partu* (Strassburg: Johann Prüss, 1495), ISTC ib01079500, title page. The treatise also circulated as large-format broadsides and was printed in a number of other nearby cities in both Latin and German. For more on this and similar cases, see Jennifer Spinks, *Monstrous Births and Visual Culture in Sixteenth-Century Germany* (New York: Routledge, 2009). On monstrous births as symbolic premodern phenomena, see Lorraine Daston and Katharine Park, *Wonders and the Order of Nature 1150–1750* (New York: Zone, 1998), 173ff. Prüss and Grüninger are in fact directly connected through imagery: Prüss reused an image from Grüninger's printing of Brunschwig in his *Hortus sanitatis* (Strassburg: Johann Prüss, 1497), ISTC ih00487000.

20. The print survives in a number of states but was originally produced in Nuremberg and Augsburg; the former is known only from one example, now Vienna, Albertina, Inventarnummer DG1930/210. On the historiography of this image and the identification of its

subject, see Colin T. Eisler, "Who Is Dürer's Syphilitic Man?," *Perspectives in Biology and Medicine* 52, no. 1 (2009): 48–60. Likely aware of Brant's work, Dürer had created an engraving of a monstrous eight-legged pig in the same year.

21. No match has yet been found for these initials among known contemporary woodcutters, although as more archival research is undertaken on these print shops, certain suitable candidates may well come to light. The initials are anonymously referenced in broad collections of early modern signatures, such as Georg Kaspar Nagler, *Die Monogrammisten* (Munich: Franz, 1860), 2:601.

22. Hieronymus Brunschwig, *Buch der Cirurgia* (Strassburg: Johann Grüninger, 1513), VD16 B 8705; on Brunschwig's *Anatomie*, see Karl Sudhoff, "Brunschwig's *Anatomie*," *Archiv für Geschichte der Medizin* 1, no. 2 (1907): 141–56. The Low German edition is Hieronymus Brunschwig, *Buch der Cirurgia* (Rostock: Ludwig Dietz, 1518), VD16 B 8708; on this work, see Chiara Benati, "The 1518 Low German Edition of Hieronymus Brunschwig's *Buch der Cirurgia* and Its Terminology," in *Medieval German Textrelations: Translations, Editions, and Studies*, ed. Sibylle Jefferis (Göppingen: Kümmerle, 2012), 189–254. The first English edition is Hieronymus Brunschwig, *The Noble Experyence of the Vertuous Handy Warke of Surgeri* (London: Peter Treveris, 1525), USTC 501872; for more on this edition and its English context, see the penultimate section of this chapter. The Dutch edition is Hieronymus Brunschwig, *Dits dat hantwerck der cirurgien ende leert alle wonden, gehouden gesteken gheslaghen* (Utrecht: Jan Berntsz, 1535), USTC 421066. Benati notes a Czech translation of 1559, but this in fact appears to be a translation of Brunschwig's work on distillation: Hieronymus Brunschwig, *Knijhy o prawém Vmenij Dystyllowánj a neb wod pálen* (Olomouc: Jana Gúnthera, 1559), USTC 567651.

23. Hieronymus Brunschwig, *Chirurgia* (Augsburg: Alexander Weißenhorn, 1534), VD16 B 8706. This edition was popular, as suggested by its reprinting several years later as Hieronymus Brunschwig, *Chirurgia* (Augsburg: Alexander Weißenhorn, 1539), VD16 B 8707.

24. Johannes Peyligk, *Compendium philosophiae naturalis* (Leipzig: Melchior Lotter, 1499), ISTC ip00539000; Magnus Hundt, *Antropologium de hominis dignitate, natura et proprietatibus* (Leipzig: Wolfgang Stöckel, 1501), VD16 H 5904; Gregor Reisch, *Margarita philosophica* (Freiburg im Breisgau: Johann Schott, 1503), VD16 R 1033; Lorenz Freis, *Spiegel der Artzney* (Strassburg: Johann Grüninger, 1518), VD16 F 2871.

25. *In disem biechlin . . .* (Basel: Pamphilus Gengenbach, 1513), VD16 C 2049; *In disem biechlin . . .* (Cologne: Arnd von Aich, 1515), VD16 C 2051 and ZV 16650; *In disem buchlin . . .* (Augsburg: Hans Froschauer, 1515), VD16 C 2048 and C 2052. The medical contents of these books are discussed in Eckhart, "Medial Translations and Material Manifestations," 43–88. On the relationship of sixteenth-century German vernacular works such as these to contemporaneous Latin literature, see Mechtild Habermann, *Deutsche Fachtexte der frühen Neuzeit: Naturkundlich-medizinische Wissensvermittlung im Spannungsfeld von Latein und Volkssprache* (Berlin: De Gruyter, 2001).

26. Hans von Gersdorff, *Feldtbuch der Wundtartzney* (Strassburg: Johann Schott, 1517), VD16 G 1618. For an extremely full account of this book and Gersdorff's biography, including a revision of his date of death to 1520 based on archival documents, see Melanie Panse, *Hans von Gersdorffs "Feldbuch der Wundarznei": Produktion, Präsentation, und Rezeption von Wissen* (Wiesbaden: Reichert, 2012). On the use of the term *Feldbuch* and its translation, see Gundolf Keil, "Das Feldbuch als Vertreter der chirurgischen Fachprosa," *Studia Germanistica* 12, no. 20 (2018): 37–49; Chiara Benati, "The Field Surgery Manual Which Became a Medical Commonplace Book: Hans von Gersdorff's *Feldtbuch der Wundarzney* (1517) Translated into Low German," in *Bodily and Spiritual Hygiene in Medieval and Early Modern Literature*, ed. Albrecht Classen (Berlin: De Gruyter, 2017), 510–27.

27. Mentions of the towns of Grandson, Murten, and Nancy suggest that Gersdorff was involved in the Burgundian Wars. See Panse, *Hans von Gersdorffs "Feldbuch der Wundarznei,"* 27ff.

28. The image appears at the beginning of chap. 19, entitled "Von dem Chirurgico."

29. On developing military technologies in the fifteenth century, see Ralf Vollmuth, "'Von den geschosszenen Wunden': Die Behandlung von Schußwunden in deutschsprachigen chirurgischen Werken des 15. Jahrhunderts," *Orvostörténeti közlemények* 40, nos. 1/2 (1994): 5–28.

30. *Biblia latina* (Basel: Johann Amerbach, 1479), ISTC ib00561000. On this edition and other related books, see Kristian Jensen, "Printing the Bible in the Fifteenth Century: Devotion, Philology, and Commerce," in *Incunabula and Their Readers: Printing, Selling, and Using Books in the Fifteenth Century*, ed. Kristian Jensen (London: British Library, 2003), 115–38.

31. Hans von Gersdorff, *Feldtbuch der Wundartzney* (Strassburg: Johann Schott, 1526), VD16 G 1619, frontispiece.

32. On these saws and their "biting" work, see Hartnell, "Surgical Saws and Cutting-Edge Agency."

33. Vienna, MAK (Museum of Applied Arts), Inventarnummer F 1033. See a brief entry on this object in Walther Bernt, *Altes Werkzeug* (Munich: Callwey, 1939), no. 96.

34. These images are discussed in, among others, Suzanne Karr Schmidt, *Interactive and Sculptural Printmaking in the Renaissance* (Leiden: Brill, 2018), 133ff; Kusukawa, *Picturing the Book of Nature*, 7–15; Kerstin te Heesen, *Das illustrierte Flugblatt als Wissensmedium der Frühen Neuzeit: Langfristige Entwicklungen in Deutschland und neueste Daten für Ost- und Westdeutschland* (Leverkusen: Budrich, 2011), 306–12; Andrea Carlino, *Paper Bodies: A Catalogue of Anatomical Fugitive Sheets 1538–1687*, trans. Noga Arikha (London: Wellcome Institute, 1999), 88ff.

35. Such combined works are numerous. See, for instance, a well-preserved example in Vienna, Österreichische Nationalbibliothek, ALT PRUNK 70.P.12. On Wächtlin's role in developing color printing in Germany, see Alice Klein, "Hans Wechtlin and the Production of German Colour Woodcuts," in *Printing Colour 1400–1700: History, Techniques, Functions, and Receptions*, ed. Ad Stijnman and Elizabeth Savage (Leiden: Brill, 2015), 103–15.

36. For more on early modern concepts of the counterfeit, see Stephanie Leitch, "Visual Acuity and the Physiognomer's Art of Observation," *Oxford Art Journal* 38, no. 2 (2015): 189–208; Peter Parshall, "*Imago contrafacta*:

Images and Facts in the Northern Renaissance," *Art History* 16 (1993): 554–79.

37. Wendelin Hock, *Mentagra* (Strassburg: Johann Schott, 1514), VD16 H 4008. On Schott's other collaborators, see Christoph Reske, *Die Buchdrucker des 16. und 17. Jahrhunderts im deutschen Sprachgebiet: Auf der Grundlage des gleichnamigen Werks von Josef Benzing* (Wiesbaden: Harrassowitz, 2007), 874.

38. Hans von Gersdorff, *Feldtbuch der Wundartzney* (Augsburg: Heinrich Steiner, 1530), VD16 G 1621, chap. XVII; Hans von Gersdorff, *Feldtbuch der Wundartzney* (Augsburg: Heinrich Steiner, 1532), VD16 G 1623, chap. XVII.

39. Theodorus Priscianus, *Rerum medicarum* (Strassburg: Johann Schott, 1532), VD16 T 840, 115; Hildegard von Bingen, *Physica* (Strassburg: Johann Schott, 1533), VD16 H 3626, appearing just before the book's opening list of contents.

40. Hans von Gersdorff, *Feldtbuch der Wund-Artzney* (Strassburg: Johann Schott, 1540), VD16 G 1625, xliiii.

41. For more on the *Bild-Enzyklopädien*, see Stephanie Leitch, *Early Modern Print Media and the Art of Observation: Training the Literate Eye* (Cambridge: Cambridge University Press, 2024), 191–259; Ewa Chojecka, *Bayerische Bild-Enzyklopädie: Das Weltbild eines wissenschaftlich-magischen Hausbuches aus dem frühen 16. Jahrhundert* (Baden-Baden: Koerner, 1982). For a short introduction to the long history of this genre, see Rudolph, "Hausbücher (Nr. 49a)."

42. Kraków, Biblioteka Jagiellońska, BJ Rkp. Przyb. 35/64. The localization to Bavaria is made on linguistic grounds, while the possible date is taken from the start of the book's various calendrical materials.

43. Other technical medical materials are nearly always paired with folk traditions in this book. For instance, the bloodletting figure on fol. 27r is covered in green prints made from loading the leaves of healing plants with paint. Chojecka notes that similar prints that appear in the fencing portion of the manuscript appear to be knotweed, a herb commonly used in the treatment of the very wounds being sustained by the fencers: *Bayerische Bild-Enzyklopädie*, 18.

44. Inscribed around the circle in which the Wound Man stands, another verse draws attention to the same six non-naturals highlighted by the *Wundarznei*'s mnemonic poetry: "*ein artz solt anschaüen die zeit die aygnschafft, das elter die gegñt undt natur̈ und complexn*" (a doctor should look to the time, the quality, the age, the clime and nature and complexion). For earlier appearances of this verse in the *Wundarznei*, see chapter 2. The unusual inclusion of a leather instrument-case hanging from the circular frame of the scene is drawn from another image commonly included in the *Cirurgia* showing an arsenal of surgical tools hung around a wooden structure.

45. Erlangen, Friedrich-Alexander-Universität, Universitätsbibliothek, MS B 200, fols. 65v and 69r. The Rughalm family is recorded in Passau and Benedictus as studying at the University of Vienna; the manuscript could have been illustrated anywhere in this general south German-Austrian region. For more on this manuscript, see Leitch, *Early Modern Print Media and the Art of Observation*, 191ff; Pia Rudolph, "Hausbücher: Handschrift Nr. 49a.5.1.," in Bodemann et al., *Katalog der deutschsprachigen illustrierten Handschriften des Mittelalters (KdiH)*, vol. 6.

46. Vatican City, Biblioteca Apostolica Vaticana, MS Reg. Lat. 1298, fol. 41v. This is an intriguing book. It is listed in the seventeenth-century Roman library of Queen Christina of Sweden, but its previous provenance is not clear. See Jeanne Bignami Odier, "Les manuscrits de la Reine Christine au Vatican," in *Queen Christina of Sweden: Documents and Studies*, ed. Magnus von Platen (Stockholm: Norstedt & Söner, 1966), 38. One text within the manuscript reproduces the date 1546 in a hand that appears to have amended another text in the book, perhaps providing a terminus ante quem. All but one of these figures are tightly cropped paste-ins. They appear at first to be from Gersdorff's *Feldtbuch*, but on closer inspection they are of higher quality in terms of their detail; small variations (for instance, the presence of text scrolls in the brace images) reveal that they do not match any known *Feldtbuch* printings. The first image in the book, a bloodletting figure, is likewise virtually identical to that in Gersdorff but is a full-page insert rather than having been cut out of another printed book. None of the accompanying details of the original print are present—for instance, the date and title in the lower left-hand corner. All of this perhaps suggests that the images are the product of a printer with access to the original blocks.

47. Los Angeles, UCLA, Louise M. Darling Biomedical Library, MS Benjamin 8. On this manuscript, see Ferrari, *Medieval and Renaissance Manuscripts at the University of California, Los Angeles*, 12–13.

48. The 1551 edition was the *Feldtbuch*'s eleventh printing: Hans von Gersdorff, *Feldtbuch der Wundartzney* (Frankfurt: Hermann Gülfferich, 1551), VD16 G 1628. Two further Frankfurt editions followed in 1556 and 1576 under the title *Feldt und Stattbuch Wundtartzney*, but neither contains the Wound Man image.

49. These were produced in the presses of Cornelis Claesz, Jan Evertsz Cloppenburgh, and Jacob Theunisz Lootsman; they appear in the USTC as numbers 423160, 1013040, 1506228, 1508664, and 1820133. For a summary of the Dutch versions, see Panse, *Hans von Gersdorffs "Feldbuch der Wundarznei,"* 153ff.

50. *Wundartznei* (Strassburg: Christian Egenolff, 1530), VD16 C 2044. This volume contained only some of the incunable's original figures, but seven years later, in 1537, yet another Strassburg printer, Jacob Cammerlander, printed a book by the humanist writer Jacob Scholl entitled the *Fasciculus totius medicinae* (Little Bundle of All Medicine), VD16 S 3820, which contained new woodcuts of all six *Dreibilderserie* figures, including a nude, bearded Wound Man on fol. 54v.

51. *Thesoro universale della medicina* (Venice: Giovanni Antonio Vidali, 1668), USTC 1723198.

52. London, Wellcome Library, MS 990, 572. A large part of this book consists of ophthalmological procedures and images copied from the German physician Georg Bartisch's *Ophthalmodouleia* (Dresden: Matthes Stöckel, 1583), VD16 B 558. This suggests that the Wound Man was likewise copied from a printed source. That said, the manuscript is not without its own additions. For instance, in most scenarios the physicians and laymen of Bartisch's imagery have been replaced with monastic figures dressed in Franciscan garb, hence the attribution of this manuscript copy to a Franciscan house. The examination

booklet is the third edition of Joseph Schmid, *Examen chirurgicum* (Augsburg: Johann Weh, 1649), cited in the follow-on catalog to the VD16—the *Verzeichnis der im deutschen Sprachraum erschienenen Drucke des 17. Jahrhunderts* (hereafter VD17)—as 23:297229P; its Wound Man plate is inserted between pages 60 and 61.

53. Bethesda, National Library of Medicine, MS E 98, fol. 56r; Giovanni Battista Ferraro, *Trattato utile e necessario ad ogni agricoltore* (Bologna; Giovanni Antonio Remondin, 1673), Bethesda, National Library of Medicine, WZ 250 F3764t 1673, 40.

54. Useful summaries are J. Andrew Mendelsohn, Annemarie Kinzelbach, and Ruth Schilling, eds., *Civic Medicine: Physician, Polity, and Pen in Early Modern Europe* (London: Routledge, 2019); Ian Maclean, *Logic, Signs, and Nature in the Renaissance: The Case of Learned Medicine* (Cambridge: Cambridge University Press, 2002); David Gentilcore, *Healers and Healing in Early Modern Italy* (Manchester: Manchester University Press, 1998); Laurence Brockliss and Colin Jones, *The Medical World of Early Modern France* (Oxford: Clarendon, 1997).

55. Lawrence is speaking in more general terms about scientific practice as a whole, but her comments transfer interestingly to medicine as a subfield: *Charitable Knowledge: Hospital Pupils and Practitioners in Eighteenth-Century London* (Cambridge: Cambridge University Press, 2010), 20.

56. For more on these anatomical ideas, see Monique Kornell, *Flesh and Bones: The Art of Anatomy* (Los Angeles: Getty Research Institute, 2022); Andrew Cunningham, *The Anatomical Renaissance: The Resurrection of the Anatomical Projects of the Ancients* (London: Routledge, 1997). The Wound Man's history could be argued to intersect closely with contemporary shifts in anatomical understanding during the period, both in Europe and elsewhere. But given that these materials have been covered extensively—even exhaustively—in the scholarship, I do not make further reference to them in this chapter, mindful instead of treating the Wound Man on its own terms.

57. On Paracelsus and for an extensive bibliography of his life and work, see Bruce T. Moran, *Paracelsus: An Alchemical Life* (London: Reaktion, 2019).

58. Paracelsus, *Die Große Wundarznei* (Augsburg: Heinrich Steiner, 1536), VD16 P 452, chap. XVII; Andreas Vesalius, *Chirurgia magna* (Venice: Vincenzo Valgrisi, 1568), USTC 863065, fol. 214v.

59. Driving some of the most engaging investigations of this artisanal knowledge is the work of Pamela H. Smith, most recently *From Lived Experience to the Written Word: Reconstructing Practical Knowledge in the Early Modern World* (Chicago: University of Chicago Press, 2022).

60. The best example of such a Nahuatl codex is a book known today as the Codex Mexicanus, now Paris, Bibliothèque nationale de France, MS Mexicain 23–24. Its Zodiac Man, on page 12, draws from Andrés de León, *Tratados de medicina, cirugia, y anatomia* (Valladolid: Luis Sánchez, 1605), USTC 5017734, or perhaps from León's slightly earlier *Libro primero de annathomia* (Baeza: Juan Bautista de Montoya, 1591), USTC 339447. An interesting example of Arabic materials moving eastward is discussed in Vivek Gupta, "Images for Instruction: A Multilingual Illustrated Dictionary in Fifteenth-Century Sultanate India," *Muqarnas* 38, no. 1 (2021): 77–112. Persian versions of Vesalian skeletons appear in Bethesda, National Library of Medicine, P 20, item 2, fols. 558b–559a. On Chinese equivalents, see Jonathan Hay, "Culture, Ethnicity, and Empire in the Work of Two Eighteenth-Century 'Eccentric' Artists," *RES* 35 (1999): 201–23.

61. For a recent rich overview of intercultural print transmission in various contexts, see the essays in *Prints as Agents of Global Change, 1500–1800*, ed. Heather Madar (Amsterdam: Amsterdam University Press, 2021).

62. Jean Tagault, *De chirurgica institutione libri quinque* (Paris: Chrétien Wechel, 1543), USTC 140825, 143. Only one *Dreibilderserie* manuscript containing the figure is known to have been produced in France during the later Middle Ages, and its specific provenance remains unclear; for more on this, see chapter 2. On Tagault's biography, see Maurits Biesbrouck, Theodoor Goddeeris, and Omer Steeno, "Jean Tagault (c. 1486–1546), professor heelkunde in Parijs, plagiator van Vesalius' *Tabulae anatomicae sex* (1538)?," *Journal of the Royal Library of Belgium* 10 (2017): 7–63.

63. Iain Lonie, "The 'Paris Hippocratics': Teaching and Research in Paris in the Second Half of the Sixteenth Century," in *The Medical Renaissance of the Sixteenth Century*, ed. Andrew Wear, Iain Lonie, and Roger French (Cambridge: Cambridge University Press, 1985), 155–74.

64. Houllier would himself rise to become a significant medical authority, publishing alongside Tagault.

65. Initially, Wechel produced multiple editions of Galenic works, but from the 1540s, he issued a more diverse range of historical and contemporary medical books. On Chrétien Wechel, see Geneviève Guilleminot-Chrétien, "Chrétien Wechel, Rabelais et le *Tiers livre*," in *Narrations fabuleuses: Melanges en l'honneur de Mireille Huchon*, ed. Isabelle Garnier et al. (Paris: Garnier, 2022), 129–38; Elizabeth Armstrong, "The Origins of Chrétien Wechel Re-Examined," *Bibliothèque d'Humanisme et Renaissance* 23(1961): 341–46.

66. Sten Lindberg notes that Wechel must have traded blocks with Hermann Ryff and Balthasar Beck in Strassburg: *Chrestien Wechel and Vesalius: Twelve Unique Medical Broadsides from the Sixteenth Century* (Uppsala: Almqvist & Wiksells, 1954), 64. On the ability of printers to travel in sixteenth-century France, see Malcolm Walsby, "Printer Mobility in Sixteenth-Century France," in *Print Culture and Peripheries in Early Modern Europe*, ed. Benito Rial Costas (Leiden: Brill, 2013), 249–70.

67. The only other images in the book are three skeletons taken from a work by Vesalius and printed in Venice by Bernadino Vitalis, the *Tabulae anatomicae sex* (1538); this book survives today in only two copies, one of which is now Venice, Biblioteca Nazionale Marciana, 228.d.1. The degree to which these images can be seen as directly plagiarized—if indeed such a modern term is even useful in this context—is discussed by Andrea Carlino, who summarizes Sten Lindberg's findings that an earlier fugitive sheet of skeletons was produced by Wechel in 1536, perhaps with Vesalius's knowledge: *Paper Bodies*, 47ff.

68. Jean Tagault, *De chirurgica institutione libri quinque* (Venice: Vincenzo Valgrisi, 1544), USTC 857925, 143.

69. Jean Tagault, *De chirurgica institutione libri quinque* (Lyon: Guillaume Rouillé, 1545), USTC 154827. On Rouillé, see Natalie Zemon Davis, "Publisher Guillaume Rouillé: Businessman and Humanist," in *Editing Sixteenth*

Century Texts, ed. Richard J. Schoeck (Toronto: University of Toronto Press, 1966), 72–112. For an interesting parallel case, see Charles Schmitt, "The Correspondence of Jacques Daléchamps (1513–1588)," *Viator* 8 (1977): 399–434.

70. The Swiss edition is excerpted in Conrad Gessner, *Chirurgia* (Zürich: Andreas and Hans Jakob Geßner, 1555), USTC 621030. The Dutch edition is Jean Tagault, *Der chirurgijen instructie* (Antwerp: printer unknown, 1559), USTC 441128. The Frankfurt edition excerpts Tagault's work as part of Peter Uffenbach, *Thesaurus chirurgicae* (Frankfurt: Jakob Fischer and Nikolaus Hoffman, 1610), USTC 2119695. The Dordrecht edition is Jean Tagault, *Der chirurgyen instructie* (Dordrecht: Peeter Verhaghen, 1621), USTC 1027807. The Amsterdam edition is Jean Tagault, *Chirurgie* (Amsterdam: Broer Jansz, 1649), USTC 1122692, now lost.

71. Tagault, *Les institutions chirurgiques*, 245. The French and Latin editions of this work were clearly conceived in tandem by Rouillé, as the privileges included in both date to the same day, July 19, 1547.

72. Davis, "Publisher Guillaume Rouillé," 90, citing the privilege of Paolo Giovio, *Histoires* (Lyon: Guillaume Rouillé, 1558), USTC 15098. On medicine developing in the French and Italian vernaculars, see Andrea Carlino and Michel Jeanneret, eds., *Vulgariser la medicine: Du style medical en France et en Italie (XVIe et* XVII*e siècles)* (Geneva: Droz, 2009).

73. Although she does not mention Tagault, Maria Patijn discusses the use of the crossbow in healing: "The Medical Crossbow from Jan Yperman to Isaack Koedijck," in *Wounds in the Middle Ages*, ed. Anne Kirkham and Cordelia Warr (London: Routledge, 2016), 197–214. She does mention a related image from a copy of Gui de Chauliac's work printed in Venice in 1546, although here the crossbow is illustrated in a complete scene of extraction rather than a floating leg. The edition is Guy de Chauliac, *Ars chirurgica* (Venice: Lucantonio Giunta, 1546), USTC 803161, fol. 27v.

74. These Czech works are discussed in chapter 2.

75. Jacopo Berengario da Carpi, *Tractatus de fractura calve sive cranei* (Bologna: Girolamo Benedetti, 1518), USTC 813936. For an English translation and commentary, see L. R. Lind, "Berengario da Carpi on Fracture of the Skull or Cranium," *Transactions of the American Philosophical Society* 80, no. 4 (1990): 1–164.

76. Berengario da Carpi, *Tractatus de fractura calve sive cranei*, fol. CIIIv.

77. Jacopo Berengario da Carpi, *Tractatus perutilis et completus de fractura cranei* (Venice: Giovanni Antonio Nicolini da Sabio and Giovanni Battista Pederzani, 1535), USTC 813942, title page. The same printer-publisher team was also behind a particularly intricate flap anatomy of a female figure from 1539, now London, Wellcome Library, EPB/D/7340.2. My thanks to Monique Kornell for bringing this connection to my attention.

78. For an exhaustive catalog of Paré's works, see Janet Doe, *A Bibliography of the Works of Ambroise Paré* (Chicago: University of Chicago Press, 1937). On Paré's biography and times, see Jean-Pierre Poirier, *Ambroise Paré: Un urgentiste au XVIe siècle* (Paris: Pygmalion, 2005); Évelyne Berriot-Salvadore, ed., *Ambroise Paré (1510–1590): Pratique et écriture de la science à la Renaissance* (Paris: Honoré Champion, 2003); the classic Joseph-François Malgaigne, *Oeuvres complètes d'Ambroise Paré*, 3 vols. (Paris: Baillière, 1840–1841). For Paré's work on prosthetics specifically, see Heide Hausse, *The Malleable Body: Surgeons, Artisans, and Amputees in Early Modern Germany* (Manchester: Manchester University Press, 2023), 210–37.

79. This is from the dedication to the first edition of Paré's collected works: *Les oeuvres de M. Ambroise Paré* (Paris: Gabriel Buon, 1575), USTC 29582.

80. Ambroise Paré, *La maniere de traicter les playes faictes tant par hacquebutes que par fleches* (Paris: Widow of Jean de Brie, 1552), USTC 23471.

81. When and where exactly the printed trope of a limb emanating from a cloud first appears is unclear. The woodcutter may have been looking to the images which accompanied Gersdorff's *Feldtbuch*, which while not quite emanating from clouds are sometimes flanked by them. The technique is also used to present a pair of hands in the printer's mark of Vincenzo Valgrisi, publisher of the first Venetian editions of Tagault's *De chirurgia institutione*, another possible source.

82. Paré, *Les oeuvres de M. Ambroise Paré* (1575), iii.

83. The artist Paré commissioned for these engravings is not currently known, but Paule Dumaître suggests that no fewer than five—Jean le Royer, René Boivin, Etienne Delaune, Léonard Gaultier, and Stephanus Delaulne—were all at some point responsible for portraits of Paré that appear in his publications: "Les représentations d'Ambroise Paré: Gravures, peintures, sculptures, scènes d'histoire et de guerre," *Histoire des sciences médicales* 34, no. 4 (2000): 349–66.

84. London, Wellcome Library, EPB/B/4818.

85. The origins and ordering of these images suggest that among the book's sources were many different works by Paré. The first thirty-five images appear in almost precisely the same order as Paré's 1552 work on projectiles that was printed by the widow of Jean de Brie, as mentioned earlier, and at least four further images have been taken from the 1575 *Oeuvres*. Other anatomical images appear to be taken from Ambroise Paré, *La methode curative des playes et fractures de la teste humaine* (Paris: Jean le Royer, 1561), USTC 29579; Ambroise Paré, *Anatomie universelle du corps humain* (Paris: Jean le Royer, 1561), USTC 29578; Ambroise Paré, *Dix livres de la chirurgie* (Paris: Jean Le Royer, 1564), USTC 27088.

86. London, Wellcome Library, EPB/B/4818, fol. b8r.

87. Nicolas was the brother of the collector François Rasse des Neux, discussed in Malcolm Walsby, "Plantin and the French Book Market," in *International Exchange in the Early Modern Book World*, ed. Matthew McLean and Sara K. Barker (Leiden: Brill, 2016), 93.

88. Ambroise Paré, *Les oeuvres de M. Ambroise Paré* (Paris: Gabriel Buon, 1585), USTC 3626.

89. Thomas Gale, *Certaine Workes of Chirurgerie* (London: Rowland Hall, 1563), USTC 506133. On Gale, see Max Satchell, "Gale, Thomas (c. 1507–1567)," in *Oxford Dictionary of National Biography* (Oxford: Oxford University Press, 2004); Elizabeth Lane Furdell, *The Royal Doctors, 1485–1714: Medical Personnel at the Tudor and Stuart Courts* (Rochester, NY: University of Rochester Press, 2001), 85.

90. Gale, *Certaine Workes of Chirurgerie*, book II, frontispiece.

91. See chapter 2.

92. On early modern English medicine more generally, see Melissa Reynolds, *Reading Practice: The Pursuit of Natural Knowledge from Manuscript to Print* (Chicago: University of Chicago Press, 2024); Elaine Leong, *Recipes and Everyday Knowledge: Medicine, Science, and the Household in Early Modern England* (Chicago: University of Chicago Press, 2018); Elizabeth Lane Furdell, *Publishing and Medicine in Early Modern England* (Rochester, NY: University of Rochester Press, 2002); Andrew Wear, *Knowledge and Practice in English Medicine, 1550–1680* (Cambridge: Cambridge University Press, 2000); Margaret Pelling, *Sickness, Medical Occupations, and the Urban Poor in Early Modern England* (London: Routledge, 1998). Two ongoing digital projects look set to significantly extend our understanding of this field: "The Medical World of Early Modern England, Wales and Ireland, c. 1500–1715," a database of medical practitioners based at the Centre for Medical History at the University of Exeter, https://practitioners.exeter.ac.uk (accessed August 1, 2024); "Reading Early Medicine (Beta)," a database of pre-1700 English medical books being produced by Mary Fissell and Elaine Leong and currently hosted by the Max-Planck-Institut für Wissenschaftsgeschichte in Berlin, https://reademed.mpiwg-berlin.mpg.de (accessed August 1, 2024).

93. The institution was known from 1551 as the Royal College of Physicians, under which name it still functions.

94. These works are Ulrich von Hutten, *Of the Wood Called Guaiacum* (London: Thomas Berthelet, 1536), USTC 502815; Desiderius Erasmus, *A Declamacion in the Prayse and Commendation of the Most Hygh and Excellent Science of Phisyke* (London: Robert Redman, 1537), USTC 502897; Eucharius Rösslin, *The Byrth of Mankynde* (London: Thomas Raynald, 1540), USTC 503194; Guy de Chauliac, *The Questyonary of Cyrurgyens* (London: Robert Wyer, 1542), USTC 503341; Giovanni da Vigo, *The Most Excellent Workes of Chirurgerye* (London: Edward Whitchurch, 1543), USTC 503456; *Regimen sanitatis Salerni* (London: Thomas Berthelet, 1528), USTC 502087; *The Practyse of Cyrurgyons of Mountpyller* (London: Richard Bankes, 1540), USTC 503136.

95. Hieronymus Brunschwig, *The Noble Experyence of the Vertuous Handy Warke of Surgeri* (London: Peter Treveris, 1525), USTC 501872.

96. Here he is presumably referring, respectively, to the original 1497 Strassburg edition and the 1518 edition from Rostock, both noted earlier.

97. From Reisch he borrows diagrams of the brain and inner anatomy; from the Chauliac editions he borrows images of surgical instruments; and from Vérard and du Pré he borrows a style of Zodiac Man familiar from their printed Books of Hours, also known by scholars today as the Planetary Man.

98. On an earlier attempt to combine physicians and surgeons in London, see Justin Colson and Robert Ralley, "Medical Practice, Urban Politics, and Patronage: The London 'Commonalty' of Physicians and Surgeons of the 1420s," *English Historical Review* 130, no. 546 (2015): 1102–31. On practical medicine elsewhere in England, see Donna A. Seger, *The Practical Renaissance: Information Culture and the Quest for Knowledge in Early Modern England* (London: Bloomsbury, 2022).

99. These figures come from Rosemary O'Day, *The Professions in Early Modern England, 1450–1800* (London: Routledge, 2000), 193–95.

100. On uroscopy, see Robert Record, *The Urinal of Physick* (London: Reyner Wolfe, 1547), USTC 503906. On anatomy, see Thomas Vicary, *A Profitable Treatise of the Anatomie of Mans Body* (London: Henry Bamford, 1577), USTC 508458, although this work is referenced by some contemporaries as having first been printed in 1548. See Duncan Thomas, "Thomas Vicary and the *Anatomie of Mans Body*," *Medical History* 50, no. 2 (2006): 235–46.

101. On this movement in a number of different areas, see Anna-Maria Hartmann, *English Mythography in Its European Context, 1500–1650* (Oxford: Oxford University Press, 2018); Sarah Hutton, "Platonism, Stoicism, Scepticism, and Classical Imitation," in *A New Companion to English Renaissance Literature and Culture*, ed. Michael Hattaway (Oxford: Blackwell, 2010), 1:106–19; Donna Kurtz, "The Concept of the Classical Past in Tudor and Early Stuart England," *Journal of the History of Collections* 20, no. 2 (2008): 189–204; John E. Curran, *Roman Invasions: The British History, Protestant Anti-Romanism, and the Historical Imagination in England, 1530–1660* (Newark: University of Delaware Press, 2002); Lucy Gent, ed., *Albion's Classicism: The Visual Arts in Britain 1550–1660* (New Haven, CT: Yale University Press, 1995).

102. On the specifics of related Classical translations, see Vivian Nutton, "Humanist Surgery," in Wear, Lonie, and French, *The Medical Renaissance of the Sixteenth Century*, 75–99.

103. Claudius Galen, *De temperamentis* (Cambridge: John Siberch, 1521), USTC 501666; Claudius Galen, *De naturalibus facultatibus* (London: Richard Pynson, 1523), USTC 501743; Claudius Galen, *De symptomatum differentiis* (London: Richard Pynson, 1524), USTC 501787.

104. Quoted in Wear, *Knowledge and Practice in English Medicine*, 43n82, from Llwyd's translation of *The Treasury of Healthe Conteynyng Many Profitable Medycines* (London: William Copland, 1550), USTC 516498. In 1556, the United Company required all apprentices to be literate in English and Latin, although this regulation was dropped in 1557.

105. For a recent investigation into the literary roles played by science in early modern English, see Debapriya Sarkar, *Possible Knowledge: The Literary Forms of Early Modern Science* (Philadelphia: University of Pennsylvania Press, 2023).

106. This number is based on data from the Reading Early Medicine (Beta) database, cited earlier. Paul Slack suggests a figure of around 153 strictly medical titles published in England before 1605: "Mirrors of Health and Treasures of Poor Men: The Uses of the Vernacular Medical Literature of Tudor England," in *Health, Medicine, and Mortality in the Sixteenth Century*, ed. Charles Webster (Cambridge: Cambridge University Press, 1979), 237–74.

107. Plutarch, *Precepts for the Preservation of Good Healthe* (London: Richard Grafton, 1543), USTC 503449. On translations of Plutarch, see Fred Schurink, "Print, Patronage, and Occasion: Translations of Plutarch's 'Moralia' in Tudor England," *Yearbook of English Studies* 38, nos. 1/2 (2008): 86–101.

108. Christopher Langton, *An Introduction into Phisycke* (London: Edward Whitchurch, 1545), USTC 503663.

109. Christopher Langton, *A Very Brefe Treatise, Ordrely*

Declaring the Principal Partes of Physik (London: Edward Whitchurch, 1547), USTC 503917.

110. For a case study in Wyer's editorship and some details of his relatively unknown biography, see Christine Silvi, "Mise au point sur deux petits imprimés anglais: Robert Wyer, éditeur du 'Livre de Sidrac,'" *Gutenberg-Jahrbuch* 92 (2017): 123–40.

111. *The Questyonary of Cyrurgyens, with the Fourth Boke of the Terapentyke* (London: Robert Wyer, 1542), USTC 503341.

112. *Prognosticacion, Drawen Out of the Bookes of Ipocras, Avicen, and Other Notable Auctours* (London: Robert Wyer, 1545), USTC 503644.

113. Plutarch, *Practica Plutarche the Excellent Phylosopher* (London: Robert Wyer, 1545), USTC 503652; Plutarch, *The Governaunce of Good Helthe* (London: Robert Wyer, 1549), USTC 504290.

114. Claudius Galen, *Certaine Workes of Galens Called Methodus Medendi* (London: John Kingston and Henry Denham, 1567), USTC 516677. See also an entry on this work in Neil Rhodes, ed., *English Renaissance Translation Theory* (London: Modern Humanities Research Association, 2013), 312–16.

115. The term *Enchiridion* was popularized in northern Europe by Martin Luther and probably reached Gale via the English translation of Erasmus's *Enchiridion militis Christiani* (The Christian Soldier's Handbook): *A Booke Called in Latyn Enchiridion militis Christiani, and in Englysshe the Manuell of the Christen Knyght* (London: Wynkyn de Worde, 1533), USTC 502542.

116. Gale, *Certaine Workes*, book I, 9.

117. Gale, *Certaine Workes*, book I, 6.

118. Thomas Elyot, *The Boke Named The Governour* (London: Thomas Berthelet, 1531), USTC 502320, fol. 50r. As well as Field's poem, Gale's book II, the *Enchiridion*, is given a poetic preface by John Hall, and his book IV, the *Antidoarie*, is given another by William Cunningham. In the same year, 1563, Hall produced an invective against quack doctors written entirely in verse: *A Poesie in Forme of a Vision* (London: Roland Hall, 1563), USTC 516629.

119. Satchell cites Gale's will as London, National Archives, PRO, PROB 11/49, sig. 255.

120. Thomas Gale, *Certaine Workes of Chirurgerie* (London: Thomas East, 1586), USTC 510524; William Clowes, *A Prooved Practise for All Young Chirurgians* (London: Thomas Orwin, 1588), USTC 510929. On Clowes, see Celeste Chamberland, "Between the Hall and the Market: William Clowes and Surgical Self-Fashioning in Elizabethan London," *Sixteenth Century Journal* 41, no. 1 (2010): 69–89; Furdell, *The Royal Doctors, 1485–1714*, 87ff; Frederick N. L. Poynter, ed., *The Selected Writings of William Clowes* (London: Harvey & Blythe, 1948).

121. In "Between the Hall and the Market," Chamberland paints a picture of Clowes as building a reputation of intelligence and respectability in print in order to whitewash his often troublesome personality and complicated professional relations.

122. Clowes, *A Prooved Practise for All Young Chirurgians*, Piiii4r. Note that this appears in a part of the book where the running pagination at the top of the page is paused.

123. Ambroise Paré, *The Method of Curing Wounds Made by Gun-Shot* (London: Isaac Jaggard, 1617), USTC 3007488; Ambroise Paré, *The Workes of That Famous Chirurgion Ambrose Parey* (London: Thomas Cotes and Robert Young, 1634), USTC 3017258.

124. Helkiah Crooke, *ΜΙΚΡΟΚΟΣΜΟΓΡΑΦΙΑ: A Description of the Body of Man* (London: Thomas Cotes and Richard Cotes, 1631), USTC 3015323. On seventeenth-century physicians, see the classic work by Harold J. Cook, *The Decline of the Old Medical Regime in Stuart London* (Ithaca, NY: Cornell University Press, 1986). The figure also appeared in Crooke's shorter *ΣΩΜΑΤΩΓΑΦΙΑ ΑΝΘΡΩΠΙΝΗ, or A Description of the Body of Man* (London: Thomas Cotes, 1634), USTC 3017315. Clearly the figure avoided the censorship of civic and collegiate authorities who had seen wrangling over the original edition of the *ΜΙΚΡΟΚΟΣΜΟΓΡΑΦΙΑ*. On this affair, see Lauren Kassell, "Medical Understandings of the Body, c. 1500–1750," in *The Routledge History of Sex and the Body, 1500 to the Present*, ed. Sarah Toulalan and Kate Fisher (London: Routledge, 2013), 57–74.

125. *A Larum for London* (London: Edward Allde, 1602), USTC 3001037. The character of Stump is discussed in Patricia A. Cahill, *Unto the Breach: Martial Formations, Historical Trauma, and the Early Modern Stage* (Oxford: Oxford University Press, 2008), 189.

126. Daniel Lakin, *A Miraculous Cure of the Prusian Swallow-Knife* (London: John Oakes, 1642), USTC 3051502. The account first appeared in Germany, originally in Latin and later in German: *Acclamationes votivae, in nuperam sectionem, Regiomonte Borussorum factam, cum rustico, qui per imprudentiam, cultrum deglutierat* (Königsberg: Peter Händel, 1635), VD17 23:261509F; Daniel Beckher, *Historische Beschreibung des Preussischen Messerschluckers* (Königsberg: Peter Händel, 1643), VD17 23:235310R.

127. London, British Library, C.20.f.7.474-475 and English Broadside Ballad Archive no. 30317. Thanks to Thom Pritchard for drawing this work to my attention. On the contents of contemporary surgical handbills, see Roberta Mullini, "Graphic Surgical Practice in the Handbills of Seventeenth-Century London Irregulars," in *Medical Paratexts from Medieval to Modern: Dissecting the Page*, ed. Hannah C. Tweed and Diane G. Scott (London: Palgrave Macmillan Cham, 2018), 57–73.

128. Alexander Wragge-Morley, *Aesthetic Science: Representing Nature in the Royal Society of London, 1650–1720* (Chicago: University of Chicago Press, 2020).

129. John Browne, *A Compleat Discourse of Wounds* (London: E[lizabeth?] Flesher, 1678), USTC 3097607. On Browne, see Sophie Morris, "John Browne's *Treatise of the Muscles* (1681) and the Image of Mobility in Late Seventeenth-Century London," PhD diss., University College London, 2019; Ian Lyle, "Browne, John (1642–1702/3?)," in *Oxford Dictionary of National Biography* (Oxford: Oxford University Press, 2004); Kenneth F. Russell, "John Browne, 1642–1702: A Seventeenth-Century Surgeon, Anatomist, and Plagiarist," *Bulletin of the History of Medicine* 33, no. 6 (1959): 503–25.

130. Browne, *A Compleat Discourse of Wounds*, 34–35. Browne emphasizes the figure again later in the book, on page 96, when he turns to consider gunshot wounds: "when they [surgeons] enter the stage of Gunshot-Wounds, they ought so readily to be prepared with the Knowledge of them … being conducted by Hippocrates, the Master of the Ceremony, I here to commend you to the Figure, which does relate how the humane Body may

receive the impress of many kinds of war-like Instruments, no Part being shot-free from the Head to the Foot. The Figure is presented you before, near the beginning of my discourse of Wounds in generall."

131. In an intellectual sense too, Browne clearly understood images to be an important element of argumentation, and he was just as committed as his scientific contemporaries in the Royal Society to visualizing ideas. He had contributed to the society's journal, *Philosophical Transactions*, when in 1685 he offered a short description of hepatic cirrhosis in a patient at St. Thomas' Hospital accompanied by a labeled image of the dissected liver in question: "A Remarkable Account of a Liver," *Philosophical Transactions* 15, no. 178 (1685): 1266–68.

132. On White's biography, see Anne Dunan-Page, "'The Pourtraiture of John Bunyan' Revisited: Robert White and Images of the Author," *Bunyan Studies* 13 (2008): 7–39; Antony Griffiths, *The Print in Stuart Britain, 1603–1689* (London: British Museum, 1998), 203–7.

133. *Hospitium Mente-Captorum Londinense*, London, British Museum, no. 1977, U.824; John Browne, *Adenochoiradelogia, or, An Anatomick-Chirurgical Treatise of Glandules and Strumaes* (London: Thomas Newcomb, 1684), USTC 3109105.

134. Browne's own portrait by White is included at the beginning of the *Compleat Discourse* as well as in several of the surgeon's later writings. This was just one of many commissions granted to the engraver by medics in the capital and beyond, ranging from well-known experts such as Thomas Browne, George Ent, James Cooke, and Richard Morton to others decried as quacks by the medical establishment, for instance William Salmon. At least six portraits of John Browne are known from between 1677 and 1698, although several of these may simply have been adjusted by other artists from White's original. All are listed in the collections of London's National Portrait Gallery: Reference Collection, NPG D30094 to D30099.

135. Johan van Beverwijck, *Wercken der genees-konste* (Amsterdam: Widow of Jan Jacobsz. Schipper, 1672), USTC 1809520. On another of Beverwijck's publications, see Cornelia Niekus Moore, "'Not by Nature but by Custom': Johan van Beverwijck's *Van de wtnementheyt des vrouwelicken Geslachts*," *Sixteenth Century Journal* 25, no. 3 (1994): 633–51.

136. Many of White's portraits are in Oxford and are listed in C. F. Bell and Rachel Poole, "English Seventeenth-Century Portrait Drawings in Oxford Collections: Part II," *Walpole Society* 14 (1925–1926): 64ff.

137. John Ogilby, *Homer, His Odysses Translated, Adorn'd with Sculpture* (London: James Flesher, 1669), USTC 3084976. White's 1669 commission was to copy the frontispiece of an earlier, similar work, *Homer, His Iliads Translated, Adorn'd with Sculpture* (London: Thomas Roycroft, 1660), USTC 3078465; Anthony Wood, *Historia et antiquitates Universitatis Oxoniensis* (Oxford: Theatro Sheldoniano, 1674), USTC 3092377.

138. Joachim von Sandrart, *Teutsche Academie* (Nuremberg: Michael Endter, 1679), VD17 1:080147T; Jan Bisschop, *Signorum veterum icones* (Amsterdam: printer unknown, 1668–1669), USTC 1806274.

139. François Perrier, *Segmenta nobilium signorum et statuarum* (Rome: printer unknown, 1638), USTC 4008512, table 30. The sculpture and its reception history are discussed in Francis Haskell and Nicholas Penny, *Taste and the Antique: The Lure of Classical Sculpture, 1500–1900* (New Haven, CT: Yale University Press, 1981), 136–41.

140. On Scultetus's biography, see Anneliese Seiz, *Johannes Scultetus und sein Werk: Biographie und Glossar* (Stuttgart: Kohlhammer, 1974). For a shorter summary, see Werner E. Gerabek, "Scultetus, Johannes," *Neue Deutsche Biographie* 24 (2010): 101.

141. Johannes Scultetus, *ΧΕΙΡΟΠΛΟΘΗΚΗ, seu Armamentarium Chirurgicum* (Ulm: Balthasar Kühne, 1655), VD17 39:153208L.

142. Johannes Scultetus, *Wund-Artzneyisches Zeug-Hauß* (Frankfurt am Main: Johannes Gerlini, 1666), VD17 12:194393D. Multiple Wound Men appear at table LII; the doubled figures appear at table XXV, although intriguingly the plate bears an earlier date of 1658.

143. Johannes Scultetus, *ΧΕΙΡΟΠΛΟΘΗΚΗ, seu Armamentarium Chirurgicum* (The Hague: Adriaan Vlacq, 1656), USTC 1829040; Johannes Scultetus, *Magazyn, ofte, Wapen-huys* (Amsterdam: Jan Jansen Brouwer, 1657), USTC 1842475; Johannes Scultetus, *Het Vermeerderde Wapenhuis der Heel-Meesters* (Amsterdam: Janssoons van Waesberge, 1748), Amsterdam, Universiteitsbibliotheek, OTM: O 62-7225,7226.

144. Johannes Scultetus, *L'arcenal de chirurgie de Iean Scultet* (Lyon: Antoine Galien, 1672), USTC 6073811; Johannes Scultetus, *The Chyrurgeons Store-house Furnished with Forty-Three Tables Cut in Brass* (London: John Starkey, 1674), USTC 3091631.

145. Irako Mitsuaki 伊良子光顕, *Geka kinmō zui* 外科訓蒙図彙 (Kyoto: unknown publisher, 1769), Union Catalog Database of Japanese Texts (hereafter UCDJT), WID no. 1000948. Norman Ozaki notes that the work is sometimes dated 1767, which is in fact the date of the work's preface: "Conceptual Changes in Japanese Medicine during the Tokugawa Period," PhD diss., University of California at San Francisco, 1979, 127ff.

146. For recent work on these companies, see Adam Clulow and Tristan Mostert, eds., *The Dutch and English East India Companies: Diplomacy, Trade, and Violence in Early Modern Asia* (Amsterdam: Amsterdam University Press, 2018). Medicine's place in these colonial histories has received extensive treatment, most recently in Zachary Dorner, *Merchants of Medicines: The Commerce and Coercion of Health in Britain's Long Eighteenth Century* (Chicago: University of Chicago Press, 2020); Kalle Kananoja and Markku Hokkanen, eds., *Healers and Empires in Global History: Healing as Hybrid and Contested Knowledge* (Cham: Springer, 2019); Suman Seth, *Difference and Disease: Medicine, Race, and the Eighteenth-Century British Empire* (Cambridge: Cambridge University Press, 2018). For recent work specifically on the role of surgeons in colonial contexts, see Craig Koslofsky and Roberto Zaugg, eds. and trans., *A German Barber-Surgeon in the Atlantic Slave Trade: The Seventeenth-Century Journal of Johann Peter Oettinger* (Charlottesville: University of Virginia Press, 2020).

147. The seminal account in English of Japan's isolationist policies—which emphasizes such policies' coexistence with a more complex and connected stance toward East Asian nations and has inspired much subsequent work—is Ronald P. Toby, *State and Diplomacy in Early Modern Japan: Asia in the Development of the Tokugawa Bakufu* (Princeton, NJ: Princeton University Press, 1984).

148. Histories of Dejima have largely been written through the extensive record-keeping activities of the Dutch, in particular the so-called "Deshima Diaries," a series of continuous journals kept by respective Dutch heads of the trading post. The diaries and their marginalia have been published in a number of volumes, most recently in Cynthia Vialle, Isabel Tanaka-van Daalen, and Leonard Blussé, eds., *The Deshima Diaries 1641–1660* (Leiden: Brill, 2023).

149. On Andreas Cleyer, see his *Tagebuch des Kontors zu Nagasaki auf der Insel Deshima, 20 Oktober 1682–5 November 1683*, trans. Eva S. Kraft (Bonn: Bonner Zeitschrift für Japanologie, 1985). On Ten Rhijne, see Harold J. Cook, *Matters of Exchange: Commerce, Medicine, and Science* (New Haven, CT: Yale University Press, 2007), 349ff; Robert W. Carrubba and John Z. Bowers, "The Western World's First Detailed Treatise on Acupuncture: Willem Ten Rhijne's *De acupunctura*," *Journal of the History of Medicine and Allied Sciences* 29, no. 4 (1974): 371–98.

150. On Japanese medicine before sustained European contact, see Andrew Goble, *Confluences of Medicine in Medieval Japan: Buddhist Healing, Chinese Knowledge, Islamic Formulas, and Wounds of War* (Honolulu: University of Hawaii Press, 2011). On the early importation of distillation techniques, see Wolfgang Michel and Elke Werger-Klein, "Drop by Drop: The Introduction of Western Distillation Techniques into Seventeenth-Century Japan," *Journal of the Japanese Society for the History of Medicine* 50, no. 3 (2004): 463–92. On botany, see Willy F. van de Walle and Kazuhiko Kasaya, eds., *Dodonaeus in Japan: Translation and the Scientific Mind in the Tokugawa Period* (Leuven: Leuven University Press, 2001). On anatomical practice, see Timon Screech, *Edo no karada o hiraku* 江戸の身体を開く, trans. Hiroshi Takayama (Tokyo: Sakuhinsha, 1997).

151. Schamberger was permitted to stay in Edo to attend to members of the Tokugawa court. For a full account of Schamberger's life and Japanese work, see Wolfgang Michel, *Von Leipzig nach Japan: Der Chirurg und Handelsmann Caspar Schamberger (1623–1706)* (Munich: Iudicium, 1999).

152. On Japanese translation and translators in the early modern period, see Mino Saito and Miki Sato, eds., *"Tsūji": Interpreters in and around Early Modern Japan* (New York: Springer, 2023); Christopher Joby, *The Dutch Language in Japan (1600–1900)* (Leiden: Brill, 2021); Rebekah Clements, *A Cultural History of Translation in Early Modern Japan* (Cambridge: Cambridge University Press, 2015).

153. On Inoue Masashige, see Timon Screech, "A 17th-Century Japanese Minister's Acquisition of Western Pictures: Inoue Masashige (1585–1661) and His European Objects," in *Transforming Knowledge Orders: Museums, Collections, and Exhibitions*, ed. Larissa Förster (Paderborn: Wilhelm Fink, 2014), 72–106. Inoue's case is discussed alongside that of the Governor of Nagasaki, Kusakabe Hirosada (日下部博貞), who made a request for remedies for cervical tumors, in Joby, *The Dutch Language in Japan*, 259ff.

154. Dutch surgical terminology remains scattered throughout the profession in Japan to this day. The Japanese word for a scalpel, *mesu* (メス), is itself drawn from the Dutch word for knife, *mes*. On the procurement of surgical licenses, see Wolfgang Michel, "Ōtaguro Genpa no oranda geka menkyojō to sono haikei ni tsuite 太田黒玄淡の阿蘭陀外科免許状とその背景について," *Nihon Ishigaku Zasshi* 日本医史学雑誌 49, no. 3 (2003): 455–77.

155. For an interesting case study in the early modern Japanese blurring of manuscript and print traditions, see Linda H. Chance and Julie Nelson Davis, "The Handwritten and the Printed: Issues of Format and Medium in Japanese Premodern Books," *Manuscript Studies* 1, no. 1 (2016): 90–114. For a broad summary of the growth in different aspects of Japanese print culture over the course of the seventeenth century, see Mary Elizabeth Berry, *Japan in Print: Information and Nation in the Early Modern Period* (Berkeley: University of California Press, 2007).

156. All of these early works, often alongside discussion of their authors, are listed in the index of primary sources in Joby, *The Dutch Language in Japan*, 465ff. For a broader sense of secret literature and its place in early modern Japan, see Maki Morinaga, *Secrecy in Japanese Arts: "Secret Transmission" as a Mode of Knowledge* (London: Palgrave Macmillan, 2005). For European counterparts, see Alisha Rankin and Elaine Leong, *Secrets and Knowledge in Medicine and Science 1500–1800* (Farnham: Ashgate, 2011). An interesting example of a later material challenge to these Japanese secret transmissions in the medical realm is discussed in Chan Che-chia, "A Wooden Skeleton Emerges in the Knowledge Hub of Edo Japan," in *Entangled Itineraries: Materials, Practices, and Knowledges across Eurasia*, ed. Pamela H. Smith (Pittsburgh: University of Pittsburgh Press, 2019), 258–82.

157. Chinzan was known by various names throughout his life, including Tokitoshi (時敏), Shin'emon (新右衛門), Hikogorō (彦五郎), Shingobei (新五兵衛), and Eikyū (栄休). For Chinzan's biography, see Wolfgang Michel, "Narabayashi Chinzan Igaku ni mewo muketa dejima shōkan no tsūji 楢林鎮山医学に目を向けた出島商館の通詞," in *Kyūshū no rangaku—ekkyō to kōryū* 九州の蘭学 越境と交流, ed. Wolfgang Michel et al. (Kyoto: Shibunkaku Shuppan, 2009), 34–40.

158. Michel, "Narabayashi Chinzan," 38.

159. The clearest overview of *Geka sōden* in English is Gabor Lukacs, *"Kaitai Shinsho": The Single Most Famous Japanese Book of Medicine & "Geka Sōden": An Early Very Important Manuscript on Surgery* (Utrecht: Hes & De Graaf, 2008). Lukacs's opinions in this text are somewhat compromised by the fact that an important surviving manuscript of *Geka sōden*—elevated by Lukacs almost to the status of an autograph copy—happened to be in his personal collection at the time. Besides an incomplete list produced by Lukacs, *Geka sōden* manuscripts have not been the subject of sustained cataloging. Copies in Japan include: Nagasaki, University Library, 和漢古書, 1-1 and 1-2; Kyoto, University Library, キ/256; Kyoto, University Library, ケ/165; Kyoto, University Library, ケ/166; Kyoto, University Library, ケ/183; Fukuoka, Kyushu University Medical Library, ケ-118; Fukuoka, Kyushu University Medical Library, N51; Tokyo, Keio University Library, F/ケ/44; Tokyo, Keio University Library, F/オ/26; Tokyo, National Institute of Japanese Literature, Old Japanese Books 49-8; Tokyo, Institute of Medical Research Library, no shelfmark, UCDJT BID no. 1385531; Tokyo, Medical University Library, no shelfmark, UCDJT BID no. 100252613; Kawasaki, Tsurumi University Library, 494/T; Kakamigahara, Naito Museum of Pharmaceutical Science and Industry, 35333-494; Osaka, Tekijuku

Commemoration Center, no shelfmark, UCDJT BID no. 2731115. At least two copies survive in collections outside of Japan: Washington, DC, Library of Congress, R128.6 .N37 1706 (this copy was formerly in the collections of both Gabor Lukacs and Jean Blondelet, and I thank Jonathan Hill for sharing images of it before its recent sale); Los Angeles, UCLA, Louise M. Darling Biomedical Library, AC 9 WO N633k 1735.

160. Given that no autograph manuscripts are known to survive, the precise authorship of these chapters is a matter of debate. See Lukacs, "*Geka sōden*," 217ff.

161. Concordances with Paré suggest that this book was most likely a 1649 Dutch printed edition: *De chirurgie, ende alle de opera* (Amsterdam: Jan Jacobsz Schipper, 1649), USTC 1013962. Gordon Mestler suggests that oral histories of Japanese surgeons also document similar books in the care of the Arashiyama family of Hirado, who kept handwritten Dutch copies of Paré's work: "A Galaxy of Old Japanese Medical Books with Miscellaneous Notes on Early Medicine in Japan, Part V," *Bulletin of the Medical Library Association* 45, no. 2 (1957): 191.

162. Grant K. Goodman, *Japan and the Dutch 1600–1853* (Richmond: Routledge Curzon, 2000), 59.

163. Lukacs, "*Geka sōden*," 215–17. A useful corrective to Lukacs's technical errors in the treatment of Chinese medicine appears in an extended review of the work by Grégoire Espesset, "Traditional Chinese Knowledge before the Japanese Discovery of Western Science in Gabor Lukacs' *Kaitai Shinsho & Geka Sōden*," *East Asian Science, Technology, and Medicine* 40 (2014): 113–28.

164. Again, these images have long been labeled simply as copies from the texts of Paré, but as Kanbara Hiroshi has shown, their sources are in fact far more varied: "Kōi geka sōden zuhan seiritsu e no sukurutetasu no gekasho Armamentarium Chirurgicum no eikyō『紅夷外科宗伝』図版成立へのスクルテタス(Scultetus) の外科書 Armamentarium chirurgicumの影響," *Nihonshikaishi gakkai kaishi* 日本歯科医史学会会誌 18, no. 3 (1992): 229–30. See Lukacs, "*Geka sōden*," 203–7, for a table of most correspondences.

165. Casseri's images were combined with Spieghel's text in its first Venetian printing of 1627, although the edition mostly likely to have been available in Japan was printed in Amsterdam in 1645: *Opera quae extant Omnia* (Amsterdam: Johannes Blaeu, 1645), USTC 1035389. On the use of Spieghel on Dejima, see Iwao Seiichi, "A Dutch Doctor in Old Japan," *Japan Quarterly* 8 (1961): 170–78.

166. Wolfgang Michel, "Medicine and Allied Sciences in the Cultural Exchange between Japan and Europe in the Seventeenth Century," in *Theories and Methods in Japanese Studies: Current State and Future Developments*, ed. Hans Dieter Ölschleger (Göttingen: V&R, 2007), 289.

167. This estimate comes from Kanbara Hiroshi, "Fukuoka hara mitsunobu shi kazō oranda gekajutsushiki zufu emaki nitsuite no kōsatsu 福岡・原三信氏家蔵『阿蘭陀外科術式図譜絵巻』についての考察," *Nihon Ishigaku Zasshi* 日本医史学雑誌 43, no. 3 (1997): 364–65. At least four such handscrolls are currently in public collections: Tokyo, National Diet Library, 本別 10–26; Tokyo, National Diet Library, 本別 10–27; Tokyo, Medical and Dental University Museum, item no. 12-B1; Kobe, City Museum, no shelfmark ["外科手術図"].

168. The current whereabouts of Irako Mitsuaki's scroll are unknown, but it was displayed in Tokyo in 1925 as part of the Congresses of the Far Eastern Association of Tropical Medicine: *Nihon igaku rekishi shiryō mokuroku: Dairokkai kyokutō nettai igakkai futai tenrankai* 日本医學歴史資料目録: 第六回極東熱帯医學會附帯展覧會 (Tokyo: Far Eastern Association of Tropical Medicine, 1925), no. 117. Regarding the *Geka kinmō zui*, print was not the last word in this surgical tradition, which maintained the same print-manuscript dynamics as the European equivalents discussed in chapter 4. Consider a manuscript in Tokyo whose details suggest that it was in turn copied from Irako's printed work, now Tokyo, Kenkyukai Foundation Library, UCDJT BID no. 100257498. Nor was this the last Wound Man to be produced in Japan: another appeared in the pictorial *Yōka seisen zukai* (瘍科精選図解 *Selected Images of Oncological Surgery*) by Koshimura Tokuki (越村徳基), published in two volumes in 1820: UCDJT Work ID no. 525520.

169. Kobe, City Museum, no shelfmark ["外科手術図"].

170. A source for the *Kōmō zashiki* phrase is noted in Joby, *The Dutch Language in Japan*, 60.

171. Ari Larissa Heinrich, *The Afterlife of Images: Translating the Pathological Body between China and the West* (Durham, NC: Duke University Press, 2008).

EPILOGUE. NUCLEAR WOUND MAN

1. Stefan Hirschauer, "The Manufacture of Bodies in Surgery," *Social Studies of Science* 21, no. 2 (1991): 279–319.

2. "People," *Time*, February 9, 1968, 39. The article records Lewis as saying: "I'll promise not to wear a uniform if you promise not to salute." Lewis published on technical approaches to image analysis, among other subjects: "Visual Indexing of Graphic Materials," *Special Libraries* 67, no. 11 (1976): 518–27.

3. Coincidentally, several decades earlier, Mestler had published on Japanese materials relevant to the figure's history, as discussed in chapter 5.

4. Elizabeth Matthew Lewis, *An Exhibition of Selected Landmark Books and Articles in the History of Military Medicine, Together with a Graphic Display of the Wound Man through History* (West Point, NY: United States Military Academy, 1976), 26.

5. The episode is discussed at length in John Harwood, "The Wound Man: George Nelson and the 'End of Architecture,'" *Grey Room* 31 (2008): 90–115. The text of Nelson's episode later appeared in the journal *Industrial Design*, for which the Wound Man was chosen as the title page: "How to Kill People: A Problem of Design," *Industrial Design* 8, no. 1 (1961): 45–53. The article states that the original episode was written by George Nelson in collaboration with Clair Roskam, produced by John McGiffert, and directed by John Desmond.

6. Lewis, *The Wound Man through History*, iii.

7. Lewis, *The Wound Man through History*, 33.

8. Lewis, *The Wound Man through History*, 41.

Bibliography

MANUSCRIPTS CITED

Augsburg, Staats- und Stadtbibliothek, 2° Cod 158
Augsburg, Staats- und Stadtbibliothek, 2° Cod 159
Bamberg, Staatsbibliothek, Msc.Med.1
Bamberg, Staatsbibliothek, Msc.Med.6
Basel, Universitätsbibliothek, O IV 38
Berlin, Staatsbibliothek, Mgf 495
Berlin, Staatsbibliothek, Mgf 557
Berlin, Staatsbibliothek, Mgo 710
Berlin, Staatsbibliothek, Mgq 2021
Berlin, Staatsbibliothek, Mlf 782
Berlin, Staatsbibliothek, Mlq 275
Berlin, Staatsbibliothek, Mtlo 71
Bethesda, National Library of Medicine, MS E 98
Bethesda, National Library of Medicine, P 20, item 2
Bologna, Biblioteca Universitaria, MS Greci 3632
Bruges, Bibliothèque de la Ville, MS 411
Brussels, Koninklijke Bibliotheek van België, MS 19546
Budapest, Országos Széchényi Könyvtár (Széchényi-Nationalbibliothek), Cod. Germ. 56
Cambridge, Corpus Christi College, MS 218
Cambridge, Gonville and Caius College, MS 190/223
Cambridge, Trinity College, Wren Library, O.9.31
Cambridge, Trinity College, Wren Library, R.15.21
Cambridge, University Library, MS Dd.10.68
Cambridge, MA, Harvard, Houghton Library, MS Ger. 69
Cardiff, National Library of Wales, MS 3026C
Cologne, Historisches Archiv, MS Best. 7010
Copenhagen, Kongelige Bibliothek, GKS 1658 4°
Copenhagen, Kongelige Bibliothek, NKS 84 b 2°
Copenhagen, Kongelige Bibliothek, Thott 290, 2°
Darmstadt, Universitäts- und Landesbibliothek, Hs. 266
Darmstadt, Universitäts- und Landesbibliothek, Hs. 2282
Dessau-Roßlau, Anhaltische Landesbücherei, Georg Hs. 271
Dresden, Sächsische Landesbibliothek, Staats- und Universitätsbibliothek, Mscr.Dresd.C.487
Dresden, Sächsische Landesbibliothek, Staats- und Universitätsbibliothek, Mscr.Dresd.M.32
Edinburgh, University Library, MS 126
Erfurt, Universitätsbibliothek, CA. 2° 257
Erlangen, Friedrich-Alexander-Universität, Universitätsbibliothek, MS B 200
Florence, Biblioteca Nazionale Centrale, MS Landau Finaly 221
Frankfurt am Main, Universitätsbibliothek, MS Barth. 160
Frankfurt am Main, Universitätsbibliothek, MS Carm. 1
Freiburg im Breisgau, Universitätsbibliothek, Hs. 57
Freiburg im Breisgau, Universitätsbibliothek, Hs. 458
Fukuoka, Kyushu University Medical Library, N51
Fukuoka, Kyushu University Medical Library, ケ-118
Gießen, Universitätsbibliothek, Hs. 232
Gotha, Forschungsbibliothek, MS Chart. A 558
Gotha, Forschungsbibliothek, MS Chart. B 69
Grein, Stadtarchiv, Urk. Nr. 1
Heidelberg, Universitätsbibliothek, Cpg 5
Heidelberg, Universitätsbibliothek, Cpg 144
Heidelberg, Universitätsbibliothek, Cpg 300
Heidelberg, Universitätsbibliothek, Cpg 339
Heidelberg, Universitätsbibliothek, Cpg 438
Heidelberg, Universitätsbibliothek, Cpg 644
Heidelberg, Universitätsbibliothek, Cpg 848
Heidelberg, Universitätsbibliothek, Urk. Lehmann 185
Heidelberg, Universitätsbibliothek, Urk. Lehmann 186
Heiligenkreuz, Zisterzienserstift, Cod. 325
Hildesheim, Dombibliothek, Hs. 750
Innsbruck, Universitäts- und Landesbibliothek, Cod. 960
Kakamigahara, Naito Museum of Pharmaceutical Science and Industry, 35333–494
Karlsruhe, Badische Landesbibliothek, Cod. Lichtenthal 76
Kassel, Universitätsbibliothek, Landesbibliothek, und Murhardsche Bibliothek der Stadt Kassel, 2° MS Astron. 1
Kassel, Universitätsbibliothek, Landesbibliothek, und Murhardsche Bibliothek der Stadt Kassel, 2° MS Med 7
Kassel, Universitätsbibliothek, Landesbibliothek, und Murhardsche Bibliothek der Stadt Kassel, 2° MS Poet. et Roman. 1
Kawasaki, Tsurumi University Library, 494/T
Klosterneuburg, Augustiner-Chorherrenstift, Cod. 278
Kobe, City Museum, no shelfmark [“外科手術図”]

Kraków, Biblioteka Jagiellońska, BJ Rkp. Przyb. 35/64
Kyoto, University Library, キ/256
Kyoto, University Library, ケ/165
Kyoto, University Library, ケ/166
Kyoto, University Library, ケ/183
Leiden, Universiteitsbibliotheek, MS BPL 1905
Leiden, Universiteitsbibliotheek, MS VCO 6
Leipzig, Universitätsbibliothek, Fragm. Lat. 368
Leipzig, Universitätsbibliothek, MS 1122
Leipzig, Universitätsbibliothek, MS 1346
Leipzig, Universitätsbibliothek, MS 1483
Ljubljana, Semeniška knjižnica, SKLJ Rkp. 2
London, British Library, Additional MS 15582
London, British Library, Additional MS 17987
London, British Library, Arundel MS 66
London, British Library, Arundel MS 251
London, British Library, Harley MS 941
London, British Library, Sloane MS 6
London, British Library, Sloane MS 345
London, British Library, Sloane MS 702
London, British Library, Sloane MS 1977
London, Sokol Books, no shelfmark ["Medicine"]
London, Wellcome Library, MS 49
London, Wellcome Library, MS 290
London, Wellcome Library, MS 508
London, Wellcome Library, MS 990
Los Angeles, UCLA, Louise M. Darling Biomedical Library, AC 9 WO N633k 1735
Los Angeles, UCLA, Louise M. Darling Biomedical Library, MS Benjamin 8
Los Angeles, UCLA, Louise M. Darling Biomedical Library, MS Benjamin 10
Madrid, Biblioteca Nacional de España, 2.328.
Madrid, Biblioteca Nacional de España, VITR/25/7
Madrid, Real Biblioteca del Monasterio de El Escorial, MS T-I-6
Melk, Stiftsbibliothek, Cod. 737 (23, A 26)
Michelstadt, Nicolaus-Matz-Kirchenbibliothek, MS D 728
Montecassino, Archivio della Badia, Cod. 97
Munich, Bayerische Staatsbibliothek, Cgm 28
Munich, Bayerische Staatsbibliothek, Cgm 328
Munich, Bayerische Staatsbibliothek, Cgm 340
Munich, Bayerische Staatsbibliothek, Cgm 430
Munich, Bayerische Staatsbibliothek, Cgm 571
Munich, Bayerische Staatsbibliothek, Cgm 597
Munich, Bayerische Staatsbibliothek, Cgm 1507
Munich, Bayerische Staatsbibliothek, Cgm 5250(33 a)
Munich, Bayerische Staatsbibliothek, Clm 206
Munich, Bayerische Staatsbibliothek, Clm 4394
Munich, Bayerische Staatsbibliothek, Clm 14546
Munich, Bayerische Staatsbibliothek, Clm 14851
Munich, Bayerische Staatsbibliothek, Clm 18294
Munich, Bayerische Staatsbibliothek, Clm 28609
Munich, Bayerische Staatsbibliothek, Cod. icon. 394a
Munich, Universitätsbibliothek, 4° Cod. 885
Munich, Universitätsbibliothek, 8° Cod. 339
Nagasaki, University Library, 和漢古書, 1-1 and 1-2
New York, Morgan Library, MS M.763
Nuremberg, Germanisches Nationalmuseum, Hs. 3227a
Nuremberg, Germanisches Nationalmuseum, Hs. 7060
Nuremberg, Germanisches Nationalmuseum, Hs. 18792
Osaka, Tekijuku Commemoration Center, no shelfmark, UCDJT BID no. 2731115
Oxford, Bodleian Library, MS Ashmole 391(5)
Oxford, Bodleian Library, MS Ashmole 789
Oxford, Bodleian Library, MS Canon. Misc. 559
Oxford, Bodleian Library, MS Digby 46
Oxford, Bodleian Library, MS Saville 39
Padua, Biblioteca storica di Medicina e botanica Vincenzo Pinali e Giovanni Marsili, MS Fanzago 2,I,5,28
Paris, Bibliothèque de l'Arsenal, MS 1037 Rés.
Paris, Bibliothèque nationale de France, MS Allemand 106
Paris, Bibliothèque nationale de France, MS Arsenal 2894
Paris, Bibliothèque nationale de France, MS Français 9141
Paris, Bibliothèque nationale de France, MS Grec 2180
Paris, Bibliothèque nationale de France, MS Hébreu 1181
Paris, Bibliothèque nationale de France, MS Latin 6734
Paris, Bibliothèque nationale de France, MS Latin 6884
Paris, Bibliothèque nationale de France, MS Latin 7138
Paris, Bibliothèque nationale de France, MS Latin 11229
Paris, Bibliothèque nationale de France, MS Latin 15113
Paris, Bibliothèque nationale de France, MS Mexicain 23–24
Paris, Bibliothèque nationale de France, MS NAL 1487
Philadelphia, University of Pennsylvania Special Collections, Schoenberg Institute, MS LJS 449
Philadelphia, University of Pennsylvania Special Collections, Schoenberg Institute, MS LJS 463
Prague, Královská kanonie premonstrátů na Strahově, Strahovská knihovna, MS DC III 3
Prague, Lobkowicz Collection, MS VI Fc 29
Prague, Národní knihovna České republiky, MS I E 39
Prague, Národní knihovna České republiky, MS III C 2
Prague, Národní knihovna České republiky, MS XIV A 17
Prague, Národní knihovna České republiky, MS XVII D 10
Prague, Národní knihovna České republiky, MS XVII H 22
Prague, Národní knihovna České republiky, MS XIX C 49
Salzburg, Erzabtei St. Peter, Benediktinerstift, MS A VI 17
Schwäbisch Hall, Stadtarchiv, HV HS 40
Solothurn, Zentralbibliothek, Cod. S 474
St. Gallen, Kantonsbibliothek, VadSlg MS 302
St. Louis, Concordia Seminary Library, no shelfmark ["Medizinisch-astrologisches Hausbuch"]
Stockholm, Kungliga Biblioteket, MS A 225
Strasbourg, Bibliothèque nationale et universitaire, MS 2929
Stuttgart, Württembergische Landesbibliothek, Cod.hist.qt.141
Stuttgart, Württembergische Landesbibliothek, Cod.med.et.phys.fol.14
Tokyo, Institute of Medical Research Library, no shelfmark, UCDJT BID no. 1385531
Tokyo, Keio University Library, F/オ/26
Tokyo, Keio University Library, F/ケ/44
Tokyo, Medical and Dental University Museum, item no. 12-B1
Tokyo, Medical University Library, no shelfmark, UCDJT BID no. 100252613
Tokyo, National Diet Library, 本別 10–26
Tokyo, National Diet Library, 本別 10–27
Tokyo, National Institute of Japanese Literature, Old Japanese Books 49-8
Třeboň, Státní Oblastní Archiv, MS A 17
Trier, Stadtbibliothek, Hs. 1899/1472 8°
Tübingen, Universitätsbibliothek, Md 2
Uppsala, Universitetsbibliotek, C 420
Vatican City, Biblioteca Apostolica Vaticana, MS Pal. Lat. 1105

Vatican City, Biblioteca Apostolica Vaticana, MS Pal. Lat. 1181
Vatican City, Biblioteca Apostolica Vaticana, MS Pal. Lat. 1183
Vatican City, Biblioteca Apostolica Vaticana, MS Pal. Lat. 1199
Vatican City, Biblioteca Apostolica Vaticana, MS Pal. Lat. 1225
Vatican City, Biblioteca Apostolica Vaticana, MS Pal. Lat. 1232
Vatican City, Biblioteca Apostolica Vaticana, MS Pal. Lat. 1241
Vatican City, Biblioteca Apostolica Vaticana, MS Pal. Lat. 1264
Vatican City, Biblioteca Apostolica Vaticana, MS Pal. Lat. 1293
Vatican City, Biblioteca Apostolica Vaticana, MS Pal. Lat. 1305
Vatican City, Biblioteca Apostolica Vaticana, MS Pal. Lat. 1325
Vatican City, Biblioteca Apostolica Vaticana, MS Pal. Lat. 1376
Vatican City, Biblioteca Apostolica Vaticana, MS Pal. Lat. 1451
Vatican City, Biblioteca Apostolica Vaticana, MS Pal. Lat. 1452
Vatican City, Biblioteca Apostolica Vaticana, MS Reg. Lat. 1298
Vatican City, Biblioteca Apostolica Vaticana, MS Reg. Lat. 1309
Vatican City, Biblioteca Apostolica Vaticana, MS Vat. Lat. 2411
Venice, Biblioteca Nazionale Marciana, MS Lat. VII 32 (=3032)
Venice, Biblioteca Nazionale Marciana, MS Lat. Zan. 320 (=1937)
Vienna, Österreichische Nationalbibliothek, Cod. 2426
Vienna, Österreichische Nationalbibliothek, Cod. 2469
Vienna, Österreichische Nationalbibliothek, Cod. 2826
Vienna, Österreichische Nationalbibliothek, Cod. 4417*
Vienna, Österreichische Nationalbibliothek, Cod. 5206
Vienna, Österreichische Nationalbibliothek, Cod. 5511
Vienna, Österreichische Nationalbibliothek, Cod. 13106
Vienna, Österreichische Nationalbibliothek, Cod. 14034
Vienna, Österreichische Nationalbibliothek, Cod. 15478
Vienna, Österreichische Nationalbibliothek, Cod. Ser. n. 2641
Vienna, Österreichische Nationalbibliothek, Cod. Ser. n. 2663
Vienna, Schottenstift, Cod. 160 (Hübl. 257)
Washington, DC, Library of Congress, R128.6 .N37 1706
Washington, DC, Library of Congress, Rosenwald Collection, MS 4
Wolfenbüttel, Herzog August Bibliothek, Cod. Guelf. 18.2 Aug 4°
Wolfenbüttel, Herzog August Bibliothek, Cod. Guelf. 29.14 Aug. 4°
Wolfenbüttel, Herzog August Bibliothek, Cod. Guelf. 30.12 Aug. 2°
Wolfenbüttel, Herzog August Bibliothek, Cod. Guelf. 1189 Helmst.
Wrocław, Biblioteka Uniwersytecka, MS I F 334
Wrocław, Biblioteka Uniwersytecka, MS R 458
Würzburg, Universitätsbibliothek, M.ch.q.30
Zürich, Zentralbibliothek, MS C 54
Zürich, Zentralbibliothek, MS C 102b
Zürich, Zentralbibliothek, MS Z VII 287

SECONDARY SOURCES

Abad, Julián Martín. *Los primeros tiempos de la imprenta en España*. Madrid: Laberinto, 2003.
Abad, Julián Martín. *Cum figuris: Texto e imagen en los incunables españoles. Catálogo bibliográfico y descriptivo*. Madrid: Arco Libros, 2018.
Aelst, José van. "Visualizing the Spiritual: Images in the Life and Teachings of Henry Suso (c. 1295–1366)." In *Speaking to the Eye: Sight and Insight through Text and Image (1150–1650)*, edited by Thérèse De Hemptinne, Veerle Fraeters, and María Eugenia Góngora, 129–51. Turnhout: Brepols, 2013.
Ahnfelt, Nils-Otto, Hjalmar Fors, and Karin Wendin. "Making and Taking Theriac: An Experimental and Sensory Approach to the History of Medicine." *British Journal for the History of Science: Themes* 7 (2022): 39–62.
Akbari, Suzanne Conklin. "Erasing the Body: History and Memory in Medieval Siege Poetry." In *Remembering the Crusades: Myth, Image, and Identity*, edited by Nicholas Paul and Suzanne Yeager, 146–73. Baltimore: Johns Hopkins University Press, 2012.
Almeida, Francisco Alonso. "A Middle English Text on Phlebotomy." *Revista canaria de estudios ingleses* 80 (2020): 29–49.
Amelung, Peter. "Zum Bilderschmuck der frühen Einblattkalender: Probleme um einen Augsburger Almanach auf das Jahr 1496 (GW 1513)." *Gutenberg-Jahrbuch* 55 (1980): 235–45.
Ammer, Jessica. *Der deutsche Cicero*. Göttingen: V&R Unipress, 2020.
Andersen, Peter, and Nikolaus Henkel, eds. *Sebastian Brant (1457–1521): Europäisches Wissen in der Hand eines Intellektuellen der Frühen Neuzeit*. Berlin: De Gruyter, 2023.
Anderson, Emily R. "Printing the Bespoke Book: Euclid's *Elements* in Early Modern Visual Culture." *Nuncius* 35, no. 3 (2020): 536–60.
Anglo, Sydney. *The Martial Arts of Renaissance Europe*. New Haven, CT: Yale University Press, 2000.
Arbesmann, Rudolph. "The Concept of 'Christus Medicus' in St. Augustine." *Traditio* 10 (1954): 1–28.
Areford, David S. *The Viewer and the Printed Image in Late Medieval Europe*. Aldershot: Ashgate, 2010.
Armstrong, Elizabeth. "The Origins of Chrétien Wechel Re-examined." *Bibliothèque d'Humanisme et Renaissance* 23 (1961): 341–46.
Armstrong, Lilian. *Studies of Renaissance Miniaturists in Venice*. 2 vols. London: Pindar, 2003.
Armstrong, Lilian. "The Decoration and Illustration of Venetian Incunabula: From Hand Illumination to the Design of Woodcuts." In *Printing R-Evolution and Society 1450–1500*, edited by Cristina Dondi, 775–818. Venice: Ca' Foscari, 2020.
Arrizabalaga, Jon. *The Articella in the Early Press, c. 1476–1534*. Cambridge: Wellcome Unit/CSIC, 1998.
Arrizabalaga, Jon. "El libro científico en la primera imprenta castellana (1485–1520)." In *Historia de la ciencia y de la técnica en la Corona de Castilla*, edited by

Luis García Ballester, 2:619–50. Valladolid: Junta de Castilla y León, 2002.

Arrizabalaga, Jon. "Medical Genres in the Early Printing Press." In *Écritures médicales: Discours et genres, de la tradition antique à l'époque moderne*, edited by Laurence Moulinier-Brogi and Marilyn Nicoud, 311–34. Lyon-Avignon: CIHAM, 2019.

Aue, Hartmann von. *Ereck: Textgeschichtliche Ausgabe mit Abdruck sämtlicher Fragmente und der Bruchstücke des mitteldeutschen "Erek,"* edited by Andreas Hammer, Victor Millet, and Timo Reuvekamp-Felber. Berlin: De Gruyter, 2017.

Auer, Erltraud, and Bernhard Schnell. "'Der Wundenmann': Ein traumatologisches Schema in der Tradition der 'Wundarzenie' des Ortolf von Baierland: Untersuchung und Edition." In *"ein teutsch puech machen": Untersuchungen zur landessprachlichen Vermittlung medizinischen Wissens*, edited by Gundolf Keil, 349–401. Wiesbaden: Reichert, 1993.

Auerbach, Erich. "Figura." *Archivum Romanicum* 22 (1938): 436–89.

Auerbach, Erich. *Time, History, and Literature: Selected Essays of Erich Auerbach*, edited by James I. Porter, translated by Jane O. Newman. Princeton, NJ: Princeton University Press, 2016.

Augustyn, Wolfgang. "Zu einem astronomisch-medizinischen Handbuch aus dem Spätmittelalter (München, Bayerische Staatsbibliothek, cod. lat. mon. 4394): Ein Vorbericht." In *Rondo: Beiträge für Peter Diemer zum 65. Geburtstag*, edited by Wolfgang Augustyn and Iris Lauterbach, 33–43. Munich: Zentralinstitut für Kunstgeschichte, 2010.

Baader, Gerhard. "Die Entwicklung der medizinischen Fachsprache in der Antike und im frühen Mittelalter (1970)." In *Medizin im mittelalterlichen Abendland*, edited by Gerhard Baader and Gundolf Keil, 417–42. Darmstadt: Wissenschaftliche Buchgesellschaft, 1982.

Baader, Gerhard, and Gundolf Keil, eds. *Medizin im mittelalterlichen Abendland*. Darmstadt: Wissenschaftliche Buchgesellschaft, 1982.

Bachoffner, Pierre. "Jérôme Brunschwig, chirurgien et apothicaire strasbourgeois, portraituré en 1512." *Revue d'histoire de la pharmacie* 298 (1993): 269–78.

Baierland, Ortolf von. *Das Arzneibuch Ortolfs von Baierland*, edited by Gundolf Keil and Ortrun Riha. Wiesbaden: Reichert, 2014.

Baird, Davis. *Thing Knowledge: A Philosophy of Scientific Instruments*. Berkeley: University of California Press, 2004.

Baldasso, Renzo. "Printing for the Doge: On the First Quire of the First Edition of the *Liber elementorum Euclidis*." *La Bibliofilía* 115, no. 3 (2013): 525–52.

Bale, Anthony. *Feeling Persecuted: Christians, Jews, and Images of Violence in the Middle Ages*. London: Reaktion, 2010.

Ballester, Luis García. *Medicine in a Multicultural Society: Christian, Jewish, and Muslim Practitioners in the Spanish Kingdoms, 1222–1610*. Aldershot: Ashgate, 2001.

Barker, Sheila. "The Making of a Plague Saint: Saint Sebastian's Imagery and Cult before the Counter-Reformation." In *Piety and Plague from Byzantium to the Baroque*, edited by Franco Mormando and Thomas Worcester, 90–131. Kirksville, MO: Truman State University Press, 2007.

Barnes, Robin B. *Astrology and Reformation*. Oxford: Oxford University Press, 2016.

Barnhouse, Lucy C. "From Helpful Gardens to Hateful Words: Moral and Physical Healthscaping in the Late Medieval Rhineland." In *Disease and the Environment in the Medieval and Early Modern Worlds*, edited by Lori Jones, 52–64. New York: Routledge, 2022.

Bauer, Matthias Johannes. "Teaching How to Fight with Encrypted Words: Linguistic Aspects of German Fencing and Wrestling Treatises of the Middle Ages and Early Modern Times." In *Late Medieval and Early Modern Fight Books: Transmission and Tradition of Martial Arts in Europe (14th–17th Centuries)*, edited by Daniel Jaquet, Karin Verelst, and Timothy Dawson, 47–61. Leiden: Brill, 2016.

Bauer, Matthias, and Christoph Ernst. *Diagrammatik: Einführung in ein kultur- und medienwissenschaftliches Forschungsfeld*. Bielefeld: Transcript, 2010.

Baumann, Brigitte, and Helmut Baumann. *Die Mainzer Kräuterbuch-Inkunabeln*. Stuttgart: Hiersemann, 2010.

Baumgarten, Elisheva. "Ask the Midwives: A Hebrew Manual on Midwifery from Medieval Germany." *Social History of Medicine* 32, no. 4 (2019): 712–33.

Beckwith, Sarah. *Christ's Body: Identity, Culture, and Society in Late Medieval Writings*. New York: Routledge, 1996.

Bell, C. F., and Rachel Poole. "English Seventeenth-Century Portrait Drawings in Oxford Collections: Part II." *Walpole Society* 14 (1925): 43–80.

Bellingradt, Daniel, and Anna Reynolds, eds. *The Paper Trade in Early Modern Europe: Practices, Materials, Networks*. Leiden: Brill, 2021.

Benati, Chiara. "The 1518 Low German Edition of Hieronymus Brunschwig's *Buch der Cirurgia* and Its Terminology." In *Medieval German Textrelations: Translations, Editions, and Studies*, edited by Sibylle Jefferis, 189–254. Göppingen: Kümmerle, 2012.

Benati, Chiara. "Charms and Blessings in the Middle Low German Medical Tradition." In *Medieval German Tristan and Trojan War Stories*, edited by Sibylle Jefferis, 115–44. Göppingen: Kümmerle, 2017.

Benati, Chiara. "The Field Surgery Manual Which Became a Medical Commonplace Book: Hans von Gersdorff's *Feldtbuch der Wundarzney* (1517) Translated into Low German." In *Bodily and Spiritual Hygiene in Medieval and Early Modern Literature*, edited by Albrecht Classen, 510–27. Berlin: De Gruyter, 2017.

Benati, Chiara. "*À la guerre comme à la guerre* but with Caution: Protection Charms and Blessings in the Germanic Tradition." *Brathair* 17, no. 1 (2017): 155–91.

Bender, John, and Michael Marrinan. *The Culture of Diagram*. Stanford, CA: Stanford University Press, 2010.

Benham, Jenny. "Wounding in the High Middle Ages: Law and Practice." In *Wounds in the Middle Ages*, edited by Anne Kirkham and Cordelia Warr, 151–74. London: Routledge, 2014.

Benskin, Michael. "For Wound in the Head: A Late Mediaeval View of the Brain." *Neuphilologische Mitteilungen* 86, no. 2 (1985): 199–215.

Bergmann, Heinz, and Gundolf Keil. "Das Münchner Pest-Laßmännchen: Standardisierungstendenzen in der spätmittelalterlichen deutschen Pesttherapie." In *Fachprosa-Studien: Beiträge zur mittelalterlichen Wissenschafts- und Geistesgeschichte*, edited by Gundolf

Keil, with Peter Assion, Willem Frans Daems, and Heinz-Ulrich Roehl, 318–30. Berlin: Schmidt, 1982.
Berliner, Rudolf. "Arma Christi." *Münchner Jahrbuch der bildenden Kunst* 6 (1955): 35–152.
Bernt, Walther. *Altes Werkzeug*. Munich: Callwey, 1939.
Berriot-Salvadore, Évelyne, ed. *Ambroise Paré (1510–1590): Pratique et écriture de la science à la Renaissance*. Paris: Honoré Champion, 2003.
Berry, Mary Elizabeth. *Japan in Print: Information and Nation in the Early Modern Period*. Berkeley: University of California Press, 2007.
Bertram, Gitta, Nils Büttner, and Claus Zittel, eds. *Gateways to the Book: Frontispieces and Title Pages in Early Modern Europe*. Leiden: Brill, 2021.
Bestul, Thomas H. *Texts of the Passion: Latin Devotional Literature and Medieval Society*. Philadelphia: University of Pennsylvania Press, 1996.
Biesbrouck, Maurits, Theodoor Goddeeris, and Omer Steeno. "Jean Tagault (c. 1486–1546), professor heelkunde in Parijs, plagiator van Vesalius' *Tabulae anatomicae sex* (1538)?" *Journal of the Royal Library of Belgium* 10 (2017): 7–63.
Bildhauer, Bettina. *Medieval Blood*. Chicago: University of Chicago Press, 2009.
Bildhauer, Bettina. *Medieval Things: Agency, Materiality, and Narratives of Objects in Medieval German Literature and Beyond*. Columbus: Ohio State University Press, 2020.
Bingen, Hildegard von. *Scivias*, edited by Barbara Newman, translated by Columba Hart and Jane Bishop. New York: Paulist, 1990.
Binski, Paul. "The Crucifixion and the Censorship of Art around 1300." In *The Medieval World*, edited by Peter Linehan and Janet L. Nelson, 342–60. London: Routledge, 2001.
Black, Winston. "Christ's Pharmacy: Theriac and Drug Jars in the Medieval Iconography of Disease Management." In *Materialities of Disease in the Global Medieval World: Images, Objects, and Remains*, edited by Lori Jones. York: Arc Humanities Press, forthcoming.
Blackhall, Sheena. *The Wound Man: Poems in Scots and English*. Aberdeen: Lochlands, 2015.
Blair, Ann M. "Reflections on Technological Continuities: Manuscripts Copied from Printed Books." *Bulletin of the John Rylands Library* 91, no. 1 (2015): 7–33.
Bober, Harry. "The Zodiacal Miniature of the *Très Riches Heures* of the Duke of Berry: Its Sources and Meaning." *Journal of the Warburg and Courtauld Institutes* 11 (1948): 1–34.
Bodemann, Ulrike. "Astrologie/Astronomie (Nr. 11)." In *Katalog der deutschsprachigen illustrierten Handschriften des Mittelalters (KdiH)*, edited by Norbert H. Ott, Ulrike Bodemann, and Gisela Fischer-Heetfeld, vol. 1. Munich: Beck, 1991.
Bogen, Steffen. "Der Körper des Diagramms: Präsentationsfiguren, mnemonische Hände, vermessene Menschen." In *Bild und Körper im Mittelalter*, edited by Kristin Marek, Raphaèle Preisinger, Marius Rimmele, and Katrin Kärcher, 61–81. Munich: Fink, 2006.
Bogen, Steffen. "Das Diagramm als Spiel: Semiotische Entdeckungen im Spielebuch von Alfons dem Weisen (1283 n. Chr.) mit einigen Beobachtungen zu Gudea als Architekt (2000 v. Chr.)." In *Diagramm und Text: Diagrammatische Strukturen und die Dynamisierung von Wissen und Erfahrung*, edited by Eckart Conrad Lutz, Vera Jerjen, and Christine Putzo, 385–412. Wiesbaden: Reichert, 2014.
Bogen, Steffen, and Felix Thürlemann. "Jenseits der Opposition von Text und Bild: Überlegungen zu einer Theorie des Diagramms und des Diagrammatischen." In *Die Bildwelt der Diagramme Joachims von Fiore: Zur Medialität religiös-politischer Programme im Mittelalter*, edited by Alexander Patschovsky, 1–22. Berlin: De Gruyter, 2003.
Boot, Christine. "*an aderlaszen ligt grosz gesunthait*: Zur Repräsentanz von Ortolfs Phlebotomie in deutschsprachigen Aderlaßtexten." In *"ein teutsch puech machen": Untersuchungen zur landessprachlichen Vermittlung medizinischen Wissens*, edited by Gundolf Keil, 112–57. Wiesbaden: Reichert, 1993.
Booton, Diane E. *Publishing Networks in France in the Early Era of Print*. London: Routledge, 2018.
Borland, Jennifer. "Gendering Treatment: Cupping by Female Practitioners in Late Medieval Visual Culture." In *Gender and the "Natural" Environment in the Middle Ages: Bodies, Boundaries, and Belief*, edited by Patricia Skinner and Theresa L. Tyers, 36–62. Cardiff: University of Wales Press, 2023.
Bos, Gerrit, and Y. Tzvi Langermann. *The Alexandrian Summaries of Galen's "On Critical Days."* Leiden: Brill, 2015.
Bouras-Vallianatos, Petros. "Cross-Cultural Transfer of Medical Knowledge in the Medieval Mediterranean: The Introduction and Dissemination of Sugar-Based Potions from the Islamic World to Byzantium." *Speculum* 96, no. 4 (2021): 963–1008.
Bowden, Sarah, Nine Miedema, and Stephen Mossman, eds. *Verletzungen und Unversehrtheit in der deutschen Literatur des Mittelalters*. Tübingen: Narr Francke, 2020.
Bowden, Sarah, and Annette Volfing, eds. *Punishment and Penitential Practices in Medieval German Writing*. Woodbridge: Boydell & Brewer, 2018.
Boxer, Carly B. "Uroscopy Diagrams, Judgment, and the Perception of Color in Late Medieval England." *Word & Image* 38, no. 4 (2022): 327–47.
Brain, Peter. *Galen on Bloodletting*. Cambridge: Cambridge University Press, 1986.
Braunstein, Philippe. *Les Allemands à Venise (1380–1520)*. Rome: École française, 2016.
Breen, Katharine. *Machines of the Mind: Personification in Medieval Literature*. Chicago: University of Chicago Press, 2021.
Brévart, Francis B. "Johann Blaubirers Kalender von 1481 und 1483: Traditionsgebundenheit und experimentelle Innovation." *Gutenberg-Jahrbuch* 63 (1988): 74–83.
Brévart, Francis B. "The German 'Volkskalender' of the Fifteenth Century." *Speculum* 63, no. 2 (1988): 312–42.
Brinkhus, Gerd, David Juste, and Helga Lengenfelder. *Iatromathematisches Kalenderbuch / Die Kunst der Astronomie und Geomantie. Farbmikrofiche-Edition der Handschrift Tübingen, Universitätsbibliothek, Md 2*. Munich: Lengenfelder, 2005.
Brockliss, Laurence, and Colin Jones. *The Medical World of Early Modern France*. Oxford: Clarendon, 1997.
Bronstein, Judith, Edna J. Stern, and Elisabeth Yehuda. "Franks, Locals and Sugar Cane: A Case Study of Cultural Interaction in the Latin Kingdom of Jerusalem." *Journal of Medieval History* 45, no. 3 (2019): 316–30.

Brown, Horatio F. *The Venetian Printing Press*. London: Nimmo, 1891.

Brunsch, Swen H. "Schmerzmittel im Mittelalter." *Der Schmerz* 21, no. 4 (2007): 331–38.

Bumke, Joachim. *Der "Erec" Hartmanns von Aue: Eine Einführung*. Berlin: De Gruyter, 2006.

Burkart, Eric. "Die Aufzeichnung des Nicht-Sagbaren: Annäherung an die kommunikative Funktion der Bilder in den Fechtbüchern des Hans Talhofer." *Das Mittelalter* 19, no. 2 (2014): 253–301.

Burkart, Eric. "The Autograph of an Erudite Martial Artist: A Close Reading of Nuremberg, Germanisches Nationalmuseum, Hs. 3227a." In *Late Medieval and Early Modern Fight Books: Transmission and Tradition of Martial Arts in Europe (14th–17th Centuries)*, edited by Daniel Jaquet, Karin Verelst, and Timothy Dawson, 451–80. Leiden: Brill, 2016.

Burkart, Eric. "Body Techniques of Combat: The Depiction of a Personal Fighting System in the Fight Books of Hans Talhofer (1443–1467 CE)." In *Killing and Being Killed: Bodies in Battle, Perspectives on Fighters in the Middle Ages*, edited by Jörg Rogge, 109–30. Bielefeld: Transcript, 2017.

Burkart, Eric. "Mensch—Waffe—Körperwissen: Die bildliche und textliche Repräsentation von embodied knowledge in vormodernen Kampfbüchern." In *Objekte des Krieges: Präsenz & Repräsentation*, edited by Romana Kaske and Julia Saviello, 49–66. Berlin: De Gruyter, 2019.

Burnett, Charles. "Lunar Astrology: The Varieties of Texts Using Lunar Mansions, with Emphasis on Jafar Indus." *Micrologus* 12 (2004): 43–133.

Burnett, Charles, and Danielle Jacquart, eds. *Constantine the African and ʿAlī ibn al-ʿAbbās al-Maǧūsī: The "Pantegni" and Related Texts*. Leiden: Brill, 1994.

Busse Berger, Anna Maria. *Medieval Music and the Art of Memory*. Berkeley: University of California Press, 2005.

Butler, Sara M. *Forensic Medicine and Death Investigation in Medieval England*. London: Routledge, 2014.

Bylebyl, Jerome J. "Interpreting the Fasciculo Anatomy Scene." *Journal of the History of Medicine and Allied Sciences* 45, no. 3 (1990): 285–316.

Bynum, Caroline Walker. *The Resurrection of the Body in Western Christianity, 200–1336*. New York: Columbia University Press, 1995.

Bynum, Caroline Walker. "Violent Imagery in Late Medieval Piety." *Bulletin of the German Historical Institute* 30 (2002): 3–36.

Bynum, Caroline Walker. *Wonderful Blood: Theology and Practice in Late Medieval Northern Germany and Beyond*. Philadelphia: University of Pennsylvania Press, 2007.

Cadden, Joan. *The Meanings of Sex Difference in the Middle Ages: Medicine, Science, and Culture*. Cambridge: Cambridge University Press, 1993.

Cahill, Patricia A. *Unto the Breach: Martial Formations, Historical Trauma, and the Early Modern Stage*. Oxford: Oxford University Press, 2008.

Camille, Michael. "The Image and the Self: Unwriting Late Medieval Bodies." In *Framing Medieval Bodies*, edited by Sarah Kay and Miri Rubin, 62–99. Manchester: Manchester University Press, 1994.

Campbell, Eldridge, and James Colton, trans. *The Surgery of Theodoric ca. A.D. 1267*. New York: Appleton-Century-Crofts, 1955–1960.

Capwell, Tobias, ed. *The Noble Art of the Sword: Fashion and Fencing in Renaissance Europe*. London: Wallace Collection, 2012.

Carey, Hilary M. "What Is the Folded Almanac? The Form and Function of a Key Manuscript Source for Astro-Medical Practice in Later Medieval England." *Social History of Medicine* 16, no. 3 (2003): 481–509.

Carlino, Andrea. *La fabbrica del corpo: Libri e dissezione nel Rinascimento*. Turin: Einaudi, 1994.

Carlino, Andrea. *Paper Bodies: A Catalogue of Anatomical Fugitive Sheets 1538–1687*, translated by Noga Arikha. London: Wellcome Institute, 1999.

Carlino, Andrea, and Michel Jeanneret, eds. *Vulgariser la medicine: Du style medical en France et en Italie (XVIe et XVIIe siècles)*. Geneva: Droz, 2009.

Carrubba, Robert W., and John Z. Bowers. "The Western World's First Detailed Treatise on Acupuncture: Willem Ten Rhijne's *De acupunctura*." *Journal of the History of Medicine and Allied Sciences* 29, no. 4 (1974): 371–98.

Carruthers, Mary. *The Craft of Thought: Meditation, Rhetoric, and the Making of Images, 400–1200*. Cambridge: Cambridge University Press, 1998.

Carruthers, Mary. *The Book of Memory: A Study of Memory in Medieval Culture*. Cambridge: Cambridge University Press, 2008.

Carruthers, Mary. "*Ars oblivionalis, ars inveniendi*: The Cherub Figure and the Arts of Memory." *Gesta* 48, no. 2 (2009): 99–119.

Carter, Victor, Lotte Hellinga, and Tony Parker. "Printing with Gold in the Fifteenth Century." *British Library Journal* 9, no. 1 (1983): 1–13.

Černá, Alena. *Staročeské knihy lékařské*. Brno: Host, 2006.

Chajes, Jeffrey H. "We-ʿatah ʾatsayyer lekha ʿagulah u-mi-sham tavin mah she-tsarikh le-havin: ha-tarshim ha-qabbali ka-tsiyyur ʾepisṭemi ועתה אצייר לך עגולה ומשם תבין מה שצריך להבין: התרשים הקבלי כציור אפיסטמי." *Peʿamim* 150/152 (2018): 235–88.

Chamberland, Celeste. "Between the Hall and the Market: William Clowes and Surgical Self-Fashioning in Elizabethan London." *Sixteenth Century Journal* 41, no. 1 (2010): 69–89.

Chance, Linda H., and Julie Nelson Davis. "The Handwritten and the Printed: Issues of Format and Medium in Japanese Premodern Books." *Manuscript Studies* 1, no. 1 (2016): 90–114.

Che-chia, Chan. "A Wooden Skeleton Emerges in the Knowledge Hub of Edo Japan." In *Entangled Itineraries: Materials, Practices, and Knowledges across Eurasia*, edited by Pamela H. Smith, 258–82. Pittsburgh: University of Pittsburgh Press, 2019.

Chinca, Mark. "Women and Hunting-Birds Are Easy to Tame: Aristocratic Masculinity and the Early German Love-Lyric." In *Masculinity in Medieval Europe*, edited by Dawn M. Hadley, 199–213. London: Routledge, 1999.

Chojecka, Ewa. *Bayerische Bild-Enzyklopädie: Das Weltbild eines wissenschaftlich-magischen Hausbuches aus dem frühen 16. Jahrhundert*. Baden-Baden: Koerner, 1982.

Chrisman, Miriam Usher. *Lay Culture, Learned Culture: Books and Social Change in Strasbourg, 1480–1599*. New Haven, CT: Yale University Press, 1982.

Christoph, Siegfried R. "Violence Stylized." In *Violence in Medieval Courtly Literature: A Casebook*, edited by Albrecht Classen, 115–25. New York: Routledge, 2004.

Cianci, Eleonora. *The German Tradition of the "Three Good Brothers" Charm*. Göppingen: Kümerle, 2013.
Cifuentes i Comamala, Lluís. "Vernacular Surgery in the Medieval and Early Modern Latin West: Works, Individuals, and Research Methodologies." *Medicina nei secoli* 36, no. 1 (2024): 103–32.
Cilliers, Louise. "Vindicianus's *Gynaecia*: Text and Translation of the Codex Monacensis." *Journal of Medieval Latin* 15 (2005): 153–236.
Cîtrome, Jeremy J. *The Surgeon in Medieval English Literature*. New York: Palgrave Macmillan, 2006.
Clark, Charles West. "The Zodiac Man in Medieval Medical Astrology." PhD diss., University of Colorado, 1979.
Clarke, Edwin, and Kenneth Dewhurst. *An Illustrated History of Brain Function*. Berkeley: University of California Press, 1972.
Clasper, Jon. "The Management of Military Wounds in the Middle Ages." In *Wounds in the Middle Ages*, edited by Anne Kirkham and Cordelia Warr, 17–42. Aldershot: Ashgate, 2014.
Classen, Albrecht. *The Poems of Oswald von Wolkenstein: An English Translation of the Complete Works*. New York: Palgrave Macmillan, 2009.
Clements, Rebekah. *A Cultural History of Translation in Early Modern Japan*. Cambridge: Cambridge University Press, 2015.
Cleyer, Andreas. *Tagebuch des Kontors zu Nagasaki auf der Insel Deshima, 20 Oktober 1682–5 November 1683*, translated by Eva S. Kraft. Bonn: Bonner Zeitschrift für Japanologie, 1985.
Clulow, Adam, and Tristan Mostert, eds. *The Dutch and English East India Companies: Diplomacy, Trade, and Violence in Early Modern Asia*. Amsterdam: Amsterdam University Press, 2018.
Coatsworth, Elizabeth, and Gale Owen-Crocker. *Clothing the Past: Surviving Garments from Early Medieval to Early Modern Western Europe*. Leiden: Brill, 2018.
Cohen, Esther. "The Animated Pain of the Body." *American Historical Review* 105, no. 1 (2000): 36–68.
Cohen, Esther. *The Modulated Scream: Pain in Late Medieval Culture*. Chicago: University of Chicago Press, 2010.
Cohen, Esther. "'If You Prick Us, Do We Not Bleed?': Reflections on the Diminishing of the Other's Pain." In *Knowledge and Pain*, edited by Esther Cohen, Leona Toker, Manuela Consonni, and Otniel E. Dror, 25–41. Amsterdam: Rodopi, 2012.
Cohn, Henry J. "Götz von Berlichingen and the Art of Military Autobiography." In *War, Literature, and the Arts in Sixteenth-Century Europe*, edited by J. R. Mulryne and Margaret Shewring, 22–40. New York: Palgrave Macmillan, 1989.
Collins, Minta. *Medieval Herbals: The Illustrative Traditions*. London: British Library, 2000.
Colson, Justin, and Robert Ralley. "Medical Practice, Urban Politics, and Patronage: The London 'Commonalty' of Physicians and Surgeons of the 1420s." *English Historical Review* 130, no. 546 (2015): 1102–31.
Connell, Brian, Amy Gray Jones, Rebecca Redfern, and Don Walker. *A Bioarchaeological Study of Medieval Burials on the Site of St. Mary Spital: Excavations at Spitalfields Market, London E1, 1991–2007*. London: Museum of London Archaeology, 2012.
Constable, Giles. *Three Studies in Medieval Religious and Social Thought*. Cambridge: Cambridge University Press, 1995.
Cook, Harold J. *The Decline of the Old Medical Regime in Stuart London*. Ithaca, NY: Cornell University Press, 1986.
Cook, Harold J. *Matters of Exchange: Commerce, Medicine, and Science*. New Haven, CT: Yale University Press, 2007.
Cooper, Lisa H., and Andrea Denny-Brown, eds. *The Arma Christi in Medieval and Early Modern Material Culture*. Abingdon: Taylor & Francis, 2014.
Coppens, Christian. *De vele levens van een boek: De Fasciculus medicinae opnieuw bekeken*. Brussels: Koninklijke Academie voor Geneeskunde van België, 2009.
Coppens, Christian. "'For the Benefit of Ordinary People': The Dutch Translation of the *Fasciculus medicinae*, Antwerp 1512." *Quaerendo* 39, no. 2 (2009): 168–205.
Costas, Benito Rial, ed. *Print Culture and Peripheries in Early Modern Europe: A Contribution to the History of Printing and the Book Trade in Small European and Spanish Cities*. Leiden: Brill, 2013.
Couto-Ferreria, Erica, and Lorenzo Verderame, eds. *Cultural Constructions of the Uterus in Pre-Modern Societies, Past and Present*. Newcastle: Cambridge Scholars, 2018.
Creager, Angela N. H., Mathias Grote, and Elaine Leong, eds. "Learning by the Book: Manuals and Handbooks in the History of Science." *British Journal for the History of Science: Themes* 5 (special issue) (2020).
Crossgrove, William. "The Vernacularization of Science, Medicine, and Technology in Late Medieval Europe." *Early Science and Medicine* 5 (2000): 47–63.
Cunningham, Andrew. *The Anatomical Renaissance: The Resurrection of the Anatomical Projects of the Ancients*. London: Routledge, 1997.
Curran, John E. *Roman Invasions: The British History, Protestant Anti-Romanism, and the Historical Imagination in England, 1530–1660*. Newark: University of Delaware Press, 2002.
Dahl, Camilla Luise, and Isis Sturtewagen. "The Cap of St. Birgitta." In *Medieval Clothing and Textiles 4*, edited by Robin Netherton and Gale R. Owen-Crocker, 99–129. Woodbridge: Boydell & Brewer, 2008.
Dane, Joseph. *Blind Impressions: Methods and Mythologies in Book History*. Philadelphia: University of Pennsylvania Press, 2013.
D'Anzi, Maria Rosaria, ed. *Hanothomya del corpo humano: Volgarizzamento da Mondino de Liuzzi*. Rome: ARACNE, 2012.
Da Rold, Orietta. *Paper in Medieval England: From Pulp to Fictions*. Cambridge: Cambridge University Press, 2020.
Daston, Lorraine. "Epistemic Images." In *Vision and Its Instruments: Art, Science, and Technology in Early Modern Europe*, edited by Alina Payne, 13–35. University Park, PA: Penn State University Press, 2015.
Daston, Lorraine, and Katharine Park. *Wonders and the Order of Nature 1150–1750*. New York: Zone, 1998.
Davis, Natalie Zemon. "Publisher Guillaume Rouillé: Businessman and Humanist." In *Editing Sixteenth Century Texts*, edited by Richard J. Schoeck, 72–112. Toronto: University of Toronto Press, 1966.
Delaurenti, Béatrice. *La Contagion des émotions:* Compassio, *une énigme médiévale*. Paris: Garnier, 2016.

Demaitre, Luke. *Medieval Medicine: The Art of Healing from Head to Toe*. Santa Barbara, CA: Praeger, 2013.
Dendle, Peter, and Alain Touwaide, eds. *Health and Healing from the Medieval Garden*. Woodbridge: Boydell & Brewer, 2008.
De Renzi, Silvia. "Medical Expertise, Bodies, and the Law in Early Modern Courts." *Isis* 98, no. 2 (2007): 315–22.
Derolez, Albert. *The Library of Raphael de Marcatellis, Abbot of St. Bavon's, Ghent, 1437–1508*. Ghent: Story-Scientia, 1979.
De Young, Gregg. "Mathematical Diagrams from Manuscript to Print: Examples from the Arabic Euclidean Transmission." *Synthese* 186 (2012): 21–54.
Didi-Huberman, Georges. *L'image survivante: Histoire de l'art et temps des fantômes selon Aby Warburg*. Paris: Minuit, 2002.
Dines, Ilya. "The Theophilus Manuscript Tradition Reconsidered in the Light of New Manuscript Discoveries." In *Zwischen Kunsthandwerk und Kunst: Die "Schedula diversarum artium,"* edited by Andreas Speer, 3–10. Berlin: De Gruyter, 2014.
Dittmeyer, Daria. *Gewalt und Heil: Bildliche Inszenierungen von Passion und Martyrium im späten Mittelalter*. Cologne: Böhlau, 2014.
Doe, Janet. *A Bibliography of the Works of Ambroise Paré*. Chicago: University of Chicago Press, 1937.
Doležalová, Lucie. "*Fugere artem memorativam*? The Art of Memory in 15th c. Bohemia and Moravia (A Preliminary Survey)." *Studia Mediaevalia Bohemica* 2 (2010): 221–60.
Doležalová, Lucie. "Personal Multiple-Text Manuscripts in Late Medieval Central Europe: The 'Library' of Crux of Telč (1434–1504)." In *The Emergence of Multiple-Text Manuscripts*, edited by Alessandro Bausi, Michael Friedrich, and Marilena Maniaci, 145–70. Berlin: De Gruyter, 2020.
Dondi, Cristina. "Books of Hours: The Development of the Texts in Printed Form." In *Incunabula and Their Readers: Printing, Selling, and Using Books in the Fifteenth Century*, edited by Kristian Jensen, 53–70. London: British Library, 2003.
Dondi, Cristina. "The European Printing Revolution." In *The Book: A Global History*, edited by Michael F. Suarez and Henry R. Woudhuysen, 80–92. Oxford: Oxford University Press, 2013.
Dondi, Cristina, ed. *Printing R-Evolution and Society 1450–1500*. Venice: Ca' Foscari, 2020.
Dondi, Cristina, Abhishek Dutta, Matilde Malaspina, and Andrew Zisserman. "The Use and Reuse of Printed Illustrations in 15th-Century Venetian Editions." In *Printing R-Evolution and Society 1450–1500*, edited by Cristina Dondi, 839–70. Venice: Ca' Foscari, 2020.
Dondi, Cristina, and Neil Harris. "Oil and Green Ginger: The *Zornale* of the Venetian Bookseller Francesco de Madiis, 1484–1488." In *Documenting the Early Modern Book World: Inventories and Catalogues in Manuscript and Print*, edited by Malcolm Walsby and Natasha Constantinidou, 341–406. Leiden: Brill, 2013.
Dorner, Zachary. *Merchants of Medicines: The Commerce and Coercion of Health in Britain's Long Eighteenth Century*. Chicago: University of Chicago Press, 2020.
Draelants, Isabelle. "*Depingo ut ostendam, depictum ita est expositio*: Diagrams as an Indispensable Complement to the Cosmological Teaching of the *Liber Nemroth de astronomia*." In *Inscribing Knowledge in the Medieval Book: The Power of Paratexts*, edited by Rosalind Brown-Grant, Patrizia Carmassi, Gisela Drossbach, Anne D. Hedeman, Victoria Turner, and Iolanda Ventura, 56–92. Berlin: De Gruyter, 2019.
Drimmer, Sonja. "The Manuscript Copy and the Printed Original in the Digital Present." *Digital Philology* 9, no. 2 (2020): 93–119.
Dubé, Waltraut F. "Medieval Medicine in Middle High German Epics." PhD diss., Indiana University, 1981.
Dumaître, Paule. "Les représentations d'Ambroise Paré: Gravures, peintures, sculptures, scènes d'histoire et de guerre." *Histoire des sciences médicales* 34, no. 4 (2000): 349–66.
Dunan-Page, Anne. "'The Pourtraiture of John Bunyan' Revisited: Robert White and Images of the Author." *Bunyan Studies* 13 (2008): 7–39.
Durling, Richard J. "An Early Manual for the Medical Student and the Newly-Fledged Practitioner: Martin Stainpeis' *Liber de modo studendi seu legendi in medicina* ([Vienna] 1520)." *Clio Medica* 5 (1970): 7–33.
Dyer, Joseph. "Didactic Images in a Thirteenth-Century French Music Theory Treatise: The *Scientia artis musice* of Hélie Salomon." *Plainsong and Medieval Music* 28, no. 1 (2019): 1–27.
Eagleton, Catherine. *Monks, Manuscripts, and Sundials: The Navicula in Medieval England*. Leiden: Brill, 2010.
Ealy, Nicholas. *Narcissism and Selfhood in Medieval French Literature: Wounds of Desire*. New York: Palgrave Macmillan, 2019.
Eamon, William. *Science and the Secrets of Nature: Books of Secrets in Medieval and Early Modern Culture*. Princeton, NJ: Princeton University Press, 1994.
Eastwood, Bruce, and Gerd Graßhoff. *Planetary Diagrams for Roman Astronomy in Medieval Europe, ca. 800–1500*. Philadelphia: American Philosophical Society, 2004.
Ebermann, Oskar. *Blut- und Wundsegen in ihrer Entwicklung dargestellt*. Berlin: Mayer & Müller, 1903.
Eckhart, Pia. "Medial Translations and Material Manifestations: The *Fasciculus medicinae* in Physician-Patient Interaction." In *Between Manuscript and Print: Transcultural Perspectives, ca. 1400–1800*, edited by Sylvia Brockstieger and Paul Schweitzer-Martin, 43–88. Berlin: De Gruyter, 2023.
Edge, Joanne. *Onomantic Divination in Late Medieval Britain: Questioning Life, Predicting Death*. Woodbridge: Boydell & Brewer, 2024.
Edwards, Cyril, trans. *The Nibelungenlied: The Lay of the Nibelungs*. Oxford: Oxford University Press, 2010.
Egidi, Margreth, Markus Greulich, and Marie-Sophie Masse, eds. *Hartmann von Aue, 1230–1517: Kulturgeschichtliche Perspektiven der handschriftlichen Überlieferung*. Stuttgart: Hirzel, 2020.
Egmond, Florike. *Eye for Detail: Images of Plants and Animals in Art and Science 1500–1630*. London: Reaktion, 2016.
Ehingen, Jörg von. *The Diary of Jörg von Ehingen*, edited and translated by Malcolm Letts. London: Humphrey Milford, 1929.
Ehlert, Trude, and Rainer Leng. "Frühe Koch- und Pulverrezepte aus der Nürnberger Handschrift GNM 3227a (um 1389)." In *Medizin in Geschichte, Philologie, und Ethnologie*, edited by Dominik Groß and Monika

Reininger, 289–320. Würzburg: Königshausen & Neumann, 2003.
Eisenstein, Elizabeth L. *The Printing Press as an Agent of Change*. Cambridge: Cambridge University Press, 1979.
Eisenstein, Elizabeth L. "An Unacknowledged Revolution Revisited." *American Historical Review* 107, no. 1 (2002): 87–105.
Eisermann, Falk. "Mixing Pop and Politics: Origins, Transmission, and Readers of Illustrated Broadsides in Fifteenth-Century Germany." In *Incunabula and Their Readers: Printing, Selling, and Using Books in the Fifteenth Century*, edited by Kristian Jensen, 159–77. London: British Library, 2003.
Eisermann, Falk. "The Gutenberg Galaxy's Dark Matter: Lost Incunabula, and Ways to Retrieve Them." In *Lost Books: Reconstructing the Print World of Pre-Industrial Europe*, edited by Flavia Bruni and Andrew Pettegree, 31–54. Leiden: Brill, 2016.
Eisermann, Falk, and Volker Honemann. "Die ersten typographischen Einblattdrucke." *Gutenberg-Jahrbuch* 75 (2000): 88–131.
Eisler, Colin T. "Who Is Dürer's Syphilitic Man?" *Perspectives in Biology and Medicine* 52, no. 1 (2009): 48–60.
Elliott, Brent. "The World of the Renaissance Herbal." *Renaissance Studies* 25, no. 1 (2011): 24–41.
Elmes, Melissa Ridley. "Public Displays of Affliction: Women's Wounds in Sir Thomas Malory's *Morte Darthur*." *Modern Philology* 116, no. 3 (2019): 187–210.
Eming, Jutta. "Gewalt im Geistlichen Spiel: Das *Donaueschinger* und das *Frankfurter Passionsspiel*." *German Quarterly* 78 (2005): 1–22.
Enders, Jody. *The Medieval Theater of Cruelty: Rhetoric, Memory, Violence*. Ithaca, NY: Cornell University Press, 1999.
Engammare, Max, ed. *Calendrier des Bergers*. Paris: Fondation Martin Bodmer, 2008.
Eschenbach, Wolfram von. *Willehalm*, translated by Werner Schröder. Berlin: De Gruyter, 2019.
Espesset, Grégoire. "Traditional Chinese Knowledge before the Japanese Discovery of Western Science in Gabor Lukacs' *Kaitai Shinsho & Geka Sōden*." *East Asian Science, Technology, and Medicine* 40 (2014): 113–28.
Evans, Michael. "The Geometry of the Mind: Scientific Diagrams and Medieval Thought." *Architectural Association Quarterly* 12, no. 4 (1980): 32–55.
Even-Ezra, Ayelet. *Lines of Thought: Branching Diagrams and the Medieval Mind*. Chicago: University of Chicago Press, 2020.
Falque, Ingrid. "'*Daz man bild mit bilde us tribe*': Imagery and Knowledge of God in Henry Suso's *Exemplar*." *Speculum* 92, no. 2 (2017): 447–92.
Faral, Edmond, ed. *Les arts poétiques du XIIe et du XIIIe siècle*. Paris: Édouard Champion, 1924.
Der Fasciculus medicinae des Johannes de Ketham, Alemannus: Facsimile des Venetianer Erstdruckes von 1491. Commentary by Karl Sudhoff. Milan: Lier, 1924.
Fendrych, Miroslav. "České rukopisné rostlináře." *Časopis Národního muzea: Oddíl přírodovědný* 131 (1962): 186–97.
Ferckel, Christoph. "Zur Gynäkologie und Generationslehre im *Fasciculus medicinae* des Johannes de Ketham." *Archiv für Geschichte der Medizin* 6, no. 3 (1912): 205–22.
Ferrari, Mirella. *Medieval and Renaissance Manuscripts at the University of California, Los Angeles*. Berkeley: University of California Press, 1991.
Fichtner, Gerhard. "Christus als Arzt: Ursprünge und Wirkungen eines Motivs." *Frühmittelalterliche Studien* 16, no. 1 (1982): 1–18.
Finckh, Ruth. *Minor mundus homo: Studien zur Mikrokosmos-Idee in der mittelalterlichen Literatur*. Göttingen: V&R Unipress, 1999.
Fischer-Homberger, Esther. *Medizin vor Gericht: Gerichtsmedizin von der Renaissance bis zur Aufklärung*. Bern: Huber, 1983.
Fleming, Fergus. *The Man with the Golden Typewriter: Ian Fleming's James Bond Letters*. London: Bloomsbury, 2015.
Flood, John L. "'*Volentes sibi comparare infrascriptos libros impressos . . .*': Printed Books as a Commercial Commodity in the Fifteenth Century." In *Incunabula and Their Readers: Printing, Selling, and Using Books in the Fifteenth Century*, edited by Kristian Jensen, 139–151. London: British Library, 2003.
Folz, Hans. *Die Reimpaarsprüche*, edited by Hanns Fischer. Munich: Beck, 1961.
Foscati, Alessandra. "Healing with the Body of Christ: Religion, Medicine, and Magic." In *Il "Corpus Domini": Teologia, antropologia, e politica*, edited by Laura Andreani and Agostino Paravicini Bagliani, 209–27. Florence: SISMEL, 2015.
Fowler, Caroline. *The Art of Paper: From the Holy Land to the Americas*. New Haven, CT: Yale University Press, 2019.
Franklin, Andrea. "Woodcuts." In *Book Parts*, edited by Dennis Duncan and Adam Smyth, 209–22. Oxford: Oxford University Press, 2019.
Fransen, Sietske, and Katherine M. Reinhart, eds. "The Practice of Copying in Making Knowledge in Early Modern Europe." *Word & Image* 35, no. 3 (special issue) (2019).
Freedman, Paul. *Out of the East: Spices and the Medieval Imagination*. New Haven, CT: Yale University Press, 2008.
Frohne, Bianca, and Jenni Kuuliala. "The Trauma of Pain in Later Medieval Miracle Accounts." In *Trauma in Medieval Society*, edited by Wendy J. Turner and Christina Lee, 215–36. Leiden: Brill, 2018.
Frutos Gonzalez, Virginia. *Flos medicine (Regimen sanitatis Salernitanum): Estudio, edición crítica, y traducción*. Valladolid: Universidad de Valladolid, 2010.
Führkötter, Adelgundis, and Angela Carlevaris, eds. *Hildegardis Bingensis: Scivias*. Turnhout: Brepols, 1978.
Fürbeth, Frank. *Johannes Hartlieb: Untersuchungen zu Leben und Werk*. Tübingen: Niemeyer, 1992.
Furdell, Elizabeth Lane. *The Royal Doctors, 1485–1714: Medical Personnel at the Tudor and Stuart Courts*. Rochester, NY: University of Rochester Press, 2001.
Furdell, Elizabeth Lane. *Publishing and Medicine in Early Modern England*. Rochester, NY: University of Rochester Press, 2002.
Gadebusch Bondio, Mariacarla, ed. *Blood in History and Blood Histories*. Florence: SISMEL, 2005.
Gamba, Eleonora. "Pietro da Montagnana: La vita, gli studi, la biblioteca di un *homo trilinguis*." PhD diss., Università degli Studi di Padova, 2016.
García, Nuria Aranda. "Book Illustration in the Late Fifteenth and Early Sixteenth Centuries: The First

Editions of the Siete Sabios de Roma." In *Illustration and Ornamentation in the Iberian Book World, 1450–1800*, edited by Alexander Samuel Wilkinson, 240–58. Leiden: Brill, 2022.

Gent, Lucy, ed. *Albion's Classicism: The Visual Arts in Britain 1550–1660*. New Haven, CT: Yale University Press, 1995.

Gentilcore, David. *Healers and Healing in Early Modern Italy*. Manchester: Manchester University Press, 1998.

Gernert, Folke. *Fictionalizing Heterodoxy: Various Uses of Knowledge in the Spanish World from the Archpriest of Hita to Mateo Alemán*. Berlin: De Gruyter, 2019.

Gilchrist, Roberta. *Sacred Heritage: Monastic Archaeology, Identities, Beliefs*. Cambridge: Cambridge University Press, 2020.

Gil-Sotres, Pedro. "Derivation and Revulsion: The Theory and Practice of Medieval Phlebotomy." In *Practical Medicine from Salerno to the Black Death*, edited by Luis García-Ballester, Roger French, Jon Arrizabalaga, and Andrew Cunningham, 110–55. Cambridge: Cambridge University Press, 2004.

Giordano, Carmela. "Ruolo e funzione delle immagini nei testi scientifici del medioevo tedesco: Considerazioni su due Hausbücher." In *Testo e immagine nel medioevo germanico*, edited by Maria Grazia Saibene and Marina Buzzoni, 268–76. Milan: Parole, 2001.

Goble, Andrew. *Confluences of Medicine in Medieval Japan: Buddhist Healing, Chinese Knowledge, Islamic Formulas, and Wounds of War*. Honolulu: University of Hawaii Press, 2011.

Goehl, Konrad, and Johannes Gottfried Mayer. "Variationen über den Phlebotomie-Traktat 'Venarum minutio': Die Vorlage des sogenannten '24-Paragraphen-Textes.'" In *Editionen und Studien zur lateinischen und deutschen Fachprosa des Mittelalters*, edited by Konrad Goehl and Johannes Gottfried Mayer, 45–66. Würzburg: Königshausen & Neumann, 2000.

Goehl, Konrad, and Johannes Gottfried Mayer. "Der Aderlaßmann aus Michelstadt: Ein Plakat aus dem Mittelalter." In *Bewahren und Erforschen: Beiträge aus der Nicolaus-Matz-Bibliothek (Kirchenbibliothek) Michelstadt*, edited by Wolfgang Schmitz, 56–74. Michelstadt: Stadt Michelstadt, 2003.

Goldie, Matthew Boyd. *Scribes of Space: Place in Middle English Literature and Late Medieval Science*. Ithaca, NY: Cornell University Press, 2019.

González Jiménez, Manuel, Manuel Fuertes de Gisbert, María Teresa López de Guereño, Laura Fernández, César Bordóns, Jesús Basulto, and José Antioni Camúñez, eds. *Libro de los juegos de ajedrez, dados, y tablas de Alfonso X el Sabio*. 2 vols. Valencia: Scriptorium, 2010.

Goodman, Grant K. *Japan and the Dutch 1600–1853*. Richmond: Routledge Curzon, 2000.

Grafton, Anthony T. "The Importance of Being Printed." *Journal of Interdisciplinary History* 11, no. 2 (1980): 265–86.

Green, Jonathan. *Printing and Prophecy: Prognostication and Media Change 1450–1550*. Ann Arbor: University of Michigan Press, 2012.

Green, Monica H. "Gynäkologische und geburtshilfliche Illustrationen in mittelalterlichen Manuskripten: Sprechende Bilder halfen den Frauen." *Die Waage* 30, no. 4 (1991): 161–67.

Green, Monica H. "Gender, Health, Disease: Recent Work on Medieval Women's Medicine." *Studies in Medieval and Renaissance History* 3, no. 1 (2005): 1–46.

Green, Monica H. *Making Women's Medicine Masculine: The Rise of Male Authority in Pre-Modern Gynaecology*. Oxford: Oxford University Press, 2008.

Green, Monica H. "Rethinking the Manuscript Basis of Salvatore De Renzi's Collectio Salernitana: The Corpus of Medical Writings in the 'Long' Twelfth Century." In *La "Collectio Salernitana" di Salvatore De Renzi*, edited by Danielle Jacquart and Agostino Paravicini Bagliani, 15–60. Florence: SISMEL, 2008.

Green, Monica H. "Moving from Philology to Social History: The Circulation and Uses of Albucasis's Latin *Surgery* in the Middle Ages." In *Between Text and Patient: The Medical Enterprise in Medieval and Early Modern Europe*, edited by Florence Eliza Glaze and Brian K. Nance, 331–72. Florence: SISMEL, 2011.

Griebler, Andrew. *Botanical Icons: Critical Practices of Illustration in the Premodern Mediterranean*. Chicago: University of Chicago Press, 2024.

Griffiths, Antony. *The Print in Stuart Britain, 1603–1689*. London: British Museum, 1998.

Groebner, Valentin. *Ungestalten: Die visuelle Kultur der Gewalt im Mittelalter*. Munich: Hanser, 2003; translated into English as *Defaced: The Visual Culture of Violence in the Late Middle Ages*, trans. Pamela Selwyn (New York: Zone, 2008).

Grosmont, Henry of. *Le livre de seyntz medicines: The Book of Holy Medicines*, translated by Catherine Batt. Tempe: Arizona Center for Medieval and Renaissance Studies Press, 2014.

Gross, Hilde-Marie. "Illustrationen in medizinischen Sammelhandschriften: Eine Auswahl anhand von Kodizes der Überlieferungs- und Wirkungsgeschichte des 'Arzneibuchs' Ortolfs von Baierland." In *"ein teutsch puech machen": Untersuchungen zur landessprachlichen Vermittlung medizinischen Wissens*, edited by Gundolf Keil, 172–348. Wiesbaden: Reichert, 1993.

Gross, Hilde-Marie, and Gundolf Keil. "'*Wiltu die wunde wol bewarn*': Ein Leitfaden feldärztlicher Notversorgung aus dem spätmittelalterlichen Schlesien." In *Medizin-, Pharmazie-, und Wissenschaftsgeschichte vom Mittelalter bis zur Gegenwart*, edited by Regine Pfrepper, 1–26. Aachen: Shaker, 2007.

Guardiola, Ginger Lee. "Within and Without: The Social and Medical Worlds of the Medieval Midwife, 1000–1500." PhD diss., University of Colorado at Boulder, 2002.

Guilleminot-Chrétien, Geneviève. "Chrétien Wechel, Rabelais et le Tiers livre." In *Narrations fabuleuses: Melanges en l'honneur de Mireille Huchon*, edited by Isabelle Garnier, Claude La Charité, Romain Menini, Anne-Pascale Pouey-Mounou, and Anne Réach-Ngô, 129–38. Paris: Garnier, 2022.

Gumbert, J. P. *Bat Books: A Catalogue of Folded Manuscripts Containing Almanacs or Other Texts*. Turnhout: Brepols, 2016.

Gupta, Vivek. "Images for Instruction: A Multilingual Illustrated Dictionary in Fifteenth-Century Sultanate India." *Muqarnas* 38, no. 1 (2021): 77–112.

Haage, Bernhard Dietrich. *Studien zur Heilkunde im "Parzival" Wolframs von Eschenbach*. Göppingen: Kümmerle, 1992.

Habermann, Mechtild. *Deutsche Fachtexte der frühen Neuzeit: Naturkundlich-medizinische Wissensvermittlung im Spannungsfeld von Latein und Volkssprache*. Berlin: De Gruyter, 2001.

Habicht, Tanja-Isabel, and Björn Reich. "Die Farbe der Erinnerung." In *Farbe im Mittelalter: Materialität—Medialität—Semantik*, edited by Ingrid Bennewitz and Andrea Schindler, 1:537–50. Berlin: Akademie, 2011.

Haeseli, Christa M. *Magische Performativität: Althochdeutsche Zaubersprüche in ihrem Überlieferungskontext*. Würzburg: Königshausen & Neumann, 2011.

Hagedorn, Dierk. "German Fechtbücher from the Middle Ages to the Renaissance." In *Late Medieval and Early Modern Fight Books: Transmission and Tradition of Martial Arts in Europe (14th–17th Centuries)*, ed. Daniel Jaquet, Karin Verelst, and Timothy Dawson, 247–79. Leiden: Brill, 2016.

Hagenmaier, Winfried. *Die deutschen mittelalterlichen Handschriften der Universitätsbibliothek und die mittelalterlichen Handschriften anderer öffentlicher Sammlungen (Kataloge der Universitätsbibliothek Freiburg im Breisgau 1,4)*. Wiesbaden: Harrassowitz, 1988.

Hall, Bert S. "The Didactic and the Elegant: Some Thoughts on Scientific and Technological Illustrations in the Middle Ages and Renaissance." In *Picturing Knowledge: Historical and Philosophical Problems Concerning the Use of Art in Science*, edited by Brian Baigrie, 3–39. Toronto: University of Toronto Press, 1996.

Hallbäck, Dan-Axel. "A Medieval(?) Bone with a Copper Plate Support, Indicating an Open Surgical Treatment." *Ossa* 34 (1976): 63–82.

Hamburger, Jeffrey F. *Nuns as Artists: The Visual Culture of a Medieval Convent*. Berkeley: University of California Press, 1997.

Hamburger, Jeffrey F. "Heinrich Seuse, 'Das Exemplar' (Nr. 36.)." In *Katalog der deutschsprachigen illustrierten Handschriften des Mittelalters (KdiH)*, edited by Ulrike Bodemann, Kristina Freienhagen-Baumgardt, and Peter Schmidt, vol. 4/1. Munich: Beck, 2012.

Hamburger, Jeffrey F. *Haec figura demonstrat: Diagramme in einem Pariser Exemplar von Lothars von Segni "De missarum mysteriis" aus dem frühen 13. Jahrhundert*. Berlin: De Gruyter, 2013.

Hamburger, Jeffrey F. *Diagramming Devotion: Berthold of Nuremberg's Transformation of Hrabanus Maurus's Poems in Praise of the Cross*. Chicago: University of Chicago Press, 2020.

Hamburger, Jeffrey F. *Color in Cusanus*. Stuttgart: Hiersemann, 2021.

Hamburger, Jeffrey F. "Between Basel and Lyon: Bernhard Richel, Martin Huss, and a Possible Printer's Vade Mecum (The Morgan Library & Museum, MS M.158)." *Gutenberg-Jahrbuch* 97 (2022): 16–37.

Hamburger, Jeffrey F., David S. Roxburgh, and Linda Safran, eds. *The Diagram as Paradigm: Cross-Cultural Approaches*. Washington, DC: Dumbarton Oaks Publications, 2022.

Hamburger, Jeffrey F., Robert Suckale, and Gude Suckale-Redlefsen, eds. *Painting the Page in the Age of Print: Central European Manuscript Illumination of the Fifteenth Century*. Toronto: PIMS, 2018.

Hamburger, Jeffrey F., and Maria Theisen, eds. *Unter Druck: Mitteleuropäische Buchmalerei im 15. Jahrhundert*. Peterberg: Imhof, 2018.

Harari, Yuval Noah. *Renaissance Military Memoirs: War, History and Identity, 1450–1600*. Woodbridge: Boydell & Brewer, 2004.

Harris, Neil. "Costs We Don't Think About: Rubrication and Illumination. An Unusual Copy of Franciscus de Platea, *Opus restitutionum* (1474), and a Few Other Items." In *Printing R-Evolution and Society 1450–1500*, edited by Cristina Dondi, 511–40. Venice: Ca' Foscari, 2020.

Hartmann, Anna-Maria. *English Mythography in Its European Context, 1500–1650*. Oxford: Oxford University Press, 2018.

Hartnell, Jack. "Surgical Saws and Cutting-Edge Agency." In *The Agency of Things in Medieval and Early Modern Art: Materials, Power, and Manipulation*, edited by Grażyna Jurkowlaniec, Ika Matyjaszkiewicz, and Zuzanna Sarnecka, 157–69. New York: Routledge, 2017.

Hartnell, Jack. "Tools of the Puncture: Skin, Knife, Bone, Hand." In *Flaying in the Pre-Modern World: Practice and Representation*, edited by Larissa Tracy, 20–50. Woodbridge: Boydell & Brewer, 2017.

Hartnell, Jack. "Wording the Wound Man." *British Art Studies* 6 (2017). https://doi.org/10.17658/issn.2058-5462/issue-06/jhartnell/000 (accessed August 1, 2024).

Harwood, John. "The Wound Man: George Nelson and the 'End of Architecture.'" *Grey Room* 31 (2008): 90–115.

Haskell, Francis, and Nicholas Penny. *Taste and the Antique: The Lure of Classical Sculpture, 1500–1900*. New Haven, CT: Yale University Press, 1981.

Hasty, Will. *Art of Arms: Studies of Aggression and Dominance in Medieval German Court Poetry*. Heidelberg: C. Winter, 2002.

Haubrichs, Wolfgang. "leid, harm und sêr: Zur Geschichte eines semantischen Komplexes der Verletzung." In *Verletzungen und Unversehrtheit in der deutschen Literatur des Mittelalters*, ed. Sarah Bowden, Nine Miedema, and Stephen Mossman, 17–34. Tübingen: Narr Francke, 2020.

Haug, Walter, and Burghart Wachinger, eds. *Die Passion Christi in Literatur und Kunst des Spätmittelalters*. Berlin: Niemeyer, 1993.

Hausse, Heide. *The Malleable Body: Surgeons, Artisans, and Amputees in Early Modern Germany*. Manchester: Manchester University Press, 2023.

Hauter, Ashwak. "Madness, Pain, and *Ikhtilāṭ al-ʿaql*: Conceptualizing Ibn Abī Ṣādiq's Medico-Philosophical Psychology." *Early Science and Medicine* 25, no. 5 (2020): 453–79.

Hay, Jonathan. "Culture, Ethnicity, and Empire in the Work of Two Eighteenth-Century 'Eccentric' Artists." *RES* 35 (1999): 201–23.

Heesen, Kerstin te. *Das illustrierte Flugblatt als Wissensmedium der Frühen Neuzeit: Langfristige Entwicklungen in Deutschland und neueste Daten für Ost- und Westdeutschland*. Leverkusen: Budrich, 2011.

Heiduk, Matthias, Klaus Herbers, and Hans-Christian Lehner, eds. *Prognostication in the Medieval World: A Handbook*. Berlin: De Gruyter, 2020.

Heinrich, Ari Larissa. *The Afterlife of Images: Translating the Pathological Body between China and the West*. Durham, NC: Duke University Press, 2008.

Heinrichs, Erik A. *Plague, Print, and the Reformation:*

The German Reform of Healing 1473–1573. Abingdon: Routledge, 2018.

Hellinga, Lotte. *Incunabula in Transit: People and Trade*. Leiden: Brill, 2018.

Hénaff, Arthur. "Le *Tübinger Hausbuch*: La miscellanée scientifique à l'épreuve de l'image." *Micrologus* 27 (special issue: "Les miscellanées scientifiques au Moyen Âge") (2019): 429–42.

Herrera, María Teresa. *Compendio de la humana salud*. Madrid: ARCOS/LIBROS, 1990.

Herrero, María Nieves Sánchez González, and María Concepción Vázquez Benito. *Tratado de fisonomía: Tratado de la forma de la generación de la criatura*. Salamanca: DLE, 2009.

Herrlinger, Robert. *Geschichte der medizinischen Abbildung*. Munich: Heinz Moos, 1967.

Hill, Boyd H., Jr. "A Medieval German Wound Man: Wellcome MS 49." *Journal of the History of Medicine and Allied Sciences* 20, no. 4 (1965): 334–57.

Hiller, Diana. "Some Italian Wall Paintings of the Sunday Christ: Monitory and Redemptory Iconographies and the Effect of Position." *Parergon* 37, no. 1 (2020): 79–112.

Hiroshi Kanbara. "Kōi geka sōden zuhan seiritsu e no sukurutetasu no gekasho Armamentarium Chirurgicum no eikyō『紅夷外科宗伝』図版成立へのスクルテタス (Scultetus) の外科書 Armamentarium chirurgicum の影響." *Nihonshikaishi gakkai kaishi* 日本歯科医史学会会誌 18, no. 3 (1992): 229–30.

Hiroshi, Kanbara. "Fukuoka hara mitsunobu shi kazō oranda gekajutsushiki zufu emaki nitsuite no kōsatsu 福岡・原三信氏家蔵『阿蘭陀外科術式図譜絵巻』についての考察." *Nihon Ishigaku Zasshi* 日本医史学雑誌 43, no. 3 (1997): 364–65.

Hirschauer, Stefan. "The Manufacture of Bodies in Surgery." *Social Studies of Science* 21, no. 2 (1991): 279–319.

Hitthaler-Frank, Theresa. *Hebammen, Ärzte und ihr "Rosengarten": Ein medizinisches Handbuch und die Umbrüche in der Obstetrik des 15. und 16. Jahrhunderts*. Berlin: Peter Lang, 2021.

Hoffman, Godehard. *Das Gabelkreuz in Santa Maria im Kapitol zu Köln und das Phänomen der "Crucixifi dolorosi" in Europa*. Worms: Wernersche, 2006.

Hoffmann, Leonhard. "Almanache des 15. und 16. Jahrhunderts und ihre Käufer." *Beiträge zur Inkunabelkunde* 3, no. 8 (1983): 130–43.

Holladay, Joan A. *Genealogy and the Politics of Representation in the High and Late Middle Ages*. Cambridge: Cambridge University Press, 2019.

Holste, Thomas. *Der Theriakkrämer: Ein Beitrag zur Frühgeschichte der Arzneimittelwerbung*. Hannover: Wellm, 1976.

Honecker, Martin. "Christus medicus." In *Der kranke Mensch in Mittelalter und Renaissance*, edited by Peter Wunderli, 27–43. Düsseldorf: Drosde, 1986.

Honemann, Volker, Sabine Griese, Falk Eisermann, and Marcus Ostermann, eds. *Einblattdrucke des 15. und frühen 16. Jahrhunderts: Probleme, Perspektiven, Fallstudien*. Tübingen: Niemeyer, 2000.

Huey, Caroline. *Hans Folz and Print Culture in Late Medieval Germany*. New York: Routledge, 2017.

Hunt, Tony. "The Poetic Vein: Phlebotomy in Middle English and Anglo-Norman Verse." *English Studies* 77, no. 4 (1996): 311–22.

Hutton, Sarah. "Platonism, Stoicism, Scepticism, and Classical Imitation." In *A New Companion to English Renaissance Literature and Culture*, edited by Michael Hattaway, 1:106–19. Oxford: Blackwell, 2010.

Hyman, Aaron M. *Rubens in Repeat: The Logic of the Copy in Colonial Latin America*. Los Angeles: GRI, 2021.

Infelise, Mario. "Book Publishing and the Circulation of Information." In *A Companion to Venetian History, 1400–1797*, edited by Eric R. Dursteler, 651–74. Leiden: Brill, 2013.

Israel, Uwe. "Brokers as German-Italian Cultural Mediators in Renaissance Venice." In *Migrating Words, Migrating Merchants, Migrating Law: Trading Routes and the Development of Commercial Law*, edited by Stefania Gialdroni, Albrecht Cordes, Serge Dauchy, Dave De ruysscher, and Heikki Pihlajamäki, 95–117. Leiden: Brill, 2020.

Jacquart, Danielle. "Les sciences dans la bibliothèque de Saint-Victor." In *L'école de Saint-Victor de Paris: Influence et rayonnement du Moyen Âge à l'époque moderne*, edited by Dominique Poirel, 197–225. Turnhout: Brepols, 2010.

Jancke, Gabriele, with Marc Jarzebowski, Klaus Krönert, and Yvonne Aßmann. *Selbstzeugnisse im deutschsprachigen Raum: Autobiographien, Tagebücher und andere autobiographische Schriften 1400–1620*. https://www.geschkult.fu-berlin.de/e/jancke-quellenkunde/index.html (accessed August 1, 2024).

Jaquet, Daniel. "Fighting in the Fightschools Late XVth, Early XVIth Century." *Acta Periodica Duellatorum* 1, no. 1 (2013): 47–66.

Jaquet, Daniel. "Six Weeks to Prepare for Combat: Instruction and Practices from the Fight Books at the End of the Middle Ages, a Note on Ritualised Single Combats." In *Killing and Being Killed: Bodies in Battle, Perspectives on Fighters in the Middle Ages*, edited by Jörg Rogge, 131–64. Bielefeld: Transcript, 2017.

Jaquet, Daniel, Karin Verelst, and Timothy Dawson, eds. *Late Medieval and Early Modern Fight Books: Transmission and Tradition of Martial Arts in Europe (14th–17th Centuries)*. Leiden: Brill, 2016.

Jaritz, Gerhard. "Aderlaß und Schröpfen im Chorfrauenstift Klosteneuburg (1445–1533)." *Jahrbuch des Stiftes Klosterneuburg* 9 (1975): 67–108.

Jensen, Kristian. "Printing the Bible in the Fifteenth Century: Devotion, Philology, and Commerce." In *Incunabula and Their Readers: Printing, Selling, and Using Books in the Fifteenth Century*, edited by Kristian Jensen, 115–38. London: British Library, 2003.

Jensen, Kristian, ed. *Incunabula and Their Readers: Printing, Selling, and Using Books in the Fifteenth Century*. London: British Library, 2003.

Jerjen, Vera. "Struktur und Erfahrung im 'Welschen Gast' Thomasins von Zerclaere." In *Diagramm und Text: Diagrammatische Strukturen und die Dynamisierung von Wissen und Erfahrung*, edited by Eckart Conrad Lutz, Vera Jerjen, and Christine Putzo, 349–72. Wiesbaden: Reichert, 2014.

Jeudy, Colette, and Ludwig Schuba. "Erhard Knab und die Heidelberger Universität im Spiegel von Handschriften und Akteneinträgen." *Quellen und Forschungen aus italienischen Archiven und Bibliotheken* 61 (1981): 60–108.

Jezler, Peter, Peter Niederhäuser, and Elke Jezler, eds. *Ritterturnier: Geschichte einer Festkultur*. Luzern: Quaternio, 2014.

Jiménez, Aurelio Pérez. "Las mansiones lunares: Adaptación árabe de una doctrina astrológica antigua." In *El Cielo del Islám*, edited by Fátima Roldán Castro, 239–64. Seville: Universidad de Sevilla, 2014

Joby, Christopher. *The Dutch Language in Japan (1600–1900)*. Leiden: Brill, 2021.

Johnsson, J.W.S. "Zur Geschichte der Rothaarigen Mannes im Manuskript Ny k. S. 846 in der Königlichen Bibliothek zu Kopenhagen." *Janus* 30 (1926): 304–17.

Jones, Martin H., and Timothy McFarland, eds. *Wolfram's "Willehalm": Fifteen Essays*. Rochester, NY: Camden House, 2002.

Jones, Peter Murray. *Medieval Medicine in Illuminated Manuscripts*. London: British Library, 1998.

Jones, Peter Murray. "Image, Word, and Medicine in the Middle Ages." In *Visualizing Medieval Medicine and Natural History, 1200–1550*, edited by Jean A. Givens, Karen M. Reeds, and Alain Touwaide, 1–24. Aldershot: Ashgate, 2006.

Jones, Peter Murray. "The Surgeon as Story-Teller." *Poetica* 72 (2009): 77–92.

Jones, Richard. *Sweet Waste: Medieval Sugar Production in the Mediterranean Viewed from the 2002 Excavation at Tawahin Es-Sukkar, Safi, Jordan*. Glasgow: Potingair, 2016.

Juste, Davide. *Les manuscrits astrologiques latins conservés à la Bayerische Staatsbibliothek de Munich*. Paris: CNRS, 2011.

Kaeuper, Richard W. *Chivalry and Violence in Medieval Europe*. Oxford: Oxford University Press, 1999.

Kaeuper, Richard W. *Medieval Chivalry*. Cambridge: Cambridge University Press, 2016.

Kalning, Pamela, Matthias Miller, and Karin Zimmermann. *Die Codices Palatini germanici in der Universitätsbibliothek Heidelberg (Cod. Pal. germ. 496–670)*. Wiesbaden: Harrassowitz, 2014.

Kananoja, Kalle, and Markku Hokkanen, eds. *Healers and Empires in Global History: Healing as Hybrid and Contested Knowledge*. Cham: Springer, 2019.

Kassell, Lauren. "Medical Understandings of the Body, c. 1500–1750." In *The Routledge History of Sex and the Body, 1500 to the Present*, edited by Sarah Toulalan and Kate Fisher, 57–74. London: Routledge, 2013.

Kaye, Joel. *A History of Balance, 1250–1375: The Emergence of a New Model of Equilibrium and Its Impact on Thought*. Cambridge: Cambridge University Press, 2014.

Keil, Gundolf. "Zum Problem lateinisch-landessprachiger Verflechtung: Der 'Wunden-mann' des Kodex Wellcome 49." *Nachrichtenblatt der Deutschen Gesellschaft für Geschichte, Medizin, und Technik* 25, no. 2 (1975): 79–80.

Keil, Gundolf. "Ortolfs chirurgischer Traktat und das Aufkommen der medizinischen Demonstrationszeichnung." In *Text und Bild, Bild und Text*, edited by Wolfgang Harms, 137–49. Stuttgart: Metzler, 1990.

Keil, Gundolf. "Ein Schlesisches Aderlassbüchlein des 15. Jahrhunderts: Untersuchungen zum funktionsbedingten Gestaltwandel des Vierundzwanzig-Paragraphen-Textes." In *Fachtexte des Spätmittelalters und der Frühen Neuzeit: Tradition und Perspektiven der Fachprosa- und Fachsprachenforschung*, edited by Lenka Vaňková, 75–118. Berlin: De Gruyter, 2017.

Keil, Gundolf. "Das Feldbuch als Vertreter der chirurgischen Fachprosa." *Studia Germanistica* 12, no. 20 (2018): 37–49.

Keil, Gundolf, Friedrich Lenhardt, and Christoph Weisser, eds. *Vom Einfluss der Gestirne auf die Gesundheit und den Charakter des Menschen*. 2 vols. Luzern: Faksimile, 1983.

Kellett, Rachel E. *Single Combat and Warfare in German Literature of the High Middle Ages: Stricker's* Karl der Grosse *and* Daniel von dem Blühenden Tal. London: Manley, 2008.

Kellett, Rachel E. "'... Vnnd schüß im vnder dem schwert den ort lang ein zů der brust': The Placement and Consequences of Sword-Blows in Sigmund Ringeck's Fifteenth-Century Fencing Manual." In *Wounds and Wound Repair in Medieval Culture*, edited by Larissa Tracy and Kelly DeVries, 128–50. Leiden: Brill, 2015.

Kellett, Rachel E. "Only a Flesh-Wound? The Literary Background to Medieval German Fight Books." In *Late Medieval and Early Modern Fight Books: Transmission and Tradition of Martial Arts in Europe (14th–17th Centuries)*, edited by Daniel Jaquet, Karin Verelst, and Timothy Dawson, 62–87. Leiden: Brill, 2016.

Kemper, Tobias A. *Die Kreuzigung Christi: Motivgeschichtliche Studien zu lateinischen und deutschen Passionstraktaten des Spätmittelalters*. Berlin: Niemeyer, 2006.

Keys, Thomas E. "The Earliest Medical Books Printed with Moveable Type." *Library Quarterly* 10, no. 2 (1940): 220–30.

Kibre, Pearl. "Hippocrates Latinus: Repertorium of Hippocratic Writings in the Latin Middle Ages (V)." *Traditio* 35 (1979): 273–302.

King, Helen. *Hippocrates' Woman: Reading the Female Body in Ancient Greece*. London: Routledge, 1998.

Kinzelbach, Annamarie. *Chirurgen und Chirugie-Praktiken: Wundärzte als Reichsstadtbürger 16. bis 18. Jahrhundert*. Mainz: Donata Kinzelbach, 2015.

Klapisch-Zuber, Christiane. *L'ombre des ancêtres: Essai sur l'imaginaire médiéval de la parenté*. Paris: Fayard, 2000.

Klapisch-Zuber, Christiane. *L'arbre des familles*. Paris: La Martinière, 2003.

Klebs, Arnold C. *Incunabula scientifica et medica*. Bruges: Saint Catherine Press, 1938.

Klein, Alice. "Hans Wechtlin and the Production of German Colour Woodcuts." In *Printing Colour 1400–1700: History, Techniques, Functions, and Receptions*, edited by Ad Stijnman and Elizabeth Savage, 103–15. Leiden: Brill, 2015.

Klein, Dorothea. "Geschlecht und Gewalt: Zur Konstitution von Männlichkeit im 'Erec' Hartmanns von Aue." In *Literarische Leben: Rollenentwürfe in der Literatur des Hoch- und Spätmittelalters*, edited by Matthias Meyer and Hans-Jochen Schiewer, 433–63. Tübingen: Max Niemeyer, 2002.

Klestinec, Cynthia. *Theaters of Anatomy: Students, Teachers, and Traditions of Dissection in Renaissance Venice*. Baltimore: Johns Hopkins University Press, 2011.

Knüsel, Christopher. "The Physical Evidence of Warfare: Subtle Stigmata?" In *Warfare, Violence, and Slavery in Prehistory*, edited by Mike Parker Pearson and I.J.N. Thorpe, 49–65. Oxford: BAR, 2005.

Kornell, Monique. *Flesh and Bones: The Art of Anatomy*. Los Angeles: Getty Research Institute, 2022.

Koslofsky, Craig, and Roberto Zaugg, eds. and trans. *A German Barber-Surgeon in the Atlantic Slave Trade: The Seventeenth-Century Journal of Johann Peter Oettinger*. Charlottesville: University of Virginia Press, 2020.

Krause, Carl von, ed. *Deutsche Liederdichter des 13. Jahrhunderts.* Tübingen: Niemeyer, 1952.

Kremer, Richard L. "Incunable Almanacs and Practica as Practical Knowledge Produced in Trading Zones." In *The Structures of Practical Knowledge*, edited by Matteo Valleriani, 333–69. Cham: Springer, 2017.

Kruse, Britta-Juliane. *Verborgene Heilkünste: Geschichte der Frauenmedizin im Spätmittelalter.* Berlin: De Gruyter, 2012.

Künzel, Max. "Beilngrieser Aderlaßmännlein." *Würzburger medizinhistorische Mitteilungen* 19 (2000): 153–75.

Kupfer, Marcia, Adam S. Cohen, and Jeffrey H. Chajes, eds. *The Visualization of Knowledge in Medieval and Early Modern Europe.* Turnhout: Brepols, 2020.

Kurtz, Donna. "The Concept of the Classical Past in Tudor and Early Stuart England." *Journal of the History of Collections* 20, no. 2 (2008): 189–204.

Kusukawa, Sachiko. "Andreas Nolthius' *Almanach* for 1575." *Journal of the History of Astronomy* 42, no. 1 (2011): 91–110.

Kusukawa, Sachiko. *Picturing the Book of Nature: Image, Text, and Argument in Sixteenth-Century Human Anatomy and Medical Botany.* Chicago: University of Chicago Press, 2012.

Landau, David, and Peter Parshall. *The Renaissance Print 1470–1550.* New Haven, CT: Yale University Press, 1994.

Langum, Virginia. "'The Wounded Surgeon': Devotion, Compassion, and Metaphor in Medieval England." In *Wounds and Wound Repair in Medieval Culture*, edited by Larissa Tracy and Kelly DeVries, 269–90. Leiden: Brill, 2015.

Lawrence, Susan C. *Charitable Knowledge: Hospital Pupils and Practitioners in Eighteenth-Century London.* Cambridge: Cambridge University Press, 2010.

Lechtermann, Christina. "Die geometrischen Diagramme der Geometria Culmensis." *Das Mittelalter* 22, no. 2 (2017): 314–31.

Leedham-Green, Elisabeth, Dennis E. Rhodes, and Frank H. Stubbings. *Garrett Godfrey's Accounts, c. 1527–1533.* Cambridge: Cambridge Bibliographical Society, 1992.

Leerdam, Andrea van. "Popularising and Personalising an Illustrated Herbal in Dutch." *Nuncius* 36, no. 2 (2021): 356–93.

Leerdam, Andrea van. *Woodcuts as Reading Guides: How Images Shaped Knowledge Transmission in Medical-Astrological Books in Dutch (1500–1550).* Amsterdam: Amsterdam University Press, 2024.

Lehmann, Johann Georg. *Urkundliche Geschichte der Grafschaft Hanau-Lichtenberg.* 2 vols. Hanau-Lichtenberg: Schneider, 1863.

Leitch, Stephanie. "Visual Acuity and the Physiognomer's Art of Observation." *Oxford Art Journal* 38, no. 2 (2015): 189–208.

Leitch, Stephanie. *Early Modern Print Media and the Art of Observation: Training the Literate Eye.* Cambridge: Cambridge University Press, 2024.

Leng, Rainer. "Fecht- und Ringbücher (Nr. 38.)." In *Katalog der deutschsprachigen illustrierten Handschriften des Mittelalters (KdiH)*, edited by Ulrike Bodemann, Peter Schmidt, and Christine Stöllinger-Löser, vol. 4/2. Munich: Beck, 2010. http://kdih.badw.de/datenbank/stoffgruppe/38 (accessed August 1, 2024).

Lenhardt, Friedrich. *Blutschau: Untersuchungen zur Entwicklung der Hämatoskopie.* Pattensen: Wellm, 1986.

Leong, Elaine. *Recipes and Everyday Knowledge: Medicine, Science, and the Household in Early Modern England.* Chicago: University of Chicago Press, 2018.

Leslie, Michael, ed. *A Cultural History of Gardens in the Medieval Age.* London: Bloomsbury, 2013.

Lewis, Elizabeth Matthew. *An Exhibition of Selected Landmark Books and Articles in the History of Military Medicine, Together with a Graphic Display of the Wound Man through History.* West Point, NY: United States Military Academy, 1976.

Liebenow, Peter K., ed. *Das Künzelsauer Fronleichnamspiel.* Berlin: De Gruyter, 1969.

Lima, Manuel. *The Book of Trees: Visualizing Branches of Knowledge.* New York: Princeton Architectural Press, 2014.

Lind, L. R. "Berengario Da Carpi on Fracture of the Skull or Cranium." *Transactions of the American Philosophical Society* 80, no. 4 (1990): 1–164.

Lindberg, Sten G. *Chrestien Wechel and Vesalius: Twelve Unique Medical Broadsides from the Sixteenth Century.* Uppsala: Almqvist & Wiksells, 1954.

Lipton, Sara. *Dark Mirror: The Medieval Origins of Anti-Jewish Iconography.* New York: Metropolitan, 2014.

Lonie, Iain. "The 'Paris Hippocratics': Teaching and Research in Paris in the Second Half of the Sixteenth Century." In *The Medical Renaissance of the Sixteenth Century*, edited by Andrew Wear, Iain Lonie, and Roger French, 155–74. Cambridge: Cambridge University Press, 1985.

Lukacs, Gabor. *"Kaitai Shinsho": The Single Most Famous Japanese Book of Medicine, and "Geka Sōden": An Early Very Important Manuscript on Surgery.* Utrecht: Hes & De Graaf, 2008.

Lüthy, Christoph, and Alexis Smets. "Words, Lines, Diagrams, Images: Towards a History of Scientific Imagery." *Early Science and Medicine* 14 (2009): 398–439.

Macdougall, Simone C. "The Surgeon and the Saints: Henri de Mondeville on Divine Healing." *Journal of Medieval History* 26, no. 3 (2000): 253–68.

MacKinney, Loren C. "The Beginnings of Western Scientific Anatomy: New Evidence and a Revision in Interpretation of Mondeville's Role." *Medical History* 6, no. 3 (1962): 233–39.

MacKinney, Loren C. *Medical Illustrations in Medieval Manuscripts.* London: Wellcome Historical Medical Library, 1965.

Maclean, Ian. *Logic, Signs, and Nature in the Renaissance: The Case of Learned Medicine.* Cambridge: Cambridge University Press, 2002.

MacMurdie, Meekyung. "Proven Recipes: Geometry and the Art of Arabic Medicine." In *The Diagram as Paradigm: Cross-Cultural Approaches*, edited by Jeffrey F. Hamburger, David J. Roxburgh, and Linda Safran, 331–57. Washington, DC: Dumbarton Oaks Publications, 2022.

Madar, Heather, ed. *Prints as Agents of Global Change, 1500–1800.* Amsterdam: Amsterdam University Press, 2021.

Maerlant, Jacob van. *Der naturen bloeme*, edited by Herman Thys. Antwerp: De Vries-Brouwers, 2011.

Majno, Guido. *The Healing Hand: Man and Wound in the Ancient World.* Cambridge, MA: Harvard University Press, 1975.

Malgaigne, Joseph-François. *Oeuvres complètes d'Ambroise Paré*. 3 vols. Paris: Baillière, 1840–1841.
Malik, Richard, Jacqueline Norris, Joanna White, and Bozena Jantulik. "Wound Cat." *Journal of Feline Medicine and Surgery* 8 (2006): 135–40.
Marcelis, K. *De afbeelding van de aderlaat- en de zodiakman in astrologisch-medische handschriften van de 13de en 14de eeuw*. Brussels: Paleis der Academien, 1986.
Marchetti, Francesca. "Le illustrazioni di uno Iatrosophion bizantino del XV secolo, cod. 3632 della Biblioteca Universitaria di Bologna." PhD diss., Università di Bologna, 2011.
Marchetti, Francesca. "Educating the Midwife: The Role of Illustrations in Late Antique and Medieval Obstetrical Texts." In *Pregnancy and Childbirth in the Premodern World: European and Middle Eastern Cultures from Late Antiquity to the Renaissance*, edited by Costanza Gislon Dopfel, Alessandra Foscati, and Charles Burnett, 3–28. Turnhout: Brepols, 2019.
Margolis, Oren. *Aldus Manutius: The Invention of the Publisher*. London: Reaktion, 2023.
Marrow, James H. *Passion Iconography in Northern European Art of the Late Middle Ages and Early Renaissance*. Kortrijk: Van Ghemmert, 1979.
Marshall, Louise. "Reading the Body of a Plague Saint: Narrative Altarpieces and Devotional Images of St. Sebastian in Renaissance Art." In *Reading Texts and Images: Essays on Medieval and Renaissance Art and Patronage*, edited by Bernard J. Muir, 237–72. Exeter: University of Exeter Press, 2002.
Märtl, Claudia, Gisela Drossbach, and Martin Kintzinger, eds. *Konrad von Megenberg (1309–1374) und sein Werk: Das Wissen der Zeit*. Munich: Beck, 2006.
Mayer, Johannes. "Die Blutschau in der spätmittelalterlichen deutschen Diagnostik: Nachträge zu Friedrich Lenhardt aus der handschriftlichen Überlieferung des 'Arzneibuchs' Ortolfs von Baierland." *Sudhoffs Archiv* 72, no. 2 (1988): 225–33.
McCall, Taylor. "Illuminating the Interior: The Illustrations of the Nine Systems of the Body and Anatomical Knowledge in Medieval Europe." PhD diss., Cambridge University, 2017.
McCall, Taylor. "*Reliquam dicit pictura*: Text and Image in an Illustrated Anatomical Manual (Cambridge, Gonville and Caius College MS 190/223)." *Transactions of the Cambridge Bibliographical Society* 16 (2017): 1–22.
McCall, Taylor. "Functional Abstraction in Medieval Anatomical Diagrams." In *Abstraction in Medieval Art: Beyond the Ornament*, edited by Elina Gertsman, 285–308. Amsterdam: Amsterdam University Press, 2021.
McCall, Taylor. "Anatomical Icon: The Dissection Scene across Manuscript and Print." *KNOW: A Journal on the Formation of Knowledge* 6, no. 1 (special issue: "Anatomical Things") (2022): 7–46.
McCall, Taylor. *The Art of Anatomy in Medieval Europe*. London: Reaktion, 2023.
McCann, Daniel. *Soul-Health: Therapeutic Reading in Later Medieval England*. Cardiff: University of Wales Press, 2018.
McCracken, Peggy. *The Curse of Eve, the Wound of the Hero: Blood, Gender, and Medieval Literature*. Philadelphia: University of Pennsylvania Press, 2003.
McDonald, William C. "Turnus in Veldeke's *Eneide*: The Effects of Violence." In *Violence in Medieval Courtly Literature: A Casebook*, edited by Albrecht Classen, 83–95. New York: Routledge, 2004.
McGinn, Bernard. *Mystik im Abendland*, vol. 4, *Fülle: Die Mystik im mittelalterlichen Deutschland (1300–1500)*. Freiburg: Herder, 2008.
McKitterick, David. "What Is the Use of Books without Pictures? Empty Space in Some Early Printed Books." *La Bibliofilía* 116, nos. 1–3 (2014): 67–82.
McNamer, Sarah. *Affective Meditation and the Invention of Medieval Compassion*. Philadelphia: University of Pennsylvania Press, 2010.
McVaugh, Michael R. "Bedside Manners in the Middle Ages." *Bulletin of the History of Medicine* 71, no. 2 (1997): 201–23.
McVaugh, Michael R. "Therapeutic Strategies: Surgery." In *Western Medical Thought from Antiquity to the Middle Ages*, edited by Mirko D. Grmek, 273–90. Cambridge, MA: Harvard University Press, 1998.
McVaugh, Michael R. "Surface Meanings: The Identification of Apostemes in Medieval Surgery." In *Medical Latin: From the Late Middle Ages to the Eighteenth Century*, edited by Wouter Bracke and Herwig Deumens, 13–29. Brussels: Koninklijke Academie voor Geneeskunde, 2000.
McVaugh, Michael R. *The Rational Surgery of the Middle Ages*. Florence: SISMEL, 2006.
McVaugh, Michael R. "Academic Medicine and the Vernacularization of Medieval Surgery: The Case of Bernat de Berriac." In *El saber i les llengües vernacles a l'època de Llull i Eiximenis*, edited by Anna Alberni, Lola Badia, Lluís Cifuentes, and Alexander Fidora, 257–84. Barcelona: Publicacions de l'Abadia de Montserrat, 2012.
McVaugh, Michael R. "Spaces of Anatomy: Fistulas, the Knee, and the 'Three-Dimensional' Body." In *Medicine and Space: Body, Surroundings, and Borders in Antiquity and the Middle Ages*, edited by Patricia A. Baker, Han Nijdam, and Karine van 't Land, 23–36. Leiden: Brill, 2012.
Meier-Staubach, Christel. "Die Quadratur des Kreises: Die Diagrammatik des 12. Jahrhunderts als symbolische Denk- und Darstellungsform." In *Die Bildwelt der Diagramme Joachims von Fiore: Zur Medialität religiös-politischer Programme im Mittelalter*, edited by Alexander Patschovsky, 23–53. Berlin: De Gruyter, 2003.
Mellyn, Elizabeth W. "Passing on Secrets: Interactions between Latin and Vernacular Medicine in Medieval Europe." *I Tatti Studies* 16, nos. 1/2 (2013): 289–310.
Mendelsohn, J. Andrew, Annemarie Kinzelbach, and Ruth Schilling, eds. *Civic Medicine: Physician, Polity, and Pen in Early Modern Europe*. London: Routledge, 2019.
Mentzel-Reuters, Arno. "Das Nebeneinander von Handschrift und Buchdruck im 15. und 16. Jahrhundert." In *Buchwissenschaft in Deutschland: Ein Handbuch*, edited by Ursula Rautenberg, 411–42. Berlin: De Gruyter, 2010.
Merback, Mitchell B. *The Thief, the Cross, and the Wheel: Pain and the Spectacle of Punishment in Medieval and Renaissance Europe*. London: Reaktion, 1999.
Merback, Mitchell B. "Reverberations of Guilt and Violence, Resonances of Peace: A Comment on Caroline

Walker Bynum's Lecture." *Bulletin of the German Historical Institute* 30 (2002): 37–50.
Messerli, Alfred, and Michael Schilling, eds. *Die Intermedialität des Flugblatts in der Frühen Neuzeit*. Stuttgart: Hirzel, 2015.
Messner, Florian, and Ulrike Töchterle. "The Highest Art of Smithery: Research on a Tyrolean Sword." In *The Sword: Form and Thought*, edited by Lisa Deutscher, Mirjam Kaiser, and Sixt Wetzler, 102–16. Woodbridge: Boydell & Brewer, 2019.
Mestler, Gordon E. "A Galaxy of Old Japanese Medical Books with Miscellaneous Notes on Early Medicine in Japan, Part V." *Bulletin of the Medical Library Association* 45, no. 2 (1957): 164–219.
Michel, Wolfgang. *Von Leipzig nach Japan: Der Chirurg und Handelsmann Caspar Schamberger (1623–1706)*. Munich: Iudicium, 1999.
Michel, Wolfgang. "Ōtaguro Genpa no oranda geka menkyojō to sono haikei ni tsuite 太田黒玄淡の阿蘭陀外科免許状とその背景について." *Nihon Ishigaku Zasshi* 日本医史学雑誌 49, no. 3 (2003): 455–77.
Michel, Wolfgang. "Medicine and Allied Sciences in the Cultural Exchange between Japan and Europe in the Seventeenth Century." In *Theories and Methods in Japanese Studies: Current State and Future Developments*, edited by Hans Dieter Ölschleger, 285–302. Göttingen: V&R, 2007.
Michel, Wolfgang. "Narabayashi Chinzan Igaku ni mewo muketa dejima shōkan no tsūji 楢林鎮山医学に目を向けた出島商館の通詞." In *Kyūshū no rangaku—ekkyō to kōryū* 九州の蘭学 越境と交流, edited by Wolfgang Michel, Torii Yumiko, and Kawashima Mahito, 34–40. Kyoto: Shibunkaku Shuppan, 2009.
Michel, Wolfgang, and Elke Werger-Klein. "Drop by Drop: The Introduction of Western Distillation Techniques into Seventeenth-Century Japan." *Journal of the Japanese Society for the History of Medicine* 50, no. 3 (2004): 463–92.
Millares Carlo, Agustín. *Introducción a la historia del libro y de las bibliotecas*. Mexico City: Fondo de Cultura Económica, 1993.
Minuzzi, Sabrina. "La stampa medico-scientifica nell'Europa del XV secolo: Con cenni sulla fruizione dei libri di materia medica e ricettari." In *Printing R-Evolution and Society 1450–1500*, edited by Cristina Dondi, 199–251. Venice: Ca' Foscari, 2020.
Minuzzi, Sabrina. "15th-Century Practical Medicine in Print: Beyond the Profession, towards the *miscere utile dulci*." *Nuncius* 36, no. 2 (2021): 199–263.
"Les miscellanées scientifiques au Moyen Âge." *Micrologus* 27 (special issue) (2019).
Mitchell, Piers D. *Medicine in the Crusades: Warfare, Wounds, and the Medieval Surgeon*. Cambridge: Cambridge University Press, 2004.
Monaco, Francesca Roversi, ed. *Teoria e pratica medica nel basso Medioevo: Teodorico Borgognoni, vescovo, chirurgo, ippiatra*. Florence: SISMEL, 2019.
Mondeville, Henri de. *Die Chirurgie des Heinrich von Mondeville*, edited by Julius Pagel. Berlin: Hirschwald, 1892.
Moorat, Samuel A. J. *Catalogue of Western Manuscripts on Medicine and Science in the Wellcome Historical Medical Library*. London: Wellcome Library, 1962.
Moore, Cornelia Niekus. "'Not by Nature but by Custom': Johan van Beverwijck's *Van de wtnementheyt des vrouwelicken Geslachts*." *Sixteenth Century Journal* 25, no. 3 (1994): 633–51.
Moran, Bruce T. "Preserving the Cutting Edge: Traveling Woodblocks, Material Networks, and Visualizing Plants in Early Modern Europe." In *The Structures of Practical Knowledge*, edited by Matteo Valleriani, 393–419. Cham: Springer, 2017.
Moran, Bruce T. *Paracelsus: An Alchemical Life*. London: Reaktion, 2019.
Morel, P. Gallup. *Die Regesten der Benediktiner-Abtei Einsiedeln*. Chur: Hitz, 1848.
Moretti, Franco. *Graphs, Maps, Trees: Abstract Models for a Literary Theory*. New York: Verso, 2004.
Morgenstern, Arthur. "Das Aderlaßgedicht des Johannes von Aquila und seine Stellung in der Aderlaßlehre des Mittelalters." PhD diss., Universität Leipzig, 1917.
Morinaga, Maki. *Secrecy in Japanese Arts: "Secret Transmission" as a Mode of Knowledge*. London: Palgrave Macmillan, 2005.
Moritz, Tilman G. *Autobiographik als ritterschaftliche Selbstverständigung: Ulrich von Hutten, Götz von Berlichingen, Sigmund von Herberstein*. Göttingen: V&R Unipress, 2019.
Morris, Sophie. "John Browne's *Treatise of the Muscles* (1681) and the Image of Mobility in Late Seventeenth-Century London." PhD diss., University College London, 2019.
Mossman, Stephen. *Marquard von Lindau and the Challenges of Religious Life in Late Medieval Germany: The Passion, the Eucharist, the Virgin Mary*. Oxford: Oxford University Press, 2010.
Mueller, Markus. *Beherrschte Zeit: Lebensorientierung und Zukunftsgestaltung durch Kalenderprognostik zwischen Antike und Neuzeit: Mit einer Edition des Passauer Kalendars (UB/LMB 20 Ms. astron. 1)*. Kassel: Kassel University Press, 2009.
Müller, Jan-Dirk. "Writing—Speech—Image: The Competition of Signs." In *Visual Culture and the German Middle Ages*, edited by Kathryn Starkey and Horst Wenzel, 35–52. New York: Palgrave Macmillan, 2005.
Müller, Kathrin. *Visuelle Weltaneignung: Astronomische und kosmologische Diagramme in Handschriften des Mittelalters*. Göttingen: V&R Unipress, 2009.
Mullini, Roberta. "Graphic Surgical Practice in the Handbills of Seventeenth-Century London Irregulars." In *Medical Paratexts from Medieval to Modern: Dissecting the Page*, edited by Hannah C. Tweed and Diane G. Scott, 57–73. London: Palgrave Macmillan Cham, 2018.
Murdoch, John. *Album of Science: Antiquity and the Middle Ages*. New York: Scribner's & Sons, 1984.
Murphy, Hannah. *A New Order of Medicine: The Rise of Physicians in Reformation Nuremberg*. Pittsburgh: University of Pittsburgh Press, 2019.
Nagler, Georg Kaspar. *Die Monogrammisten*. 5 vols. Munich: Franz, 1858–1879.
Naylor, Ian. "Medicines for Surgical Practice in Fourteenth-Century England: The Judgement against John Le Spicer." In *Wounds in the Middle Ages*, edited by Anne Kirkham and Cordelia Warr, 175–96. Aldershot: Ashgate, 2014.
Needham, Paul. "Review: *The Printing Press as an Agent of Change*." *Fine Print* 6 (1980): 23–35.
Needham, Paul. "Prints in the Early Printing Shops."

In *The Woodcut in Fifteenth-Century Europe*, edited by Peter Parshall, 38–91. New Haven, CT: Yale University Press, 2009.

Nelson, George. "How to Kill People: A Problem of Design." *Industrial Design* 8, no. 1 (1961): 45–53.

Netz, Reviel. *The Shaping of Deduction in Greek Mathematics: A Study in Cognitive History*. Cambridge: Cambridge University Press, 1999.

Neuhaus, Klaus. "Der Wundenmann: Tradition und Struktur einer Abbildungsart in der medizinischen Literatur." PhD diss., Westfälische Wilhelms-Universität, 1982.

Nicaise, Edouard. *Chirurgie de maitre Henri de Mondeville*. Paris: Alcan, 1893.

Nichols, Stephen G., and Siegfried Wenzel, eds. *The Whole Book: Cultural Perspectives on the Medieval Miscellany*. Ann Arbor: University of Michigan Press, 1996.

Nicolle, David. "Wounds, Military Surgery, and the Reality of Crusading Warfare: The Evidence of Usāmah's Memoires." In David Nicolle, *Warriors and Their Weapons around the Time of the Crusades*, 599–612. Burlington: Ashgate, 2002.

Nielsen, Melinda. *An Illustrated Speculum humanae salvationis: Green Collection MS 000321*. Leiden: Brill, 2022.

Nihon igaku rekishi shiryō mokuroku: Dairokkai kyokutō nettai igakkai futai tenrankai 日本医學歷史資料目録: 第六回極東熱帯医學會附帯展覧會. Tokyo: Far Eastern Association of Tropical Medicine, 1925.

Nijdam, Han. "Measuring Wounds in the *Lex Frisionum* and the Old Frisian Registers of Fines." In *Philologia Frisica Anno 1999*, edited by Piter Boersma, 180–203. Leeuwarden: Fryske Akademy, 2000.

Nijdam, Han. "Compensating Body and Honor: The Old Frisian Compensation Tariffs." In *Medicine and the Law in the Middle Ages*, edited by Wendy J. Turner and Sara M. Butler, 25–57. Leiden: Brill, 2014.

Noacco, Cristina, and Christophe Imbert, eds. *Le château allégorique: Image mentale et paysage d'autorité de l'Antiquité à nos jours*. Rennes: Presses Universitaires de Rennes, 2021.

Norri, Johani. *Dictionary of Medical Vocabulary in English, 1375–1550*. New York: Routledge, 2016.

North, John. "Diagram and Thought in Medieval Science." In *Villard's Legacy: Studies in Medieval Technology, Science and Art*, edited by Marie-Thérèse Zenner, 265–87. Burlington: Ashgate, 2004.

Nótári, Tamás. "Physicians, Patients, and Treatments in Early Medieval German (Especially Bavarian) Legislation." *Fundamina* 23, no. 1 (2017): 61–88.

Nothaft, C. Philipp E. *Scandalous Error: Calendar Reform and Calendrical Astronomy in Medieval Europe*. Oxford: Oxford University Press, 2018.

Nuovo, Angela. *The Book Trade in the Italian Renaissance*. Leiden: Brill, 2013.

Nutton, Vivian. "Humanist Surgery." In *The Medical Renaissance of the Sixteenth Century*, edited by Wear Andrew, Lonie Iain, and French Roger, 75–99. Cambridge: Cambridge University Press, 1985.

Nutton, Vivian. "Medicine at the German Universities, 1348–1500: A Preliminary Sketch." In *Practical Medicine from the Black Death to the French Disease*, edited by Roger French, Jon Arrizabalaga, Andrew Cunningham, and Luis García-Ballester, 85–109. Aldershot: Ashgate, 1998.

Nutton, Vivian. "Books, Printing, and Medicine in the Renaissance." *Medicina nei secoli* 17, no. 2 (2005): 421–42.

Nutz, Beatrix, and Harald Stadler. "Gebrauchsgegenstand und Symbol: Die Unterhose (Bruoch) aus der Gewölbezwickelfüllung von Schloss Lengberg, Osttirol." In *Neue Alte Sachlichkeit: Studienbuch Materialität des Mittelalters*, edited by Jan Keupp and Romedio Schmitz-Esser, 221–50. Ostfildern: Jan Thorbecke, 2015.

Nuvoloni, Laura. "Un'aggiunta al catalogo di Antonio Maria da Villafora: Il *Corona florida medicinae* di Antonio Gazio (1491) della University Library di Cambridge." In *Miniatura: Lo sguardo e la parola*, edited by Federica Toniolo and Gennaro Toscano, 330–35. Milan: Cinisello Balsamo, 2012.

Obrist, Barbara. "Le diagramme Isidorien des saisons, son contenu physique et les représentations figuratives." *Mélanges de l'École française de Rome* 108 (1996): 95–164.

Obrist, Barbara. "Visual Representation and Science: Visual Figures of the Universe between Antiquity and the Early Thirteenth Century." *Spontaneous Generations* 6, no. 1 (2012): 15–23.

Obrist, Barbara. "Démontrer, montrer, et l'évidence visuelle: Les figures cosmologiques, de la fin de l'Antiquité à Guillaume de Conches et au début du XIIIe siècle." In *Diagramm und Text: Diagrammatische Strukturen und die Dynamisierung von Wissen und Erfahrung*, edited by Eckart Conrad Lutz, Vera Jerjen, and Christine Putzo, 45–78. Wiesbaden: Reichert, 2014.

O'Daly, Irene. "Diagrams of Knowledge and Rhetoric in Manuscripts of Cicero's *De inventione*." In *Manuscripts of the Latin Classics 800–1200*, edited by Erik Kwakkel, 77–106. Leiden: Leiden University Press, 2015.

O'Day, Rosemary. *The Professions in Early Modern England, 1450–1800*. London: Routledge, 2000.

Odier, Jeanne Bignami. "Les manuscrits de la Reine Christine au Vatican." In *Queen Christina of Sweden: Documents and Studies*, edited by Magnus von Platen, 33–43. Stockholm: Norstedt & Söner, 1966.

Ogilvie, Brian W. *The Science of Describing: Natural History in Renaissance Europe*. Chicago: University of Chicago Press, 2006.

Olariu, Dominic. "The Misfortune of Philippus de Lignamine's Herbal, or New Research Perspectives in Herbal Illustrations from an Iconological Point of View." In *Early Modern Print Culture in Central Europe*, edited by Stefan Kiedroń, Anna-Maria Rimm, and Patrycja Poniatowska, 39–62. Wrocław: Wydawnictwo Uniwersytetu Wrocławskiego, 2014.

Olsan, Lea. "Charms and Prayers in Medieval Medical Theory and Practice." *Social History of Medicine* 16, no. 3 (2003): 343–66.

Olsan, Lea. "The Three Good Brothers Charm: Some Historical Points." *Incantatio* 1, no. 1 (2011): 48–78.

O'Neill, Ynez Violé. "Another Look at the 'Anatomia porci.'" *Viator* 1 (1970): 115–24.

O'Neill, Ynez Violé. "The *Fünfbilderserie*: A Bridge to the Unknown." *Bulletin of the History of Medicine* 51, no. 4 (1977): 538–49.

O'Neill, Ynez Violé. "Diagrams of the Medieval Brain: A Study in Cerebral Localization." In *Iconography at the Crossroads*, edited by Brendan Cassidy, 91–105. Princeton, NJ: Princeton Department of Art and Archaeology, 1993.

Orlemanski, Julie. *Symptomatic Subjects: Bodies, Medicine, and Causation in the Literature of Late Medieval England*. Philadelphia: University of Pennsylvania Press, 2019.

Osler, William. *Incunabula Medica: A Study of the Earliest Printed Medical Books 1467–1480*. New York: Garrison & Morton, 1923.

Ott, Norbert H. "Nonverbale Kommentare: Zur Kommentarfunktion von Illustrationen in mittelalterlichen Handschriften." In *Schrift—Text—Edition*, edited by Christiane Henkes, Walter Hettche, Gabriele Radecke, and Elke Senne, 113–23. Berlin: De Gruyter, 2011.

Outhwaite, Patrick. *Christ the Physician in Late-Medieval Religious Controversy: England and Central Europe, 1350–1434*. Woodbridge: Boydell & Brewer, 2024.

Ouy, Gilbert. *Les manuscrits de l'abbaye de Saint-Victor*. Turnhout: Brepols, 1999.

Overbey, Karen Eileen, and Jennifer Borland. "Diagnostic Performance and Diagrammatic Manipulation in the Physician's Folding Almanacs." In *The Agency of Things in Medieval and Early Modern Art: Materials, Power, and Manipulation*, edited by Grażyna Jurkowlaniec, Ika Matyjaszkiewicz, and Zuzanna Sarnecka, 144–56. London: Routledge, 2017.

Ozaki, Norman T. "Conceptual Changes in Japanese Medicine during the Tokugawa Period." PhD diss., University of California at San Francisco, 1979.

Pac, Grzegorz. "The Attire of the Virgin Mary and Female Rulers in Iconographical Sources of the Ninth to Eleventh Centuries: Analogues, Interpretations, Misinterpretations." In *Medieval Clothing and Textiles 12*, edited by Robin Netherton and Gale R. Owen Crocker, 1–26. Woodbridge: Boydell & Brewer, 2016.

Page, Jamie. "Masculinity and Prostitution in Late Medieval German Literature." *Speculum* 94, no. 3 (2019): 739–73.

Pallarés Jiménez, Miguel Ángel. *La imprenta de los incunables de Zaragoza y el comercio internacional del libro a finales del siglo XV*. Zaragoza: IFC, 2008.

Panse, Melanie. *Hans von Gersdorffs "Feldbuch der Wundarznei": Produktion, Präsentation, und Rezeption von Wissen*. Wiesbaden: Reichert, 2012.

Panse, Melanie. "Den Leser in Text und Bild begleiten: Formen der Wissensvermittlung in medizinischen Schriften des ausgehenden Mittelalters." In *Lehre und Schule im Mittelalter—Mittelalter in Schule und Lehre*, edited by Ursula Kundert, 126–38. Berlin: De Gruyter, 2012.

Park, Katharine. *Secrets of Women: Gender, Generation, and the Origins of Human Dissection*. New York: Zone, 2006.

Parshall, Peter. "*Imago contrafacta*: Images and Facts in the Northern Renaissance." *Art History* 16 (1993): 554–79.

Parshall, Peter. "The Modem Historiography of Early Printmaking." In *The Woodcut in Fifteenth-Century Europe*, edited by Peter Parshall, 9–15. New Haven, CT: Yale University Press, 2009.

Parshall, Peter, and Rainer Schoch. *Origins of European Printmaking: Fifteenth-Century Woodcuts and Their Public*. New Haven, CT: Yale University Press, 2005.

Patijn, Maria. "The Medical Crossbow from Jan Yperman to Isaack Koedijck." In *Wounds in the Middle Ages*, edited by Anne Kirkham and Cordelia Warr, 197–214. London: Routledge, 2016.

Pavlicek, Ota, ed. *Studying the Arts in Late Medieval Bohemia: Production, Reception, and Transmission of Knowledge*. Turnhout: Brepols, 2021.

Pedraza-Gracia, Manuel-José. "Illustrating and Publishing on the Hand-Press in Spain from the Fifteenth to the Eighteenth Century: The Ownership of Icono-Typographic Resources." In *Illustration and Ornamentation in the Iberian Book World, 1450–1800*, edited by Alexander Samuel Wilkinson, 61–86. Leiden: Brill, 2022.

Peirce Edition Project. *The Essential Peirce: Selected Philosophical Writings (1893–1913)*, vol. 2. Bloomington: Indiana University Press, 1998.

Pelling, Margaret. *Sickness, Medical Occupations, and the Urban Poor in Early Modern England*. London: Routledge, 1998.

Pesenti, Tiziana. "Editoria medica tra Quattro e Cinquecento: L'*Articella* e il *Fasciculus medicine*." In *Trattati scientifici nel Veneto fra il XV e XVI secolo*, edited by Ezio Riondato, 1–29. Venice: Pozza, 1985.

Pesenti, Tiziana. *Fasiculo de medicina in volgare: Venezia, Giovanni e Gregorio de Gregori, 1494*. 2 vols. Treviso: Antilia, 2001.

Petzold, Kay Joe. "Die Kanaan-Karten des R. Salomo Ben Isaak (Raschi)—Bedeutung und Gebrauch mittelalterlicher hebräischer Karten-Diagramme." *Das Mittelalter* 22, no. 2 (2017): 332–50.

Pfister, Silvia. *Parodien astrologisch-prophetischen Schrifttums 1470–1590: Textform—Entstehung—Vermittlung—Funktion*. Baden-Baden: Koerner, 1990.

Pfolsprundt, Heinrich von, *Buch der Bündth-Ertznei*, edited by Heinrich von Haeser and Albrecht Middeldorpf. Berlin: Reimer, 1868.

Pfotenhauer, Bettina. *Nürnberg und Venedig im Austausch: Menschen, Güter, und Wissen an der Wende vom Mittelalter zur Neuzeit*. Regensburg: Schnell & Steiner, 2016.

Pigg, Daniel F. "Masculinity Studies." In *Handbook of Medieval Studies: Terms—Methods—Trends*, edited by Albrecht Classen, 1:829–35. Berlin: De Gruyter, 2010.

Pincikowski, Scott E. *Bodies of Pain: Suffering in the Works of Hartmann von Aue*. New York: Routledge, 2002.

Pincikowski, Scott E. "Violence and Pain at the Court: Comparing Violence in German Heroic and Courtly Epics." In *Violence in Medieval Courtly Literature: A Casebook*, edited by Albrecht Classen, 97–114. New York: Routledge, 2004.

Pinkus, Assaf. *Visual Aggression: Images of Martyrdom in Late Medieval Germany*. University Park, PA: Penn State University Press, 2021.

Plebani, Tiziana. *Venezia 1469: La legge e la stampa*. Venice: Marsilio, 2004.

Poirier, Jean-Pierre. *Ambroise Paré: Un urgentiste au XVIe siècle*. Paris: Pygmalion, 2005.

Porras, Stephanie. *The First Viral Images: Maerten de Vos, Antwerp Print, and the Early Modern Globe*. University Park, PA: Penn State University Press, 2023.

Porter, James I. "Disfigurations: Erich Auerbach's Theory of *Figura*." *Critical Inquiry* 44 (2017): 80–113.

Pouchelle, Marie-Christine. *Corps et chirurgie à l'apogée du Moyen Âge*. Paris: Flammarion, 1983.

Poynter, Frederick N. L., ed. *The Selected Writings of William Clowes*. London: Harvey & Blythe, 1948.

Puglisi, Catherine R., and William L. Barcham, eds. *New Perspectives on the Man of Sorrows*. Kalamazoo: Medieval Institute, 2013.

Rampling, Jennifer M. "Depicting the Medieval Alchemical Cosmos: George Ripley's *Wheel of Inferior Astronomy*." *Early Science and Medicine* 18, nos. 1/2 (2013): 45–86.

Rankin, Alisha. *Panaceia's Daughters: Noblewomen as Healers in Early Modern Germany*. Chicago: University of Chicago Press, 2013.

Rankin, Alisha, and Elaine Leong. *Secrets and Knowledge in Medicine and Science 1500–1800*. Farnham: Ashgate, 2011.

Ransom, Lynn. "The '*Speculum theologie*' and Its Readership: Considering the Manuscript Evidence." *Papers of the Bibliographical Society of America* 93, no. 4 (1999): 461–83.

Rappl, Stephanie. *Text und Bild in der "Elsässischen Legenda aurea": Der Cgm 6 (Bayerische Staatsbibliothek München) und der Cpg 144 (Universitätsbibliothek Heidelberg)*. Hamburg: Kovač, 2015.

Rasmussen, Ann Marie. "Masculinity and the *Minnerede*: Berlin, Staatsbibliothek Preussischer Kulturbesitz, Ms. germ. oct. 186 (Livonia, 1431)." In *Triviale Minne? Konventionalität und Trivialisierung in spätmittelalterlichen Minnereden*, edited by Ludger Lieb and Otto Neudeck, 119–38. Berlin: De Gruyter, 2006.

Rautenberg, Ursula. "Das Werk als Ware: Der Nürnberger Kleindrucker Hans Folz." *Internationales Archiv fur Sozialgeschichte der deutschen Literatur* 24 (1999): 1–40.

Rautenberg, Ursula. *Das Titelblatt: Die Entstehung eines typographischen Dispositivs im frühen Buchdruck*. Erlangen: FAU, 2004.

Rautenberg, Ursula. "Die Entstehung und Entwicklung des Buchtitelblatts in der Inkunabelzeit in Deutschland, den Niederlanden und Venedig: Quantitative und qualitative Studien." *Archiv für Geschichte des Buchwesens* 62 (2008): 1–105.

Regensburg, Berthold von. *Predigten*, edited by Franz Pfeiffer and Joseph Strobl. Vienna: Braumüller, 1880.

Reichert, Hermann, ed. *Das Nibelungenlied: Text und Einführung*, 2nd ed. Berlin: De Gruyter, 2017.

Reiss, Athene. *The Sunday Christ: Sabbatarianism in English Medieval Wall Painting*. Oxford: Archaeopress, 2000.

Reske, Christoph. *Die Buchdrucker des 16. und 17. Jahrhunderts im deutschen Sprachgebiet: Auf der Grundlage des gleichnamigen Werks von Josef Benzing*. Wiesbaden: Harrassowitz, 2007.

Reynolds, Melissa. *Reading Practice: The Pursuit of Natural Knowledge from Manuscript to Print*. Chicago: University of Chicago Press, 2024.

Rhodes, Dennis E. *Silent Printers: Anonymous Printing at Venice in the Sixteenth Century*. London: British Library, 1995.

Rhodes, Neil, ed. *English Renaissance Translation Theory*. London: Modern Humanities Research Association, 2013.

Ridderbos, Bernhard. "The Man of Sorrows: Pictorial Images and Metaphorical Statements." In *The Broken Body: Passion Devotion in Late-Medieval Culture*, edited by Alasdair A. MacDonald, Bernhard Ridderbos, and Rita M. Schlusemann, 145–81. Groningen: Egbert Forsten, 1998.

Rieder, Paula M. *On the Purification of Women: Churching in Northern France, 1100–1500*. New York: Palgrave MacMillan, 2006.

Rigaux, Dominique. *Le Christ du Dimanche: Histoire d'une image médiévale*. Paris: Harmattan, 2005.

Riha, Ortrun. "Der Aderlaß in der mittelalterlichen Medizin." *Medizin, Gesellschaft, und Geschichte* 8 (1989): 92–118.

Riha, Ortrun. *Wissensorganisation in medizinischen Sammelhandschriften: Klassifikationskriterien und Kombinationsprinzipien bei Texten ohne Werkcharakter*. Wiesbaden: Reichert, 1992.

Riha, Ortrun. *Ortolf von Baierland und seine lateinischen Quellen: Hochschulmedizin in der Volkssprache*. Wiesbaden: Reichert, 1992.

Riha, Ortrun, *Mittelalterliche Heilkunst: Das Arzneibuch Ortolfs von Baierland (um 1300)*. Baden-Baden: Deutscher Wissenschaftsverlag, 2014.

Riha, Ortrun. "Verwundungen aus der Sicht mittelalterlicher Chirurgen: Möglichkeiten und Grenzen der Behandlung." In *Verletzungen und Unversehrtheit in der deutschen Literatur des Mittelalters*, edited by Sarah Bowden, Nine Miedema, and Stephen Mossman, 175–88. Tübingen: Narr Francke, 2020.

Říhová, Milada. "*Regimen sanitatis* pro krále Václava." *Acta Universitatis Carolinae: Historia Universitatis Carolinae Pragensis* 35, nos. 1/2 (1995): 13–28.

Rimmele, Marius. "Geordnete Unordnung: Zur Bedeutungsstiftung in Zusammenstellungen der Arma Christi." In *Das Bild im Plural: Mehrteilige Bildformen zwischen Mittelalter und Gegenwart*, edited by David Ganz and Felix Thürlemann, 219–42. Berlin: Reimer, 2010.

Rischpler, Susanne. *"Biblia Sacra figuris expressa": Mnemotechnische Bilderbibeln des 15. Jahrhunderts*. Wiesbaden: Reichert, 2001.

Ritchey, Sara. "The Wound's Presence and Bodily Absence: Activating the Spiritual Senses in a Fourteenth-Century Manuscript." In *Sensory Reflections: Traces of Experience in Medieval Artifacts*, edited by Fiona Griffiths and Kathryn Starkey, 163–80. Berlin: De Gruyter, 2019.

Ritchey, Sara. *Acts of Care: Recovering Women in Late Medieval Health*. Ithaca, NY: Cornell University Press, 2021.

Ritchey, Sara, and Sharon Strocchia, eds. *Gender, Health, and Healing, 1250–1550*. Amsterdam: Amsterdam University Press, 2021.

Ritter, François. "Les successeurs de l'imprimeur Jean Prüss (Père)." *Gutenberg-Jahrbuch* 26 (1951): 101–9.

Rizzi, Andrea, ed. *Trust and Proof: Translators in Renaissance Print Culture*. Leiden: Brill, 2017.

Robertson, Kellie. "Scaling Nature: Microcosm and Macrocosm in Later Medieval Thought." *Journal of Medieval and Early Modern Studies* 49, no. 3 (2019): 609–31.

Roby, Courtney. "Galen on the Patient's Role in Pain Diagnosis: Sensation, Consensus, and Metaphor." In *Homo Patiens: Approaches to the Patient in the Ancient World*, edited by Georgia Petridou and Chiara Thumiger, 304–22. Leiden: Brill, 2016.

Rogge, Jörg. "Kämpfer als Schreiber: Bemerkungen zur Erzählung von Kampferfahrung und Verwundung in deutschen Selbstzeugnissen des späten Mittelalters." In *Kriegserfahrungen erzählen: Geschichts- und literaturwissenschaftliche Perspektiven*, edited by Jörg Rogge, 73–106. Bielefeld: Transcript, 2016.

Romero-Barranco, Jesús. *The Late Middle English Version*

of Constantinus Africanus's "Venerabilis anatomia" in London, Wellcome Library, MS 290 (ff. 1r–41v). Newcastle: Cambridge Scholars, 2015.

Rothenberger, Eva. "Die Performanz des Schmerzes: Poetische Inszenierungsstrategien von *passio* und *compassio* bei Oswald von Wolkenstein." In *Geistliche Liederdichter zwischen Liturgie und Volkssprache: Übertragungen, Bearbeitungen, Neuschöpfungen in Mittelalter und Früher Neuzeit*, edited by Andreas Kraß and Matthias Standke, 107–24. Berlin: De Gruyter, 2020.

Rozenski, Steven, and Claire Taylor Jones. "Christ's Passion Shown in a Vision: A Newly Identified Acephalous Fragment from Cambridge, Massachusetts, Houghton Library MS Ger. 69, Fol. 101r–106v." *Journal of Medieval Religious Cultures* 45, no. 2 (2019): 113–38.

Rubin, Jonathan. "The Use of the 'Jericho Tyrus' in Theriac: A Case Study in the History of the Exchanges of Medical Knowledge between Western Europe and the Realm of Islam in the Middle Ages." *Medium Aevum* 83, no. 2 (2014): 234–53.

Rubin, Miri. *Corpus Christi: The Eucharist in Late Medieval Culture*. Cambridge: Cambridge University Press, 1991.

Rublack, Ulinka. "The Right to Dress: Sartorial Politics in Germany, c. 1300–1750." In *The Right to Dress: Sumptuary Laws in a Global Perspective, c. 1200–1800*, edited by Giorgio Riello and Ulinka Rublack, 37–73. Cambridge: Cambridge University Press, 2019.

Rückert, Heinrich, ed. *Der wälsche Gast des Thomasin von Zirclaria*. Quedlinburg: Basse, 1852.

Rudolph, Pia. "Hausbücher (Nr. 49a)." In *Katalog der deutschsprachigen illustrierten Handschriften des Mittelalters (KdiH)*, edited by Ulrike Bodemann, Kristina Freienhagen-Baumgardt, Norbert H. Ott, Pia Rudolph, Peter Schmidt, and Nicola Zotz, vol. 6. Munich: Beck, 2015. https://kdih.badw.de/datenbank/stoffgruppe/49a (accessed August 1, 2024).

Rudolph, Pia. *Im Garten der Gesundheit: Pflanzenbilder zwischen Natur, Kunst und Wissen in gedruckten Kräuterbüchern des 15. Jahrhunderts*. Cologne: Böhlau 2020.

Rudolph, Pia. "Medizin (Nr. 87)." In *Katalog der deutschsprachigen illustrierten Handschriften des Mittelalters (KdiH)*, vol. 9, edited by Kristina Freienhagen-Baumgardt, Pia Rudolph, and Nicola Zotz. Munich: Beck, 2022. https://kdih.badw.de/datenbank/stoffgruppe/87 (accessed August 1, 2024).

Rudy, Kathryn. *Piety in Pieces: How Medieval Readers Customized Their Manuscripts*. Cambridge: Open Book Publishers, 2016.

Rudy, Kathryn. *Image, Knife, and Gluepot: Early Assemblage in Manuscript and Print*. Cambridge: Open Book Publishers, 2019.

Russell, Kenneth F. "John Browne, 1642–1702: A Seventeenth-Century Surgeon, Anatomist, and Plagiarist." *Bulletin of the History of Medicine* 33, no. 6 (1959): 503–25.

Rütten, Thomas. "Karl Sudhoff and 'The Fall' of German Medical History." In *Locating Medical History: The Stories and Their Meanings*, edited by Frank Huisman and John Harley Warner, 95–114. Baltimore: Johns Hopkins University Press, 2004.

Ruys, Juanita Feros. "An Alternative History of Medieval Empathy: The Scholastics and *compassio*." *Emotions: History, Culture, Society* 2, no. 2 (2018): 192–213.

Sabaté, Flocel. *Memory in the Middle Ages: Approaches from Southwestern Europe*. Leeds: Arc Humanities, 2020.

Saint Victor, Hugh of. *On the Sacraments of the Christian Faith (De sacramentis)*, translated by Roy J. Deferrari. Cambridge, MA: Medieval Academy, 1951.

Saito, Mino, and Miki Sato, eds. *"Tsūji": Interpreters in and around Early Modern Japan*. New York: Springer, 2023.

Salisbury, Eve. *Narrating Medicine in Middle English Poetry: Poets, Practitioners, and the Plague*. London: Bloomsbury, 2022.

Salmón, Fernando. "Academic Discourse and Pain in Medieval Scholasticism." In *Medicine and Medical Ethics in Medieval and Early Modern Spain: An Intercultural Approach*, edited by Samuel S. Kottek and Luis García Ballester, 136–53. Jerusalem: Magnes, 2009.

Salmón, Fernando. "The Body Inferred: Knowing the Body through the Dissection of Texts." In *A Cultural History of the Human Body in the Medieval Age*, edited by Linda Kalof, 77–98. London: Bloomsbury, 2010.

Salzberg, Rosa. *Ephemeral City: Cheap Print and Urban Culture in Renaissance Venice*. Manchester: Manchester University Press, 2014.

Sandgren, Eva Lindqvist. "Birgittinska bönboksbilder." *Nordisk Tidskrift för Bildtolkning* 2 (2014): 19–48.

Sarkar, Debapriya. *Possible Knowledge: The Literary Forms of Early Modern Science*. Philadelphia: University of Pennsylvania Press, 2023.

Saurma-Jeltsch, Lieselotte. *Spätformen mittelalterlicher Buchherstellung: Bilderhandschriften aus der Werkstatt Diebold Laubers in Hagenau*. 2 vols. Wiesbaden: Reichert, 2002.

Scarry, Elaine. *The Body in Pain: The Making and Unmaking of the World*. Oxford: Oxford University Press, 1988.

Schalick, Walton O. "To Market, to Market: The Theory and Practice of Opiates in the Middle Ages." In *Opioids and Pain Relief: A Historical Perspective*, edited by Marcia L. Meldrum, 5–20. Seattle: IASP, 2003.

Schmid, Alfred. *Conrad Türsts Iatro-mathematisches Gesundheitsbüchlein für den Berner Schultheissen Rudolf von Erlach*. Bern: Haupt, 1947.

Schmidt, Peter. *Gedruckte Bilder in handgeschriebenen Büchern: Zum Gebrauch von Druckgraphik im 15. Jahrhundert*. Cologne: Böhlau, 2003.

Schmidt, Suzanne Karr. *Interactive and Sculptural Printmaking in the Renaissance*. Leiden: Brill, 2018.

Schmidt, Suzanne Karr, and Kimberly Nichols. *Altered and Adorned: Using Renaissance Prints in Daily Life*. New Haven, CT: Yale University Press, 2011.

Schmidt, Suzanne Karr, and Edward H. Wouk, eds. *Prints in Translation, 1450–1750: Image, Materiality, Space*. London: Routledge, 2017.

Schmitt, Charles. "The Correspondence of Jacques Daléchamps (1513–1588)." *Viator* 8 (1977): 399–434.

Schmitt, Jean-Claude. "Qu'est-ce qu'un diagramme? A propos du *Liber floridus* de Lambert de Saint-Omer (ca. 1120)." In *Diagramm und Text: Diagrammatische Strukturen und die Dynamisierung von Wissen und Erfahrung*, edited by Eckart Conrad Lutz, Vera Jerjen, and Christine Putzo, 79–94. Wiesbaden: Reichert, 2014.

Schneider, Karin. *Die deutschen Handschriften der Bayerischen Staatsbibliothek München: Cgm 501–690*. Wiesbaden: Harrassowitz, 1978.

Schnell, Bernhard. *Arzneibücher—Kräuterbücher—Wörter-*

bücher: Kleine Schriften zur Text- und Überlieferungsgeschichte mittelalterlicher Gebrauchsliteratur. Würzburg: Königshauses & Neuman, 2019.
Schnell, Bernhard, and Marlis Stähli, eds. *Heinrich Laufenberg: Regimen der Gesundheit*. Munich: Lengenfelder, 1998.
Schuba, Ludwig. *Die medizinischen Handschriften der Codices Palatini Latini in der Vatikanischen Bibliothek*. Wiesbaden: Reichert, 1981.
Schuler, Carol M. "The Seven Sorrows of the Virgin: Popular Culture and Cultic Imagery in Pre-Reformation Europe." *Simiolus* 21, nos. 1/2 (1992): 5–28.
Schultz-Balluff, Simone. "Das Wissen über Wunden: Zu Verwendungsweisen, Semantisierung, und Konzeptualisierung von ahd. *wunti*/as. *wunda*/mhd. *wunde*." In *Verletzungen und Unversehrtheit in der deutschen Literatur des Mittelalters*, ed. Sarah Bowden, Nine Miedema, and Stephen Mossman, 35–80. Tübingen: Narr Francke, 2020.
Schurink, Fred. "Print, Patronage, and Occasion: Translations of Plutarch's 'Moralia' in Tudor England." *Yearbook of English Studies* 38, nos. 1/2 (2008): 86–101.
Scott, Kathleen L. *Later Gothic Manuscripts 1390–1490*. 2 vols. London: Harvey Miller, 1998.
Screech, Timon. *Edo no karada o hiraku* 江戸の身体を開く, translated by Hiroshi Takayama. Tokyo: Sakuhinsha, 1997.
Screech, Timon. "A 17th-Century Japanese Minister's Acquisition of Western Pictures: Inoue Masashige (1585–1661) and His European Objects." In *Transforming Knowledge Orders: Museums, Collections, and Exhibitions*, edited by Larissa Förster, 72–106. Paderborn: Wilhelm Fink, 2014.
Sears, Elizabeth. "Sensory Perception and Its Metaphors in the Time of Richard of Fournival." In *Medicine and the Five Senses*, edited by William F. Bynum and Roy Porter, 17–39. Cambridge: Cambridge University Press, 1993.
Seebohm, Almuth. *Apokalypse, Ars moriendi, medizinische Traktate, Tugend- und Lasterlehren: Die erbaulich-didaktische Sammelhandschrift London, Wellcome Institute for the History of Medicine, Ms. 49*. Munich: Helga Lengenfelder, 1995.
Seger, Donna A. *The Practical Renaissance: Information Culture and the Quest for Knowledge in Early Modern England*. London: Bloomsbury, 2022.
Seiichi, Iwao. "A Dutch Doctor in Old Japan." *Japan Quarterly* 8 (1961): 170–78.
Seiz, Anneliese. *Johannes Scultetus und sein Werk: Biographie und Glossar*. Stuttgart: Kohlhammer, 1974.
Seth, Suman. *Difference and Disease: Medicine, Race, and the Eighteenth-Century British Empire*. Cambridge: Cambridge University Press, 2018.
Seyed-Gohrab, Ali-Asghar. "Description (*Wasf*) and Ekphrasis in Anvari's Poetry." In *Studies on the Poetry of Anvari*, edited by Daniela Meneghini, 111–26. Venice: Cafoscarina, 2006.
Sherman, Claire Richter. *Writing on Hands: Memory and Knowledge in Early Modern Europe*. Washington, DC: Folger Shakespeare Library, 2000.
Siegel, Rudolph. *Galen on the Affected Parts: Translation from the Greek Text with Explanatory Notes*. Basel: Karger, 1976.
Sigerist, Henry E. *Hieronymus Brunschwig and His Work: A Fifteenth-Century Surgeon*. New York: Abrahamson, 1946.
Silva, Chelsea. "Opening the Medieval Folding Almanac." *Exemplaria* 30 (2018): 49–65.
Silvi, Christine. "Mise au point sur deux petits imprimés anglais: Robert Wyer, éditeur du 'Livre de Sidrac.'" *Gutenberg-Jahrbuch* 92 (2017): 123–40.
Singer, Charles, and Luke Demaitre, trans. *The Fasciculus medicinae of Johannes de Ketham, Alemanus: Facsimile of the First (Venetian) Edition of 1491*. Birmingham: Classics of Medicine Library, 1988.
Singer, Johannes, ed. *Strickers "Karl der Große."* Berlin: De Gruyter, 2016.
Sinka, Margit M. "Wound Imagery in the Medieval German Epic: Structural Significance of Wounds." PhD diss., University of North Carolina, 1974.
Sinka, Margit M. "Wound Imagery in Gottfried von Strassburg's 'Tristan.'" *South Atlantic Bulletin* 42, no. 2 (1977): 3–10.
Siraisi, Nancy G. *Medieval and Early Renaissance Medicine: An Introduction to Knowledge and Practice*. Chicago: University of Chicago Press, 1990.
Slack, Paul. "Mirrors of Health and Treasures of Poor Men: The Uses of the Vernacular Medical Literature of Tudor England." In *Health, Medicine, and Mortality in the Sixteenth Century*, edited by Charles Webster, 237–74. Cambridge: Cambridge University Press, 1979.
Šmahel, František. *Alma mater Pragensis: Studie k počátkům Univerzity Karlovy*. Prague: Karolinum, 2016.
Smallwood, T. M. "A Charm-Motif to Cure Wounds Shared by Middle Dutch and Middle English." In *Cultuurhistorische Caleidoscoop*, edited by Christian De Backer, 477–505. Ghent: Stichting Mens en Kultuur, 1992.
Smith, Margaret M. *The Title-Page: Its Early Development, 1460–1510*. London: British Library, 2000.
Smith, Pamela H. *From Lived Experience to the Written Word: Reconstructing Practical Knowledge in the Early Modern World*. Chicago: University of Chicago Press, 2022.
Solomon, Michael R. *Fictions of Well-Being: Sickly Readers and Vernacular Medical Writing in Late Medieval and Early Modern Spain*. Philadelphia: University of Pennsylvania Press, 2010.
Spink, Martin S., and Geoffrey L. Lewis, eds. and trans. *Albucasis on Surgery and Instruments: A Definitive Edition of the Arabic Text with English Translation and Commentary*. London: Wellcome Institute, 1973.
Spinks, Jennifer. *Monstrous Births and Visual Culture in Sixteenth-Century Germany*. New York: Routledge, 2009.
Sposato, Peter, and Samuel Claussen. "Chivalric Violence." In *A Companion to Chivalry*, edited by Robert W. Jones and Peter Coss, 99–118. Woodbridge: Boydell & Brewer, 2019.
Spyra, Ulrike. *Das "Buch der Natur" Konrads von Megenberg: Die illustrierten Handschriften und Inkunabeln*. Cologne: Böhlau, 2005.
Stafford, Grace. "Veiling and Head-Covering in Late Antiquity: Between Ideology, Aesthetics, and Practicality." *Past & Present* 263, no. 1 (2024): 3–46.
Stannard, Jerry. *Herbs and Herbalism in the Middle Ages and Renaissance*. London: Routledge, 1999.
Starkey, Kathryn. *Courtier's Mirror: Cultivating Elite*

Identity in Thomasin von Zerclaere's "Welscher Gast." Notre Dame, IN: University of Notre Dame Press, 2013.

Stechow, Wolfgang. "Shooting at Father's Corpse." *Art Bulletin* 24, no. 3 (1942): 213–25.

Stehlíková, Dana. *Od andělíky po zimostráz: Latinský Herbář Křišťana z Prachatic a počátky staročeských herbářů.* Brno: Centrum pro studium demokracie a kultury, 2017.

Stijnman, Ad, and Elizabeth Savage. "Materials and Techniques for Early Colour Printing." In *Printing Colour 1400–1700: History, Techniques, Functions, and Receptions*, edited by Ad Stijnman and Elizabeth Savage, 11–22. Boston: Brill, 2015.

Stok, Fabio. "Vindiciano e la teoria dei temperamenti." *Medicina nei secoli* 24, no. 1 (2012): 517–32.

Stolberg, Michael. *Gelehrte Medizin und ärztlicher Alltag in der Renaissance.* Berlin: De Gruyter, 2020.

Stoudt, Debra L. "The Medical Manuscripts of the Bibliotheca Palatina." In *Manuscript Sources of Medieval Medicine: A Book of Essays*, edited by Margaret R. Schleissner, 159–81. New York: Routledge, 1995.

Suckale, Robert. "Arma Christi: Überlegungen zur Zeichenhaftigkeit mittelalterlicher Andachtsbilder." *Städel-Jahrbuch* 6 (1977): 177–208.

Sudhoff, Karl. *Tradition und Naturbeobachtung in den Illustrationen medizinischer Handschriften und Frühdrucke vornehmlich des 15. Jahrhunderts.* Leipzig: Barth, 1907.

Sudhoff, Karl. "Brunschwig's Anatomie." *Archiv für Geschichte der Medizin* 1, no. 2 (1907): 141–56.

Sudhoff, Karl. *Deutsche medizinische Inkunabeln.* Leipzig: Barth, 1908.

Sudhoff, Karl. "Der 'Wundenmann' in Frühdruck und Handschrift und sein erklärender Text: Ein Beitrag zur Quellengeschichte des 'Ketham.'" *Archiv für Geschichte der Medizin* 1, no. 5 (1908): 351–61.

Sudhoff, Karl. "Eine Pariser 'Ketham'-Handschrift aus der Zeit König Karls VI. (1380–1422)." *Archiv für Geschichte der Medizin* 2, no. 2 (1908): 84–100.

Sudhoff, Karl. "Laßtafelkunst in Drucken des 15. Jahrhunderts." *Archiv für Geschichte der Medizin* 1, nos. 3/4 (1908): 219–88.

Sudhoff, Karl. "Abermals eine neue Handschrift der anatomischen Fünfbilderserie." *Archiv für Geschichte der Medizin* 3, no. 6 (1910): 353–68.

Sudhoff, Karl. "Zwei deutsche Reklamezettel zur Empfehlung von Arzneimitteln—Petroleum und Eichenmistel—gedruckt um 1500." *Archiv für Geschichte der Medizin* 3, no. 6 (1910): 397–402.

Sudhoff, Karl. "Neue Beiträge zur Vorgeschichte des 'Ketham.'" *Archiv für Geschichte der Medizin* 5, nos. 4/5 (1911): 280–301.

Sudhoff, Karl. *Beiträge zur Geschichte der Chirurgie im Mittelalter: Graphische und textliche Untersuchungen in mittelalterlichen Handschriften.* 2 vols. Leipzig: Barth, 1914–1918.

Swan, Claudia. "The Uses of Realism in Early Modern Illustrated Botany." In *Visualizing Medieval Medicine and Natural History, 1200–1550*, edited by Jean A. Givens, Karen M. Reeds, and Alan Touwaide, 239–49. Burlington: Ashgate, 2006.

Taape, Tillmann. "Distilling Reliable Remedies: Hieronymus Brunschwig's *Liber de arte distillandi* (1500) between Alchemical Learning and Craft Practice." *Ambix* 61, no. 3 (2014): 236–56.

Taape, Tillmann. "Common Medicine for the Common Man: Picturing the 'Striped Layman' in Early Vernacular Print." *Renaissance Quarterly* 74, no. 1 (2021): 1–58.

Taavitsainen, Irma. *Middle English Lunaries: A Study of the Genre.* Helsinki: Société Néophilologique, 1988.

Tenger, Zeynep, and Paul Trolander. "From Print versus Manuscript to Sociable Authorship and Mixed Media: A Review of Trends in the Scholarship of Early Modern Publication." *Literature Compass* 7, no. 11 (2010): 1035–48.

Thomas, Duncan. "Thomas Vicary and the *Anatomie of Mans Body*." *Medical History* 50, no. 2 (2006): 235–46.

Thorndike, Lynn. "Some Little Known Astronomical and Mathematical Manuscripts." *Osiris* 8 (1948): 41–72.

Thorndike, Lynn, and Pearl Kibre. *A Catalogue of Incipits of Scientific Writings in Latin.* Cambridge: Cambridge University Press, 1963.

Thurston, John. "How to Do It: How to Acquire a Coat of Arms." *British Medical Journal* 315, no. 7123 (1997): 1682–84.

Timmermann, Achim. *Real Presence: Sacrament Houses and the Body of Christ, c. 1270–1600.* Turnhout: Brepols, 2009.

Timmermann, Achim. "Good and Bad Prayers, before Albertus Pictor: Prolegomena to the History of a Late Medieval Image." *Baltic Journal of Art History* 5 (2013): 131–77.

Timmermann, Achim. "Vain Labor(?): Things, Strings, and the Human Condition in the Art of Giovanni Baleison." *RES: Anthropology and Aesthetics* 65, no. 66 (2014): 224–41.

Toby, Ronald P. *State and Diplomacy in Early Modern Japan: Asia in the Development of the Tokugawa Bakufu.* Princeton, NJ: Princeton University Press, 1984.

Tomíček, David. *Víra, rozum a zkušenost v lékařství pozdně středověkých Čech.* Ústí nad Labem: UJEP, 2009.

Trotter, David. *Traitier de cyrurgie: Édition de la traduction en ancien français de la Chirurgie d'Abū-ʾl Qāsim Halaf Ibn ʿAbbās al-Zahrāwī du manuscrit BnF, Français 1318.* Berlin: De Gruyter, 2005.

Tufte, Edward R. *The Visual Display of Quantitative Information.* Cheshire, CT: Graphics Press, 1983.

Turner, Wendy J., and Sara M. Butler, eds. *Medicine and the Law in the Middle Ages.* Leiden: Brill, 2014.

Tweed, Hannah C., and Diane G. Scott, eds. *Medical Paratexts from Medieval to Modern: Dissecting the Page.* London: Palgrave Macmillan Cham, 2018.

Tzouriadis, Iason-Eleftherios. "'What Is the Riddle of Steel?': Problems of Classification and Terminology in the Study of Late Medieval Swords." In *The Sword: Form and Thought*, edited by Lisa Deutscher, Mirjam Kaiser, and Sixt Wetzler, 3–11. Woodbridge: Boydell & Brewer, 2019.

Undorf, Wolfgang. "Lost Books, Lost Libraries, Lost Everything? A Scandinavian Early Modern Perspective." In *Lost Books: Reconstructing the Print World of Pre-Industrial Europe*, edited by Flavia Bruni and Andrew Pettegree, 101–19. Leiden: Brill, 2016.

Valls, Helen E. "Illustrations as Abstracts: The Illustrative Programme in a Montpellier Manuscript of Roger Frugardi's *Chirurgia*." *Medicina nei secoli* 8 (1996): 67–83.

Vance, Eugene. "Roland and the Poetics of Memory."

In *Textual Strategies: Perspectives in Post-Structuralist Criticism*, edited by Josué V. Harari, 374–403. Ithaca, NY: Cornell University Press, 1979.
Van de Walle, Willy F., and Kazuhiko Kasaya, eds. *Dodonaeus in Japan: Translation and the Scientific Mind in the Tokugawa Period*. Leuven: Leuven University Press, 2001.
Van der Lugt, Maaike. "Nature as Norm in Medieval Medical Discussions of Maternal Breastfeeding and Wet-Nursing." *Journal of Medieval and Early Modern Studies* 49, no. 3 (2019): 563–88.
Vanková, Lenka, ed. *Fachtexte des Spätmittelalters und der Frühen Neuzeit als Objekt der Fachsprachen- und Fachprosaforschung: Tradition und Perspektiven der Fachprosa- und Fachsprachenforschung*. Berlin: De Gruyter, 2014.
Van 't Land, Karine. "The Solution of Continuous Things: Wounds in Late Medieval Medicine and Surgery." In *Wounds in the Middle Ages*, edited by Anne Kirkham and Cordelia Warr, 89–109. Aldershot: Ashgate, 2014.
Verboon, Annemieke R. "Brain Ventricle Diagrams: A Century after Walther Sudhoff: New Manuscript Sources from the XVth Century." *Sudhoffs Archiv* 98, no. 2 (2014): 212–33.
Verboon, Annemieke R. "The Medieval Tree of Porphyry: An Organic Structure of Logic." In *The Tree: Symbol, Allegory, and Structural Device in Medieval Art and Thought*, edited by Andrea Worm and Pippa Salonis, 83–101. Turnhout: Brepols, 2014.
Vialle, Cynthia, Isabel Tanaka-van Daalen, and Leonard Blussé, eds. *The Deshima Diaries 1641–1660*. Leiden: Brill, 2023.
Voigts, Linda E., and Robert P. Hudson. "*A drynke þat men callen dwale to make a man to slepe whyle men kerven him*: A Surgical Anaesthetic from Late Medieval England." In *Health, Disease, and Healing in Medieval Culture*, edited by Sheila Campbell, Bert Hall, and David Klausner, 34–56. New York: Palgrave, 1992.
Voigts, Linda E., and Michael R. McVaugh. *A Latin Technical Phlebotomy and Its Middle English Translation*. Philadelphia: American Philosophical Society, 1984.
Vollmuth, Ralf. "'Von den geschosszenen Wunden': Die Behandlung von Schußwunden in deutschsprachigen chirurgischen Werken des 15. Jahrhunderts." *Orvostörténeti közlemények* 40, nos. 1/2 (1994): 5–28.
Vulić, Kathryn. "The Vernon Paternoster Diagram, Medieval Graphic Design, and the *Parson's Tale*." In *Chaucer: Visual Approaches*, edited by Susanna Fein and David Raybin, 59–85. University Park, PA: Penn State University Press, 2016.
Wallis, Faith. *Medieval Medicine: A Reader*. Toronto: University of Toronto Press, 2010.
Wallis, Faith. "What a Medieval Diagram Shows: A Case Study of *Computus*." *Studies in Iconography* 36 (2015): 1–40.
Wallis, Faith. "Pre-Modern Surgery: Wounds, Words, and the Paradox of 'Tradition.'" In *The Palgrave Macmillan Handbook of the History of Surgery*, edited by Thomas Schlich, 49–70. London: Palgrave Macmillan, 2018.
Walsby, Malcolm. "Printer Mobility in Sixteenth-Century France." In *Print Culture and Peripheries in Early Modern Europe*, edited by Benito Rial Costas, 249–70. Leiden: Brill, 2013.
Walsby, Malcolm. "Plantin and the French Book Market." In *International Exchange in the Early Modern Book World*, edited by Matthew McLean and Sara K. Barker, 80–101. Leiden: Brill, 2016.
Walsby, Malcolm. "The Creation of the Title Page in French Incunabula." *Gutenberg-Jahrbuch* 97 (2022): 38–46.
Walter, Katie L. "Peril, Flight, and the Sad Man: Medieval Theories of the Body in Battle." In *War and Literature*, edited by Laura Ashe and Ian Patterson, 21–40. Woodbridge: Boydell & Brewer, 2014.
Ward, John O. "What the Middle Ages Missed of Cicero, and Why." In *Brill's Companion to the Reception of Cicero*, edited by William H. F. Altman, 307–26. Leiden: Brill, 2015.
Watson, Gilbert. *Theriac and Mithridatium: A Study in Therapeutics*. London: Wellcome Historical Medical Library, 1966.
Wear, Andrew. *Knowledge and Practice in English Medicine, 1550–1680*. Cambridge: Cambridge University Press, 2000.
Wee, John. "Discovery of the Zodiac Man in Cuneiform." *Journal of Cuneiform Studies* 67 (2015): 217–33.
Weidemann, Bodo. "'Kunst der Gedächtnüß' und 'De mansionibus', zwei frühe Traktate des Johann Hartlieb." PhD diss., Freie Universität Berlin, 1964.
Wen, Xinyi. "When Jupiter Meets Saturn: Aby Warburg, Karl Sudhoff, and Astrological Medicine in the Age of Disenchantment." *Journal of the History of Ideas* 84, no. 2 (2024): 321–55.
Wenzel, Horst, and Christina Lechtermann, eds. *Beweglichkeit der Bilder: Text und Imagination in den illustrierten Handschriften des "Welschen Gastes" von Thomasin von Zerclaere*. Cologne: Böhlau, 2002.
White, Eric Marshall. "Binding Waste as Book History: Patterns of Survival among the Early Mainz Donatus Editions." In *Printing R-Evolution and Society 1450–1500*, edited by Cristina Dondi, 253–77. Venice: Ca' Foscari, 2020.
Whitehead, Christiania. *Castles of the Mind: A Study of Medieval Architectural Allegory*. Cardiff: University of Wales Press, 2003.
Whittington, Karl. "Picturing Christ as Surgeon and Patient in British Library MS Sloane 1977." *Mediaevalia* 35 (2014): 83–115.
Whittington, Karl. *Trecento Pictoriality: Diagrammatic Painting in Late Medieval Italy*. London: Harvey Miller, 2023.
Wickersheimer, Ernest. *Maître Jean Gispaden: Chirurgien annécien et grenoblois de la fin du XVe siècle*. Genève: Kundig, 1926.
Wierschin, Martin. *Meister Johann Liechtenauers Kunst des Fechtens*. Munich: Beck, 1965.
Williams, Ulla, Werner Williams-Krapp, and Konrad Kunze, eds. *Die Elsässische "Legenda Aurea."* 3 vols. Tübingen: Niemeyer, 1980.
Williams-Krapp, Werner. "Bild und Text: Zu den illustrierten Handschriften der *Legenda aurea* des französischen und deutschsprachigen Raums." *Archiv für Kulturgeschichte* 97 (2015): 89–107.
Willson, H. B. "Blood and Wounds in the 'Nibelungenlied.'" *Modern Language Review* 55, no. 1 (1960): 40–50.
Wilson, Adrian, and Joyce Lancaster Wilson. *A Medieval Mirror: "Speculum humanae salvationis" 1324–1500*. Berkeley: University of California Press, 1985.

Wirth, Karl-August. "Von mittelalterlichen Bildern und Lehrfiguren im Dienste der Schule und des Unterrichts." In *Studien zum städtischen Bildungswesen des späten Mittelalters und der frühen Neuzeit*, edited by Bernd Moeller, Hans Patze, and Karl Stackmann, 256–370. Göttingen: V&R Unipress, 1983.

Witherden, Sian. "Balancing Form, Function, and Aesthetic: A Study of Ruling Patterns for Zodiac Men in Astro-Medical Manuscripts of Late Medieval England." *Journal of the Early Book Society* 20 (2017): 79–110.

Wolkenstein, Oswald von. *Das poetische Werk*, translated by Wernfried Hofmeister. Berlin: De Gruyter, 2011.

Worm, Andrea, and Pippa Salonis, eds. *The Tree: Symbol, Allegory, and Structural Device in Medieval Art and Thought*. Turnhout: Brepols, 2014.

Wragge-Morley, Alexander. *Aesthetic Science: Representing Nature in the Royal Society of London, 1650–1720*. Chicago: University of Chicago Press, 2020.

Wright, Aaron E. "'*Die gotlich sterk gab daz der teutschen zungen*': Folz, Schedel, and the Printing Press in Fifteenth-Century Nuremberg." *Fifteenth Century Studies* 19 (1992): 319–49.

Yates, Donald. "A Fourteenth-Century Latin Poem on the Art of the Physician." *Bulletin of the History of Medicine* 54, no. 3 (1980): 447–50.

Yearl, Mary K. K. "Medieval Monastic Customaries on *Minuti* and *Infirmi*." In *The Medieval Hospital and Medical Practice*, edited by Barbara S. Bowers, 175–94. Aldershot: Ashgate, 2007.

Yearl, Mary K. K. "Bloodletting as Recreation in the Monasteries of Medieval Europe." In *Between Text and Patient: The Medical Enterprise in Medieval and Early Modern Europe*, edited by Florence Eliza Glaze and Brian K. Nance, 217–44. Florence: SISMEL, 2011.

Yoeli-Tlalim, Ronit. *ReOrienting Histories of Medicine: Encounters along the Silk Roads*. London: Bloomsbury, 2021.

Zahnd, Urs Martin, ed. *Die autobiographischen Aufzeichnungen Ludwig von Diesbachs: Studien zur spätmittelalterlichen Selbstdarstellung im oberdeutschen und schweizerischen Raume*. Bern: Stämpfli, 1986.

Zaina, Alberto. "Il precetto festivo tra ammonizione e devozione: Il 'Cristo della domenica' negli affreschi bresciani." *Brixia Sacra* 12, nos. 3/4 (2008): 33–63.

Zaun, Stefanie, and Hans Geisler. "Die Harnfarbbezeichnungen im *Fasciculus medicine* und ihre italienischen und spanischen Übersetzungen." In *Farbe im Mittelalter: Materialität—Medialität—Semantik*, edited by Ingrid Bennewitz and Andrea Schindler, 969–85. Berlin: Akademie, 2011.

Zerclêre, Thomasin von. *Thomasin von Zirclaria: Der Welsche Gast (The Italian Guest)*, translated by Marion Gibbs and Winder McConnell. Kalamazoo, MI: Medieval Institute, 2009.

Ziegler, Joseph. *Medicine and Religion c. 1300: The Case of Arnau de Vilanova*. Oxford: Clarendon, 1998.

Zimmermann-Homeyer, Catarina. *Illustrierte Frühdrucke lateinischer Klassiker um 1500: Innovative Illustrationskonzepte aus der Strassburger Offizin Johannes Grüningers und ihre Wirkung*. Wiesbaden: Harrassowitz, 2018.

Zimmermann-Homeyer, Catarina. "Spuren eines drucktechnischen Experiments in den Holzschnitten der Terenz-Ausgaben des Straßburger Frühdruckers Johann Prüß." *Gutenberg-Jahrbuch* 94 (2019): 129–50.

Zimmermann-Homeyer, Catarina. "Illustrated Almanacs: Imaging Strategies in Bloodletting Calendars of the Incunabula Period." *Gutenberg Jahrbuch* 97 (2022): 118–45.

Zorzi, Marino. "Stampatori tedeschi a Venezia." In *Venezia e la Germania: Arte, politica, commercio*, edited by Susanna Biadene, 115–40. Milan: Electa, 1986.

Index

Note: **bold** page numbers refer to illustrations.

Image Credits

Almost all of the institutions and individuals listed below generously offered photographs of their collections for this book free of charge or with minimal fees. They did this by sharing their images through open-access repositories with Creative Commons licenses and by embracing the new legal frameworks emerging in various countries and regions designed to democratize historical works in the public domain. I thank them for their forward-thinking support of scholarly work in this way, and for acknowledging the essential role that the free exchange of images plays in developing the public understanding of their historic collections.

Albertina, Wien, Public Domain Mark 1.0 (fig. 5.3)
Archiv & Bibliothek des Schottenstifts (fig. 1.17)
Bayerische Staatsbibliothek München, 2 Inc.c.a. 1453 (fig. 4.12)
Bayerische Staatsbibliothek München, 2 Inc.c.a. 3452 (figs. 5.1, 5.2)
Bayerische Staatsbibliothek München, Cgm 571 (fig. 1.6)
Bayerische Staatsbibliothek München, Cgm 597 (figs. 2.10, 2.13)
Bayerische Staatsbibliothek München, Cgm 1507 (fig. 3.9)
Bayerische Staatsbibliothek München, Clm 28609 (fig. 1.5)
Bayerische Staatsbibliothek München, Einbl.Kal. 1490 p (fig. 4.9)
Bayerische Staatsbibliothek München, Rar. 185 (fig. 4.3)
Biblioteka Jagiellońska, Kraków, Public Domain (fig. 5.9)
Biblioteka Uniwersytecka we Wrocławiu, Public Domain Mark 1.0 (fig. 1.13)
Bibliothèque interuniversitaire de santé, Paris, Open License (figs. 5.17, 5.27)
Bibliothèque Mazarine, Paris (fig. 4.18)
Bibliothèque municipale, Valenciennes, Public Domain (fig. 4.4)
Bibliothèque nationale et universitaire de Strasbourg, CC0 1.0 (fig. 3.17)
© Bodleian Libraries, University of Oxford, CC-BY-NC 4.0 (fig. 1.19)
Boston Public Library, Public Domain Mark 1.0 (fig. 4.14)
The British Library, Additional MS 15582, Public Domain (fig. 1.16)
The British Library, Harley MS 941, Public Domain (fig. 1.7)
The British Library, IA.23743, Public Domain (fig. 4.14)
The British Library, Sloane MS 1977, Public Domain (fig. 3.10)
Das Buch der Natur, Digitalisiert durch die Universitätsbibliothek J.C. Senckenberg Frankfurt am Main [2011], urn:nbn:de:hebis:30:2-11707, Public Domain Mark 1.0 (fig. 3.16)
By permission of the Master and Fellows of Gonville and Caius College, Cambridge (fig. 1.15)
College of Arms, MS Grants 162, p. 217. Reproduced by permission of the Kings, Heralds and Pursuivants of Arms (fig. 0.2)
Courtesy of the National Library of Medicine, Public Domain (figs. 4.15, 5.12)
ETH-Bibliothek Zürich, Zürich, Rare 8909, https://doi.org/10.3931/e-rara-2164, Public Domain Mark 1.0 (fig. 4.7)
Friedrich-Alexander-Universität Universitätsbibliothek, Erlangen, Public Domain Mark 1.0 (figs. 4.2, 4.10, 5.6, 5.9)
HAB Wolfenbüttel: 167.9 Poet <http://diglib.hab.de/inkunabeln/167-9-poet/start.htm>, Public Domain (fig. 4.7)
HAB Wolfenbüttel: Cod. 29.14 Aug. 4°, Public Domain (fig. 3.18)
HAB Wolfenbüttel: Cod. Guelf. 30.12 Aug. 2° <http://diglib.hab.de/mss/30-12-aug-2f/start.htm>, Public Domain (fig. 3.2)
HAB Wolfenbüttel: Cod. Guelf. 1189 Helmst. <http://diglib.hab.de/inkunabeln/1189-helmst-2/start.htm>, Public Domain (fig. 4.5)
Harvey Cushing/John Hay Whitney Medical Library, Public Domain Mark 1.0 (fig. 4.16)
Hortus sanitatis, deutsch, Digitalisiert durch die Universitätsbibliothek J.C. Senckenberg, Frankfurt am Main [2016], urn:nbn:de:hebis:30:2-264947, Public Domain Mark 1.0 (fig. 4.2)
Huis van het boek, The Hague (fig. 4.9)
The Huntington Library, San Marino, California, Call Number 86926 (fig. 4.17)
Image from the collections of the Biblioteca Nacional de España, CC BY 4.0 (figs. 3.12, 4.17)
Institut für Archäologien, Innsbruck (fig. 3.8)
Jonathan A. Hill, Bookseller (fig. 5.28)

KBR - Manuscripts Department - MS 19546 (fig. 1.8)
Klosterneuburg, Stiftsbibliothek (fig. 1.20)
Koninklijke Bibliotheek, The Hague (fig. 5.22)
Královská kanonie premonstrátů na Strahově (fig. 2.4)
Leiden University Libraries, Public Domain Mark 1.0 (fig. 4.23)
Llyfrgell Genedlaethol Cymru - National Library of Wales, Public Domain (fig. 1.19)
The Lobkowicz Library and Archives, Nelahozeves Castle, Czech Republic (fig. 2.1)
Mainzer Diözesanbrevier, Digitalisiert durch die Universitätsbibliothek J.C. Senckenberg Frankfurt am Main [2011], urn:nbn:de:hebis:30:2-14120, Public Domain Mark 1.0 (fig. 1.24)
© MAK/Aslan Kudrnofsky (fig. 5.7)
The Master and Fellows of Trinity College, Cambridge, MS O.9.31 (fig. 4.21)
The Metropolitan Museum of Art, New York, Public Domain (fig. 3.14)
Milestones of Science Books, Ritterhude (fig. 4.18)
Muzeum Narodowe w Warszawie, Public Domain (fig. 3.11)
Národní knihovna České republiky, CC BY-NC-SA 4.0 (figs. 1.18, 2.5, 2.12, 4.19)
National Széchényi Library, Budapest, Cod. Germ. 56, fol. 37v (fig. 4.20)
Padua, Biblioteca storica di Medicina e botanica Vincenzo Pinali e Giovanni Marsili (fig. 1.16)
Paris, Bibliothèque de l'Arsenal, Public Domain (fig. 1.2)
Paris, Bibliothèque nationale de France, Public Domain (figs. 1.7, 1.10, 1.16, 1.22, 2.5, 2.12, 2.15, 3.18, 4.1, 4.7, 4.11, 5.13)
Patrimonio Nacional. Real Biblioteca del Monasterio de El Escorial, MS T-I-6 (fig. 1.4)
Photograph © The Warburg Institute (fig. 0.3)
Photograph courtesy of the Main Library, Kyoto University, *Geka kinmō zui* (fig. 5.26)
Photograph courtesy of the Main Library, Kyoto University, *Geka sōden kinsō shitsuboku no bu* (figs. 5.27, 5.30)
Photographic credit: The Morgan Library & Museum, New York (fig. 3.5)
Renzo Dionigi (fig. 3.15)
© Rheinisches Bildarchiv Köln, rba_d022645_02_Detail (fig. 3.13)
Royal Danish Library, NKS 84 b folio, fol. 4r (fig. 2.9 , 2.19)
Royal Danish Library, Thott 290, 2º, fols. 134v and 93v (fig. 3.7)
Sammelband in 9 Teilen, Digitalisiert durch die Universitätsbibliothek J.C. Senckenberg Frankfurt am Main, urn:nbn:de:hebis:30:2-438439, Public Domain Mark 1.0 (fig. 5.5)
Semeniška knjižnica, Ljubljana, Public Domain Mark 1.0 (fig. 4.24)
Source: National Diet Library, Tokyo (figs. 5.29, 5.30)
Staatsbibliothek Bamberg, CC BY-SA 4.0 (fig. 2.7)
Staatsbibliothek zu Berlin, Public Domain Mark 1.0 (figs. 1.23, 2.5, 5.4)
Staats- und Stadtbibliothek Augsburg: 2° Cod 158, CC BY-NC-SA 4.0 (fig. 3.16)
Staats- und Stadtbibliothek Augsburg: 4 Ink 162, CC BY-NC-SA 4.0 (fig. 4.6)
Staats- und Stadtbibliothek Augsburg: Med 3998, CC BY-NC-SA 4.0 (fig. 5.11)
Stadtarchiv Dessau-Roßlau, Anhaltische Landesbücherei, Sign. Georg 271 (fig. 1.15)
© Stift Melk (fig. 1.3)
Su concessione della Alma Mater Studiorum Università di Bologna, Biblioteca Universitaria di Bologna (fig. 2.2)
TECHNOSEUM - Landesmuseum für Technik und Arbeit in Mannheim, Public Domain Mark 1.0 (fig. 5.25)
Universitätsbibliothek Basel, Public Domain Mark 1.0 (fig. 4.20)
Universitätsbibliothek Freiburg, Hs. 458, Public Domain Mark 1.0 (fig. 3.18)
Universitätsbibliothek Gießen, Public Domain Mark 1.0 (fig. 4.8)
Universitätsbibliothek Heidelberg / 80 B 392 RES / table 30, Public Domain Mark 1.0 (fig. 5.23)
Universitätsbibliothek Heidelberg / MS Cpg 339 / vol. II / 425v, Public Domain Mark 1.0 (fig. 3.6)
Universitätsbibliothek Heidelberg / MS Cpg 644 / 1v, Public Domain Mark 1.0 (fig. 2.3)
Universitätsbibliothek Heidelberg / MS Cpg 644 / 78v, Public Domain Mark 1.0 (fig. 2.17)
Universitätsbibliothek Heidelberg / MS Pal. Lat. 1181 / Inside cover, 1r, Public Domain Mark 1.0 (fig. 1.12)
Universitätsbibliothek Heidelberg / MS Pal. Lat. 1225 / 423r, Public Domain Mark 1.0 (fig. 1.1)
Universitätsbibliothek Heidelberg / MS Pal. Lat. 1264 / 244r, 224v, Public Domain Mark 1.0 (fig. 1.11)
Universitätsbibliothek Heidelberg / MS Pal. Lat. 1293 / 1r, Public Domain Mark 1.0 (fig. 2.4)
Universitätsbibliothek Heidelberg / MS Pal. Lat. 1305 / 130r, Public Domain Mark 1.0 (fig. 1.18)
Universitätsbibliothek Heidelberg / MS Pal. Lat. 1325 / 346v, Public Domain Mark 1.0 (fig. 2.4)
Universitätsbibliothek Heidelberg / MS Pal. Lat. 1325 / 349v, Public Domain Mark 1.0 (fig. 2.10)
Universitätsbibliothek Heidelberg / MS Pal. Lat. 1325 / 360v, Public Domain Mark 1.0 (fig. 2.17)
Universitätsbibliothek Heidelberg / MS Pal. Lat. 1452 / 127v, Public Domain Mark 1.0 (fig. 1.23)
Universitätsbibliothek Heidelberg / MS Urk. Lehmann 186 / 2r, Public Domain Mark 1.0 (fig. 3.1)
Universitätsbibliothek Kassel, Public Domain Mark 1.0 (figs. 1.24, 2.12)
Universitätsbibliothek Leipzig, Public Domain Mark 1.0 (figs. 1.21, 1.23)
Universitätsbibliothek Tübingen, Public Domain (fig. 2.11)
Universitäts- und Landesbibliothek Darmstadt, CC0 1.0 (fig. 4.9)
Vadianische Sammlung der Ortsbürgergemeinde St. Gallen (fig. 3.3)
Vienna, Österreichische Nationalbibliothek, Cod. 2469, fol. 41r (fig. 1.9)
Vienna, Österreichische Nationalbibliothek, Cod. 4417*, fol. 19v (fig. 3.19)
Vienna, Österreichische Nationalbibliothek, Cod. 14034, fol. 4v (fig. 4.22)
Vienna, Österreichische Nationalbibliothek, Cod. 15478, fol. 291v (fig. 3.4)
Vienna, Österreichische Nationalbibliothek, Cod. ALT PRUNK 70.P.12 (fig. 5.8)
Wellcome Collection, London, Public Domain (figs. 0.1, 2.10, 2.16, 5.11, 5.14, 5.16, 5.18, 5.19, 5.21, 5.24)
Württembergische Landesbibliothek Stuttgart, Public Domain Mark 1.0 (fig. 4.9)
Zentralbibliothek Solothurn (fig. 2.14)